AF822684

THE RISE OF SURGERY

From Empiric Craft to Scientific Discipline

THE RISE OF SURGERY

From Empiric Craft to Scientific Discipline

by

Owen H. Wangensteen, M.D., Ph.D.

Chairman and Regents' Professor Emeritus
Department of Surgery
University of Minnesota

and

Sarah D. Wangensteen, B.A.

Senior Medical Historian Emeritus
History of Medicine
University of Minnesota

UNIVERSITY OF MINNESOTA PRESS □ MINNEAPOLIS

Copyright © 1978 by the University of Minnesota.
All rights reserved.
Printed in the United States of America
at North Central Publishing Company, St. Paul.
Published by the University of Minnesota Press, 2037 University
Avenue Southeast, Minneapolis, Minnesota 55455,
and published in Canada by Burns & MacEachern
Limited, Don Mills, Ontario

Library of Congress Cataloging in Publication Data

Wangensteen, Owen H., 1898–
The rise of surgery.

Bibliography: p.
Includes indexes.
1. Surgery—History. I. Wangensteen, Sarah D., joint author. II. Title. [DNLM: 1. Surgery—History. W011.1 W246r]
RD19.W36 617'.09 77-87933
ISBN 0-8166-0832-6

The University of Minnesota
is an equal opportunity
educator and employer.

Dedication

May the spirit of inquiry, the love of learning, and appreciation of the History of Medicine create in our medical schools an intellectual atmosphere that will heighten greater medicine's commitment and accountability in its service to mankind.

Preface

If all of Medicine from Anatomy to Zoology were taught with a view to the historic background of each discipline privileged to carry a badge of its own, our students would be better taught. Harvey Cushing's plea that the teacher is more important than the curriculum sounds a perceptive note in pedagogy. When the faculties of our schools of medicine come to recognize the importance of history in understanding the evolution and growth of the many disciplines they undertake to teach, our teachers will be seen more often among the students in our libraries, to the definite gain of all.

As the title indicates, the thrust of this effort is primarily to assess factors that contributed to or retarded surgical advance. The work lays no claim to being a formal systematic history of surgery. Imperative emergency surgery dates from antiquity; elective surgery, almost nonexistent prior to general acceptance of prophylactic surgical antisepsis in the mid-1880s, is largely a product of the last fifteen years of the nineteenth century. Surgery's advance before that time can be assessed solely through careful scrutiny of the successes and failures in operations of dire necessity. In quest of the sequences responsible for surgery's rise, it became apparent to the authors that the answers were most likely to be found by study of such operations over many centuries, with special emphasis on surgery's progress from a lowly empiric craft to a scientific discipline. This mode of address to the history of surgery's progress has hitherto been neglected by both historians and surgeons.

The empiric and chaotic status of wound management at mid-nineteenth century is confounding. There were, to be certain, as this pursuit reveals, some suggestions why operative procedures succeeded in some hands and failed in others. Needed, obviously, were well-controlled examinations of different modes of management. The despairing Russian surgeon Nikolai Pirogoff (1854), unhappy and confused over the unpredictable outcome of his operations, said that favorable results were solely a matter of luck, a deduction he would have done well to examine. One link in surgery's progress was yet to come, a knowledge of the great importance of microbiology, surgery's finest benefactor.

The three A's of surgery, anesthesia, prophylactic antisepsis, and antibiotics, each lent surgery a strong forward thrust. Interestingly, the first two came from long neglected Cinderellas of medicine: dentistry and obstetrics. W. T. G. Morton and Horace Wells, dentists, gave us anesthesia (1844–46); Ignacz Semmelweis (1847), Hungarian-born obstetrician, struggling for and denied an ongoing position in the faculty of the University of Vienna, provided prophylactic antisepsis, the very core of the modern-day surgical ritual. Lister (1867) was the first among surgeons to recognize bacteria as the source of wound infection. Alexander Fleming (1929), microbiologist at St. Mary's Hospital in London, ardent student of surgical wounds and infections, offered the first convincing glimpse of the lytic property of the penicillium mold in destroying bacterial cultures. His observation paved the way for the development of penicillin, which put in the hands of the medical profession in mid-World War II days an effective remedy against spreading cellulitic infections. Domagk and the Tréfouëls supplied sulfanilamide in 1935, also an effective antibacterial agent against spreading infections. Prior thereto, in his wrestle with wound infection, the surgeon's role was essentially that of pus evacuator.

Controlled clinical trials, today's crucial test for adoption of new therapeutic suggestions, the innovation of Britain's distinguished naval surgeon James Lind, have finally supplanted blind groping and speculation. Six years before his 1753 publication on scurvy, Lind took twelve sailors with scurvy to sea, demonstrating very quickly the curative value of two oranges and a lemon added daily to the basic diet, later observing also their worth in prophylaxis. His achievement in simplicity of experiment and significance of results stands as a durable landmark, unsurpassed after more than two centuries, probably the first well-controlled and documented clinical study in medicine. The failure of surgeons to recognize the worth of controlled clinical trials in evaluating antiseptic agents and the "little circumstances" of successful surgeons, prolonged worthless procedures in wound management for centuries.

Osler was fond of quoting Barclay, who likened research to the Reapers, Gleaners, and Geese sequence. Osler lamented that those pursuing research in the 1890s were sorting out problems not yet resolved by the Reapers and the Gleaners, suggesting that unanswered problems needed new approaches for solution. The tremendous progress made in greater medicine since Osler sounded his note of despair indicates that there are periodic lulls in the advance of most disciplines. Progress is invariably discontinuous, not progressively forward. Application of new talents from other disciplines is obviously the first remedy in the solution of stagnant enigmatic problems. The current trend toward research centers, crossing the lines of tightly compartmentalized disciplines, involving every available skill and talent bearing upon a problem, promises to eke out of existing knowledge full utilization of all usable information. For stationary or apathetic periods in medicine's history, as this study reveals, such an address to baffling problems can prove extremely helpful. From mediocre beginnings, surgery through its accomplishments in the past quarter century has become a visible force in greater medicine, listened to with attention by faculties and the public.

The fragmentation and development of many new independent disciplines in surgery as in other areas of medicine is a reflection of the growing importance of research for surgery's advance. Can surgery survive as a unified body, is today a very proper and timely question. The need for free intercommunication between the many subdivisions of the mother discipline is evident on every hand. Transpollination, the catalyst and creator of life, would appear to be the only reliable effective agent to ensure surgery's survival as a unified medical specialty.

If this narration heightens only perceptibly student and faculty interest in the importance of history for the learning process, the long years occupied in search for and collection of sources relating to surgical management of wounds in peace and war will be fully justified, more than fulfilling the most sanguine hopes of its authors.

September 1978
Owen H. Wangensteen
Sarah D. Wangensteen

Acknowledgments

Anyone endeavoring to write on aspects of medical history owes an incalculable debt to John Shaw Billings and the Surgeon General's *Index-Catalogue* of medical literature which he founded (1880). The National Library of Medicine, the world's finest collection of great and useful medical books, is Billings's imperishable monument. The authors were privileged to acquire familiarity with its extensive collections during the early 1950s on the crowded shelves of the old red brick Army Medical Library on Seventh and Independence Avenue, Washington, D.C., the forerunner of the National Library of Medicine. This superb facility, created by Congress in 1956, was functionalized in 1962 at its present site in Bethesda, Maryland, in juxtaposition to the National Institutes of Health. The wonderful spirit of cooperation of its competent staff has been a source of inspiration to the authors throughout this study.

We have worked jointly and consecutively over long years in many other distinguished medical libraries in this country and abroad in search of materials relating to surgery's origins. Libraries in this country to which we are particularly beholden include our Medical Historical Collections at Minnesota, the John Crerar in Chicago, the New York Academy of Medicine, the College of Physicians in Philadelphia, the Cushing at Yale, the Moody at the University of Texas in Galveston, and Harvard's Countway. In London, visits to the Henry S. Wellcome, the Royal College of Surgeons, the Royal Society of Medicine, the Royal College of Physicians, and the British Museum proved very rewarding, as did research in the university libraries of Edinburgh and Glasgow and medical libraries in Liverpool and Leeds. We found much pertinent material in the Bibliothèque Nationale and the libraries of the Faculty of Medicine and the Academy of Medicine in Paris, and also among the venerable collection of books at the University of Montpellier. At the History of Medicine Library in Vienna, the Semmelweis Memorial, and other great libraries in Budapest we were hospitably welcomed and rewarded in our search.

This broad exposure to many of the world's great medical libraries provides evidence that librarians are a unique, wonderful, and selfless group of people, conscious of the privilege and responsibility of presiding over their treasures, and ready and willing to make them available to sincere inquirers. This long pursuit, in the company of fascinating and helpful colleagues who demonstrate a full commitment to a lifelong stay in academia, constitutes one of the magnetic attractions of the academic life. Without direct access to documents and rare pamphlets and books generally unavailable, the present effort would have suffered.

The authors wish to acknowledge grateful thanks to a number of journals that have generously permitted us to use or quote from articles previously published for the authors, notably the following: *Bulletin of the History of Medicine*, published by the Johns Hopkins Press; *Surgery*, published by C. V. Mosby Company; *Surgery, Gynecology and Obstetrics*, an organ of the American College of Surgeons; the *Annals of the Royal College of Surgeons of England; Proceedings of the International Congress for the History of Medicine*; and the *Bulletin of the New York Academy of Medicine*. We also wish to thank Lloyd M. Nyhus and Christopher Wastell for permission to use some material from a chapter contributed by the authors to the third edition of their *Surgery of the Stomach and Duodenum*, published by Little, Brown, 1977.

We are grateful for the permission to reproduce many illustrations from various museums, publications, and private individuals, and have given credit lines in such instances. In other cases the illustrations are reproduced from the authors' own files, previous papers, or the large picture collection of the Minnesota Bio-Medical Library. We regret that in a few instances the original sources of these cannot be identified.

Many accomplished librarians and scholars gave us important help in locating source materials over the years of this pursuit. It would be a serious oversight if we did not express our great indebtedness to Mary H. Mueller, Jessie F. Richardson, Judith A. Overmier, and others at the University of Minnesota; to Estelle Brodman and Frank B. Rogers of the old Army Medical Library, and to Dorothy T. Hanks and Peter D. Olch of the National Library of Medicine; to Gertrude Annan, librarian emeritus of the New York Academy of Medicine; and Lisabeth M. Holloway, librarian of the College of Physicians in Philadelphia. In London, valuable assistance was provided by Charles Talbot, Noel Poynter, and Eric J. Freeman at the Wellcome; William LeFanu, Eustace Cornelius, and Jessie Dobson at the Royal College of Surgeons; Philip Wade at the Royal Society of Medicine; Leonard M. Payne and Charles Newman at the Royal College of Physicians; John Shepherd at the Liverpool Institute; A. Batty Shaw of the Norwich Hospital in Norfolk; Marie-José Huart, Pierre Huard, and the late Charles Coury at the libraries of the Faculty of Medicine in Paris; Josef Antall and Ferenc Nemethy in Budapest. Erna Lesky, medical historian in Vienna, has given generously of her time and talent in support of this inquiry. The authors also wish to express their thanks to Rudolf Nissen of Basel, superb surgeon, extremely knowledgeable in the history of nineteenth- and twentieth-century surgery, whose friendship with the senior author began at the Charité in Berlin in the Sauerbruch period fifty years ago. Leonard G. Wilson, Minnesota's Professor of the History of Medicine, has given sage advice in many informal colloquia.

The National Library of Medicine provided helpful support of the project over several years in its beginnings. Generous support came also from the Ralph and Marian Falk Research Foundation, the Margaret Weyerhaeuser Foundation, the Alice M. O'Brien Foundation, and the Josiah Macy, Jr. Foundation.

Our studies profited in the early 1960s from the help of Jacqueline Smith, now of Minnesota's Wilson Library; from John Witta; and in more recent years from Charles F. Klinger, who has a Doctor's degree in medieval history, and whose assistance has been extremely valuable. All three have shared with the authors the pleasures of journal authorship.

It is also a duteous pleasure to acknowledge painstaking assistance from three competent and loyal secretaries, Susan K. Greengard, Miriam Stormo, and Rosemary Braun, in preparation of the manuscript for publication, including several revisions. The authors received valuable assistance in proofreading from Lorraine Hannon. We wish to thank Martin E. Finch of our University's Biomedical Graphic Communications for help in preparing the illustrative material. The University of Minnesota Press and its competent staff complimented the authors by undertaking publication of our manuscript.

Over the years many professional colleagues have proved extremely helpful sounding boards in conferences, panels, discussions, and letter exchanges. To countless such friends the authors express their appreciative thanks.

Aids for the Reader

For brevity, we have occasionally used only the last names of persons infrequently or cursorily mentioned in the text. Full names and titles, when known, will be found in the chapter notes or in the name index. Any student of early medical literature will understand why we cannot always supply complete appellations, particularly from early French sources in which too often only patronymics are given. When sons and relatives of surgeons followed their forbear's craft, as they frequently did, even a qualifying "senior" or "son" may not be sufficient to establish identity. Moreover, in secondary accounts an obscure surgeon has sometimes been carelessly identified as a familiar personage of similar name even though of a different period, making an attempt to find the original source extremely difficult. We have tried to call attention in the notes to some of these errors, hoping to pass on to future scholars some of the generous assistance we have been privileged to receive from helpful authorities in many lands over two decades. Because of its length we have been obliged to omit from the name index many names appearing only in the notes. This omission applies particularly to authors and editors of biographical and secondary sources. We regret this curtailment but hope it will not hamper the interested reader, for the names and full citations can readily be located in the pertinent note.

Table of Contents

THE RISE OF SURGERY

From Empiric Craft to Scientific Discipline

CHAPTER 1

Overview

SURGERY'S DECISIVE RISE in achievement had to await the arrival of microbiology, a development of the last quarter of the nineteenth century. Elective surgery came only with the demonstration and acceptance of the pathogenicity of bacteria. Until then surgeons were concerned primarily with wounds of trauma and with the management of conditions compelling operative interference — an impaled arrow, a foot crushed under a cart wheel, a live baby in the womb of a dead mother. Assessment of the recorded accomplishment in such urgent situations over many centuries is, in the authors' belief, the key to a new and revealing appraisal of surgery's early advances.

As the story unfolds, it becomes apparent that the overall performance in operations of necessity, measured by the patients' survival, was indeed poor; yet there were a few surgeons, separated in space and time, who achieved records of success, notably in the amputation of extremities and removal of stones from the urinary bladder, not surpassed until the dawn of the twentieth century. Many of these achievements are not even mentioned in well-known tracts on the history of surgery. The surgeon sometimes attributed his good results to "little circumstances" or "minute particulars." Actually, however, important components of his accomplishment were techniques that left the wound partially open, the use of cautery and other primitive methods of debridement, and the observance of high standards of surgical cleanliness. These will be among significant practices explored in the first chapters of this book, as a prelude to the important revelations of nineteenth-century scientists and the emergence of surgery as a scientific discipline in the twentieth century.

This assessment of surgery's progress over the centuries represents essentially two approaches: an appraisal of achievements in operations of emergency and dire necessity, followed by an inquiry into factors that led surgery from empiricism to an acceptance of scientific observations and discoveries in other disciplines, notably microbiology, uplifting surgery in the public image to one of respect and admiration. It was a long and arduous journey, a story that deserves to be better known by the profession and by a broader audience.

For centuries many surgeons were committed to seeing what they believed; innovators, always in the minority, believing what they saw, as did that knight-errant of surgery Ambroise Paré in 1536, abandoned their theories when their observations conflicted with what they had been taught or believed. This is, obviously, a subtle distinction, but a significant difference in address to challenging problems. Tradition has always been a restraining barrier to innovation. Wrote the Nobel Laureate Maurice Maeterlinck (1907), "At every cross-way on the road that leads to the future, [tradition] has placed, against each of us, ten thousand men to guard the past."[1]

Twenty generations of men and women have come and disappeared in the four centuries since the great Renaissance triumvirate of Girolamo Fracastoro (1546), Paré (1545), and Andreas Vesalius (1543) left their durable imprints on medicine's progress. Their perceptive discoveries on the nature of contagion, the improvement of wound management, and the fabric of the human body constituted important beacons for later investigators in surgery and other medical disciplines. The forecasts of Fracastoro were enlightened by the experiments of Francesco Redi (1683) and Antonj van Leeuwenhoek (1693) in the seventeenth century and Lazaro Spallanzani (1776) in the eighteenth century and found verification by a succession of keen and original observers including Jacob Henle (1840), Ignacz Semmelweis (1847), Louis Pasteur (1860–79), Joseph Lister (1867–96), and Robert Koch (1876–90). Their studies achieved the revolution in surgical wound management which is the focus of this volume.

Important lessons in the great surgical accomplishments of an earlier era are too often ignored. It is not commonly appreciated that a succession of surgeons during the eighteenth and nineteenth centuries recognized and proclaimed the importance

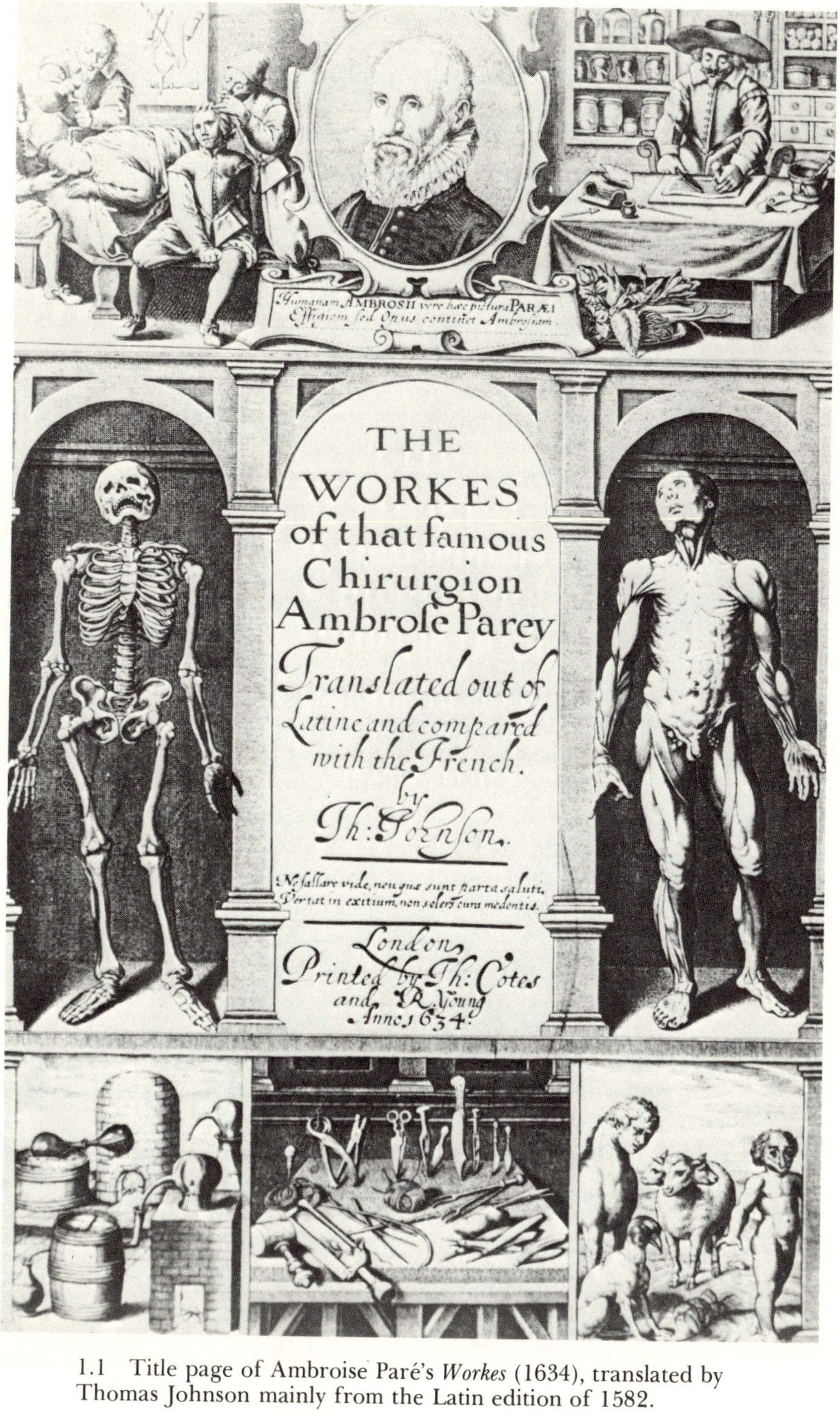

1.1 Title page of Ambroise Paré's *Workes* (1634), translated by Thomas Johnson mainly from the Latin edition of 1582.

of direct contact as the principal factor in the transference of infection. Among these were Claude Pouteau (1769), John Rollo (1797), Jacques Delpech (1815), John Thomson (1816), H. Home Blackadder (1818), and Alexandre-F. Ollivier (1822). The principle was implemented by the Hungarian-born Semmelweis (1847) on the obstetrical wards of Vienna's Allgemeines Krankenhaus. His prophylactic antiseptic wound practices antedated recognition of the pathogenicity of bacteria. A few French surgeons during the eighteenth century and Astley Cooper in the early nineteenth century had remarkable results with surgery for strangulating intestinal obstructions. Ephraim McDowell's unprecedented achievement (1809) with ovariotomy is well known, as is J. Marion Sims's success (1852) with repair of vesicovaginal fistula, an extracavitary operation in which use of silver sutures apparently was solely responsible for the auspicious outcome — when prophylactic antisepsis came into vogue, catgut and silk sutures proved equally successful.

Testing the worth of a proposed remedial measure by argument rather than by trial was common in early times, a practice unfortunately continued throughout most of the nineteenth century among university medical academicians and in the profession generally. Thus ovariotomy was proscribed by vote after four months of debate in the French Imperial Academy of Medicine (1856–57), although bold surgeons in America and Great Britain were already using the operation to save patients with huge ovarian cysts. A single dissenting voice in the Academy declared that the operation deserved further examination. Lengthy discussions in English medical meetings and journals denounced surgical intervention for intestinal obstructions. American surgeons boasted of their rejection of Lister's antiseptic practices without subjecting them to trial. Factual reporting of successes and failures came only late in the 1800s when surgeons at last began to accept accountability for operative mortality, a development that antisepsis made a more agreeable obligation.

One of the great innovations in surgery was anesthesia, an American contribution in the 1840s. Before use of anesthesia, speed of operation was the sole reliance of most surgeons, a practice that continued until late in the nineteenth century when Theodor Kocher and William S. Halsted demonstrated the superiority of careful and methodical operative techniques, including the gentle management of tissues. Anesthesia was widely hailed and rapidly utilized everywhere, but it did not contribute significantly to the extension of elective surgery until the long delayed adoption of prophylactic surgical antisepsis.

Lister, probably the first surgeon to appreciate the bacterial origin of wound infections, emphasized the instillation of antiseptics into wounds (1867) and the spraying of the operative field with dilute solutions of phenol (1871). Some leaders in the public health field in the mid-1870s, while admitting the existence of bacteria, believed their presence was merely coincidental, bearing no causal relationship to contagion or wound infection. It is to be remembered that hospital gangrene was a frequent occurrence, as was erysipelas, before Listerian practices found general recognition. As many as 80 percent of all patients operated upon and all with wounds and ulcers were affected with hospital gangrene in Johann Nussbaum's clinic in Munich as late as 1874; Nussbaum treated the complication with the cautery.

The interval from 1875 to 1890 was a fruitful period in the advance of surgery. By 1880 the germ theory of wound infection had been fully proved, owing largely to Koch's innovative morphologic and cultural studies, his improved staining techniques for identifying and documenting bacterial proliferation, and also his experimental production of infection by injection studies in mice and rabbits (1878). In addressing the tenth International Medical Congress in Berlin (1890), Koch observed that before 1875 bacteria were generally believed to be nonpathogenic and that many prestigious surgeons in America and Britain disavowed any faith or confidence in Listerian practices until the mid-1880s.

When Ernst Bergmann (1882) came to the Ziegelstrasse Clinic, now in East Berlin, to succeed Bernhard Langenbeck, he was visited by a contemporary from Dorpat, who asked, "What is new in surgery?" Replied Bergmann, "Today we wash our hands *before* operation!" That simple, terse reply rationalized the great change that came about in surgery in the last quarter of the nineteenth century, underscoring not the Listerian practice of placing antiseptics into wounds to control infection but a return to the earlier prophylactic antisepsis of Semmelweis, a practice first introduced for abdominal surgery by the Freiburg gynecologist Alfred Hegar (1876–77). Elective surgery of the other body cavities — the thorax and the calvarium — began in the mid-1880s.

Pasteur's pupil Charles E. Chamberland (1878–79) and Koch (1881) had shown that wherever applicable thermal measures were superior to chemical antiseptic practices in promoting sterility of microbiologic matériel. Their suggestions were implemented in clinical surgery by Gustav Neuber (1883) of Kiel, Bergmann, and Curt Schimmelbusch (1889–92) of Berlin. Heat was substituted for chemicals in the sterilization of instruments and matériel for operation, a practice that the French surgeons Léon Tripier (1883) and Paul Redard (1886) also adopted. This development is usually referred to as the beginning of asepsis, for want of a more appropriate designation. The Budapest surgeon A. Puky first employed the term in 1879.[2] It is clear, however, that he used it as synonymous with instillation of antiseptics into wounds and did not appreciate the prophylactic surgical antisepsis of Semmelweis. Since very few wounds are bacteria-free, the concept of aseptic wounds is essentially a microbiologic myth. The real objective is to achieve healing without evidence of suppuration. The English microbiologist Stephen D. Elek (1956) has shown that intradermal or subcutaneous injections of 10,000 staphylococci may not be followed by infection; yet, in the presence of a buried suture, as few as 100 organisms may provoke suppuration.

One of the great contributions to surgery in the final decades of the nineteenth century was the surgical rubber glove. Whereas the London physician Thomas Watson (1842) suggested the wearing of a clean glove impervious to fluid for the protection of parturients at delivery, the early promotion of surgical rubber gloves was to prevent accoucheurs from acquiring syphilis from obscure genital chancres in parturients. The importance of Watson's suggestion for the protection of patients was not fully appreciated until late in the nineteenth century.

The wearing of a face mask covering mouth and nose by the operating team, an innovation of Johann Mikulicz-Radecki (1897) of Breslau, was based on the significant work of his microbiologist colleague Carl Flügge (1897), who demonstrated the great threat of droplet infection of wounds during speech. Felix Würtz (1563) had envisioned the hazards of droplet infection long years before and had cautioned surgeons against breathing into wounds.

As prophylactic antisepsis found acceptance, hospital admissions for surgical procedures multiplied. Elective surgery of the body cavities was essentially new, and the techniques had to be acquired through experience. W. B. O'Shaughnessy (1831–32) had outlined the fluid and electrolyte requirements of patients suffering from the severe diarrhea of cholera, findings that Sidney Ringer (1880–82) later subjected to physiological scrutiny. Surgeons had to learn how to deal with these problems when the normal function of organ systems was temporarily interrupted by operations upon the digestive tract, causing distention, anorexia, and oliguria. Strange as it may seem, the need in such cases for rational parenteral fluid therapy was recognized only in the mid-1920s as a result of the studies of the Boston pediatrician J. L. Gamble.

One of the great surprises to the authors in this pursuit was the primacy of the Hippocratic writings in emphasizing the wisdom of a period of delay (fifteen days) before performing open external drainage for empyema. This observation was made more than twenty centuries before the discovery of bacteria. For over fifty years it has been generally believed that closed needle or catheter drainage of empyema was an innovation of Evarts Graham and Richard D. Bell. However, the French surgeon Charles E. Sédillot (1841) urged adoption of the Hippocratic principle of delayed opening of empyemas by external drainage. In 1918 Graham and Bell affirmed the hazard of mediastinal shifts occasioned by the equalizing of intrapleural and atmospheric pressure.

The problem of wound infection continues to shadow the surgeon. It is still the most common cause of death after operations of large magnitude. Fracastoro (1546) recognized the importance of direct contact in the conveyance of infection, but atmospheric sources of contagion and wound infection dominated the thinking of most students of the problem until about 1885. Today several British students of wound management continue to pursue the commendable but elusive objective of eliminating bacteria in operating room air in the hope of completely eradicating infection in elective operations. The struggle to achieve a sterile operation still confronts surgeons and hospital sanitary engineers. The necessity to thwart nosocomial infections is recognized, an endeavor in which observance of hygienic principles and isolation are the mainstays. As theologian John Wesley observed in the mid-1700s, "Cleanliness is indeed next to godliness," although he was probably thinking more of the spirit than of the body.[3]

Total silence of the operating team during operation may prove to be even more important than control of the particle content of the operating atmosphere and possibly as effective as John Charnley's laminar airflow over the operative field (1964). The "Surgical Flamingo," William Fergusson (1867), Lister's predecessor at King's College Hospital in London, embarrassed onlookers at operations by observing total silence, not replying to questions. Sir William found it necessary to explain to visitors upon conclusion of operations that he and his assistants actually were on speaking terms. This practice bears emulation today, even though it deemphasizes the current method of utilizing operations in progress for teaching medical students and surgical trainees. Welfare of the patient must be the paramount consideration.

Alexander Fleming's bold announcement following World War I (1919) that the instillation of antiseptics into wounds did more harm to the tissues than to the bacteria helped clarify the thesis that prophylaxis was the key to successful wound management. The effective treatment of established wound infection had to await the availability of the sulfonamides and antibiotics, which lent a new dimension to the surgeon's success in his wrestle with wound infection, reinforcing the thesis of Paul Ehrlich (1910) that systemic therapeutic measures would be found to control infection. A consistently successful *therapia sterilisans* still eludes and baffles investigators. It remains a sanguine hope and possibly a promise of the future.

An unanticipated disclosure in our study of the long record of operations of dire necessity is that mere rearrangement of indications for such an operative procedure as cesarean section has improved the accomplishment phenomenally in the last two decades of this century. When the operation was performed only after days of difficult, protracted labor, it was accompanied by a formidable mortality rate, despite adequate antisepsis. Today, when it is regularly performed for such an indication as fetal intrauterine malposition, the operation has been done without mortality in large series in several American obstetrical clinics. The reporting of maternal deaths attending labor by obstetricians in the New England area has served to focus the profession's attention upon preventable causes. This practice obviously can be adopted in several areas in surgery with beneficial consequences.

As late as the sixteenth century surgeons generally "were still roughly classed with the horde of barbers, bath-keepers, executioners, and vagrant mounte-banks."[4] Physicians in Paris in the seventeenth century, however, were lettered. Medical students, aspiring to become physicians, listened to a daily succession of philosophic lectures in Latin by the faculty, who were believed to be erudite enough to lecture on any subject. The students rarely saw a patient. After two years of indoctrination, each student was subjected to incredibly prolonged examinations, pitting his wits against as many as nine members of the faculty at a time. Many of the examination questions were not only trivial but absurd.[5] The French surgeons of the day fared better in their training. They were taught in French and acquired their professional skills through apprenticeship to experienced and established surgeons, a practice continued in many areas throughout most of the nineteenth century.

The College of St. Côme, composed of barber-surgeons of the long robe and lay barbers of the short robe, was founded in Paris under Jean Pitard early in the thirteenth century in protest against the physicians, who held that the practical experience of surgeons had no validity. At this time surgeons identified with the Paris Faculty of Medicine were obliged to take an oath acknowledging the supremacy of medicine over surgery, a humiliating formality, not abolished until 1750. Jean Louis Petit, a very innovative surgeon, was the first to refuse its observance in 1700.

By the beginning of the twelfth century the fame and influence of the University of Salerno and its medical school, which dated back three centuries, were felt throughout Europe. A century and more later universities sprang up in Bologna, Padua, Milan, Montpellier, and Paris and in Britain and Central Europe. Students ambitious for professional careers flocked to the doors of universities.

In the thirteenth century in Italy several surgeons who had been privileged to have a university education began to put in writing information on surgical practices, making accessible to larger audiences what previously had been communicated chiefly by word of mouth. Bruno, in his treatise *Chirurgia magna* (1252), emphasized the dry management of wounds. Theodoric (1205–96), whose *Cyrurgia* appeared in print in 1498, held that wounds can heal without suppuration, a thesis which was unpopular in its time but was confirmed four centuries later by prophylactic antiseptic practices. Saliceto (ca. 1210–77), surgical scholar, wrote the first anatomy for surgeons. Unlike Saliceto, Lanfranc (d. 1315) favored the cautery over the knife. Henri de Mondeville (1260–1320), like Theodoric, believed that wounds could heal without suppuration. Guy de Chauliac (ca. 1298–1368) of Avignon, the most erudite surgeon of his time, wrote his *Grande chirurgie* in 1363; he favored open management of contaminated wounds, a practice not fully appreciated until World War I. He also included suggestions about complemental pharmacy in his management of wounds.

University medical schools made available to aspiring physicians an opportunity for training in medical theories. The more

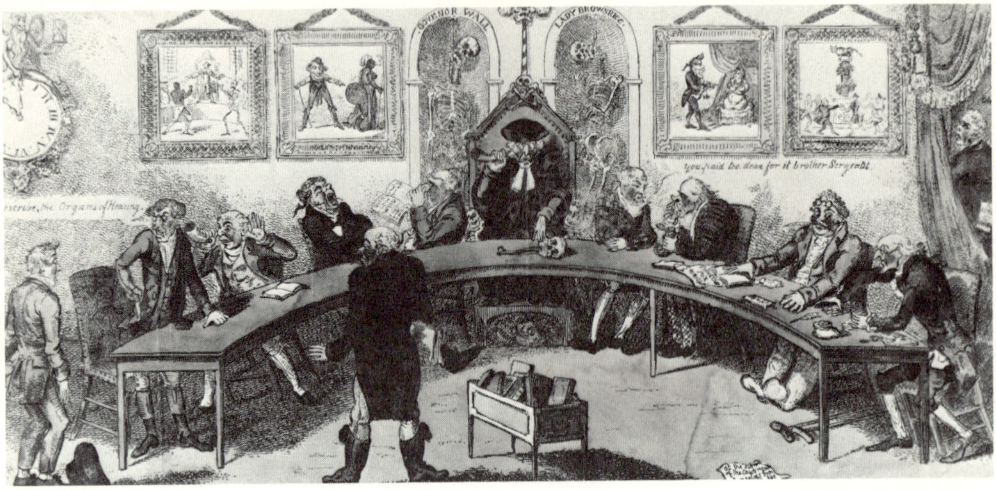

1.2 Cruikshank's caricature of young English surgeon in qualification examination (1811). Courtesy National Library of Medicine, Bethesda, Maryland.

practical aspects of medical teaching came later with the development of hospitals and medical clinics.

The frailties of the doctrines, practices, and sterile pedantry of the physicians were lampooned by Molière (1622–73), whose satires on the customs of the day greatly amused Louis XIV and, in consequence, Molière's plays came to enjoy royal patronage and support. The pompous pretenses and vacuity of the dogmas of physicians were held up to public ridicule and scorn in a succession of comedies by Molière. In his last satire, *The Hypochondriac*, Molière exposed the teachings of the physicians and their examinations for the doctorate. His work ultimately constituted an important force in the reform of medical education, as did the striking caricatures of Cruikshank in England nearly two centuries later.

The French physicians of the eighteenth and nineteenth centuries came generally from a higher social order than did the surgeons, many of whom were recruited from conditions bordering on abject poverty. The famous Paris surgeon Guillaume Dupuytren liked to startle auditors in his large medical classes at the Hôtel-Dieu by saying that had he not, out of necessity, been obliged to light his study candle with the tallow of the dissecting room, he never would have become "Monsieur *le Baron* Dupuytren."[6]

Paré, a barber-surgeon with three years of experience on the surgical wards of the Hôtel-Dieu and a long military service under five kings, became the foremost surgeon of the sixteenth century, contributing much to the improvement and elevation of the public image of the surgeon and of surgery. Even so, not knowing Latin and having no university training, he was unqualified for membership in the Paris Faculty of Medicine, a circumstance that led later to his interesting debates with Étienne Gourmelen, a surgeon and the dean of the Faculty of Medicine, in the years 1574–76. Paré taunted Gourmelen as a surgeon steeped in book learning but lacking in practical experience. Paré's writings reveal him to be a shrewd and a wise surgeon who learned from his own experience and was ready to discard theories when they were in conflict with his observations — a surgeon who believed what he observed.

Lack of erudition has always been laid up against the surgeon. Being ignorant of Latin, Paré wrote in French. John Hunter, self-tutored save for a period of apprenticeship to his brother William, wrote of a critic, "Jesse Foot accuses me of not understanding the dead languages; but I could teach him that on the dead body which he never knew in any language dead or living." The famous Leeds-Cambridge internist T. Clifford Allbutt came strongly to the defense of surgeons in his memorable tract on the historical relations of medicine and surgery, pointing out that the philosophic dissertations and discussions of physicians of early years were, in essence, what William James called "filling your belly with east wind."[7]

The episode of Louis XIV's fistula-in-ano, and the success of Charles-François Félix in dealing with it, gave surgery a much needed lift in the medical hierarchy and also in public esteem. A seed or a fecalith lodged in the crypts of the rectal columns and anal valves at the juncture of the rectum and the anal canal may cause inflammation and abscess formation in the pararectal tissues, with subsequent fistula, a painful situation. For this condition, from February until November 18, 1686 (when an operation was performed), the forty-eight-year-old king was treated by a variety of nonoperative measures including emetics, purges, applications of leeches, and bleeding, prescriptions of his physicians which today would be adjudged harmful and valueless. Guy Fagon, the king's physician, recommended that Félix relieve the king of his distressful ailment by operation.[8] Provision was made in a Paris hospital for Félix to acquire knowledge and deftness in the procedure, and patients afflicted with fistula-in-ano were sent there for surgery. Tradition has it that a number of these did not survive Félix's operations and that the bodies were disposed of at night and the deaths were attributed to poisoning. The trials went on for approximately two months. In mid-November Félix said he was ready, as was the king.

Félix inserted his bistoury, simplified from the semicircular instrument of Galen to a modest curve, into the external opening that communicated with the rectal canal. He slit the rectal tissue and the external sphincter; the operation, except for the absence of adequate anesthesia, was carried out along lines acceptable to present-day surgeons. The only change in modern management would be the passage of a flexible grooved director through the external opening, following which the tissue engaged over the probe would be divided with a knife.[9] The king bore the ordeal well, receiving a fairly large assembly of his court that evening. The convalescence was a bit trying, but by early January the royal patient was well.[10] Fagon, Félix, and the other participants were bountifully rewarded by the king. The effect upon the status of surgeons was felt far beyond the borders of Paris and France and was bitterly resented by the physicians. It was truly a great achievement for French surgery. A few decades later the founding of the French Academy of Surgery (1731) by Georges Mareschal, Félix's successor, and François de La Peyronie of Montpellier again augmented considerably the status of surgeons and surgery in France. When Louis XV (1724) provided Mareschal with five chairs for surgical instruction at St. Côme, the members of the Paris Faculty of Medicine revolted, recognizing therein a challenging threat to their assumed superiority, even though based on sterile pedagogy.[11]

The hallmark of social acceptance of a profession is recognizable and consistent achievement. A few military surgeons, notably Paré and Dominique Larrey, Napoleon's great army surgeon, were warmly appreciated by their leaders for devoted service to the armies in the care of the wounded and were adored by the soldiers, who felt that the very presence of these exceptional surgeons on the battlefield inspired confidence.

Florence Nightingale made strong pleas for hospital statistics (1860, 1862) and factual reports on successes and failures of surgical operations (1863), accounts that surgeons were reluctant to provide. James Paget, a distinguished St. Bartholomew surgeon and surgical pathologist, in his "Address on Surgery" (1862) disavowed any suggestion of accountability for mortality attending operative procedures, holding that coincidental factors were responsible for the deaths.

When prophylactic surgical antisepsis was adopted by surgeons in the final years of the nineteenth century, there gradually emerged in the hospitals a rising spirit of optimism for the future of surgery, an attitude shared also by hospital boards. Throughout Britain, whose surgeons were among the last to capitulate to the teachings of Semmelweis, Pasteur, Lister, and Koch, there became evident a spontaneous desire of hospital boards to provide surgeons better facilities in which to perform their operations; theatres with marble floors and walls and with teakwood seats for spectators came to supplant the traditional operating rooms with sawdust-covered floors reminiscent of slaughterhouse arenas.

In the post-World War II years surgeons began to take serious note of research in related fields, and surgeons in academic halls began to participate actively in research. The startling innovations that came about elicited the manifest approval of the public, which was ready to acknowledge that surgery was a productive and creative force contributing significantly to the advance of greater medicine. Research has been the powerful catalyst in the development of intracardiac and transplantation surgery. It is to continued liberal support of investigation, energized by creative minds for practical application, that we must look for surgery's progress. Surgical academicians have come to recognize the importance of active participation in research as the surest means of advancing their discipline. Research centers, which employ diverse talents from many disciplines, will undoubtedly provide the answers to many challenging problems in future decades. The role of such centers in renal transplantation demonstrates their utility.

Over the past century repeated pleas have been made by leaders in medicine for a close alignment between medicine and surgery, notably by E. H. Sieveking of London (1862), T. Clifford Allbutt of Leeds and Cambridge (1905), and Harvey Cushing (1921, 1929). With the extension of surgery into many new areas since World War II and consequent fragmentation, a more important query confronting surgery today is, can it survive as a unified body? The answer would appear to be free communication between its many disciplines. Tight compartmentalization breeds sterility; the only hope is transpollination, the catalyst of life.

(For notes, see pp. 583–84.)

CHAPTER 2

Wound Management in Amputation

THE ORIGINS OF SURGERY are lost in obscurity. Human skulls from the Neolithic period (10,000–7000 B.C.) provide evidence that primitive man performed trephination, an operation which removed circular bits of the cranium, usually less than an inch in diameter. There is no doubt that polished stones with sharp flintlike edges were used for the excisions, long before bronze and iron instruments were available. Skulls with such perforations have been found scattered geographically from the Mediterranean to Peru. Trephining probably was first attempted for depressed skull fractures; since it gave the victim obvious relief, it was tried for other ills believed to originate within the calvarium. The procedure was almost invariably extradural, and the patient's survival of the ordeal was probably not unusual. The amputation of limbs severely torn by wild beasts or crushed by falling trees or rocks undoubtedly also was undertaken by prehistoric man as a desperate expedient.

The need for amputations and for the care of wounds of trauma increased greatly after the introduction of gunpowder in warfare in Europe before the middle of the fourteenth century. Elective surgery came only with the development and acceptance of prophylactic antiseptic wound practices; until then, with few exceptions, operations were performed only in such life-threatening situations as a mangled or gangrenous extremity, a respiratory obstruction, a vesical stone, or strangulated hernia. The contamination of open wounds was augmented by the aggressive intervention of the surgeon in direct ratio to his neglect of cleanliness. His incised wounds met the same fate. His desperate and often bizarre empiric efforts against the unknown causes of wound suppuration are therefore understandable. Yet in performing amputations, surely among the earliest major operations ever attempted,[1] surgeons gradually evolved techniques of wound management that facilitated and quickened healing. (These and other important operations of necessity by which surgery advanced are described in subsequent chapters.) The study of our professional origins has important lessons to teach which, in our deep involvement with the present, are often set aside as matters of secondary concern. A look back into the causes potentiating as well as those retarding advances in a discipline can be instructive and sobering.

We will not attempt to probe in detail the contributions of Egyptian medicine, which in some areas has a well-documented and intriguing story. For instance, the Smith, Ebers, and Brugsch papyri, written probably between the sixteenth and the fourteenth centuries B.C., provide considerable information on individual medical case records dating back to the times of the great pyramids (ca. 3000 B.C.). Egyptian physicians were members of the priesthood. Their therapy was shrouded in mystery and included prayers, incantations, and magical drug prescriptions believed to be, in part, of divine direction. Surgery was employed in the management of abscesses and small tumors, for which the knife was used. Ophthalmic, ear, and dental operations were occasionally performed. In general, however, the emphasis was upon conservative measures; surgery was an action of last resort. When the Greeks entered the land of the Nile in the seventh century B.C., Egyptian medicine was well on the decline.[2]

Tradition assigns the Hippocratic writings to a single person, Hippocrates of Cos, born about 460 B.C. Hippocrates is certainly the most widely known and admired physician of antiquity, but the writings of the Hippocratic school, assembled by scholars of Alexandria in the third century B.C., undoubtedly represent the thinking and practices of generations of physicians. Which sections are truly those of Hippocrates remains obscure, yet certain of the treatises are "impressed with the marks of an outstanding genius" and these apparently were written during the latter half of the fifth century B.C.[3]

Hippocrates has long been regarded as the father of both medicine and surgery. Many medical historians have stated that the Hippocratic writings on surgery have not been surpassed, given the limitations under which they were produced. Greasy dressings were avoided, and only clean water or wine was used for wound irrigation. The Hippocratic "wait and see" policy, still much in vogue with physicians, certainly was sound practice when surgery was in its infancy. Julius L. Pagel stated that Hippocrates' surgery was largely that of fractures and dislocations, of rectal fistulas and hemorrhoids, of ulcers and chronic wounds, not fresh wounds. If Pagel had specified *incised* wounds, instead of fresh wounds, his statement would have been more meaningful.[4]

Warfare, wounds, and surgeons are intimately interlinked through all of history. The traditional counsel to those who would be surgeons was to follow the army.[5] Before the use of gunpowder in combat, the amputation of an injured limb, especially above the knee, was undoubtedly a rare occurrence. When Theodor Billroth, great scholar and innovative surgeon, wrote his historic tract on the nature and treatment of gunshot wounds, he considered Hieronymus Brunschwig's account of such therapy as the earliest (1497). A commentary written in 1460 by Heinrich Pfolspeundt, a Bavarian army surgeon, has since come to light. It also includes a discussion of treating gunshot wounds.[6]

Amputations, chiefly for gangrene following vascular occlusion, were described in the Hippocratic writings. The operations were made through devitalized rather than living tissue to avoid the great risk of hemorrhage.[7] Two thousand years later, in seventeenth-century England, this precaution was still observed. Whereas the British naval surgeon John Woodall recommended amputation through healthy tissue, most of the discussion of the subject in his *Surgeons Mate* (1639) concerned division through the upper level of the dead tissue. Woodall explained that such excision was painless and that after a limb had been removed the surgeon could whittle away the dead tissue until it was almost gone; two or three men sufficed to help with the operation. Most of the lower extremity amputations of this period, of course, were below the knee. As an additional defense of amputating through dead tissue, Woodall related the instance of a healthy cleric who pared a corn on his toe with a knife until it bled and died of infection two days later.

Woodall labeled amputation the "most lamentable part" of surgery and advised the surgeon not to neglect his prayers before undertaking the operation: "For it is no small presumption to Dismember the Image of God." That amputation continued

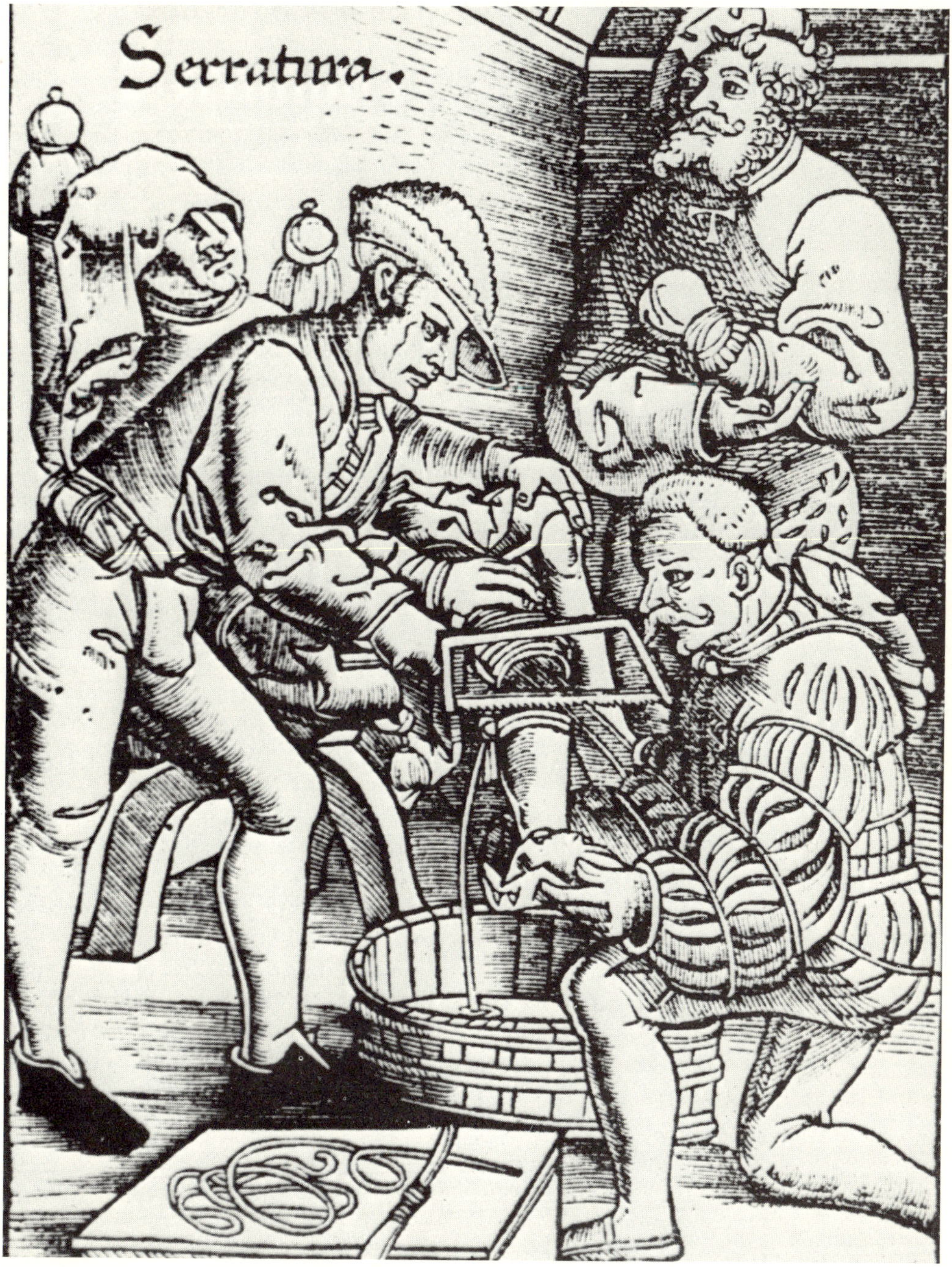

2.1 Amputation of leg, early sixteenth century. Tight bands, no tourniquet. From Hans Gersdorff, *Feldtbuch der Wundtartzney* (Strasbourg, 1517). Courtesy National Library of Medicine.

to be a procedure involving great risk was noted as late as 1869 by James Y. Simpson of Edinburgh. In discussing the high mortality rate of the operation, Simpson said, "The man laid on an operating-table in one of our surgical hospitals is exposed to more chances of death than the English soldier on the field of Waterloo."[8]

The main problems concerning amputation through the ages relate to (1) control of hemorrhage, whether to use styptic agents, cautery, or ligature; (2) selection of the type of amputation, whether circular or with long or short skin flaps; and (3) the important matter of wound closure. The wound may be left open or closed primarily. In case of closure, questions were whether to use bandage, adhesive tape, or suture. In open wound management decisions concerning irrigation and use of medicated dressings date back for many centuries. Satisfying answers to some of these questions came only with acceptance of prophylactic surgical antisepsis.

Styptics and Caustics

Much has been written about the use of styptics for the arrest of hemorrhage. Although vitriol, alum, turpentine, and other agents may have some virtue in stopping oozing from tiny vessels, the experience of surgeons is that their value in the control of bleeding is measured essentially by the degree of pressure employed in their application and the snugness of the overlying bandages.

John Hunter, England's great surgical scientist of the late eighteenth century, was partial to oil of turpentine, calling it "the best, if not the only true styptic." The "royal styptic," a French import lauded by Richard Wiseman, an English military surgeon of the seventeenth century, was apparently an oil of turpentine preparation. It probably had greater virtue as an antiseptic than as a styptic. Moreover, Wiseman conceded that the army surgeon "in the heat of Fight" would find the cautery more effective.[9]

The Paris surgeon Pierre Dionis, who was appointed in 1673 by Louis XIV to give public demonstrations in anatomy and surgery at the Jardin-du-Roi, announced in his lecture on amputations that vitriol was at that time being used to stop bleeding in all such operations at the Hôtel-Dieu, the oldest and largest hospital in the city. Dionis said that he himself preferred the ligature and resorted to buttons of vitriol only if the ligature failed.

Among the frequent anecdotes with which this popular surgeon enlivened his teachings was one about a man named Rabel, who claimed to have a styptic that could prevent any wounded soldier from bleeding to death. Rabel's enthusiasm for his vulnerary water was so persuasive that Louis's minister of war finally allowed Rabel to demonstrate the remedy in a thigh amputation on a soldier at the Hôtel des Invalides before an assembly of physicians and surgeons. Despite Rabel's frantic and repeated applications of styptic and fresh bandages, the patient bled to death.[10]

Cautery

An ancient aphorism concerning the power of the cautery proclaimed, "Those diseases which medicine does not cure, iron cures; those which iron cannot cure, fire cures; those which fire cannot cure, are to be reckoned incurable." From surgery's beginnings and well into the nineteenth century, the cautery heated over a bed of hot coals was quite regularly prepared before an operation. Used primarily to control hemorrhage, it served also as an antiputrefactive agent and was probably the first application of the principle of debridement. Hot oil and even boiling water were other early thermal devices to control hemorrhage.

Cautery as Hemostatic Agent

Paul of Aegina in the seventh century[11] and the Arabs Albucasis (ca. 936–1013) and Avicenna (980–1037) advocated the cautery for hemostatic as well as other therapeutic purposes. In the finest of his treatises, *On Surgery and Instruments*, Albucasis devoted the opening book to the virtues of the actual cautery. He considered it more efficacious than caustics ("potential" cauteries), which might spread beyond the site cauterized, whereas "fire . . . on account of the nobility of its nature . . . has no such effect unless it is overdone." The last indication for cautery enumerated by Albucasis was to arrest bleeding following injury or operative procedures. Although gold, bronze, and other metals were sometimes used, Albucasis preferred an iron cautery.[12]

The ingenious German surgeon Fabricius Hildanus (1560–1634) used a heavy red-hot knife to effect amputation in 1600, severing all tissue save the bone, thereby also controlling bleeding. Had surgeons who employed this method been able to complete their operations by the no-touch technique, as advised by

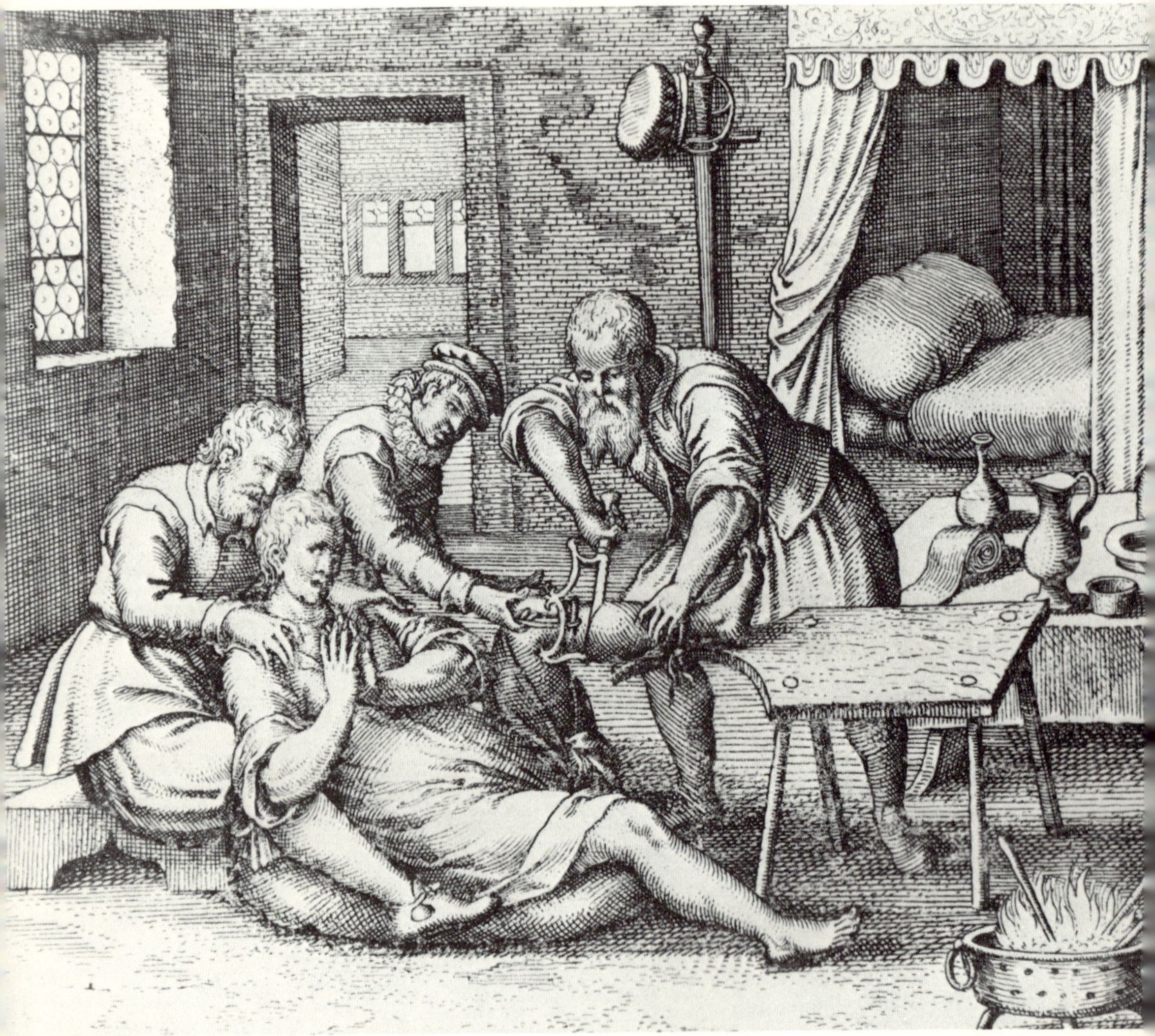

2.2 Early seventeenth-century leg amputation. Features cautery for hemostasis. From Fabricius Hildanus, *De gangraena et sphacelo* (Oppenheim, 1617). Courtesy National Library of Medicine.

Arbuthnot Lane in the early 1900s, antiseptic surgery would not have been so long aborning.[13]

Many who witnessed the use of the cautery in preanesthetic days, including surgeons, shared the dismay and anguish of the patient upon whom such techniques were practiced — little wonder that Paré's substitution of the ligature in amputation in 1564 was hailed as a great humanitarian advance. The popularity of the cautery as a surgical instrument has fluctuated over the centuries. Dionis (1707) declared that surgeons no longer used actual cauteries and that he displayed such instruments to his students "rather to excite horror with regard to their cruelty, than to advise their use." Half a century later a Montpellier physician remarked that surgical operations were not usually undertaken until the cautery was ready.[14] When the French Royal Academy of Surgery (1754) offered a prize for the best essay on the uses of the actual cautery, Guillaume Louis presented a long historical summary of the surgical applications of the instrument, adding briefly in the conclusion, "Fire will always be a means of stopping hemorrhage in very urgent cases."[15]

Today the cautery is once again a respectable tool, for most modern surgeons effect hemostasis from incisions almost solely with electrocautery. Forerunners of the modern electric device were the galvanocautery of Albrecht T. Middeldorpf (1854) and the electrical cautery of C. Pacquelin (1876). Cushing and W. T. Bovie made a significant contribution in 1928 when they introduced the surgical diathermy apparatus, which supplies a cutting current for the incision and a coagulating current to seal small blood vessels.[16]

Cautery as Antiputrefactive

Cauterization for hemostasis, although abhorrent to patient and surgeon, promoted the healing of contaminated wounds by minimizing suppuration. Such thermal debridement as a first or last weapon to destroy devitalized tissue in wounds and to control the spread of infection harks back at least to Hippocrates and Celsus. When Leonides amputated a breast in the first century, he used the cautery to stop the hemorrhage after each incision, then fulgurated all the parts to desiccation, eradicating all visible traces of a cancer.[17]

Roger (1170) and Roland (1230) of the School of Salerno are commonly credited with the thesis that provoking suppuration encourages healing, a phenomenon honored generations later by surgeons in the pre-Listerian era who hailed the appearance of "laudable pus." The fourteenth-century French surgeons Henri de Mondeville and Guy de Chauliac employed the cautery to combat the anticipated but unknown agencies which contributed to wound sepsis.[18] Over the years other surgeons learned the virtue of the cautery in arresting secondary bleeding in wounds, a complication frequently caused by infection.

When the Italian Giovanni de Vigo advised boiling oil of elder to achieve hemostasis and to counteract the alleged poison of gunshot injury in 1514, he became an early proponent of wound sterilization or debridement by heat, although his method obviously failed to distinguish between viable and devitalized tissue. Treatment with boiling oil was not original with de Vigo,[19] but his name is irrevocably attached to it through the well-known experience of that great French surgeon Paré, who so convincingly rejected it. Paré (ca. 1510–90) began as a barber's apprentice and eventually became first surgeon to Henry III, a leading writer on military surgery, and certainly one of the most memorable medical figures of all time. When he joined the army at age twenty-six, he was keenly aware of his inexperience. He remembered what he had read in de Vigo and copied the surgeons about him who poured "oyle of Elders scalding hot" mixed with treacle into gunshot wounds. One day in 1536 at the siege of Turin he ran out of hot oil and treated the remaining wounded with "a digestive made of the yolke of an egge, oyle of Roses, and Turpentine." Next morning the patients "dressed with a digestive onely" were free of pain and their wounds were not inflamed or swollen as were the others. Paré thereupon abandoned the hot oil treatment and substituted the turpentine remedy, a mature innovation for a young surgeon. After many trials of the turpentine remedy he concluded that gunshot wounds were not poisoned and should not be cauterized, and in 1545, at age thirty-five, he published his historic book, *La méthode de traicter les playes*, in which he repudiated the conventional boiling oil treatment.[20] In this early work he also described many of the practices which he later championed. Paré wrote originally for the aspiring barber-surgeon. To understand Paré, it must be remembered that he was essentially a man of practice, and if his observations and experience were not in accord with theory, he trusted his experience.

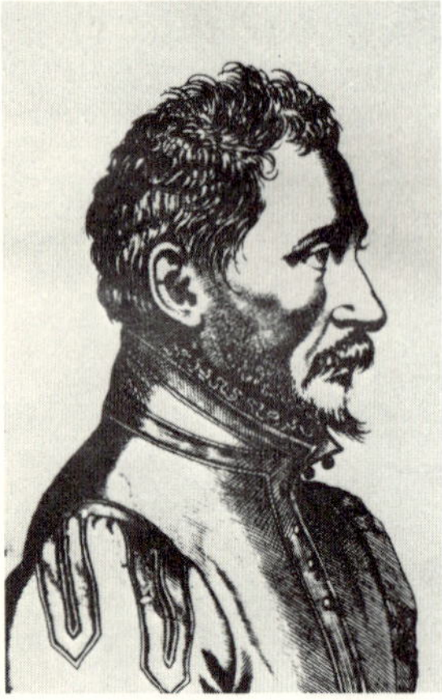

2.3 Engraving of Ambroise Paré (ca. 1510–90), great French military surgeon, at age 45. This earliest-known portrait of Paré first appeared in his *Anatomie universelle du corps humain* (1561).

Despite his disapproval of boiling oil and the cautery for hemostasis in amputation, Paré illustrated thirty-eight cauteries in his well-known *Workes*. Moreover, he did use the cautery for

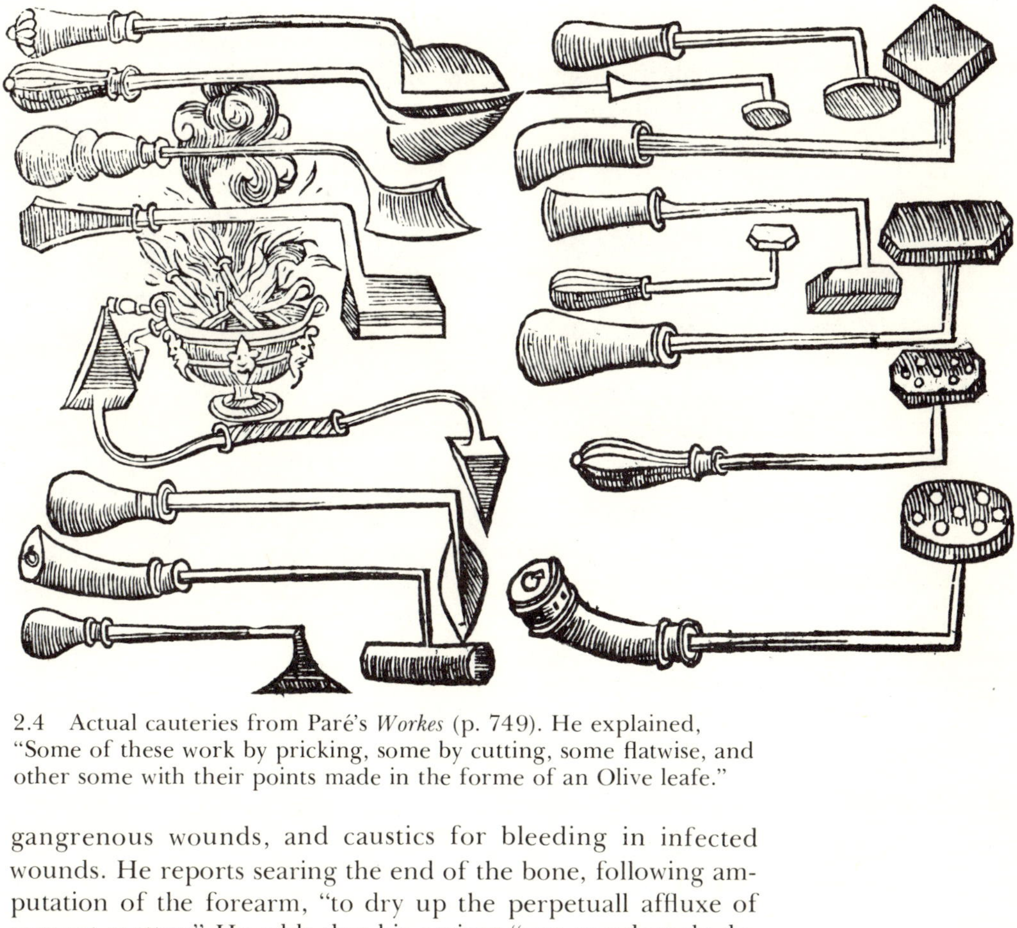

2.4 Actual cauteries from Paré's *Workes* (p. 749). He explained, "Some of these work by pricking, some by cutting, some flatwise, and other some with their points made in the forme of an Olive leafe."

gangrenous wounds, and caustics for bleeding in infected wounds. He reports searing the end of the bone, following amputation of the forearm, "to dry up the perpetuall affluxe of corrupt matter." He adds that his patient "was wondrously delighted by the application of such actuall cauteries, a certaine tickling running the whole length of the arme by reason of a gentle diffusion of the heate by applying the causticke; which same thing I have observed in many other; especially in such as lay upon the like occasion in the Hospitall of *Paris*."[21]

Many a surgeon confronted with the control of hemorrhage during an amputation was wont to quote the advice of Peter Lowe of Scotland in 1597: "Where there is putrefaction

. . . stay the flux of blood by Cauters actuals, and where there is no putrefaction . . . use the ligator." Wiseman too spoke of the cautery's antiputrefactive quality. Woodall said he had used the cautery to sear dead tissue in amputations for more than fifty years but had not seen the procedure tried by others in England. He occasionally applied it at the first dressing following amputation and quite regularly at the second. It was safe, he claimed, for both surgeons and patients, "only I advise it to be privately absconded for the reputation sake."[22] In other words, the cautery under certain circumstances was unacceptable to patients and was not generally employed by Woodall's contemporaries.

The cautery proved to be a particularly effective means to combat *pourriture d'hôpital* (hospital gangrene), that disastrous contagion so dreaded before the days of antibiotic therapy. Said John Bell (1826), "When [hospital gangrene] rages in a great hospital it is like a plague. . . . No operation dare be performed, every cure stands still, every wound becomes a sore, and every sore is apt to run into gangrene." At the Hôtel-Dieu they dared not pronounce the name, "for it sounded like a death-bell; at the hearing of that ominous word, the patients gave themselves up for lost."

A discussion of *pourriture d'hôpital* showing remarkable discernment of the sources of infection was published in 1783, shortly after the death of its distinguished author-surgeon, Pouteau of Lyons. He stated that the best therapy for *pourriture* was destruction of the infected part "by fire." His tool for the purpose was the actual cautery, but he conceded that boiling oil or a caustic might be substituted if the "cowardliness of the patient, or perhaps of the surgeon" made cauterization too repellent.[23]

Fifty years later, when the hordes of wounded from Napoleon's hapless campaign in the Peninsular War poured into Montpellier, sometimes as many as 500 a day, hospital gangrene reigned in the overcrowded hospital of Saint-Éloi. First to bring the disease were 150 men with infected bullet wounds from the siege of Pampeluna (1813). Delpech, of the surgical clinic of the University, thought it would be instructive for the students to try the cautery on all the wounds. To his surprise, all these patients recovered. When the epidemic deepened, Delpech and his associates undertook an intensive study of *pourriture*, including experiments and conferences to assess strategy. Like Pouteau, whose writings were the one practical source of information, Delpech concluded that no other treatment had the "speed and constancy" of the cautery. His monograph, published in 1815,[24] was a keen analysis of the mode of spread of the disease and told a dismaying story of the Montpellier experience, with a diatribe against Napoleon for his ruthless sacrifice of young men in warfare. Among the victims could be numbered several of Delpech's zealous medical students who lost their lives combatting the epidemic of *pourriture* and typhus.

Until Nussbaum capitulated to Lister's antiseptic wound practices in 1875, he too was an ardent advocate of the cautery in the control of hospital gangrene. In 1848 Amédée Bonnet of Lyons described the cautery as the most valuable antiputrefactive device for the control of infected wounds after operations. He particularly advised it for infection or pricks sustained during anatomical dissections or in phlebotomy, saying that every year students died or were maimed because such lesions were treated only by cataplasms or leeches. For cellulitic gangrene, Bonnet made deep incisions the length of the gangrenous tissue, followed by wide cauterization, a practice also employed by Léon Labbé of La Pitié in Paris.[25]

The cautery continued to be used well into the twentieth century as an antiputrefactive tool. Berkeley Moynihan, illustrious member of the famous Leeds school of surgeons, wrote on penetrating or perforating wounds of the knee joint in World War I, stating "A preliminary sterilisation of the tract with the actual cautery is an undoubted advantage." As late as 1935 electrical cautery was employed to control infection in 230 patients with injuries of the hands and fingers in Berlin hospitals, a treatment advised by August Bier.[26]

Cautery as Counterirritant

Albucasis recommended the cautery as a counterirritant to tighten up the periarticular ligaments in recurrent dislocations of the shoulder. Interestingly enough, this great tenth-century surgeon's techniques of reducing a dislocated shoulder are not unlike current practices. He also applied the cautery over the skin areas that covered the ligamentous structures of hernias in the belief that hernias would respond favorably to the resultant contracture of surrounding ligaments.[27]

Two famous surgeons of Napoleon's army, Baron Pierre-F. Percy and Larrey, employed the light cautery for erysipelas and phlegmonous inflammation. On one occasion Larrey applied as many as fifty cauteries to an erysipelatous extremity in six minutes, one every seven seconds, and his patient recovered.[28]

When Lister was James Syme's resident in Edinburgh in 1854,

he wrote of Syme's success in applying the cautery over the integuments of painful joints in four patients, saying "It is by no means so painful a remedy as is generally supposed, and . . . its good effects are more than can be attributed to the mere discharge of pus from the sore which it produces, seeing that a great improvement commonly occurs within a few hours . . . I believe many limbs and lives have been sacrificed that might have been saved by actual cautery, and by it alone." The practice was enthusiastically endorsed by Mitchell Banks of Liverpool in 1892.[29] Today, probably the only use of cautery for these purposes persists in the hands of veterinary surgeons, who apply it over injuries of joints in race horses, a practice known as firing. Lister apparently disregarded the antiputrefactive effect of the cautery recognized by Paré, Wiseman, Bonnet, and Nussbaum.

The Ligature and the Tourniquet

After abandoning de Vigo's boiling oil therapy for wounds, Paré needed some measure other than heat to control hemorrhage, and the ligature was his answer to the problem. He first described the use of the ligature in his *Dix livres* in 1564, but he probably had employed it as early as 1552 (in an autobiographical account Paré relates that he amputated a leg without cautery at the siege of Danvilliers). His adoption of the ligature in amputation has been called "the greatest improvement that has ever been made in operative surgery." Paré himself lays no claim to such priority and remarks that a number of surgeons before him — among them Celsus, Avicenna, Guy de Chauliac, de Vigo, Vesalius, Tagault, and Croce — had insisted on ligating bleeding vessels rather than applying the cautery.[30]

It would be strange indeed if the ligature had not been employed in amputation before Paré,[31] especially in the light of its long use for wounds generally, but certainly in his hands the method took on new vigor. Before the seventeenth century amputation above the knee was virtually unknown. The arteries and veins with which the early surgeons dealt in amputations were therefore of small caliber, readily controlled by the cautery. William Clowes in 1588 was apparently the first to perform a successful thigh amputation for gangrene, an accomplishment often credited to Fabricius, who wrote of performing one in 1614.[32]

Paré's lasting contribution was the substitution of the ligature for the cautery in the control of hemorrhage from large vessels

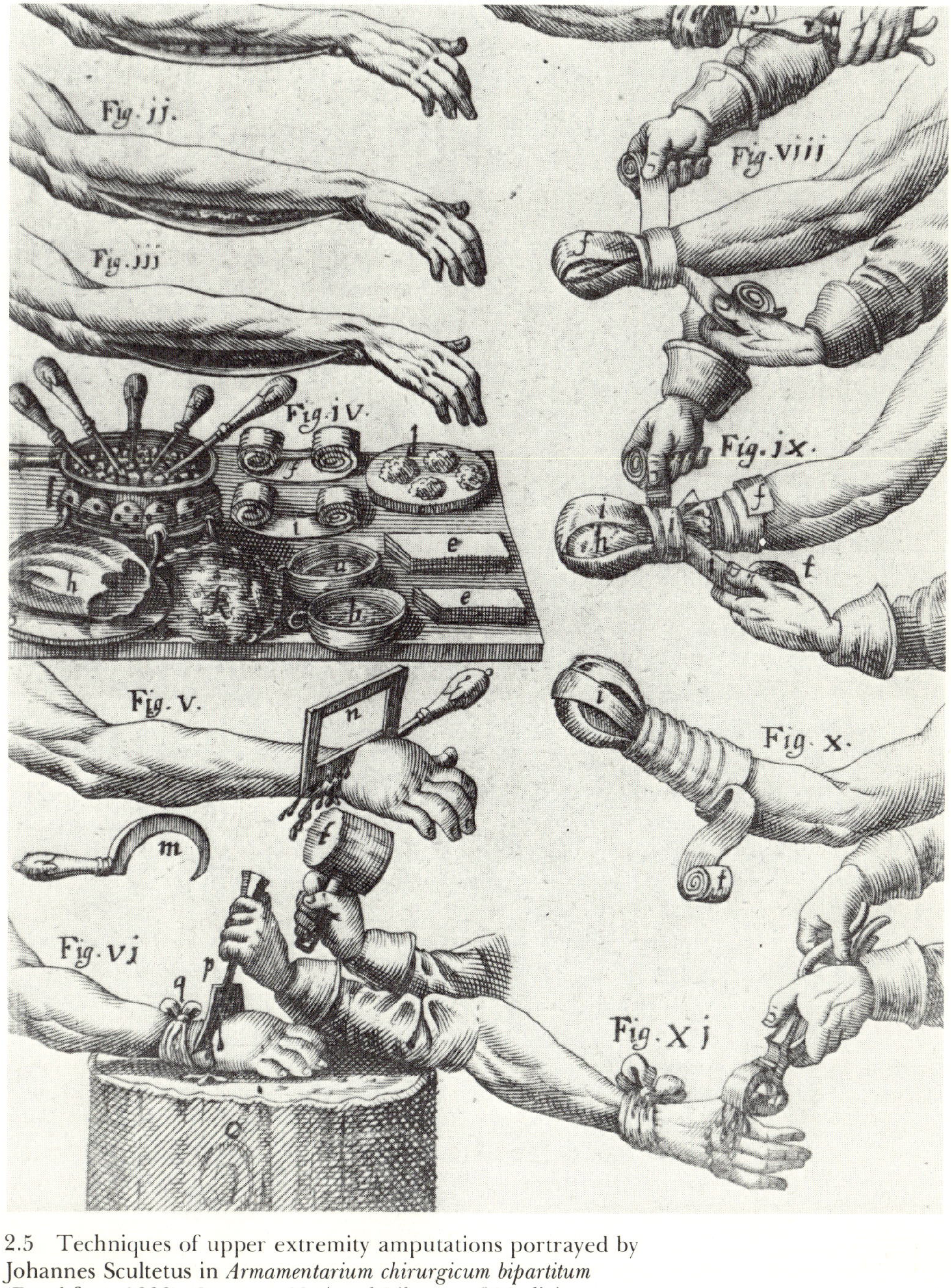

2.5 Techniques of upper extremity amputations portrayed by Johannes Scultetus in *Armamentarium chirurgicum bipartitum* (Frankfurt, 1666). Courtesy National Library of Medicine.

in amputation. There can be no doubt that ligature provides the most reliable mode of hemostasis in such operations. Paré often ligated the large vessels in continuity before severing the soft parts and the bone. When the vessels were cut, before placement of the ligature, he used a "crowes beake" to expose and draw out the divided vessels. His ultimate resource in effecting hemostasis in a deep wound was that of Brunschwig (1497), who passed a ligature about the cut vessels with a curved needle, a maneuver also employed by de Vigo and Marianus Sanctus and still practiced by modern surgeons. The adjacent tissue was transfixed before the divided vessel was ligated, minimizing the possibility that the tie might slip off. Paré stated that in amputating for gangrene he cut above the gangrenous part through the healthy tissue, certainly an unusual practice for that day.[33]

Historians have long puzzled over the slow acceptance of the ligature in amputation. Why it did not find ready adoption is apparent to surgeons who have engaged in the arduous and baffling wrestle with hemorrhage. One important consideration disregarded by both historians and surgeons is the number of ligatures necessary to effect complete hemostasis. In a German statistical study of amputation in 1890 it was reported that fifty-three ligatures were the average for a thigh amputation.[34] Many of these obviously were applied to small vessels from which bleeding in earlier days would have been controlled by prolonged pressure or, more quickly, by cautery. Even in thigh amputation for arteriosclerotic gangrene, more than twenty-five bleeding vessels often need to be ligated or sealed by electrocoagulation.

Another major factor militating against early espousal of the ligature was the lack of skilled assistants. The surgeon of those days usually operated alone and his assistants (whom Paré, Dionis, and others referred to as "servants") held the limb to be amputated and restrained the patient during the operation.[35] Observers willing to participate were probably pressed into service. The surgeon had little if any help with the operative procedure itself.

Woodall needed five assistants for amputation through live flesh, Dionis used six. The French military surgeon Hugues Ravaton (1768) speaks of having four surgeon-aides when performing an arm amputation — two to restrain the patient, another to offer him pain-relieving cordials, and the fourth to hand instruments and aid with application of the dressing.[36] Fergusson, at King's College Hospital, required four assistants. The English surgeon John Crosse on a visit to Paris in 1815 watched the famous Baron Dupuytren perform an emergency operation for strangulated hernia upon a patient in her bed at the Hôtel-Dieu. The operation being unscheduled, there were scarcely enough students to hold the candles to light the operation.[37]

Fabricius has left us a graphic description of a sixteenth-century amputation: "I was about to cut off the thigh [leg] of a man of forty yeares of age, and ready to use the saw, and Cauteries. For the sick man no sooner began to roare out, but all ranne away, except only my eldest Sonne, who was then but little, and to whom I had committed the holding of his thigh, for forme only; and but that my wife then great with child, came running out of the next chamber, and clapt hold of the Patients Thorax, both he and myselfe had been in extreme danger."[38] Undoubtedly this was not an uncommon scene before anesthesia was available. As a matter of convenience, therefore, it is apparent why surgeons employed the cautery to staunch bleeding from vessels of the forearm, hand, leg, or foot during amputation, nor is it surprising that Jacques Guillemeau (1550–1612), Paré's favorite pupil and biographer, abandoned the ligature in amputation after Paré's death because of the difficulties involved. Why Guillemeau did not forswear the cautery in amputation is patently clear in his book: "The legge now being extirpated . . . we must as then stoppe, and restraygne [the bleeding], which we must doe throughe the imposition of the fingers [on] the mouthes, or apertiōs of the Vaynes, which we must ether bind or els cauterise the one or the other according as the same shal be needfull, and requisite. . . . Supposing to take houlde [on] the vaynes with the Crowesbill, and soe to bind them, doe most commonlye chaunce to breake betweene the Crowesbill . . . we are in the end constrayned to use the actuall Cauterye." If the limb to be amputated was gangrenous, Guillemeau found the hemorrhage was "farre more stopped, through the applicatione of glowinge cauteryes" than by ligation.[39]

The ligature was not frequently used in amputation until refinement of the tourniquet and was therefore essentially an eighteenth-century development.[40]

Guy de Chauliac, among other early surgeons, wrapped a tight band above and below the site of amputation to reduce pain and minimize bleeding by compressing the soft tissues against the bone.[41] In the sixteenth century, Leonardo Botallo advised putting three bands around a major extremity to be removed, amputating between the lower two; Fabricius tightened a band above the site of amputation, twisting it with a stick to control bleeding. Johannes Scultetus of Ulm depicted a screw compressor in his famous seventeenth-century illustrated surgery. These methods were not quickly adopted by surgeons. Dionis's double twist-stick was employed in much the same manner that Red Cross aides and Boy Scouts today deal with hemorrhage in emergencies;[42] it was the best forerunner of Petit's tourniquet of 1718.

Petit's tourniquet (1718, 1731) presented an advantage over Scultetus' screw compressor in that it provided for fixation of the tourniquet upon the lower abdomen. Thus the instrument was prevented from slipping and amputation could be done at a higher level. Petit's method put direct pressure upon the main artery of the extremity to be amputated and provided the hemostasis that was needed to justify reintroduction of the ligature in amputation. It was certainly one of the most important surgical discoveries before the advent of anesthesia. Petit said he devised his tourniquet when he noted that a tight ligature and styptics caused gangrene. Fifty years later, to control hemorrhage in wounds of the extremities Ravaton relied on tourniquet, ligature, tamponade of the wound, and firm compression by external wrappings with *André de la Croix*, a type of adhesive plaster. He kept "a relaxed tourniquet" available should secondary hemorrhage occur.[43] Ravaton made no allusion to the cautery for control of bleeding. The influence of Petit had made its mark, and Paré's enthusiasm for the ligature had been fully justified.

John Hunter said that in his opinion "an amputation below the knee in most cases would not kill by its haemorrhage, even if left to itself; but this experiment can only be ascertained by accident." Hunter's thesis waited almost two centuries for verification in the experiments of Irving Enquist, Clarence Dennis, and their associates. They found that blood loss attending division of the saphenous artery in the dog averaged 323 ml. and was rarely exsanguinating.[44] Perhaps the "accident" Hunter looked for was supplied in an observation by the Prussian army surgeon Johann Schmucker in 1774. He told of the amputation by cannon ball of the arm of one patient and the thigh of another. Both stumps healed without surgical reamputation or great loss of blood. This statement may be responsible for the occasionally observed interpretation that Schmucker considered it less dangerous for a patient to have his thigh amputated by gunfire than by surgery.[45]

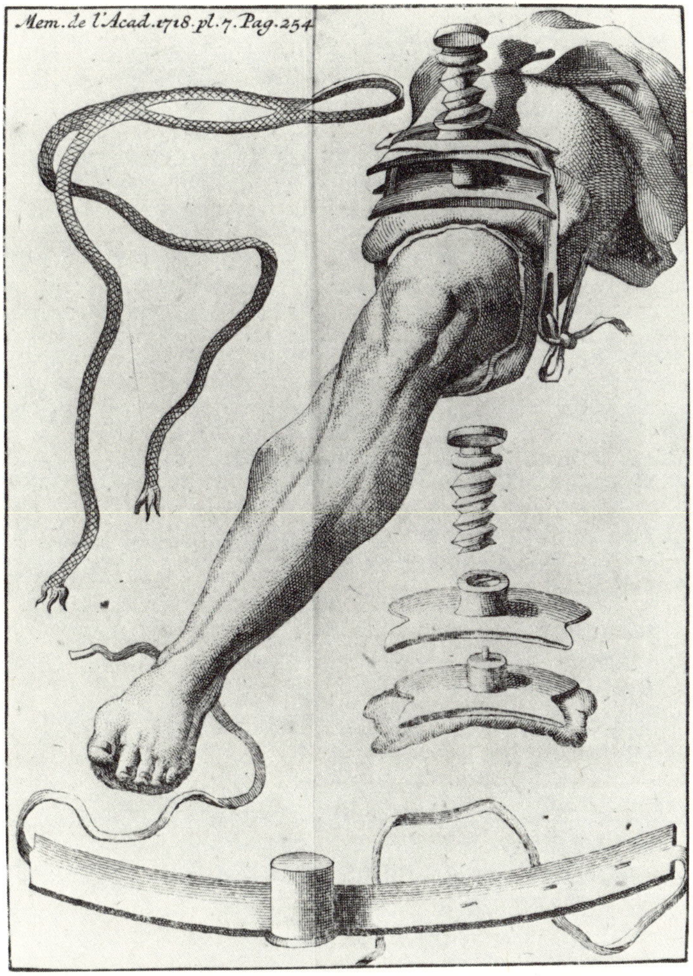

2.6 J.-L. Petit's introduction of screw compressor tourniquet for amputation (1718). From Petit, "D'un nouvel instrument de chirurgie," *Mém. Acad. roy. sci.* (1718), p. 254. Courtesy National Library of Medicine.

The Great Amputationists

A large number of military surgeons favored early amputation for fracture from gunshot, but it was a debatable issue. In 1756 the French Royal Academy of Surgery offered a prize for the best presentation on the subject. The award went to the French army surgeon Jean Faure, who favored amputation for comminuted fracture but maintained that the operation should be delayed. He stated that only thirty or forty men survived out of the

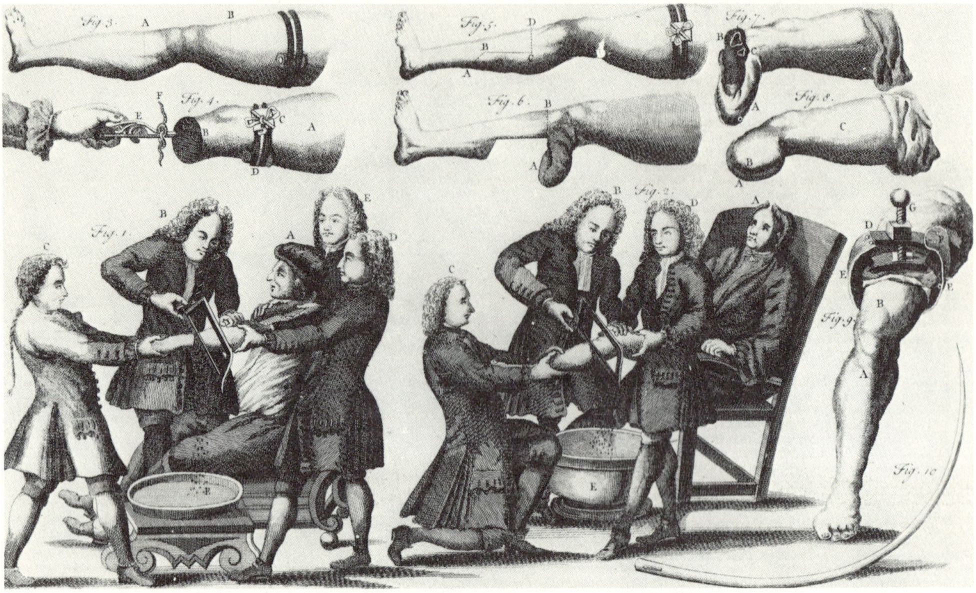

2.7 Forearm and leg amputations. From English translation of Lorenz Heister, *General system of surgery* (London, 1743). Courtesy National Library of Medicine.

three hundred who underwent immediate amputation after the Battle of Fontenoy (1745), whereas he had saved all of the ten English soldiers wounded there by deferring amputation for twenty-nine to fifty-two days. Among Faure's severest critics was another army surgeon, Boucher, who insisted that survival was highest when amputation was done directly after injury. Boucher said that one-third of all wounded would survive after immediate operation; he himself had seen four survivors among nine amputees in a hospital shortly after Fontenoy.[46]

Larrey was a proponent of early amputation during his days as a surgeon and hero of the Napoleonic Wars. His *Mémoires* contain the often quoted statement that on the road to Moscow, at the Battle of Borodino, "I performed in the first 24 hours, about 200 [amputations]." That would mean an amputation every seven minutes! The fate of his patients is not definitely known, but Larrey suggests that 75 percent recovered.[47]

In the revolution of July 1830 Larrey did 10 amputations of thigh and leg with 4 deaths (40 percent) and 6 of arm or shoulder with 3 deaths (50 percent). It is to be remembered that forty years later, during the Siege of Paris, the best of the French surgeons had an appalling mortality with amputation, nearly

100 percent from September 1870 through February 1871.[48] Such episodes of severe endemic infections attended by great mortality in the era when chemical wound antisepsis was on trial are well documented. Larrey's success with battlefield amputations, therefore, is undoubtedly a far more accurate criterion of his accomplishment than the events of July 1830.

Writing of his observations in military hospitals in Belgium after Waterloo, Thomson found it regrettable that Larrey had written so little on thigh fractures by musket balls. "Are we to infer, from his silence on this subject, that his success in the treatment of these injuries had not been very great?" Thomson quoted the British army surgeon George Guthrie to the effect that two-thirds of all patients with gunshot wounds of the thigh died, with or without amputation. Thomson held that such wounds were almost invariably fatal. He remarked that Ravaton had not seen a single recovery and that J. U. Bilguer of the Prussian army regarded gunshot fractures of the thigh as fatal. Larrey is best known to surgeons as a superb amputationist, having probably amputated more extremities than any other surgeon in history. Were all the amputations necessary? The Edinburgh military surgeon Blackadder accused Larrey of "operating mania."[49] However, other well-known military surgeons of that day — Percy, Thomson, and John Hennen — supported Larrey's mode of therapy.[50]

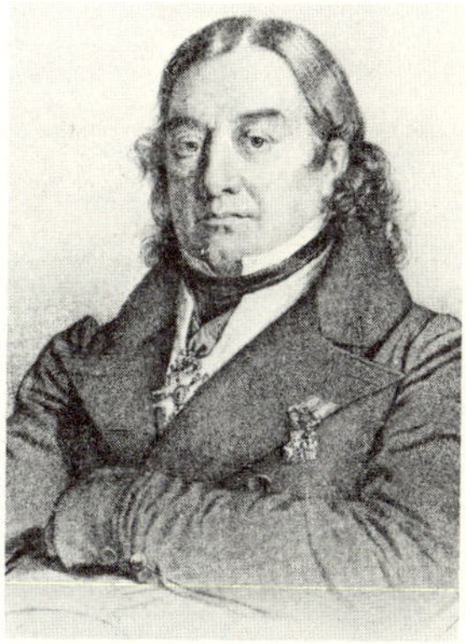

2.8 Dominique Larrey (1766–1842), Napoleon's famous military surgeon.

Guthrie, during his long and distinguished career as Britain's leading military surgeon in the Napoleonic Wars, favored immediate amputation for all compound fractures by gunshot of the lower extremity; for similar fractures of the upper extremity, Guthrie felt immediate amputation was not so compelling. The Paris surgeon, J.-F. Malgaigne, once an ardent advocate of primary amputation for fractures with wounds, changed his mind after learning that J. N. Marjolin at the Salpetrière in 1814 observed only one recovery after fourteen thigh amputations for compound fracture.[51]

In his dissertation of 1797 Larrey reviewed the question of amputation and discussed the following items: (1) Which considerations demand amputation on the battlefield? (2) Which suggest delay? (3) Which suggest conservative management? He concluded that when an extremity is badly damaged immediate amputation is lifesaving in a large number of cases. In writing after his campaign days were over, Larrey (1817) remarked that most patients with primary amputations recovered; those with delayed amputations, by contrast, did poorly.[52]

Whether to perform immediate or delayed amputation after

injury continued to be a favorite subject of debate for decades among military and civilian surgeons. The full ritual of surgical antisepsis ultimately silenced the arguments and became the important agency for saving untold numbers of limbs.

Operating Time in Amputation

Before the days of anesthesia surgeons often employed soporifics to steel the patient for the ordeal. Nevertheless, there was obviously great need for hurry in operations, an objective perpetuated by many surgeons until a quarter of a century ago.

Who is the greatest amputationist? He who does it in minimal time? Jacques Lisfranc, who used a thousand cadavers a year to teach operative surgery at La Pitié in Paris, could amputate the thigh of a cadaver in ten seconds. He advised surgeons against the practice of having one knee on the floor during the procedure because of the time lost in reassuming the erect position. Oliver Wendell Holmes abandoned attendance at Lisfranc's clinic when he heard him lament there were no more opportunities to amputate the "magnificent thighs" of the Emperor's Old Guard.[53]

Benjamin Bell (1749-1806), a distinguished surgeon of the Edinburgh Royal Infirmary, could divide all but the bone in a thigh amputation in six seconds. Larrey's time on the average in the field was approximately three minutes. Larrey was a master of disarticulation at the shoulder joint and reported having done it in seventeen seconds, not counting the time taken for ligature and wound closure. When Robert Liston (1794-1847) of University College Hospital in London amputated, "the gleam of his knife was followed so instantaneously by the sound of sawing as to make the two actions appear almost simultaneous."[54] Fergusson said that any competent surgeon should be able to perform an amputation in from thirty seconds to three minutes. He took twelve to twenty seconds to amputate at the hip joint. James R. Wood of New York could amputate a thigh in nine seconds.[55] The senior author participated in several thigh amputations in the 1920s performed by A. A. Law, one of his teachers at the University of Minnesota, who employed the transfixion method and regularly severed the extremity in less than thirty seconds.

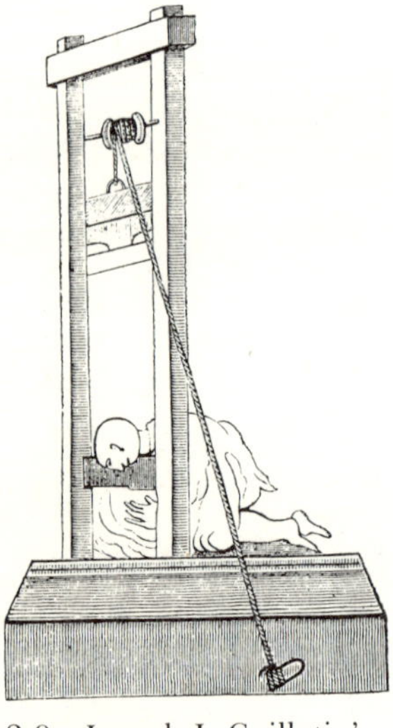

2.9 Joseph-I. Guillotin's decapitation device used during French Revolution.

These heroics are now a part of history. Certainly the far more important desideratum is the salvage score of primary amputation.

Very likely apocryphal is the anecdote of the author's former physiology professor, Frederick H. Scott, who as a student of

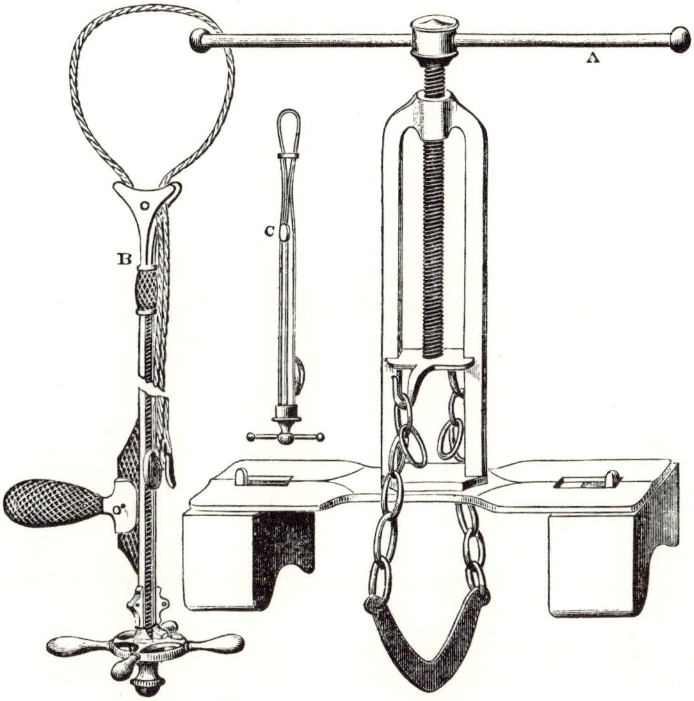

2.10 Jacques Maisonneuve's slow severance of soft tissues in amputation "to minimize infection." Employed in six successive amputations of leg and forearm without a death. From Maisonneuve, "Nouvelle méthode d'amputation, dite méthode diaclastique ou par rupture," *Gaz. méd.*, Paris (1858), 13:290–94.

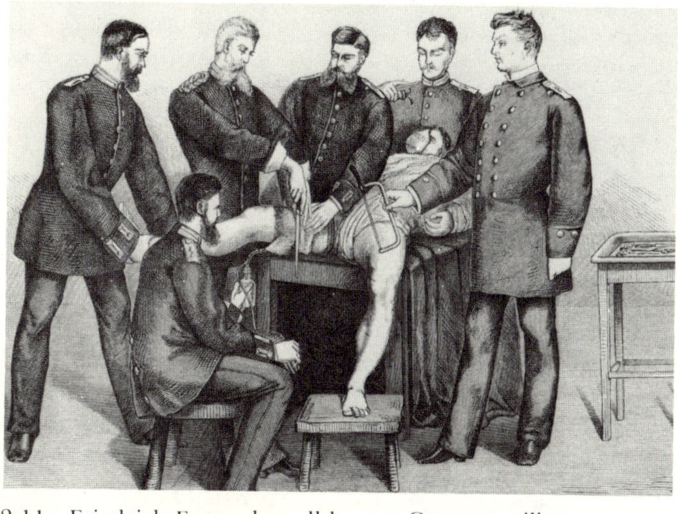

2.11 Friedrich Esmarch, well-known German military surgeon, amputating under anesthesia but without surgical antisepsis. From Esmarch, *Handbuch der kriegschirurgischen Technik* (Hannover, 1877).

Starling in London heard that a surgeon of the Liston era, in his hurry to amputate a thigh, "included two fingers of his assistant and both testes of his patient." More plausible is the description of Valentine Mott severing a piece of his own finger while performing an amputation upon a cadaver for a group of students in 1860. "Instantly putting his finger in his mouth, he sucked the wound, then wrapped it in his handkerchief . . . and went on operating." The narrator adds that one of the spectators gathered up the "piece of surgical flesh" and can now "boast of Dr. Mott in alcohol."[56]

Instruments

Early examples of a number of modern instruments are to be seen in Paré's illustrations. Forerunners of the Horsley craniotome and Sauerbruch's special shears to divide the first rib in thoracoplasty will be recognized by surgeons. Paré's "crowes beake" was a crude original of the hemostat used in amputation "to draw the vessells forth . . . so they may be tyed or bound fast." In a later refinement he added a spring to keep the jaws of the instrument open until the vessel was seized.[57]

There is a striking contrast between the instruments of the tenth-century Arab surgeon Albucasis and those of Paré, not so much in the blades as in the handles. As Paré said in his dedicatory epistle to Henry III, he was "a lover of carved workes," a passion eloquently expressed in the elaborate handles of many of his instruments. His curved amputation knife bears a female

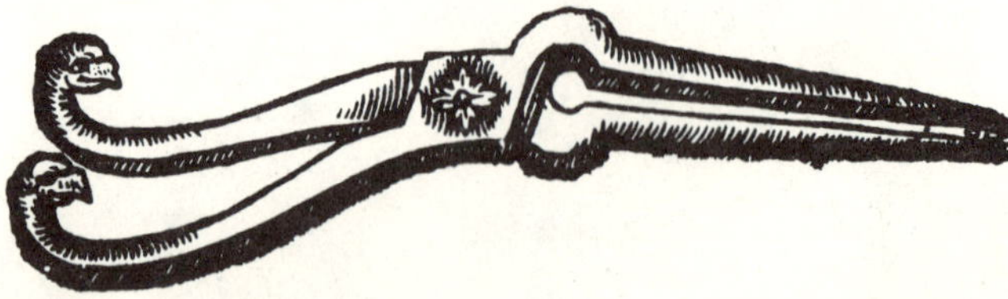

2.12 Paré's "crowes beake."

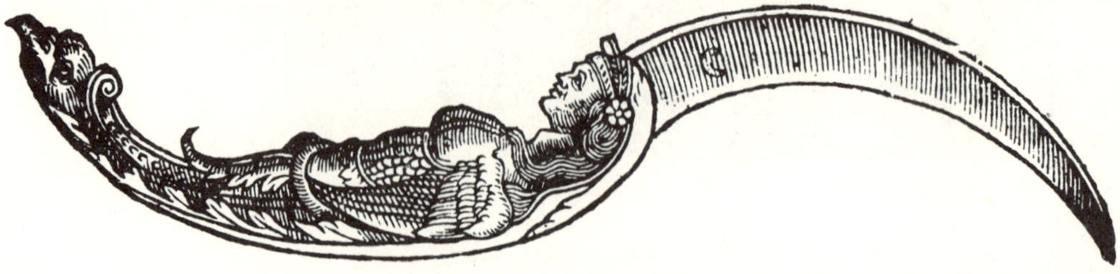

2.13 Paré's ornate amputation knife.

figure with wings on the handle, a fine example of the ornate craftsmanship he so much admired. He first referred to this instrument as a lancet, later as a bistoury.[58] Paré was partial to curved knives for amputation.

Two centuries after Paré most surgeons had supplanted curved knives with straight ones, which were more applicable to the flap operation. According to Alfred Velpeau, the sickle-shaped knife of ancient surgeons was set aside completely after the time of Antoine Louis, who had pointed out its disadvan-

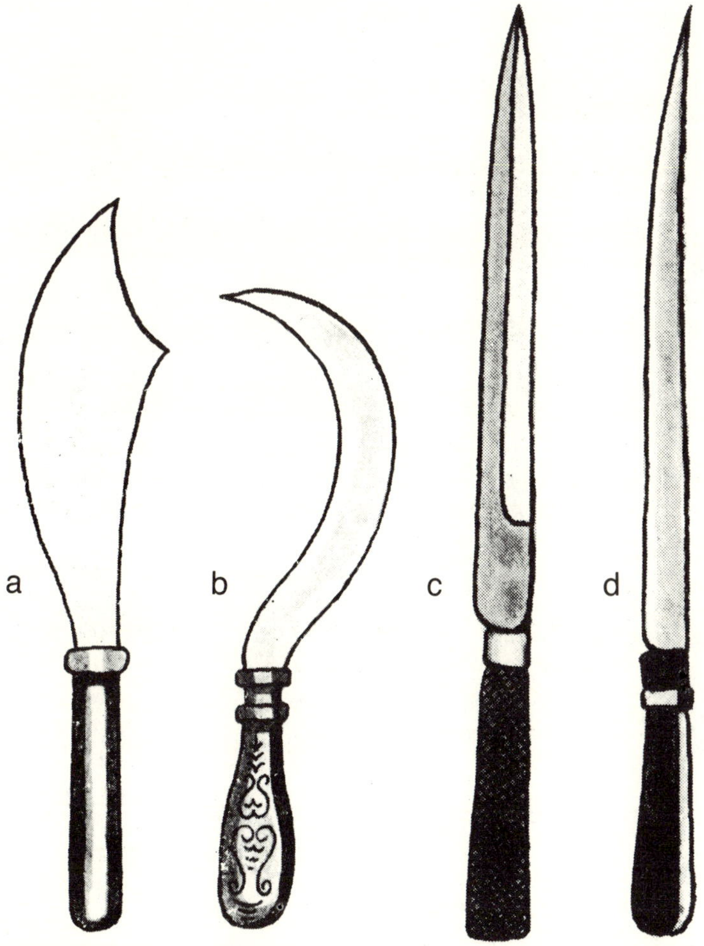

2.14 Transition from curved to straight knives for amputation: **a.** Fabricius; **b.** Scultetus; **c.** Lisfranc; **d.** Liston. From C. J. S. Thompson, *History and evolution of surgical instruments* (New York: Schuman, 1942).

tages. Velpeau said that the saw should be heavy enough to act immediately when drawn over the bone.[59]

The long use of the straight transfixion knife, the kind favored by Larrey for thigh amputation, has two possible explanations: (1) The instrument permitted great speed. (2) The pain suffered by the unanesthetized patient was undoubtedly less than with a circular percutaneous cut. Severe pain was experienced as the knife entered and as it exited on the far side, but cutting the soft tissue from within produced less pain than cutting from the outside.[60]

After the advent of anesthesia the long transfixion knife was gradually replaced by the short-bladed knife. In the 1920s there were still surgeons at the University of Minnesota Hospitals and elsewhere who used transfixion knives for thigh amputations. All other extremity amputations, however, were performed with short knives and small blades. The present generation of surgeons has been brought up on the removable knife blade, often replaced more than once during a long operation.

Skin Flaps in Amputation

The flap amputation, providing better skin cover for the divided bone, was employed in a leg amputation by James Yonge of Plymouth in 1679, its first use in major amputation. He credited an associate, C. Lowdham, with the suggestion. Yonge reported the procedure incidentally in acclaiming turpentine as a dressing for wounds.[61]

Most surgeons today have returned to the circular amputation of Celsus, in which all segments of the divided skin are optimally vascularized; in flap amputations, on the contrary, the apex of each flap has a diminished blood flow. Celsus divided the bone with a small saw proximal to the site of the amputation of skin and muscles, thus providing a cover of tissue which could be drawn together over the bone. Said Celsus, "Little by little the edges of the wound approach and the eventual cicatrix is smaller" — a suggestion not unlike that of Alexis Carrel in 1910.[62]

Wound Management after Amputation

Through the centuries the mode of closing the wound following amputation for injury has continued to be a subject of great controversy. Hippocrates, amputating through devitalized tissue, perforce found it necessary to leave the wound open to heal

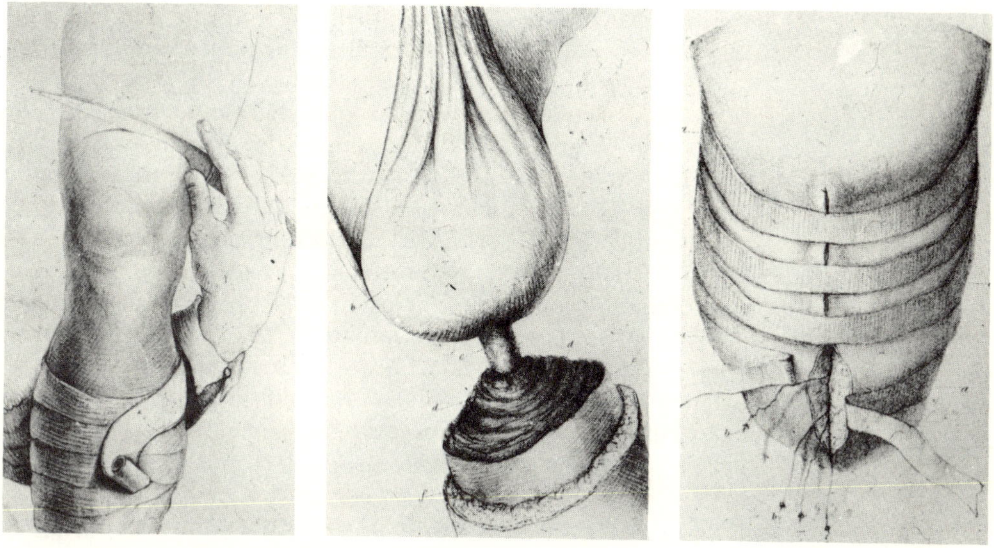

2.15 Charles Bell's circular thigh amputation (1807). Effective retraction of muscles and closure of wound with adhesive tape. The ligatures are brought out through the wound. From W. P. Cocks, *Illustrations of anatomy* (London, 1831), but undoubtedly adapted from Charles Bell's drawings in *System of operative surgery* (London, 1807), 1:374–79.

by granulation. If the patient survived, the resultant contraction of the soft tissue about the projecting segments of bone made it obligatory to remove these pieces secondarily by rongeur or saw, an experience not wholly unknown to modern surgeons. Galen (131–201 A.D.), the founder of experimental physiology and the greatest of the Greek physicians after Hippocrates, likewise amputated through "black and corrupt" tissue.[63] Not until surgeons performed amputation through viable tissue, a procedure recommended by Celsus, was primary closure possible.

Primary vs. Delayed Closure

Hugh of Lucca (ca. 1160–1257), who founded the Bologna school, his famous disciple Theodoric, and Henri de Mondeville are usually placed among the ardent proponents of primary closure of contaminated wounds, which suggests that their success was owing in part to considerable luck. Paré and others were aware that wounds of the face healed "kindly,"[64] undoubtedly owing to superior blood supply.

Primary union may seem a laudable objective, but it is not obtainable with any suggestion of regularity in contaminated wounds. Nevertheless, any compromise with this goal has been frowned upon by many historians of surgery. Ever since Theodoric made his plea for primary union of all wounds, historians have been at pains to point out what poor surgery it is to leave wounds open and seek healing by second intention. The late eminent historian Henry Sigerist (1923) took Paré to task for departing from the directive of Hugh and Theodoric.[65] It took the experience of World War I to establish definitely the superiority of open wound treatment and secondary closure of contaminated wounds, a conclusion well supported by surgeons in World War II and the Korean and Vietnam conflicts. It is no longer sound surgical doctrine to praise Theodoric's thesis of primary suture of contaminated wounds. His employment of agents that inhibit suppuration was, of course, valid, as was Paré's practice, though in theory Paré supported the use of suppuratives.

Guy de Chauliac fared badly at the hands of critics of the past generation because he insisted that nature was not the only force to influence the healing of contaminated wounds, that the intervention of the surgeon to remove foreign bodies, to provide drainage, and to utilize purifying agents (cautery, wine, turpentine, or brandy) improved the situation. Moreover, Guy applied strips of adhesive tape to the edges of such wounds and approximated them by suturing the strips together, a practice later followed by Paré. Brandy, available by the thirteenth century, was used by Guy in wounds because of "its drying and healing quality."[66] Fielding Garrison was particularly severe in his criticism of Guy's practices, suggesting that his views on therapy had retarded wound management six hundred years! Malgaigne did not share those views, nor did Édouard Nicaise, Guy's best interpreter.[67]

It is true that Guy's speculative probings of a host of wound powders, methods subsequently employed by Paracelsus and Paré, smacked of polypharmacy. Nevertheless, his approach to the contaminated wound would seem to be more in keeping with today's practice than is immediate wound closure. The time has come for surgeons and historians to be alert to Guy de Chauliac's realistic evaluations.[68]

Said Paré: "But when wee say, draw together the lippes of the wound with foure stitches, you must not so understand it, as that you must endeavour to draw them so close as to touch each other, for that is impossible; for the stitches would sooner breake out, and so the part would lye bare. Wherefore it will be sufficient to draw them indifferent close together, that so you may suffer the skinne and flesh thereunder to enjoy its former liberty which it possest before the drawing up, and so in fine by nature's assistance, the wound may be the more easily agglutinated," a method of wound closure following amputation that Paré first described in *Dix livres* (1564).[69]

Brunschwig described closing the amputation wound with sutures approximating the wound edges by bandaging.[70] Until the time of Alexander Monro I of Edinburgh and Liston, primary closure, whether by suture or adhesive tape, came to be preferred. French surgeons, who inserted small bits of linen known as *charpies* into the wound, employed such practices until the antiseptic era. The French surgeon P.-J. Roux, on a visit to English surgical clinics in 1814, was puzzled to note that wounds were being closed without *charpies*. He attributed the omission to English frugality necessitated by a shortage of lint in the country.[71]

The experience of war surgeons, which civilian surgeons have been slow to recognize, is that infection is a frequent complication when contaminated wounds are closed immediately after debridement. Larrey's early war practice taught him that primary closure after amputation for gunshot injury invited dangerous sequelae, and in later campaigns he favored open treatment of such wounds when the conditions of transport permitted.[72] The explanation came only when Billroth in 1865 showed that granulating wounds were far less susceptible than fresh wounds to invasive pyogenic organisms.[73] The protective mechanism of secondary wound closure is still not well understood. With change of the ground substance in the fresh wound from fibrinous to fibrinoid to fibroblastic tissue, the resistance of the open wound to infection becomes increasingly manifest.

Open Wound Proponents

Edward Alanson in 1782 had notable success with amputation at the Liverpool Infirmary. He almost approximated the wound edges with adhesive tape but did not actually bring them together, thus providing opportunity for drainage. His unusual success — thirty-five major amputations without a death — constituted a challenge to surgeons of many countries who sought and failed to find the answer in his mode of amputation without taking serious note of his technique of wound care. We know from his writings that his standards of surgical cleanliness were rigid.[74]

A few pre-Listerian surgeons, notably Vincenz Kern, Liston,

and Carl A. Burow, left the wound open for periods varying from a few hours to several days, then approximated the wound edges with adhesive tape. They achieved a rate of success in amputation unmatched until acceptance of the complete ritual of prophylactic antisepsis at the beginning of the twentieth century. Pouteau and William Cheselden and a few other skilled lithotomists left the perineal wound open to be washed by urine and likewise achieved records not surpassed until full capitulation to surgical antisepsis. (Their story is told in a later chapter.)

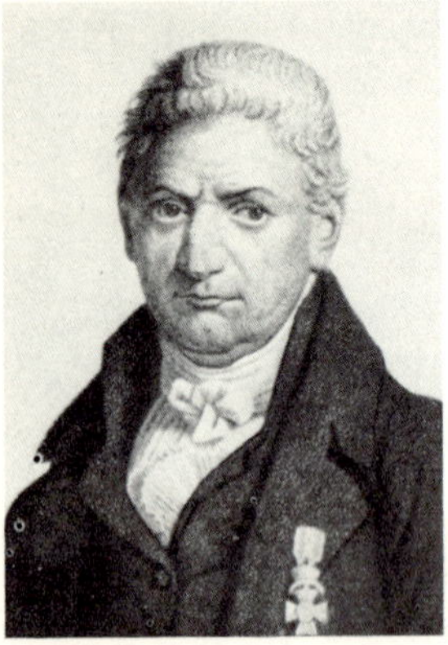

2.16 Vincenz Kern advocated open wound management in amputation (1826).

Kern and Liston waited until a "glaze" appeared upon the wound, then closed the wound with strips of adhesive tape. The contemporary reports of their methods in amputation are quite detailed. When Kern's patient was back in bed, the stump was ensheathed in a large bath towel dipped in ice water, changed first at short intervals, then at longer intervals, into the next day. "Ten to twelve hours after the operation and often earlier a glaze" appeared on the wound. When this glaze appears, Kern states, there is no further danger of secondary hemorrhage, "a truth which a thousand witnesses can affirm." Apparently, neither Kern nor Liston instilled antiseptics into wounds. Burow placed an aluminum acetate (vinegar) dressing, which is not an effective antibacterial agent, over the open wound. He reported an amputation mortality of 6 percent.[75]

Although Lisfranc did the amputation in record time, he did not hurry to close the wound, leaving it open for two to three hours to let the blood drain over its surface before closure. Charles-T. Maunoir of Geneva was wont to delay closure of amputation wounds until the bleeding was completely controlled. Dupuytren waited conventionally two or three hours before applying a final dressing. In reporting the high death rate from amputation (eleven deaths among fifteen patients) at one Paris hospital after the riots of 1832, Voison, a young surgeon, said he believed a contributory cause was the fact that the surgeons were too rushed to wait half an hour before applying dressings. Maximilian Chelius of Heidelberg stated in 1844 that many surgeons left the wound open from six to ten hours and during this time covered it with sponges or compresses dipped in cold water to guard against delayed bleeding.[76]

Liston placed a single suture in the middle of the amputation wound. His dressers applied cold-water compresses to the wound, changing these every ten minutes for seven hours. When oozing stopped and the wound had a glazed appearance, it was closed with adhesive tape. He "rode his hobby of water-dressing in the treatment of wounds rather hard," reminisced

John Erichsen in a fine account of Liston's successful open-wound therapy of the stump after amputation. "It was," said Erichsen, "the perfection of lightness compared with a poultice; the perfection of cleanliness contrasted with ointments." Wherein lies the protection of the glaze is yet not completely known. Liston's mortality record of 11.4 percent for major amputations in 1841 was a real accomplishment for his times, but it did not equal Monro's or Alanson's records of the previous century. It was, however, considerably better than the record achieved by Lister, who adopted phenol wound antisepsis in 1865, but whose mortality in amputation over the next five years was 25.2 percent.[77]

A well-known painting of Liston depicts him without the usual blood-stained operating frock and with his sleeves rolled up, an unusual but enlightened practice for 1846. It is somewhat surprising and disconcerting to learn that "in more complicated operations, when he wished to use both hands he saved much time by holding the knife by the handle in his mouth." Erichsen wrote that during his training days at University College Hospital no one thought of bringing the wound edges together until the glazing appeared. Liston's management prevailed. A London surgeon, at the first International Medical Congress in Paris, 1867, said it was the custom of several English surgeons to leave the wound open for two or three hours after a thigh amputation. Professor George Humphry, of Addenbrooke's Hospital, Cambridge, recommended leaving all wounds open and uncovered (1860).[78]

Surgical consultants to the Union Army during the Civil War advised against attempts at primary union for war wounds, but there was a definite suggestion of permissiveness in the instructions printed in *Hints for After-Treatment* by the United States Sanitary Commission of the Union Army in 1861. According to the first instruction, "When a wound is extensive, as in cases of amputation, it is far preferable to leave the wound open, with a piece of wet lint, or a thin compress, interposed between the lips, for two or three hours, until the surface has become glazed." In 1862 another group of military consultants expressed approval of the recommendation of Stephen Smith, who wrote, "In the after treatment of the amputations and resections [through the foot and at the ankle joint] it is good practice to leave the wounds open to heal by granulation."[79]

Nine years after Lister's initial publication on the management of compound fractures by carbolic acid dressing, Frederic Dennis of New York narrated the instance of two patients admitted the same evening to Ward 16 at Bellevue Hospital in 1875, each undergoing amputation of a crushed foot. One patient's wound was closed by apposition of the edges with silver sutures and strips of adhesive plaster. He had a long convalescence, complicated by hyperpyrexia (106.5° F), stump infection, and abscesses, but he ultimately recovered. The other patient's wound was left open, draining freely. The wound edges, brought together with adhesive tape a few days later, healed without complications. Dennis then reported on fourteen amputations on Wood's service, all managed by the open method and without mortality. Wrote Dennis, "Each dresser invariably washes his hands in carbolic acid water after dressing one case before undertaking another, and one who is dressing unhealthy wounds in the pavilion or making autopsies is not allowed to even assist in the daily dressing of healthy wounds."[80]

The Open Wound in Elective Surgery

In elective operations in which the potential of contamination is high, and in amputation for gangrene, in which the effective capacity of the skin as a barrier to infection is lost, open management would appear to be in order. In amputation below the knee for arteriosclerotic gangrene R. R. Kendrick (1956) obtained primary healing of wounds closed primarily in only 32 of 51 patients (63 percent). That the current wound complication rate of amputations for arteriosclerotic gangrene exceeds 30 percent, and that hospital mortalities in excess of 10 percent are usual, has pertinence for this discussion. A study by L. H. Stahlgren and Merlin Otteman (1965) from the Philadelphia General Hospital reports a mortality of 29.7 percent for thigh amputation for arteriosclerosis. Moreover, primary wound healing is achieved in only two-thirds of such patients treated by primary closure of the wounds.[81]

These occurrences have persuaded many surgeons to adopt delayed wound closure in amputations for arteriosclerotic gangrene. A few catgut sutures approximate the divided muscles over the end of the bone in thigh amputation. The wound is left open and packed lightly with gauze, kept moist with a constant drip of chloramine hypochlorite for four to five days, and then the wound edges are brought together with strips of adhesive tape. The wound usually heals readily, without evidence of suppuration. The multiple infirmities of age in this group of patients understandably exact a toll, however, despite the absence of wound complications. The main problem is to equate the risk the surgeon accepts for the patient when he closes contaminated wounds primarily. Return to delayed closure of such wounds is probably the wiser choice, a practice strictly adhered to by military field surgeons since World War I.

The Percutaneous Stitch

In 1517 Hans Gersdorff reported proudly that he had performed amputations on between one hundred and two hundred persons, many of whom survived, and that he had never closed the wound with sutures, preferring to close with adhesive tape and to use an animal bladder for a covering. Although Paré recommended four stitches to close the wound of the amputation stump, he advised the dry suture for face wounds. In this technique adhesive is applied to either side of the wound and the edges of the wound are approximated by a few sutures that bring the adhesive tape together.[82]

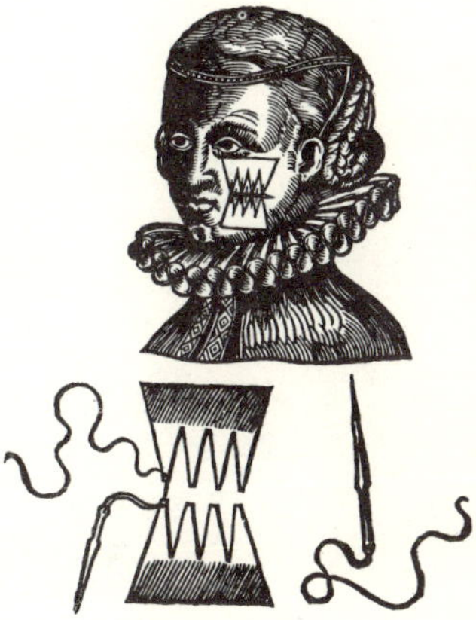

2.17 Paré's dry suture for facial wounds.

Two hundred years later Antoine Louis said that Paré's four stitches were still being used by some French surgeons to close amputations and with disastrous results. Louis censured his more enlightened fellow surgeons for not speaking out against the practice, calling their silence "deadly."[83]

Silence on this subject was scarcely the problem over the next hundred years, for ardent critics led by G. B. P. Pibrac, who popularized the dry suture, continued to point out that suturing wounds retarded healing. Many were convinced that approximation of wound edges by bandaging or adhesive tape was less likely to invite infection and had the additional advantage of being less painful than percutaneous sutures.[84] The advent of anesthesia, of course, took away the latter objection and served to revive use of the percutaneous stitch.

Today's surgeon would be wise to heed Halsted and William H. Welch of The Hopkins, who conducted studies on infection of wounds and wound healing approximately three-quarters of a century ago. Welch demonstrated that the depths of the dermis of dog and man are constant carriers of *Staphylococcus albus*. Halsted had already observed in dog experiments that omission of the percutaneous suture, which penetrates all layers of the dermis, resulted in a decreased incidence of infection. He replaced the percutaneous stitch with a running subcuticular suture, catching only the very tips of the wound edges. He also used an overlay of gutta-percha or silver foil.[85] Unmindful of Halsted's advice, surgeons, including his own lineal descendants, have returned to the percutaneous suture.

The significant role of buried nonabsorbable sutures in abetting infection in wounds was demonstrated by Elek on a few human volunteers at St. George's Hospital in 1956. When a suture mounted on a needle carrying 30,000 *Staph. aureus* organisms was pulled through the skin and subcutaneous tissue, 80 percent of the bacteria were left behind in the tissues, yet no clinical infection occurred. If, however, the suture was cut and left embedded in the tissues, as few as 100 organisms produced an abscess. Sterile sutures were harmless.[86] Inasmuch as bacteria are invariably present in elective surgical wounds of magnitude, the role of buried foreign bodies, including suture material, in provoking wound infection is clearly evident.

The hazard of penetration of the dermis by percutaneous sutures has been reiterated by M. T. F. Carpendale. He observed that closure of incised wounds in pigs by strips of adhesive tape resulted in healing without wound infection, whereas the incidence of infection was 16.7 percent in wounds closed by percutaneous sutures. Experiments in contaminated wounds in guinea pigs by Richard F. Edlich and associates in 1968 gave "strong support to the thesis that percutaneous sutures should be avoided in the closure of contaminated wounds." They found that each suture armed with two fresh needles, both passed from within out, is less likely to be accompanied by wound infection than the conventional percutaneous stitch. Benjamin Bell employed this manner of closure in 1804, undoubtedly because it was less painful.[87]

J. F. Burke and associates of Massachusetts General Hospital have come to accept an "irreducible minimum" of wound infections attending elective operations. In this occurrence the percutaneous suture undoubtedly has a role. The debates of French surgeons two centuries ago upon the theme of the percutaneous suture, which they described as a primitive or primary suture, contrasted with adhesive tape closure (*sutura sicca*), were not in vain. These considerations obviously have more than historic interest. It is strange that in the two-year study of the problem of infected wounds carried out by five American university surgical clinics under the chairmanship of John M. Howard (1964) no notice was taken of the role of the percutaneous suture.[88]

Mortality of Amputation

The heated debates sparked by Boucher and Faure (1756) in the French Academy of Surgery over whether amputation should be immediate or delayed brought into the open the astonishingly high mortality from the operation,[89] yet it is difficult to find statistical reports of the results of amputation before the fourth decade of the nineteenth century. One looks in vain through Paré's magnificent book for factual accounting of his successes and failures; the latter are usually omitted. The closest approach to a reliable statistical report of amputation that we have encountered in the early literature is in Woodall's *Surgeons Mate* (1639). Woodall stated that in twenty-four years of practice at St. Bartholomew's Hospital he had performed more than a hundred amputations with not more than twenty deaths.[90] It is to be remembered, however, that thigh amputations were then infrequent, inasmuch as Petit's tourniquet was yet to come.

The first inclusive report of mortality attending amputation would appear to be that of the anatomist surgeon Monro I in 1737. He was the leader of the Monro dynasty that helped establish Edinburgh as the great medical teaching center in the eighteenth century. Monro reported 14 consecutive major amputations done without mortality by the physicians and surgeons in the Royal Infirmary of Edinburgh. Fifteen years later he wrote that 99 amputations had been done with 8 deaths, a mortality of 8 percent.[91] This remained for years an unchallenged record and an extraordinary accomplishment compared with even later periods, when between 45 and 65 percent mortality was commonplace for amputations of the thigh.

The details of the procedure are known to us only through Monro's statement at one juncture that they followed his "Method." In this report Monro gave his oft-quoted edict on the importance of "little circumstances" for the outcome of operations. He does not mention surgical cleanliness, but for such a low mortality score in that day high standards of cleanliness must have prevailed at the Infirmary.

Ninety years later (1842–43) the mortality of amputation at the Royal Infirmary of Edinburgh was more than five times greater — 21 deaths among 43 amputations (48.8 percent), according to Simpson. The mortality for the Infirmary over a four-year period beginning in July 1839 was 48.6 percent, 35 deaths among 72 patients, as reported by T. B. Peacock.[92] A number of studies of the pre-Listerian era indicated a greater mortality attending amputation for injury than for disease. In amputation for disease there was usually no contaminated wound near or at the site of the operation, and the resultant contamination was only that incident to surgery performed without strict antiseptic or aseptic care.

The mortality rates reported by individual surgeons and clinics varied greatly, which probably is a direct reflection of the care and thought the surgeon gave to such items as hand-scrubbing and preparation of the operative field, the instruments, and the linens used in the procedure. Open wound management with delayed closure and avoidance of percutaneous sutures were other important determinants. A few widely scattered surgeons — C. Maunoir (1825) in Geneva, Paul Dubois (1830) in Paris, Stephen Hammick (1830) in Plymouth, Liston (1841) in London, and Paul Eve (1846) in Augusta — like Monro of Edinburgh and Alanson of Liverpool, were able to provide proof that all was not luck in surgery. Their records in amputations were not exceeded until prophylactic antiseptic surgical practices came to supplant placement of antiseptics in wounds.[93]

The high mortality rates attending amputation in various Paris hospitals after the revolution of July 1830 and the riots of June 1832 caught the attention of French surgeons. In an extensive five-year study of statistics from nine Paris hospitals, Malgaigne was saddened and dismayed to learn that the overall mortality for amputations was 30 percent; for major amputations, 52 percent; and for thigh amputations, 62 percent. He concluded that this appalling record must not be submerged in oblivion, and he published his findings in 1842.[94]

Malgaigne was astonished that the amputation results of the great master, Baron Dupuytren, were no better than his own. Although Dupuytren held demoralization of the patients accountable in part for the high mortality,[95] Christison's observations as a student during a visit to Dupuytren's clinic probably have some bearing on the matter: "The crowd around him was so great that I found it impossible to get near enough to hear or see his examination of his patients. The French students, moreover, were a very dirty, ill-dressed set to squeeze among. But indeed M. Dupuytren was no better. He wore a dirty white apron, superfluously protecting a dirtier pair of trousers, a greasy threadbare coat, and well-worn carpet shoes."[96]

When two of Dupuytren's protégés published a posthumous edition of his oral surgical clinics, they quoted at length from Thomson's *Lectures on Inflammation*, a French edition of which had appeared in 1827. Thomson concluded that *pourriture d'hôpital* was communicated by contact with sponges, *charpies*, and bandages. One wonders whether Dupuytren found time in his arduous, unrelenting daily schedule to read, let alone appreciate either Thomson or Blackadder, whose writings were also of great interest to Dupuytren's editors. In a nicely executed experiment Blackadder showed that *pourriture d'hôpital* was communicated from patient to patient only through direct contact with soiled wound dressings, sponges, instruments, and the like. Patients with clean wounds separated from others with the disease by a space of a few feet did not contract it when care was taken to avoid direct intercourse.[97]

Nicolai Pirogoff, Russia's most famous military surgeon of the nineteenth century, has recounted with unrestrained candor his experience in the care of the wounded. Suppuration, pyemia, erysipelas, and death stalked the hospital wards. Pirogoff himself, over a period of sixteen years, suffered an intractable diarrhea, influenced most favorably by long periods of vacation from the enervating activity of caring for surgical wounds. Little wonder that Pirogoff felt that luck and circumstance had as much influence on the outcome of operations as the surgeon's ability. Of a few thousand amputations noted in his registry Pirogoff said he could only refer with assurance to a couple of hundred whom he knew to have recovered or died.[98]

A report from H. J. Bigelow's surgical service at the Massachusetts General Hospital over a four-year period (1881–84) listed 115 compound (open) fractures and compound dislocations, in which Lister's practices were followed, with 15 deaths (13 percent) from sepsis. The achievement, a very modest one to be sure, apparently represented a distinct improvement over earlier experiences in the hospital. A decade earlier, however, Richard Volkmann of Halle had been able to report no mortality in a similar group of cases employing Listerian methods.[99]

Before antisepsis, the English mortality rates as a whole were definitely lower than those of other countries. The mortality records of German-speaking surgeons of that era are scarce. Their writings refer largely to the astonishing mortality attending amputation in the hands of French, English, and American surgeons. The German-speaking surgeons, however, were among the first to accept antiseptic surgery while its virtues were being hotly debated in England and America. They too were the first to appreciate the full impact of Pasteur's and Koch's studies and to adopt aseptic surgical techniques.

Advances in peripheral arterial surgery came as a natural sequel to the availability of anticoagulants. In World War II many limbs were spared amputation by restoration of blood vessel continuity. This achievement was greatly augmented in the Korean conflict by improved techniques of arterial suture.

Summary

The mortality rate attending major amputations remained high until the principles of prophylactic surgical antisepsis were accepted and implemented, and the mortality figures for thigh amputations were surprisingly high through all the wars of the nineteenth century. Infection continues to shadow the surgeon despite a number of significant therapeutic innovations by Semmelweis, Pasteur, Lister, Koch, Domagk, and Fleming over the past 130 years. The open method of treating potentially infected wounds has been accepted in military surgery, but how this procedure combats infection and suppuration is not completely understood. Experience and experiment must go hand in hand in resolving the problem of how to improve upon the efforts of nature in overcoming potential infection and how to speed healing of contaminated wounds, in which exploration the microbiologist and the pharmacologist are the surgeon's best aides.

Today's surgeon has much to learn from the empiricism of his predecessors. The delayed closure of wounds and the use of the cautery for hemostasis, long frowned upon by historians, are once more respectable surgical procedures. Leaving potentially infected wounds open until the wound surface has a glaze, the method of Kern and Liston, appears to have merit.

Surgeons also should heed the lessons that emerged from the debates at the French Academy of Surgery two centuries ago on the hazards of the percutaneous suture. If omission of this suture fails to eliminate or to reduce materially the incidence of wound sepsis, delayed closure of the cutaneous segment of the wound in instances in which the observed incidence of postoperative infection approximates or exceeds 10 percent is in order.

The guiding principles of wound management have evolved from centuries of experience and appear to be firmly established, but future discoveries may alter current practice. It is not the announcement of an objective but its achievement, in the final analysis, that counts. Historical appraisals of accomplishment in a technical discipline may be heightened by an assessment including the realistic and chastening lessons of experience that only active participants in such disciplines can provide.

(For notes, see pp. 586–95.)

CHAPTER 3

Debridement

PLUCKING FOREIGN BODIES out of wounds, especially an embedded arrow or other missile, is as old as surgery.[1] The difficulties were compounded by the introduction of gunpowder in warfare. Centuries of trial on the battlefields of Europe and bitter disputes among famous military surgeons preceded the acceptance of revision for war wounds. To Carl Reyher, a young Russian army surgeon of the late nineteenth century, who is generally unappreciated even today, should go much credit for establishing debridement on a scientific basis. It was actually World War I which served to focus attention upon the necessity for revision of contaminated wounds harboring devitalized tissue.

From antiquity to the introduction of antisepsis the cautery provided a useful tool to destroy necrotic tissue and to eradicate infection in wounds and was, as discussed in the preceding chapter, a primitive form of debridement. Less specific was the boiling oil therapy which Paré rejected in his monograph of 1545 — it did not distinguish between necrotic and uninjured tissue.[2]

When Paré published his collected works in 1579, representing over forty years of active experience and study, his recommendations for treatment of war injuries had assumed maturity and a unique understanding. He also knew that lodged bullets may migrate. He admonished the surgeon: "If there bee any strange bodies, as peeces of Wood, Iron, Bones, bruised flesh, congealed blood, or the like, whether they have come from without, or from within the body, and shall be by accident fastened or stucke in the wound, he must take them away, for

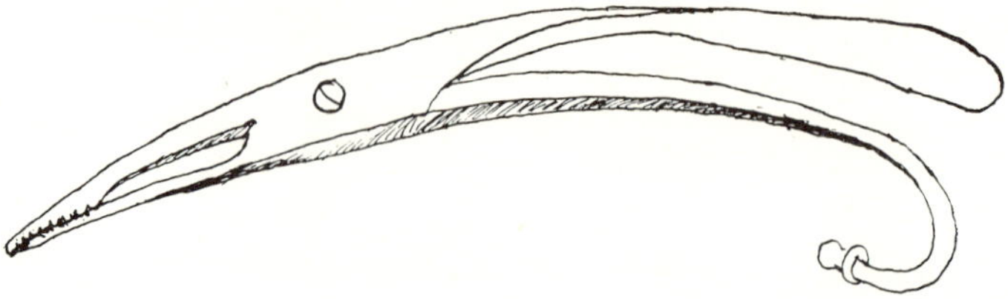

3.1 Gersdorff's forceps for removing bullets. From Thompson, *History of surgical instruments*.

otherwise there is no union to be expected. . . . It will bee fit the Chirurgion fall to worke quickely, safely, and as mildely as the thing will suffer. . . . Therefore he may pull out the strange bodies, either with his fingers, or with instruments, fit for that purpose."[3]

Preventive Debridement

The dilatation and incision of wounds to promote drainage and to obviate swelling, a form of preventive debridement, was common practice in the treatment of gunshot injuries for many centuries. Guy de Chauliac (1363) enlarged contaminated wounds to encourage drainage. Among the numerous instruments depicted by Gersdorff (1517) was a scissorslike dilator. At the first dressings, said Paré, "The wound must forthwith be enlarged, unlesse the condition of the part resist, that so there may be free passage forth both for the *sanies* [pus], or matter, as also for such things as are farced [stuffed], or otherwise contained therein." Disputes for and against preventive debridement started at least as early as the sixteenth century. Laurens Joubert, a distinguished professor of medicine at Montpellier, presented the opposing opinions in 1574. He concluded that it was often best to widen the opening of a wound.[4]

Students of semantics have traced the changing concepts of the term "debridement" from its origin in the French verb *débrider* ("to unbridle") to its present connotation and acceptance by modern surgeons. The transition was still a matter of keen controversy in 1940, as revealed in the correspondence columns of the *British Medical Journal*, where a number of prominent British surgeons arrayed their opinions on the derivation and meaning of the term.[5]

Measures to dilate or hold the wound open included the *charpie* and the *tente*. The *charpie* was a packing of lint inserted into the wound; the *tente* was a firmer, tamponlike roll, usually made of linen. The thirteenth-century Theodoric of Bologna and his illustrious French pupil, Henri de Mondeville, in their desire to achieve primary union of wounds, did not favor these devices. Mondeville said that as long as a *tente* remained in place, a wound would never close and would continually produce pus. Guy too had some reservations over the use of *tentes*.[6] In his later work (1590), Paré opposed employment of *tentes* and wound *charpies*.[7] It was almost a century more before the French military surgeon Augustin Belloste reemphasized the harmful effects of such practices,[8] and not until the nineteenth century that their use in France was seriously challenged.

Dilatation of war wounds was still practiced at the end of the eighteenth century. J.-L. Petit's "debriding" of saber wounds of the head, carrying the incision down to the pericranium, is recorded in a posthumous publication of 1774. Ravaton (1768) described a fresh, deep saber wound of the back of the neck for which wound revision akin to debridement was performed.[9]

During the American Revolutionary War the British army surgeon H. St. John Neale treated a contaminated wound as a fistula, enlarging it until the bottom of the tract equaled the size of the opening. Neale took his countryman John Hunter to task for rejecting dilatation of gunshot injuries. Hunter favored expectant treatment of such wounds, leaving them open to heal by granulation ("healing under a scab"). He was antithetic to revision other than the extraction of lodged bullets when they could be conveniently removed. Even this procedure he did not endorse in all cases.[10]

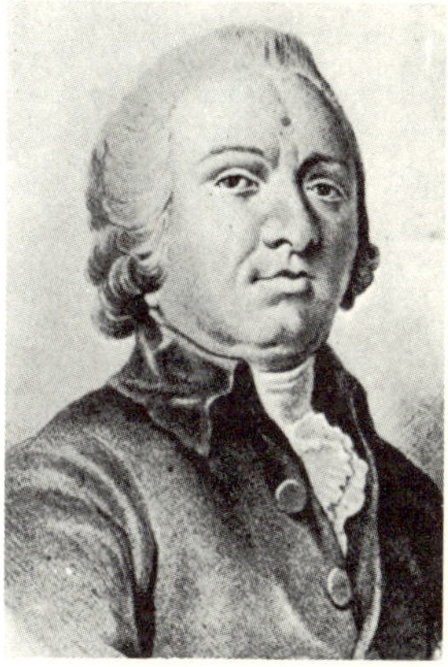

3.2 Pierre-Joseph Desault, leading French surgeon and teacher at Hôtel-Dieu, 1785–95, encouraged use of debridement.

In his manual for army surgeons (1792) Percy advised incisions with a bistoury to guard against swelling and collections from hemorrhage and suppuration causing additional tissue necrosis. He relates that young surgeons coming to Paris were repelled when they first saw him perform this procedure but were gradually won over on observing the success of the method.[11] Larrey, Napoleon's greatest military surgeon, also was a strong proponent of preventive debridement.[12]

A modern concept of debridement for contaminated wounds is credited to Pierre-Joseph Desault, who was chief of surgery at the Hôtel-Dieu from 1785 until his death in 1795. Larrey, one of his pupils, says that Desault instructed his students that it was necessary to "prune" (*refraîcher*) the contused edges of the wound with a cutting instrument, not simply to cause the wound to bleed.[13] Larrey's preference for early amputation in gunshot injuries denied him the opportunity to explore debridement fully.

The Hôtel-Dieu's internationally famous surgeon Dupuytren

(1834) called debridement "a precious resource" to prevent strangulations occasioned by the swelling of inflammation.[14] However, he often favored delayed debridement, which proved ineffective in the significant studies of Reyher several decades later.

Rejection of Debridement

Although by the middle of the nineteenth century most military surgeons tried to extract immediately any foreign bodies in a firearm wound, there were dissenting voices. P.-F. Blandin of Paris (1839), who said debridement was useful in some cases to prevent strangulation in the tissues, believed it was not needed in the removal of dead pieces, gangrenous detritus, bits of wads or clothing, or splinters. Suppuration, he said, would take care of that well enough. The German army surgeon Louis Stromeyer said that the surgeon should not touch a compound fracture of the long bones if he planned to save the limb; the presence of a projectile was no excuse for introduction of a finger, which might displace a fragment of bone.[15]

In the African campaign of 1830–39 the French army surgeon Lucien Baudens at first used preventive debridement of gunshot wounds, but he lost heart when faced with large wounds. He finally resorted to merely bandaging the wound, moistening the dressings with water, followed by several phlebotomies, after which "smooth and rapid healing occurred." Thereafter he became a keen opponent of debridement, using his bistoury only to facilitate the extraction of foreign bodies.[16] In 1848, when he was chief of surgery at the military hospital Val-de-Grâce, Baudens initiated debates on war wounds before the French National Academy of Medicine in which twelve leading surgeons participated over several months. Among the panelists, only L.-J. Bégin, a veteran surgeon of Napoleon's campaigns from the Russian steppes to Waterloo and a former chief of surgery at Val-de-Grâce (1840–42), strongly championed the merits of debridement. He was very critical of John Hunter, saying that Hunter's personal experience with war wounds was limited, for after a brief period with the army at Belle-Ile in 1761 Hunter had gone to Portugal and busied himself peacefully with studies on the digestion of lizards. P.-C. Huguier indicated that other Englishmen besides Hunter, notably the military surgeons Hennen and Thomson, also opposed debridement for contaminated wounds.[17]

The discussions revealed that many distinguished surgeons,

called upon to treat victims of the Paris revolutions of 1830 and 1848, abandoned debridement altogether, notably Huguier, Lisfranc, Roux, and Velpeau.[18] Blandin pointed out that the removal of foreign bodies, universally practiced, was actually a form of debridement. Antoine Jobert (de Lamballe) called debridement dangerous, which of course it was from the standpoint of additional contamination of wounds by unclean hands and instruments.

Jobert's gratuitous comment that English surgeons "unfortunately" were still enlarging gunshot wounds, roused an angry retort in the *Lancet* from England's great army surgeon Guthrie (1848). He said that "the enlargement of wounds, simply because they were gunshot wounds, was abandoned as injurious" by British army surgeons thirty-five to forty years before. Guthrie did, however, favor debridement to extract bone splinters.[19]

From the Napoleonic Wars until World War I debridement was used but little. Léon Legouest, a French surgeon of the Crimea, stated in 1859 that preventive debridement had been rejected by the majority of military surgeons. The British army surgeon Thomas Longmore referred to it in 1862 as a former custom that had been discarded by his compatriots since Hunter's day. He favored removal of foreign bodies and dilatation of the wound to encourage drainage and the escape of sloughs, but he did not excise dead tissue. The celebrated Russian Pirogoff related that he virtually gave up debridement after his experiences in the Crimea and the Caucasus because of the frequent supervention of pyemia and phlegmonous edema.[20] It is to be remembered that surgical antiseptic practices were yet to come. An unsterile debridement very obviously had its risks.

Reyher's Antisepsis and Debridement for Battle Wounds

It is surprising that the work of Reyher in the Russo-Turkish War of 1877 has been almost completely overlooked. This young Russian surgeon was the first to make a controlled study of debridement in contaminated gunshot wounds. He emphasized the advantages of immediate debridement upon or near the field of battle, contrasted with intermediate or delayed wound excision, and he also established the value of leaving the wound open with concomitant antiseptic treatment.

Reyher had prepared himself well for his career at a time when surgeons felt that military service offered the finest surgical experience. Following graduation in medicine at Dorpat (1870), he had enlisted as a Prussian army surgeon in the

Franco-Prussian War. Later he was an assistant to Heine in Nancy. In 1872 he joined the clinic of Bergmann in Dorpat, where he worked until 1877, with occasional interruptions for volunteer war service and a visit to London and to Lister's clinic in Edinburgh.[21] He concentrated intensively on the problem of wound sepsis, reporting in 1878 on antiseptic wound management in war surgery.[22] When at the age of thirty-two he left for the Russo-Turkish War over the protests of Bergmann,[23] he occupied a high post in the Russian army.[24]

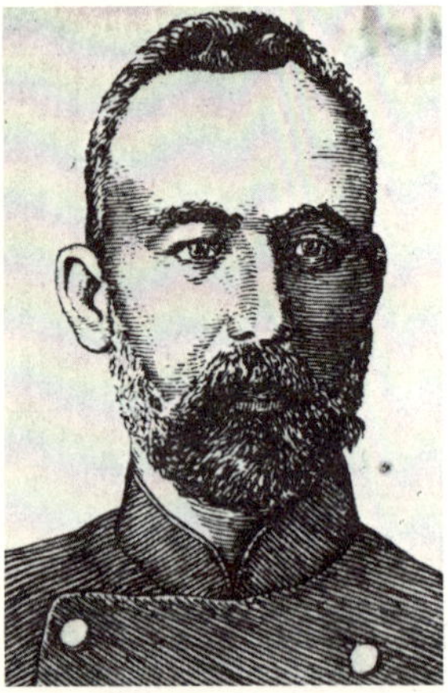

3.3 Carl Reyher established the significant role of debridement and surgical antisepsis in military surgery by controlled studies in Russo-Turkish War (1877).

When Reyher reintroduced debridement in the Russo-Turkish War, the procedure had been virtually forgotten. In a significant paper entitled "Primary Debridement for Gunshot Wounds," presented in German at the seventh International Medical Congress in London in 1881,[25] he was able to show that antiseptic treatment of wounds lowered the mortality from gunshot injuries. However, only when early debridement was added to the antiseptic management of serious wounds did he find a striking reduction in mortality. By careful statistical assessment he demonstrated that debridement added very materially to antiseptic treatment of wounds. The mortality was lowest when antiseptic therapy succeeded (9 deaths among 48 patients, or 18.7 percent). In a number of such instances, however, more aggressive surgical management was required. Reyher's best accomplishment with antisepsis, resection, and/or debridement was a mortality of 23.6 percent (13 deaths among 55 patients). Even so, he "unhesitatingly supported the thesis of primary debridement because it produced better results."

In a smaller series of cases Reyher treated 20 patients by antisepsis and resection (a type of debridement) with 2 deaths (10 percent). If delayed resection was done without antisepsis, the mortality was 66.6 percent (24 deaths in 36 cases), thus establishing the significant role of early debridement and antiseptic wound management. This was a major contribution not alone to military, but also to civilian surgery. Reyher abjured expectant antiseptic wound management on another score — the long period of wound healing involved, extending from three to nine months. In Reyher's hands, in addition to saving lives, early debridement and antiseptic wound treatment spared many amputations.

Following debridement, Reyher left the wound open, applying only a surface occlusive dressing. He employed neither primary nor delayed suture and allowed the wound edges to close by granulation. Rubber gloves, a very significant addition to wound care, probably did not become available to military surgeons until World War I, and the surgeons of Reyher's day did not have access to blood transfusions, deficiencies that may explain the high mortality with debridement for thigh and hip wounds.

In contrast to Reyher's report, other military leaders at the London congress, including Friedrich Esmarch of Kiel and H. F. L. Melladew of London, testified to the virtues of antiseptic management of wounds in civilian practice but admitted freely its failure in military practice in the Franco-Prussian War. Esmarch's advice for battlefield wounds at that conference was "Non nocere!" ("Don't touch!").[26]

When the *British Medical Journal* printed an excerpt of Reyher's presentation, it mentioned only his demonstration of the effectiveness of antiseptics in war wounds.[27] Reyher's emphasis upon debridement, the title of his paper, was completely overlooked and obviously not appreciated. "The loud and prolonged applause" following his speech, "Reyher being carried out from the Tribune in triumph,"[28] therefore, was for his establishing the effectiveness of antiseptic management for gunshot wounds in warfare. A German review of the congress ignored Reyher entirely. The only recognition of his contribution was in a brief summary by the famed military surgeon Gurlt (1882), who evinced knowledgeable insight on the important principle of wound excision that Reyher had stressed in his London address.[29]

At the next International Medical Congress, held in Copenhagen in 1884, there was considerable discussion of wound antisepsis but no mention of debridement. The first French Congress of Surgery (1885) devoted a session to war wound dressings. One French physician, Eugène Audet, a major in the military academy at Saint-Cyr, mentioned Reyher and his achievement of 21.4 percent mortality in compound gunshot fractures with antiseptics, drainage, and immobilization but did not speak of his use of debridement. The major emphasis in the discussions was on the choice of antiseptic and wound dressings. In his magnificent monograph on war surgery in 1888 Edmond Delorme recalled the impact of Reyher's 1878 paper on antiseptic management of wounds[30] but not his more significant offering in 1881 on debridement. It is patently evident, therefore, that Reyher's advice, based on personal war experience, fell on deaf ears, except for the notice it received from Gurlt. One might infer that the common reaction of surgeons to debridement was "The patient already has a wound, why make another?"

Reyher probably was the first to initiate a controlled prospective study of the management of war wounds, and he established the importance of the time factor in debridement.[31] That his suggestions went unheeded until World War I serves to emphasize how important it is that interested persons in the discipline exhibit enough credulity to initiate trials before ignoring or condemning a given hypothesis.

Innovators often live anachronistically. Born before their time, they frequently encounter little sympathy for their ideas and practices. Following the London International Medical Congress, Reyher surrounded himself with a group of capable young surgeons and introduced Listerian principles into Russian civilian surgery. In 1883 he became chief of surgery at the Semenov Hospital, one of St. Petersburg's largest. His persistence in striving to achieve reform encountered opposition from envious associates, resulting in his dismissal. These circumstances compounded with domestic infelicity apparently brought on a depression that led to Reyher's suicide on a hunting expedition on December 30, 1890, at age forty-four.[32]

The Experimental Impetus

In 1898 P. L. Friedrich, a Leipzig surgeon who apparently was familiar with Reyher's work, demonstrated in experiments with guinea pigs that the time interval for the effectiveness of debridement was delimited to approximately six hours after infection, conclusions not very different from those reached by Reyher in his military experience. Unfortunately, Friedrich did not employ bacterial cultures but implanted dust and/or garden soil into wounds. He also was able to show that dead muscle tissue in the wound aggravated the situation. Friedrich expressed doubts about the value of placing antiseptics into contaminated wounds.[33]

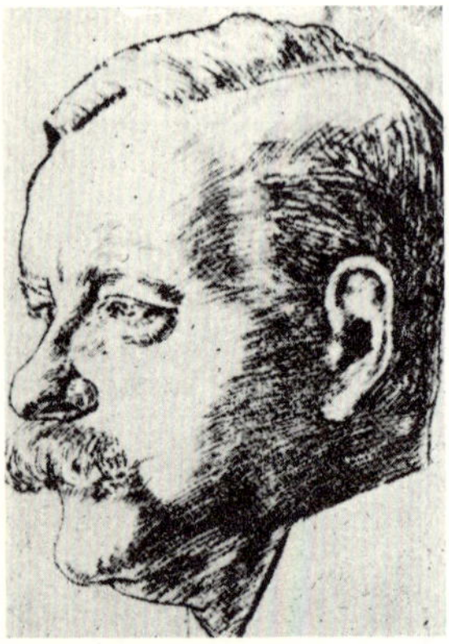

3.4 Paul L. Friedrich, in experiments on guinea pigs (1898), determined the importance of performing debridement within 4 to 6 hours to salvage infected extremities.

Shortly after Friedrich's publication on debridement, a number of papers on the superiority of open treatment for granulating wounds appeared in the German surgical literature. H. Wagner of Breslau (1903) made an especially strong and convincing case for reinstituting this mode of management.[34]

The reports of Carl Hueter (1879), L. Ferraton (1902), and A. van Emden (1915) documenting successful excision and/or cautery for wounds complicated by gas gangrene (*gangrene foudroyante*) may also have served a useful role in reviving interest in debridement. The condition, described in 1853 by Jacques Maisonneuve of the Hôtel-Dieu, became a major problem during trench warfare on the Western Front during World War I.

The fields of France and Belgium had been cultivated for centuries with animal manure used as fertilizer; the ground was laden with *Bacillus welchii* and other pathogens. A guinea pig inoculated with a few drops of the muddy water from the trenches died from gas gangrene within eighteen hours. In 1924 Thomas Cullen reintroduced the cautery to control spreading phagedenic gangrene, a grave disorder Blackadder (1818) said was known to the ancients. F. L. Meleney (1931) ascribed its origin to the symbiotic activity of microaerophilic streptococci and other organisms.[35] Fortunately, this dread complication of wounds seems to have disappeared with the arrival of chemotherapy and antibiotics.

Debridement in Twentieth-Century War Surgery

Historians of surgery writing before World War I could not appreciate or assess fully the significant difference in managing contaminated wounds by debridement followed by primary closure, contrasted with debridement followed by delayed wound closure — probably the most notable surgical lesson of World War I. In fact, the English surgeon Colonel H. M. W. Gray wrote in the *British Medical Journal* on August 28, 1915, that he had employed wound revision with primary suture since November 1914 and had been greatly impressed by the results. However, the high mortality that attended the closed treatment of wounds led surgeons to reexplore and reassess the virtue of debridement and wound closure. When Théodore Tuffier, who strongly favored delayed closure after debridement of contaminated wounds, had finished his presentation before the Société nationale de chirurgie in 1916, only two surgeons were recorded as still favoring primary suture following debridement.[36]

The Inter-Allied Surgical Conference convened in Paris in 1917 on the matter of revision of contaminated wounds.[37] After much debate the delegates established as the guiding rule for treatment, free opening of the cavity and "resection of all contused and contaminated tissues, and removal of all fragments of clothing or other foreign bodies." They agreed that primary wound closure was justifiable only when less than eight hours had elapsed since infliction of the wound. In primary amputations the wound should be left widely open, the soft parts being simply divided and the bone trimmed or rounded off, if necessary. It was concluded that circumstances which might dictate primary closure in compound fractures of warfare were rare.[38]

The French surgeon R. Lemaitre, who had served in World

War I, continued to believe that following debridement primary closure was the preferred and wiser policy. His emotional defense of the technique defies translation: "La suture primitive n'a pas besoin qu'on la défende, pas plus qu'elle ne redoute les attaques de ses adversaires: elle se défend par elle-même. Fille solide de la Chirurgie française, elle n'a besoin d'aucun père. Toute adoption inutile: elle vivra et grandira par elle-même."[39]

After the Inter-Allied Conference, excision of devitalized tissue with open wound management became standard practice. The experiences of World War II and the Korean and Vietnam conflicts lent credence to the wise decision of military surgeons of World War I. On April 26, 1943, Major General Norman Kirk, Surgeon General of the Army, sent a directive to all officers of the Medical Corps of the United States Army. The first section stated: "The guillotine or open circular method of amputation is the procedure of choice in traumatic surgery under war conditions and is especially indicated in gunshot wounds and in controlling infection. Primary suture of all wounds of extremities under war conditions is never to be done."[40]

During World War II surgeons noted a consistently high incidence of heavy seeding of wounds with microorganisms. Elliot C. Cutler reported that even after thorough and careful debridement 71 percent of contaminated war wounds were still contaminated. Yet clinical evidence of infection developed in only 8.6 percent of such cases.[41] The high-velocity missiles employed in World War II and the Korean and Vietnam conflicts frequently caused such wide shattering of tissue, including nerves and blood vessels, that primary amputation was inescapable.

In the Vietnam conflict General Leonard D. Heaton and colleagues (1966) showed that early debridement and delayed closure, accompanied by systemic administration of antibiotics, lowered the wound infection rate to compare favorably with that of elective operations in well-appointed civilian hospitals. Among 349 cases so treated in Vietnam, only 9 wound infections were observed (2.58 percent). This report documents an accomplishment exceeding the results of civilian surgeons in five university clinics in 1964, operating under the aegis of an ad hoc committee chaired by J. M. Howard, then of Hahnemann Medical College. The incidence of wound infection in clean hospital cases among the participating groups varied from 3 percent to 11.7 percent.[42]

Whereas debridement has found universal acceptance among both military and civilian surgeons, its specific role in the management of contaminated wounds has not been well defined. Some experiments conducted in this surgeon's laboratory with contaminated wounds, with and without the presence of devitalized tissue, over a three-year interval, have provided a few answers. In studying the rapidity of the peripheral spread of three organisms — *Staph. aureus*, culture 12,600, *Streptococcus pyogenes*, Group A, and *Escherichia coli*, serotype 06 — placed separately into freshly incised wounds of guinea pigs and rabbits, it was observed that the streptococcus extended peripherally considerably more rapidly than the other two organisms. The special and probably the sole role of debridement is the removal of dead tissue; energized jet irrigation of such wounds will remove debris and pus. Neither debridement nor wound irrigation with saline solution will sterilize a wound; only the appropriate antibiotics can do that. Abundant evidence emerged from these experiments to indicate that systemic administration of penicillin and saline irrigation are equally as effective as wound irrigation with penicillin. The role of devitalized tissue in accelerating the peripheral spread of bacteria from wounds was very evident in the experiments. It would appear that debridement is more effective when performed within four hours of contamination.[43]

Summary

The removal of lodged foreign bodies and the dilatation of drainage sites constituted the first application of debridement for contaminated wounds. The use of the cautery and boiling oil to destroy necrotic tissue, arrest hemorrhage, and check suppuration represented an extension of debridement in the hands of de Vigo and others, measures Paré supplanted with placement of an antiseptic (oil of turpentine) into wounds of war. A deterrent to ready acceptance of debridement had long been the thesis: "the patient already has a wound, why create another?"

Debridement gradually took on additional forms. In preventive debridement incisions were made into fascial planes to obviate strangulation and tissue necrosis from swelling beneath strong fascias. Desault introduced "pruning" or knife excision of damaged tissue in the depths of the wound. Many military surgeons continued to reject debridement until the middle of the nineteenth century. Antiseptic wound practices were yet to come and unsterile debridement obviously had its risks.

Reyher, a Russian military surgeon, spent several weeks with Lister in Edinburgh in early 1874. In the Russo-Turkish War of

1877, he made a controlled prospective study of war wounds treated by Listerian antiseptic practices and debridement; his assessment demonstrated conclusively, for the first time, the advantage to the wounded of receiving both antiseptic and debridement therapy. Reyher also recognized the importance of leaving such wounds open. In 1898 Friedrich demonstrated experimentally in guinea pigs the importance of excising dead tissue in contaminated wounds. During World War I the Inter-Allied Surgical Conference decreed excisional debridement and open wound management as standard practice for all contaminated wounds, a plan of management observed subsequently by all American military surgeons. Since the Vietnam conflict these practices have also been quite generally adopted by civilian surgeons, and with benefit to their patients.

The special function of debridement, it would appear, is to excise devitalized tissue in contaminated wounds. Energized jet irrigation can complement debridement by removing wound debris and blood clots; it does not remove dead tissue. Appropriate antibiotic therapy brought a new dimension to revision of contaminated wounds. Clinical trials are needed to determine whether energized irrigation with antibiotic solutions can supplant excision of a mass of dead tissue; it would appear unlikely.

(For notes, see pp. 596–99.)

CHAPTER 4

Lithotomy and Lithotomists

No operation of the preantiseptic era tested the surgeon's skill and mastery of wound management as did perineal lithotomy. Amputation of a limb is much simpler and can be done with far less knowledge of anatomy or sophistication in surgical techniques.

Vesical calculi were so common in France by the sixteenth century that kings appointed lithotomists to the court. Because the condition was prevalent in Lorraine in the mid-eighteenth century, the philanthropic Duke Stanislas of that province established a school for lithotomists at Lunéville where a group of surgeons developed unusual competence with perineal lithotomy.[1] Vesical calculi were said to be frequent enough among Englishmen in 1827 "to macadamise one side of Lincoln's Inn Fields." In the famous Norwich and Norfolk Hospital in England over a period of forty-four years (1772–1816) about one in every 38 admissions was for lithotomy; a total of 506 operations for vesical calculus was performed, with 70 deaths, a mortality of 16.8 percent. The calculi, meticulously preserved, were put on display tables in the hospital museum in 1851 so the "real value and beauty of this unmatched collection" could be appreciated, the most "complete record, literally graven in stone, that the world possesses of calculous experience," wrote Henry Thompson in 1863.[2] They are still to be seen in a corner of the hospital morgue.

The condition, once so prevalent among adults in Europe, the

British Isles, and the United States, has almost completely disappeared in those countries, but is still frequent among young boys in some areas of Southeast Asia, notably Thailand, and in India, Pakistan, and the Middle East. A stone discovered in 1901 among the pelvic bones of a skeleton estimated to be over seven thousand years old was an exhibit of the Royal College of Surgeons Museum in London until destroyed by a Nazi bomb in 1941. It had been found in the grave of a boy of about sixteen in Upper Egypt, where vesical calculus remains a common affliction among young boys.[3] Mahmoud Ghanem, an Alexandria surgeon, did 60 suprapubic lithotomies for vesical calculus in young boys during a sixteen-month practice at Luxor in the early 1960s. He and a surgical colleague of Luxor attribute the condition to a deficiency in body water caused by great perspiration in the hot, dry Egyptian atmosphere. Unquestionably matters of diet, water, and climate have much to do with the incidence of vesical calculus, but the reasons are somewhat obscure. Vitamin A deficiency is no longer considered an important cause.[4]

Whether vesical stones originate in the bladder or descend from the kidney remains an unsettled question. Wherever vesical calculus assumes endemic proportions today, it outnumbers renal calculus in incidence, suggesting that the stones are probably primarily vesical in origin.[5] The lesser frequency of vesical stones in females may be owing to the shortness of the female urethra, permitting extrusion of small calculi with scarcely perceptible distress.

Benjamin Franklin (1706–90), American patriot and distinguished statesman, suffered from stone in the bladder during the last eight years of his life. He had consulted John Hunter concerning the ailment during a stay in London. Riding in a carriage over bumpy pavement was especially distressing. When walking on a smooth surface, he was more comfortable when the bladder was full than when empty. Franklin, an inventor of note, said if he could be supported by a gas-filled balloon, he would be most comfortable. Spasms of pain, bloody urine, and sudden stoppage of the stream when urinating were the predominant symptoms. He had an antipathy to medicines, feeling they were often more hazardous than the maladies from which relief was sought. Franklin apparently was more comfortable when the urine was alkaline, achieved by ingestion of alkaline powders. He spent much of his last eight years in bed, observing that the horizontal position contributed to his comfort. Franklin was carried to the Constitutional Convention in 1787 in a sedan chair by four strong prisoners from the Walnut Street jail. He had brought the chair from Paris, because it was the least painful mode of transport he could find. Franklin's medical advisors counseled nonoperative treatment, advice he willingly accepted. Loss of appetite made him shrink from a plump figure to a "skeleton covered by skin." Franklin's delineation of the symptoms of vesical calculus have not been excelled.[6]

For more than two centuries, lithotomy was the most commonly discussed operation in surgical circles, and the literature is enormous. There emerges from it an incomparable variety of talent and interest. No chapter in surgery is so replete with intrigue, perfidy, and dishonest dealings with both patients and associates. Mountebanks intermingled with dedicated practitioners. Quarrels, jealousies, and struggles for the impermanent limelight of ascendancy and the glory of success enter freely into the picture. As the story evolves, it becomes apparent that open wound management, emphasized by Paré's contem-

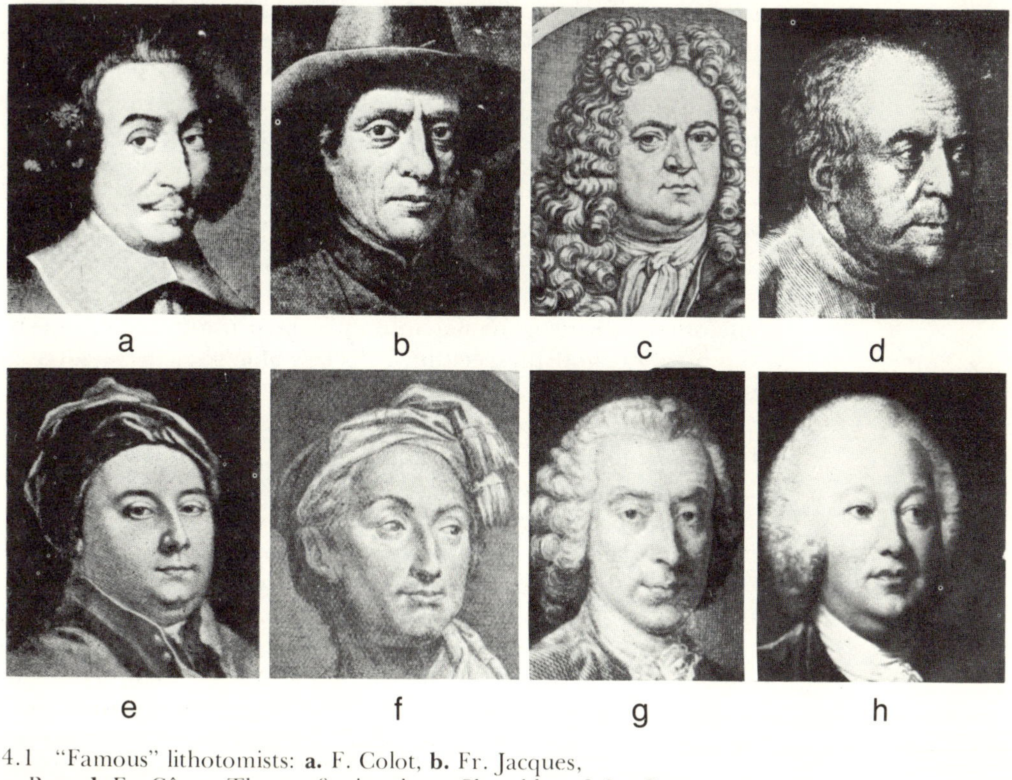

4.1 "Famous" lithotomists: **a.** F. Colot, **b.** Fr. Jacques, **c.** Rau, **d.** Fr. Côme. The professionals: **e.** Cheselden, **f.** Le Cat, **g.** Pouteau, **h.** Louis.

porary, Pierre Franco, was a dominant factor in the success of perineal lithotomy prior to asepsis.

Without anesthesia or antisepsis and employing only the helpful devices of cleanliness and superb surgical skill, a few lithotomists two centuries and more ago achieved a success rate with the intricate operation of perineal lithotomy that has never been excelled — and this was before the importance of the surgeon's knife or lithotome staying within the prostatic fascia was understood. Also significant is the fact that the two-stage perineal lithotomy often had a greater success rate in less practiced hands than was achieved by the one-stage procedure when done by some of its most experienced exponents of unrivaled expertise. These facets of the history of lithotomy reflect an important segment of surgery's progress.

Varieties of Lithotomy

The names attached to lithotomy in its various forms are numerous. The anatomist Félix Vicq d'Azyr remarked in 1780 that there were so many operations of lithotomy that "the history of the science and its nomenclature are harder to understand than the science itself."[7] The sole objective was to relieve the patient of strangury by entering the bladder and extracting the calculus with the least damage to the tissues and with minimal risk to the patient. Hemorrhage, infiltration of urine into the surrounding tissues, injury of the rectum, and severe wound and bladder infection were frequent concomitants. It was the skilled surgeon, with an intimate knowledge of the complicated anatomy of the urogenital diaphragm, the prostate and its fascia, the bladder, and the rectum, who was able to achieve success with this intricate operation.

Many students continue to enumerate all the variants of lithotomy, failing to recognize that there are essentially only two kinds: the perineal approach and the suprapubic approach. The median, lateral, bilateral, and quadrangular perineal lithotomies are all variants of the same procedure and differ only in the extent of the perineal incision and exposure provided for the real task, to enter the bladder in a manner that does not invite hemorrhage, yet permits the urine to drain freely through the wound to the exterior without collection in or dissection into the perivesical tissues. The urine draining through a properly constructed channel irrigates the wound, lessening the hazard of bacterial contamination.

Suprapubic lithotomy is by contrast a far simpler operation, but one that became popular only with the advent of anesthesia, when the struggles of the patient no longer threatened rupture of the diaphanous peritoneum, followed by extrusion of bowel into the wound.

At one period a few surgeons of distinction favored rectovesical lithotomy, entering the bladder via the rectum. The disastrous results of upper urinary tract infection and perivesical inflammation compelled discontinuance of the procedure. A few surgeons urged removal of vesical calculi in females by creating a fistula between the vagina and the bladder; the complication of persistent vesicovaginal fistula forced its suspension.

Historical Aspects of Perineal Lithotomy

The Hippocratic oath proscribed the performance of lithotomy by members of the medical profession, indicating it should be left to those practiced in its use. The real reason was undoubtedly that the procedure was attended by serious hazards that would have reflected badly upon the profession.

Celsus was the first to provide a detailed description of perineal lithotomy. His technique, median lithotomy, the oldest variety of the perineal operation, has come to be known as cutting on the gripe. It is obviously adaptable only to large vesical calculi. Two fingers of the surgeon's left hand were thrust into the patient's rectum while an assistant pressed on the lower abdomen to encourage descent of the stone. The surgeon's fingers within the rectum grasped the stone through the intervening rectal and bladder walls. A midline perineal incision was made along the median raphe. The surgeon incised the prostate with a knife immediately over the stone and extruded it with a hook introduced through the incision. Recognizing the great danger of opening the rectum, Celsus deflected the upper end of the perineal incision toward the left ischial tuberosity before incising the bladder. The wound was left open.[8] The success-failure ratio of the operation is not known.

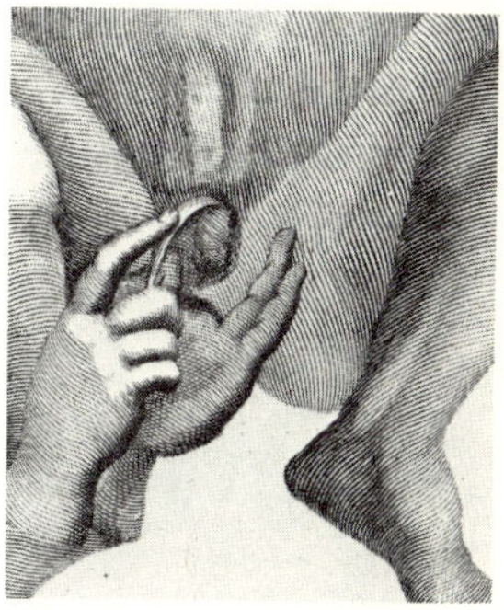

4.2 "Cutting on the gripe." From François Tolet, *Traité de la lithotomie* (Paris, 1682).

Though Guy de Chauliac and Paré both described perineal lithotomy, they apparently did not cut for stone.[9] Franco, the first surgeon to address himself seriously to the operation, began, like Paré, as a barber-surgeon. Little is known of Franco's life except that he was born in Provence about 1500, undoubtedly of humble origin. He indicates that he learned his surgery from an itinerant barber-surgeon or "stone-cutter." Franco spent some time in Switzerland, probably to escape religious persecution as a protestant Waldensian, returning to France shortly before the publication of his remarkable little book (1556), which deals chiefly with urology. He was not the gifted writer of books that Guy and Paré were but for sheer inventiveness and freshness of surgical thought they were not his equal.[10] Nor did Franco share Paré's enthusiasm for polypharmacy in wound dressings. In *Petit traite* (1556) and later in *Traité des hernies* (1561), Franco dealt with perineal lithotomy. A subtitle in the former defines his commitment, *Il faut endurer pour durer* ("To endure, it is necessary to persist"). He was also the first to describe and practice suprapubic lithotomy; however, he recognized the hazard of opening the peritoneal cavity in this procedure and remained partial to the perineal approach.[11]

In perineal lithotomy of the "small apparatus" a staff or sound was passed through the urethra into the bladder. Moreover, this was long the method employed to confirm the presence of vesical stone. With the patient in a semi-sitting posture, the tip of the sound was maneuvered to bring the stone down to the lowest point in the bladder. When the perineal incision was made, the surgeon felt for the groove on the convex side of the staff as a guide for the incision into membranous urethra and prostate. When an assistant held the urethral staff, the surgeon could include the advantage of cutting on the gripe. Scultetus in his superbly illustrated *Armamentarium chirgicum* shows the surgeon wearing a cuff at the wrist to preclude soiling his sleeve during this phase of lithotomy.[12]

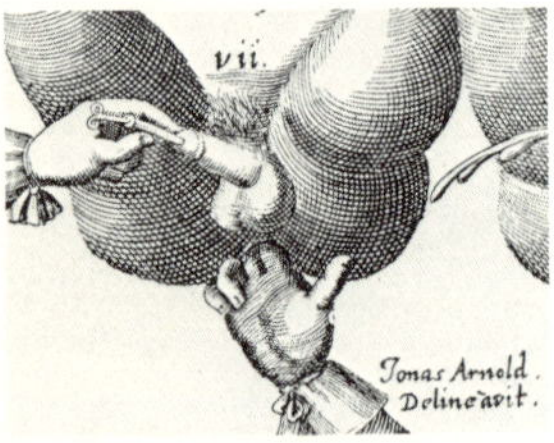

4.3 Lithotomist wearing cuff to avoid soiling sleeve. From Scultetus, *Armamentarium*.

Perineal lithotomy of the "grand apparatus" of Marianus Sanctus came next (1535),[13] the invention of his master Joannes de Romanis of Cremona, Italy. Instruments, forceps, and scoops, rather than the finger, were inserted through the perineal incision to engage and extricate the stone. In the main, it can be said that the additional apparatus not only complicated the procedure but added to the operative risk. A 1727 appraisal of the grand apparatus was that it saved only five or six out of twenty patients and that the survivors led sad lives, dripping urine, and frequently with fistulas at the incision.[14]

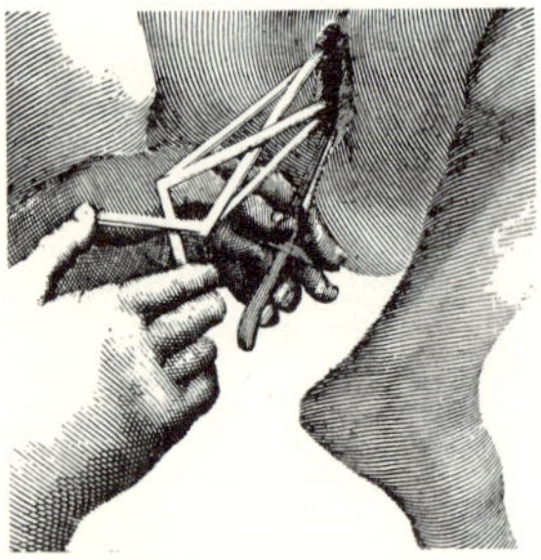

4.4 The "grand apparatus" of Marianus Sanctus. From Tolet, *Traité*.

Operations were frequently performed in the home. The patient was purged and often bled before the ordeal. Bleeding had the advantage of producing shock and diminishing considerably the patient's sensitivity to pain. After the terror and anguish of the operation were past, the patient usually had a sense of relief as urine escaped through the perineal wound without initiating attacks of vesical colic. When he later sickened from the unknown causes of wound inflammation, he was purged and leeched, often to sink progressively and succumb to complications engendered by the lithotomist's unclean hands and instruments.

Barber-Surgeon Lithotomists

From the mid-sixteenth century well into the eighteenth century a brand of self-made stone-cutters, "specialists" who acquired the art through apprenticeship, were the chief lithotomists. Among these barber-surgeon lithotomists was the family of Colot — fathers, sons, and nephews — who kept secret their procedure of lateral perineal lithotomy through eight succeeding generations,[15] nearly two hundred years, until François Colot's posthumous publication in 1727 gave a segment of his own experience. He cautioned against the dangerous effect of narcotics in lithotomy and presented illustrative cases.[16]

Jacques de Beaulieu (1651–1719), apprentice to a strolling Italian lithotomist, later donned a monklike habit and called himself Frère Jacques. When he reached Paris in 1697, he demonstrated his technique of perineal lithotomy on a cadaver at the Hôtel-Dieu. Jean Mery, serving as a witness, reported favorably on the procedure, but shortly afterward he reversed his opinion when he observed Jacques's high complication and mortality rate.[17]

Jacques's technique was described in a communication to the Royal Society of London as follows: Jacques first passed the staff into the bladder, depressing it toward the vesical neck, then felt for the tip of the sound with a finger in the perineum. Having located this, he made an incision to the left of the anus upward toward the ischial tuberosity. The bladder was pierced at its neck. The cut was extended in both directions; when urine appeared in the wound, the knife was thrust in a bit farther. Jacques then inserted a finger into the bladder to dilate the wound. Forceps were next introduced in an effort to grab the stone. Jacques did not insert any instrument into the bladder without first steeping it in oil of roses.[18] He apparently employed no dressing. According to some accounts, Jacques plunged his knife like a dagger into the perineum until it ground upon the stone, then with his finger in the anus extruded it through the perineal wound.[19]

Martin Lister, Queen Anne's physician, watched Jacques do nine lithotomies at the Hôtel-Dieu in April 1698, and was "put into some disorder with the cruelty of the Operation." However, when he visited all the patients in their beds he "found them more amazed [i.e., confused or stunned] than in pain." He decided that if Jacques's method were executed by a "Skilful Hand, it might be of good use to Mankind." On his return to England, Lister learned by letter, in August 1698, that of 71 lithotomies performed by Jacques in April (45 at the Hôtel-Dieu, 19 at La Charité, and 7 at Versailles), 38 had resulted in the patient's death (mortality, 53.5 percent). In the same period the surgeons of La Charité lost 3 patients among 22 lithotomies (mortality, 13.6 percent). Because of his high mortality rate Jacques's reputation suffered and the administrators of the two Paris hospitals denied him operating privileges. Lister's informant cautioned that the reports were questionable, for Jacques had many enemies, surgeons who publicly denounced him yet practiced his method. He learned that Jacques's only patient who died among the 7 at Versailles, for instance, was so ill preoperatively that he had not been expected to live.[20] Frère Jacques gave no postoperative treatment and left the patient to the care of relatives or attendants. This unpardonable neglect was considered partly responsible for the mortality.[21] However, as every surgeon comes to know, the best postoperative treatment is a well-performed operation, likely to assure a convalescence free of complications.

Fagon, surgeon to Louis XIV, believed that if Jacques were put under the tuition of the anatomist-surgeon J.-G. Duverney his skill would improve. This was done, but thereafter, many felt, Frère Jacques's boldness and success as an operator left him.[22] This is neither the first nor the last time critics have suggested that the "abysmal ignorance" of surgeons plays a role in their successes.

A rival of Jacques was Johan Jakob Rau (1668–1719), born in Baden, who had been apprenticed to a barber-surgeon. He was noted for his dissections and in his last years occupied the chair of anatomy at Leyden. Rau was well known as a lithotomist and quarreled with Frère Jacques when the latter visited Holland. Rau claimed to have performed 1,547 lithotomies without a death. The Dutch surgeon Pieter Camper said concerning this boast: "We will concede the number, if it is a question of treatment and not of cures; he [Rau] passes by in silence the matter of deaths. However, the record, which by order of the city fathers preserves to this day [1762] the operations for stone in the Surgical College, discloses that of 22 on whom he operated at Amsterdam, there were four deaths" (18.1 percent mortality).[23]

François Colot accused Rau of cutting for stone when there was none, saying that a stone was conveniently slipped into Rau's palm by his assistant at an appropriate time in the operation to be shown to spectators.[24] Rau never revealed his method, appar-

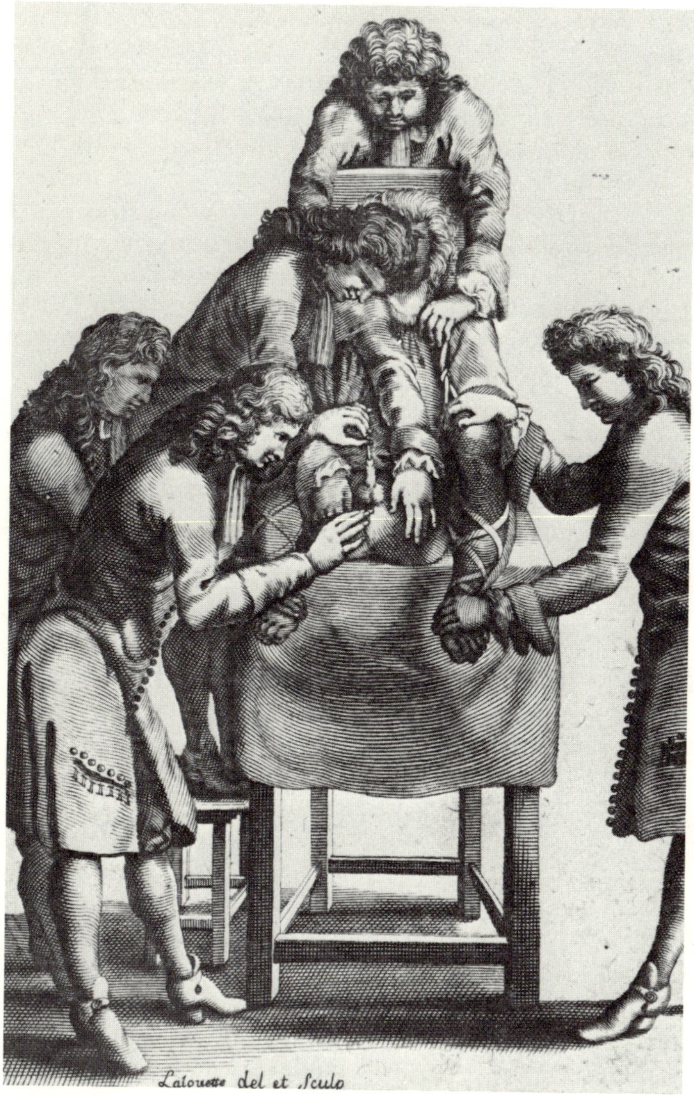

4.5 Patient restrained for lithotomy. From Tolet, *Traité*.

ently even deceiving his own pupil and assistant, B. S. Albinus. The latter published a supposed description of Rau's operation. However, those who attempted to follow his account, including the great English lithotomist Cheselden, had disastrous results. S.-F. Morand of Paris, who also experimented with it, correctly concluded that Rau must have cut through the prostate and not behind it as he led his associates to believe. Scoundrel that Rau was, he had two distinguished pupils in Albinus and Lorenz Heister.[25]

Frère Côme (1703–81), born Jean Baseilhac, came from a family of surgeons. He studied under his uncle in Lyons and later in Paris. He took orders in 1729 and decided to devote his life to the care of the poor. He devised the *lithotome caché*, first used in 1748, in which the cutting blade disappeared into a groove in the blunt segment of the gorget. When the operator probed for and located the prostate in the wound, the gorget was thrust through the prostate into the bladder and the cutting blade was extended, severing the prostate. Frère Côme left two important records of his work, including a description of suprapubic lithotomy.[26]

The success rates with perineal lithotomy of the itinerant lithotomists François Colot, Frère Jacques, Rau, and Frère Côme over a period of more than a century are very similar and do not begin to compare with the accomplishments of the professionals, typified by Cheselden, Claude-Nicolas Le Cat, Pouteau, and Jean-P. Maret.

The Professionals and Perineal Lithotomy

"The insurmountable objection to the Lateral Operation is, that we are operating in the dark," said the London surgeon Joseph C. Carpue in 1819, meaning, of course, that the exposure was limited.[27] An additional factor was that the importance of keeping the surgery within the prostatic capsule had not been recognized. Since retractors were rarely used when operations were performed without anesthesia, retraction of tissue was provided solely by the surgeon's free hand. Furthermore, the operation was done largely by the sense of touch, rather than by direct vision, a procedure which modern surgeons would consider completely unacceptable.

Lithotomy acquired the semblance of a scientific procedure in the hands of Cheselden in the first quarter of the eighteenth century. Morand, dismayed with the mortality of lithotomy with the grand apparatus as then practiced at La Charité in Paris — 32 deaths among 71 patients cut for stone (45 percent mortality) over a five-year period (1731–35) — went to London to watch Cheselden operate and observed that he employed essentially Franco's operation, later adopted by Frère Jacques.[28]

Cheselden's lateral lithotomy went through three stages of development: (1) incision into the bladder behind the prostate; (2) extension of an incision through the membranous urethra into the prostate (undoubtedly the best of Cheselden's operations); and (3) an operation in which a curved bistoury was introduced above the prostate and pulled toward the operator, cutting boldly into the substance of the prostate.[29] Great anatomist that he was, Cheselden was born a century too early to appreciate the significance of the prostatic fascia.

Perineal lithotomy provided the surgeon a fine opportunity to indulge in showmanship. Six or more cases were often scheduled for one séance. Pouteau described the scene as an *auto-da-fé*.[30] The courage and agony of the patient on the "bed of misery"[31] and the boldness and skill of the surgeon were the magnetic attractions that drew large numbers of onlookers. The spectators rarely saw into the depths of the wound. The skin incision and the seconds or minutes that intervened before the surgeon could exhibit the stone constituted the visible drama of the situation. Most operators emphasized the need for hurry. In the absence of narcosis, this attitude was understandable if not defensible. Frère Jacques performed ten perineal lithotomies in less than an hour at the Hôtel-Dieu in 1698. Morand saw Cheselden remove a stone in twenty-four seconds, and James Douglas said it seldom took Cheselden more than thirty seconds. Astley Cooper often did the operation in less than a minute. Reports of lithotomies in less than sixty seconds were frequent. The average maximum time for a lithotomy, according to a *Lancet* editorial in 1828, was about six minutes.[32]

Not all surgeons favored speed. It was the conviction of the distinguished physiologist-surgeon Charles Bell that the procedure "ought to be performed slowly and with caution." He related that once while doing a perineal lithotomy he was visited by an eminent surgeon who became impatient and said, "What can be the matter? Let me put in my finger!" Yet Bell's extraction time in the case involving two stones was only three minutes and fifteen seconds.[33]

Pouteau did not operate by the clock. He criticized the celebrated lithotomist Le Cat for meticulously recording in the provincial journals the time to the minute for completion of each operation he performed, as if, said Pouteau, "an hour-glass should be the measure of merit of an operator." Pouteau took five or six minutes to extricate the stone slowly from the bladder after the incision had been made, believing that gradual dilatations resulted, as in childbirth, in making the procedure less painful. He appraised the concern over hurry as a "desire for false glory which . . . has killed more patients than any other bad maneuver."

Pouteau's emphasis upon cleanliness in operations is well documented in his writings. He recognized the contagious nature of hospital gangrene and insisted that participants in operations, as well as those doing dressings, keep their hands clean. He also recommended disposable paper compresses for surface dressings of wounds. Pouteau's record with perineal lithotomy has probably never been excelled in a large series of consecutive cases; in 120 perineal lithotomies, he lost only three patients (2.5 percent mortality).[34]

A very different character was Le Cat of Rouen, who was as controversial and factious with the pen as he was quick with the knife, a disputatious polemicist eager for quarrels with those who did not accept his ideas. Crosse states: "Le Cat cut about half a dozen patients in twice as many minutes, and, it is said, lost nearly all of them!" Even so, his record with lithotomy is deserving of notice; over the years 1732 to 1768, Le Cat performed 150 lithotomies with an 8 percent mortality.[35] His Parisian contemporary Henri-François Le Dran wrote a detailed account of his own technique of lateral perineal lithotomy. It included transfer of the knife from his assistant's hand to his own mouth. He emphasized the importance of anatomy as a prime element in the success of perineal lithotomy, giving the sober advice, "open often the great book of the human body."[36]

Experiencing difficulty with the conventional operation, Dupuytren attempted perineal lithotomy by cutting into the bladder above the prostate. Dissection of urine into the perineal tissues caused him to lose five of seven patients operated upon in this manner (71.4 percent mortality). The most outstanding of the Lunéville lithotomists was Nicolas Saucerotte (1741–1814), who performed 1,564 lithotomies, largely in children, with 147 deaths (9.3 percent mortality).[37]

One of the most famous of the accomplished lithotomists associated with the early history of the Norwich and Norfolk Hospital was Philip M. Martineau, a member of the staff from 1777 to 1828, who held a record of 41 consecutive lithotomies without a fatality. Astley Cooper said that no surgeon in London could boast of similar success. At this period the incidence of bladder stones was higher in Norfolk than in any other county of Great Britain, a circumstance doubtless contributing to the proficiency of the region's numerous lithotomists — a group sometimes referred to as the Norwich school of lithotomy. Some important studies of bladder stones also emanated from the area, including a notable treatise by Crosse.[38]

From the foregoing it may justifiably be inferred that success with perineal lithotomy was not alone a matter of time and place but far more a reflection of the skill in dissection and the competence of the individual surgeon and undoubtedly too his standards of cleanliness. Even after anesthesia found general acceptance, a few surgeons elected not to employ it in lithotomy! Frederick Le Gros Clark in 1858 reported doing four perineal operations in two London hospitals on the same day, all without anesthesia.[39] An account of an operation in 1855 upon a sixty-six-year-old seaman for vesical calculus was given by F. J. Brown. He had invited as many lithotomists from the surrounding area of Chatham as could squeeze into the patient's small apartment to witness the procedure. On the conclusion of the operation, "the patient put on his spectacles to look at the [two] calculi, and then held a washhand basin for the accommodation of some of the gentlemen." The patient subsequently died, and the post-mortem revealed that the knife had slit not only the urethra and the prostate but also the opposite wall of the bladder and that the patient died from peritonitis and perivesical inflammation.[40]

Celsus, Franco, and Cheselden stand out in their periods as the greatest contributors to the development of lithotomy. In a supplement to *Anatomy of the Human Body* Cheselden described his technique in nine brief pages. With his usual modesty he concluded by saying, "If I have any reputation in this way [perineal lithotomy], I have earned it dearly, for no one ever endured more anxiety and sickness before an operation, yet from the time I began to operate, all uneasiness ceased; and if I have had better success than some others, I do not impute it to more knowledge, but to the happiness of a mind that was never ruffled or disconcerted, and a hand that never trembled during any operation."[41] However, the record of safety in performance of that great French surgeon Pouteau remains unchallenged. His work antedated antiseptic surgery by a century. To Pouteau must go the garland for pointing the way with an unrivaled record in an operation that commanded a formidable mortality in the hands of many.[42]

Return to Median Perineal Lithotomy

George Allarton (1863) asked a senior surgeon at one of the chief London hospitals why the median operation was not done in London. He replied, "Well, upon my word, I do not know. I have done the lateral operation 140 times with very good results, it will last my time; I leave new fangles to the young men. Cheselden did very well with the lateral operation." Allarton believed the median operation had advantages and reported 170

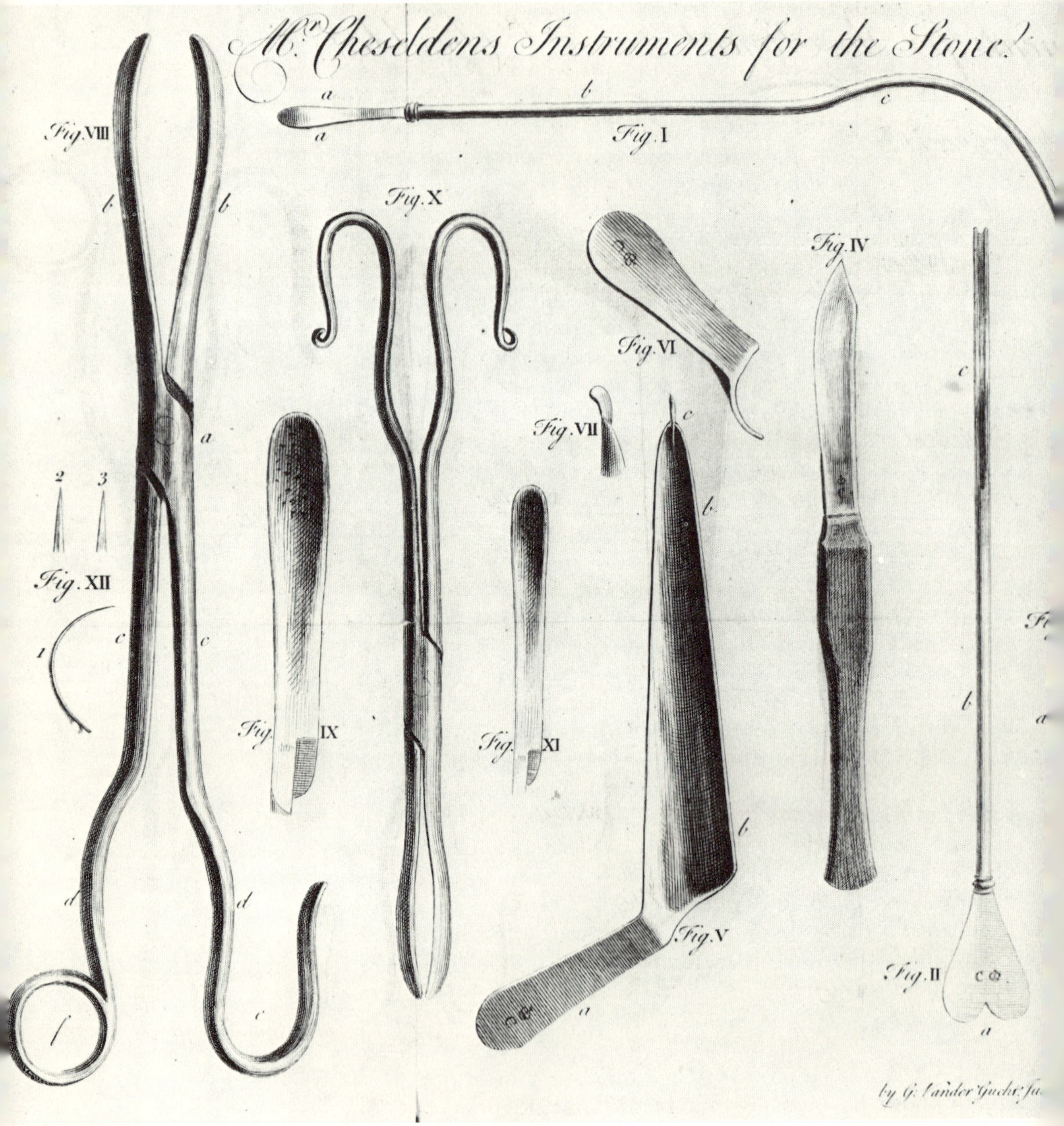

4.6 Cheselden's instruments for lithotomy. From James Douglas, *Appendix to the history of the lateral operation* (London, 1731). Courtesy National Library of Medicine.

median lithotomies by many surgeons of that day with 11 deaths (6.4 percent mortality).[43]

Joseph Lister performed a median lithotomy for vesical calculus on June 4, 1881. He swabbed the wound with zinc chloride and left it open, but he provided a drainage tube to facilitate the escape of urine. The patient recovered quickly.[44]

Perineal Lithotomy and Urinary Incontinence

Urinary incontinence, occasionally reported after perineal lithotomy in the male, was so frequent following urethrovesical lithotomy in the female that the procedure came to be abandoned. John Hunter's case books indicate that he cut five patients for stone, all of whom recovered. Case 3 was a woman of forty; following urethrolithotomy, said Hunter, "when she walked, the water dropped from her." Mullineux of Dublin suggested in 1693 that urethral dilatation without lithotomy often sufficed to remove vesical stone in the female.[45] Jean Hoin of Dijon preferred dilatation to lithotomy in the female because it did not provoke incontinence.[46] The ready distensibility and shortness of the female urethra made urethral dilatation a practical substitute.

Whereas urinary retention is not uncommon after abdominoperineal excision of the rectum for cancer in the male, urinary incontinence must be rare, for many experienced in the operation have never seen it. As in perineal lithotomy, injury to the urogenital diaphragm, which embraces the perineal urethra, cannot be completely avoided. Moreover, the studies of M. B. Wesson in 1923 and the more recent work of T. M. Oelrich are in agreement: the striated muscle within the urogenital diaphragm functions primarily as a compressor of the male urethra. It is not a true sphincter.[47]

Traditional anatomic descriptions tend to locate the sphincter of the urinary bladder in the vesical neck, where trigone and prostatic urethra meet to form the urethra. It seems strange that after centuries of perineal lithotomy for vesical stone an element of doubt still hovers over the actual location of the true internal involuntary sphincter for control of micturition.

If one may draw an inference from the frequent occurrence of incontinence attending urethrovesical lithotomy in the female, it would be that slitting the urethra, extending the incision well into the trigone, is a likely cause of the occasionally reported incontinence after perineal lithotomy in the male. The longer length and angulation of the male urethra and the compressor muscle in the urogenital diaphragm undoubtedly lessen the leaking effect of an injured internal sphincter. Jack Lapides observed that successive amputations of the male canine urethra increased urinary leakage. If 4 cm. of urethra were left beyond the urethrovesical juncture, continence was unimpaired. In both male and female dogs, amputation of the urethra 1 cm. beyond the vesical juncture was attended regularly by urinary leakage. R. T. Woodburne emphasizes the role of the elastic tissue and the smooth muscle of the urethra in sphincteric control of micturition and inclines to the belief that there is no sphincter at the vesical neck.[48] Clinicians are quite aware that functional sphincteric action may exist in the absence of a demonstrated anatomic sphincter.[49]

The Prostatic Fascia

Though attention has already been drawn to the importance of the prostatic capsule and fascia in achieving perineal lithotomy with a low operating mortality, it deserves fuller discussion. The anatomist Granville Sharp Pattison, who made the original observation in 1820, was a controversial figure. A native of Glasgow, he was then lecturing in Philadelphia and was shortly to fill the chair of anatomy at the University of Maryland. During the course of his stormy career Pattison was on the staff of several medical schools in America and, for a brief period (1827–30), at University College, London. Critics claimed that Abraham Colles of Dublin had described the prostatic fascia in 1841, but perusal of Colles's account indicates clearly that he failed to comprehend the need to delimit the incision in perineal lithotomy to the confines of the prostatic capsule.[50]

Many surgeons like Cheselden, it is true, had learned from experience the wisdom of delimiting the prostatic cut to the confines of the gland, something not easy in an unanesthetized patient and without proper wound retraction. René Garengeot attributed half of Frère Jacques's lithotomy mortality to severance of the internal pudic (pudendal) artery which lies beyond the prostatic fascia.[51] An even more frequent and often fatal complication attended cutting beyond the prostatic capsule, opening the perivesical space with ensuant collection and infiltration of urine.

More than a decade after Pattison, the French anatomist-surgeon C. P. Denonvilliers (1836, 1837), described the prostatic fascia.[52] He did not relate its significance to perineal lithotomy as had Pattison. Even so, anatomists and surgeons have come to

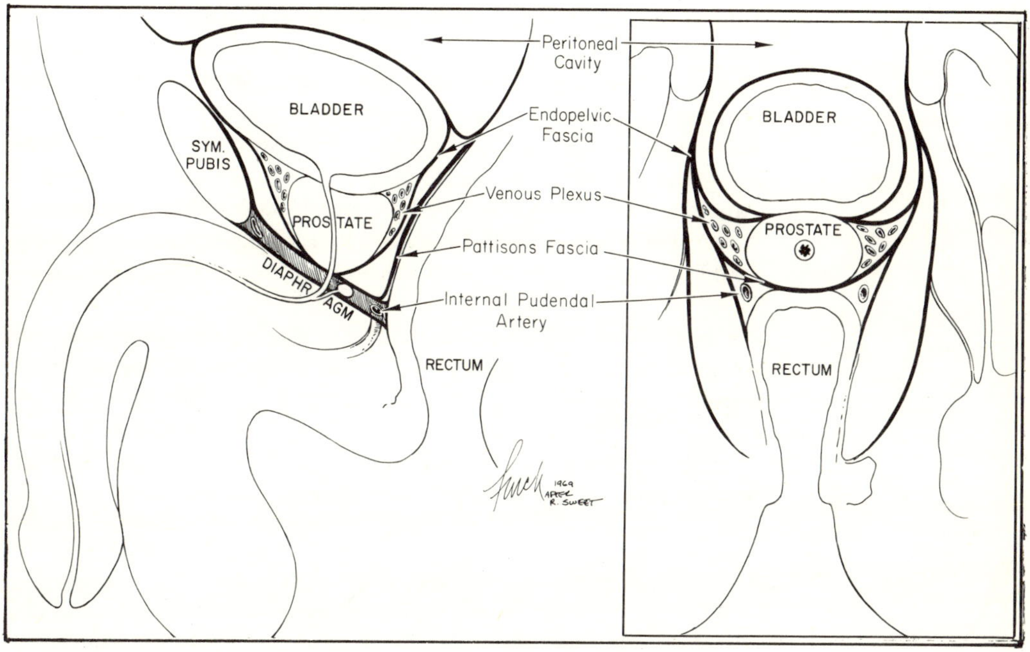

4.7 Anatomy of the prostate and its fascia, illustrating how lithotomists risked hemorrhage and urinary infiltration with inept division of prostate.

attach the name of Denonvilliers rather than Pattison to the prostatic fascia.

The Knife or the Lithotome (Gorget)

Surgical literature abounds with descriptions of special instruments with unique blades for opening the bladder through the prostatic urethra. Some lithotomists employed the gorget (lithotome), apparently believing it would be less damaging to the bladder than a knife when plunged into the patient's perineum. However, as Samuel D. Gross points out, most English, American, and European surgeons preferred the knife. A striking exception was Pouteau, who apparently used the lithotome almost exclusively. In a 1765 publication he describes and illustrates an attachment to the lithotome, a sort of carpenter's level with a bubble by which the directional slant of the thrust could be guided by the surgeon.[53]

A variant of Frère Côme's *lithotome caché* was used by many lithotomists. The Hawkins lithotome, with a cutting edge, was popular in the eighteenth century. The Austrian surgeon

Johann Hunczovsky, on a visit to London hospitals in 1783, saw Percivall Pott use this instrument in extracting a vesical calculus at St. Bartholomew's. Caesar Hawkins's son told Hunczovsky that his father had developed his method many years before. He hid a special sharp gorget in a fold of his shirt, meanwhile creating the impression that he divided the neck of the bladder with a conventional gorget displayed on the operating table. During his stay in Paris Hunczovsky observed that most surgeons, including Louis, preferred the Hawkins lithotome for section of the prostate.[54]

Charles Bell (1816) wrote that he had operated for stone with a knife for fifteen years and that all he had seen since of knife or gorget persuaded him that the knife was better. Said Astley Cooper: "If I were to be asked how many times I had known . . . of the gorget's slipping and passing between the bladder and rectum . . . , I should say at least a dozen, and in each

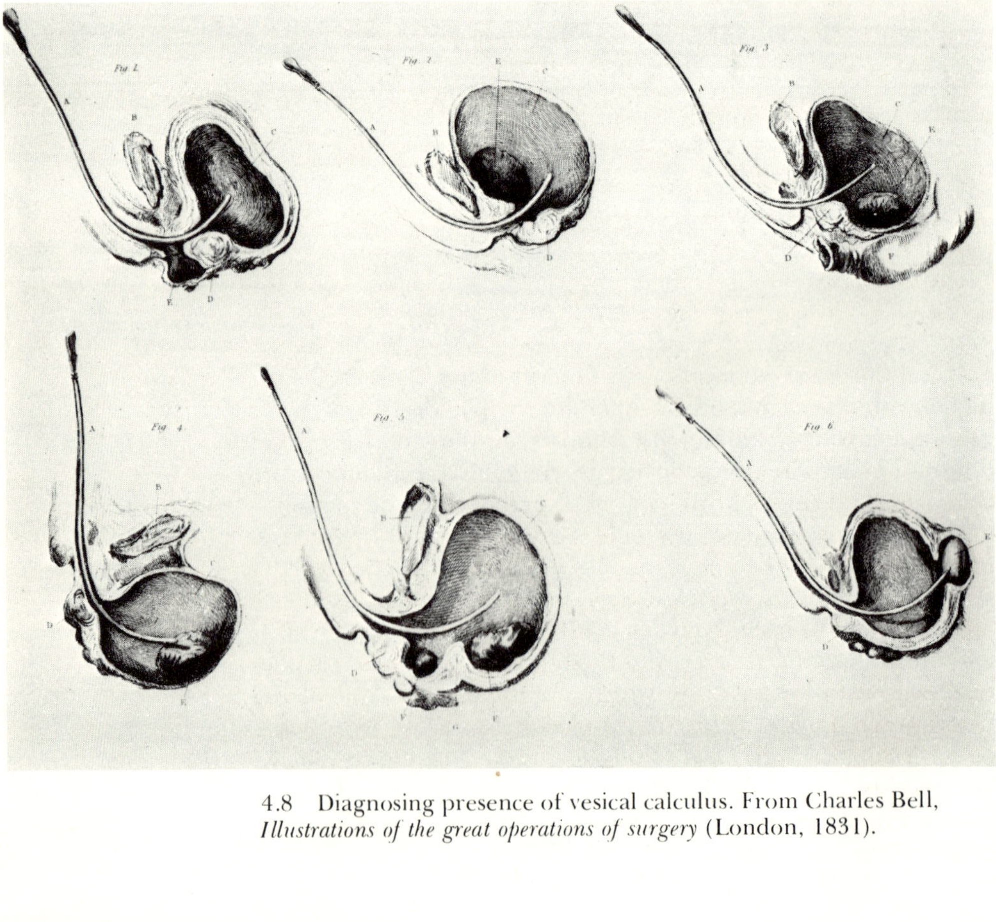

4.8 Diagnosing presence of vesical calculus. From Charles Bell, *Illustrations of the great operations of surgery* (London, 1831).

case the most lamentable and fatal consequences ensued." According to John Bell: "The gorget slips! and all the surgeons of Europe confess it!"[55]

Antonio Scarpa (1826) said that the Hawkins gorget had the special advantage of being two lines narrower (1.2 mm.) than the normal prostate in men of eighteen to twenty-five and four lines narrower in men of forty,[56] certainly a narrow margin for a potentially dangerous instrument. As surgeons improved their exposure, need for the lithotome vanished.

The Two-Stage Operation

Celsus advised against prolonged search for small vesical calculi, believing that "a small stone is later moved forward with the urine into the wound and so removed." As a recognized surgical procedure, the two-stage lithotomy (*en deux temps*) dates from Franco's advice in 1556 to defer extraction of a vesical calculus when certain difficulties arise in the operation. He used the term *en deux fois* and said that persistent attempts to remove a stone at one sitting exhausted the patient from pain and blood loss and could prove fatal. If the stone was large and could not be brought readily into the lithotomy wound, or when search for a second stone proved wearing, Franco desisted. He championed open management of the lithotomy wound, keeping it open with a *tente*, when necessary, to retard agglutination of its edges. Occasionally the stone would emerge spontaneously and be found on the dressings. If the calculus was retained, Franco found extraction at the second attempt easier and less painful. He added that "some thought it strange to leave a patient at rest for five or six days after making the incision, but men of good judgment, on hearing the reason, were satisfied or ought to be." If there had been inflammation, it subsided.[57]

In a spirited defense of the method in 1769 J.-P. Maret of Dijon said he believed it would be prudent to perform lithotomy consistently in two stages, the first sitting terminating with the vesical incision. Besides the obvious indication of hemorrhage or other crises which made deferral mandatory, Maret found that the struggles of the patient and spasmodic contraction of the bladder, incident to intravesical manipulation, were obviated by delayed extraction of the stone. Maret observed that "a simple wound resulted, with inflammation not extending beyond its lips and with light suppuration."[58] Yet even Maret did not practice the two-stage operation routinely.

Louis was apparently the first to adopt an elective two-stage perineal lithotomy and communicated his technique freely to persons who visited him, many of whom subsequently shared his enthusiasm for deliberate two-stage lithotomy. Among these were Camper, ten Haaff and G. J. van Wy, and Hunczovsky. Camper (1777) related that Louis had done several cases and had not had a death since espousing the procedure as routine for extraction of vesical stones. Hunczovsky reported he had been an eyewitness to many skillfully performed operations by the surgeons of Dijon, who were grateful for the teachings of Louis.[59]

Despite his zeal for the two-stage operation, Louis apparently left no record of his experience or results, although a Paris thesis refers to a paper on the subject by Louis being presented at a public session of the Royal Academy in 1770. Louis was a prolific writer. Moreover, according to a note by J. F. Thomassin (1791), Louis had announced that a dissertation upon the two-stage lithotomy would appear in the next memoirs of the Royal Academy of Surgery. It never appeared. The reasons are difficult to discern.[60]

Joseph Deschamps of Paris took a dim view of Louis's competence as a lithotomist, saying that after Louis left La Charité in 1761 he did not pass as a lithotomist, and that up to his death in 1791, "Louis probably had not cut more than ten patients for stone."[61] It could well have been that Louis's reluctance to publish was fear of reprisal at the hands of jealous colleagues.

The two-stage perineal lithotomy was popular only among those who had tried it. In the eyes of its critics it was a confession of surgical ineptitude.[62] "Nothing is more satisfying for a surgeon than to grasp a stone as soon as the bladder is incised, pull it out, and put it in the hand of the patient," wrote J.-P. Maret in discussing the two-stage procedure, which he favored. But he cautioned that the surgeon's reputation should not depend on removing the stone at one sitting, adding that "the public must learn to suspend judgment on matters concerning which it has no knowledge." Maret related that a local surgeon, Dechaux, waited three weeks after the incision to extract a large stone from a seventy-year-old man. The patient, Maret said, was now ninety but that Dechaux had died of grief shortly after the operation because jealous confreres ruined his reputation by calling him incompetent, even claiming he shammed a stone, necessitating the second operation.[63] John Thomson complained that for eleven years he had been the subject of "foul insinuations and professional calumnies" from his Edinburgh colleague, John Bell, for having performed a two-stage perineal lithotomy.[64]

No worse illustration of the adamant persistence of the lithotomist to complete a difficult operation in one stage is to be found than that described in 1831 by Ralph Fletcher of Gloucester: After using force to no avail, the surgeon rested, then tried again with an air of "dreadful determination to succeed. His right foot was placed . . . against a chair, which was supported by a pupil; — the scene became animated, though horrible. The straining and creaking of the forceps, as they occasionally lifted the suffering wretch from the table, (they twice pulled him off it,) — his wild, agonizing shrieks, and entreaties for forbearance, after continuing for nearly two hours, gradually became more faint. . . . When the stone was shown to him it was doubtful whether he saw it. . . . He expired a few minutes after being carried to his bed."[65]

It is difficult to assess exactly how many two-stage perineal lithotomies were done following Franco's initial suggestion. Louis, Camper, and probably Hunczovsky did many, and, if their enthusiastic testimony is to be relied upon, apparently without mortality. For deliberate two-stage lithotomy, the mortality appears to be negligible.

By persistent effort, but by no means a complete search, we have found more than forty documented cases of two-stage perineal lithotomy performed by a variety of operators.[66] Among these, two deaths occurred, but in one case the procedure was badly bungled, entailing fourteen unsuccessful passages of the lithotomy forceps at the first attempt followed by serious hemorrhage and so similarly at a second sitting.[67] A two-stage procedure cannot undo surgical complications. Our assessment would suggest that for straightforward cases the mortality was definitely under 5 percent. The reported mortality for the one-stage procedure during this period in Paris hospitals was near 20 percent.[68]

A special merit of the two-stage lithotomy is understandable in the light of Billroth's demonstration of the increased resistance of granulating tissue to pyogenic infection.[69] The exponents of the two-stage lithotomy were not aware of this advantage, but Franco and others who dared transgress against the advice of old masters to seek primary union of all wounds learned from their own experience that leaving wounds open, allowing them to close secondarily, was attended by a surprising decrease in mortality.

Open wound management, urged by Kern (1826), Liston (1841), and Burow (1859)[70] for amputation, dates back to Franco (1561) for lithotomy. The success of many of the great

French lithotomists of the eighteenth century, including Pouteau and Maret, with perineal lithotomy was owing to their adherence to Franco's principle of leaving the wound open.

Suprapubic Lithotomy

The first authentic suprapubic lithotomy for removal of vesical calculus was carried out by Franco in about 1556 on a ten-year-old boy. Unable to deliver an egg-sized stone through the perineal incision, Franco made an additional midline incision above the pubis. The bladder was opened and, unfortunately, the peritoneum too. The bladder was closed, the intestines were replaced, and the child recovered. Franco apparently did not often advise this approach because of the hazard of opening the peritoneum.[71]

François Rousset described the technique for suprapubic lithotomy (1581, 1590) but laid no claim to having performed it. He noted the nature of the attachment of the peritoneum to the dome of the bladder in the cadaver and recognized that when the bladder was filled with fluid and the penis tied with a ligature, a midline suprapubic incision need not open the peritoneum.[72]

Peter Le Mercier proposed in 1635 that the suprapubic operation for vesical calculus be "disputed on in the Phisick-Shools [sic] in Paris." He favored the operation, but like Rousset, never performed it.[73] Dionis related in 1707 that Bonnet, a surgeon at the Hôtel-Dieu in Paris, had done the high operation successfully and that [Jacques] Petit, the premier surgeon there, had observed him. Dionis considered suprapubic lithotomy less perilous an operation than was generally believed and recommended it above all approaches. He thought it should first be tried on a criminal condemned to death. Frère Côme ultimately capitulated to suprapubic lithotomy but failed to equal his success with the perineal method.[74]

Cheselden's magnificent monograph, *A Treatise on the High Operation for the Stone*, (1723) contains excerpts from and translations of the works of several pioneers in suprapubic cystostomy. Cheselden reports having performed the operation upon nine patients, two of whom died.[75] The first of these operations was done on May 5, 1722. This date is of some importance, for another London surgeon, John Douglas, did his first suprapubic operation on December 23, 1719, writing a tract entitled *Lithotomia Douglassiana* in 1720. Three of John Douglas's four cases were successful. His anatomist brother, James, of pouch of Douglas fame, had foreseen the possibility of such an operation in 1718. Cheselden failed to mention Douglas in his monograph of 1723, a circumstance which may have ignited John Douglas's ire. John Douglas accused Cheselden of plagiarism, and this circumstance has been considered a factor in Cheselden's giving up the operation. When the dust of controversy had settled with the lapse of almost a century, Deschamps placed the descriptions of the procedure by Dionis and John Douglas side by side. John Douglas apparently had followed so closely the writing of Dionis that the language was indistinguishable. It would appear, therefore, that the real plagiarist was John Douglas.[76] After Cheselden reverted to the perineal operation, James Douglas spoke very kindly of Cheselden in subsequent publications.[77]

The most enthusiastic proponent of suprapubic lithotomy prior to the arrival of antisepsis was Joseph Souberbielle. Carpue went to Paris in 1817 and had the opportunity of watching Souberbielle operate at the Hôtel-Dieu. On completion of the first operation a note was sent around stating that on August 6, 1817, between 6:00 and 7:00 in the morning, Mr. Souberbielle had operated upon a Mr. Walville, aged sixty-four, employing the high method for stone and that the operation had gone well. Carpue was asked to sign the memorandum.[78] For Carpue this was a very unusual departure and he manifested some reluctance. Noting the signatures of all the bystanders, including Baron Percy and Souberbielle, Carpue capitulated.

Subsequently, Souberbielle took Carpue about in Paris and showed him a number of patients on whom he had operated by the high method. He showed Carpue the technique of doing the operation on a cadaver and also demonstrated the lateral operation of Frère Côme. These extraordinary courtesies sound unusual indeed, but modern surgical enthusiasts, too, like Souberbielle, still revel over their success with a new venture. Souberbielle's summary of his experiences with lithotomy for the six-year period 1828–34, however, provides little justification for his enthusiasm over the suprapubic route. Among 11 patients undergoing perineal lithotomy there were no deaths; of 39 patients submitted to suprapubic lithotomy, 11 died (28.1 percent).[79]

Many young surgeons of the 1920s, for whom vesical stone was a great rarity, were astounded by J. O. Thomson's photographic exhibit of vesical calculi from 3,500 operations at the Canton Missionary Hospital in China. Most of the patients reported by Thomson had been submitted to lithotomy between 1891 and 1910. Of these, 58 percent had been operated upon by the suprapubic route, 38 percent by the perineal, and 2 percent by the vaginal route or by lithotrity and litholapaxy. Thomson reported a mortality of 3 percent for suprapubic cystostomy in patients without serious preoperative complications, and 4.9 percent for perineal lithotomy.[80]

Adoption of prophylactic antiseptic practices by the mid-1880s favored acceptance of suprapubic lithotomy. Not until then did accomplishment with the suprapubic operation begin to rival the extraordinary achievement of the great perineal lithotomists of the eighteenth century.

Lithotrity and Litholapaxy

Like lithotomy, lithotrity has a long history. Ammonius (ca. 247 B.C.) is said to have fragmented large vesical calculi by impaling them with an icepicklike device passed through a catheter. When the stone was engaged, blows with a hammer upon the pick fragmented the stone.[81]

Early in the nineteenth century Franz P. V. Gruithuisen, J.-J. Leroy d'Étiolles, Jean Z. Amussat, Jean Civiale, Charles Heurteloup, and many others contributed to the development and improvement of lithotrity. Bigelow added suction irrigation to lithotrity, naming the procedure litholapaxy.[82] It had the advantage in that the fragmented calculi usually could be removed in a single sitting. As surgeons gained experience with new instruments, lithotrity and litholapaxy lessened the need for open operations.

Crushing Large Vesical Calculi

A few successful lithotomies for vesical calculi of great size were cited by Henry Earle (1820), but he found records of few for stones weighing over 7 or 8 ounces. Paré put powerful teeth in the blades of his crushing forceps and a thumbscrew on the handle, increasing considerably the power of the instrument to crush large vesical calculi. In a modification of Paré's instrument, Le Cat employed a vise in the handles. He thus got a crush force considerably greater than that of the operator's hands and calculated it to be on the order of 370 to 400 pounds.[83] In 1851 the surgeon-historian J. E. Pétrequin of Lyons made a plea for a combination of lithotrity and lithotomy for large vesical calculi.[84]

Marcet (1819) reported the extraordinary case of Colonel Martin, a do-it-yourself patient in Bombay who had a vesical calculus. Martin, an ingenious mechanic, constructed a long, thin, curved probe of steel with a small, bulbous, filelike tip. Working with this instrument day by day over a period of time, he succeeded in pulverizing the calculus, which was gradually discharged as powder in the urine.[85]

Assessment of Methods

The subject of vesical calculus was discussed at the American Surgical Association meeting in 1887. Papers on lithotomy were presented by Dennis, John J. Packard, and Albert Vander Veer. In general, but without complete agreement, it was conceded that suprapubic had replaced perineal lithotomy. It is strange that Bigelow's litholapaxy did not enter more prominently into the discussions.[86] Mastery of the technique had yet to come. Even more significant is the fact that the American surgeons of that day employing the suprapubic approach performed not nearly so well as those doing perineal lithotomy in America fifty years earlier.[87]

Henry Thompson of London became an ardent advocate of the Bigelow method; until then he had largely favored the suprapubic operation. In an extended experience of five hundred patients treated for vesical calculi prior to 1878, Thompson reported a mortality of 7.8 percent for suprapubic lithotomy and 37.3 percent for perineal lithotomy; the majority of patients were older than twenty years. For a larger experience with perineal lithotomy, Thompson's 1886 mortality was 32 percent. He had done eleven suprapubic lithotomies with one death (9 percent).[88] It is quite clear that keen perineal lithotomists of the preceding century were not surpassed by some of the best surgeons very experienced in dealing with vesical calculi a decade after the arrival of prophylactic surgical antisepsis.

Lithotriptics

No method has yet been discovered to dissolve urinary calculi in the body. The fraudulent claim of Joanna Stephens in 1739 that

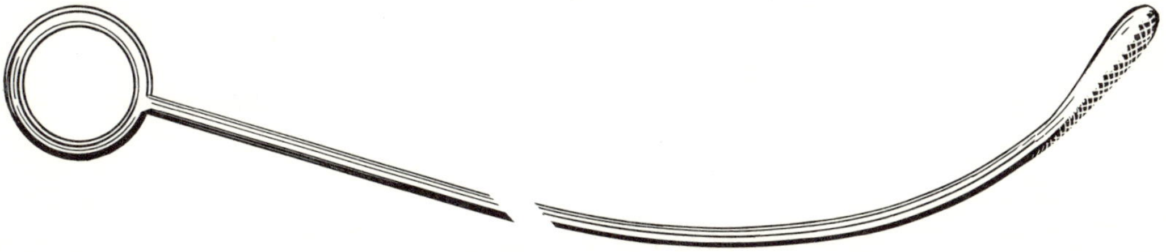

4.9 Colonel Martin's file for autolithotomy. Redrawn from Alexander Marcet, *Essay on the chemical history and medical treatment of calculous disorders*, 2d ed. (London, 1819).

she could do so by internal medication deserves mention. Many of her patients probably had cystitis rather than calculi.

Her tale beguiled influential persons, and she ultimately perpetrated her hoax upon the British government. In 1739 Parliament voted Mrs. Stephens £5,000 to reveal the nature of her mysterious compound, and she submitted the alleged ingredients of her lithotriptic agent to a Parliamentary committee: "My medicines are a Powder, a Decoction, and Pills. The Powder consists of Egg-Shells and Snails, both calcin'd. The Decoction is made by Boiling some Herbs (together with a Ball, which consists of Soap, Swines-Cresses burnt to Blackness, and Honey) in Water. The Pills consist of Snails calcin'd, Wild Carrot Seeds, Burdock-Seeds, Ashen Keys, Hips and Hawes, all burnt to Blackness, Soap and Honey." That her remedy was useless was slowly recognized when stones were revealed in autopsies of her patients.[89]

Approximately fifty years after Joanna Stephens's perpetrated fraud upon the British Parliament, William Falconer (1787), fellow of the Royal Society and physician to the General Hospital in Bath, wrote *Of the Efficacy of the Aqua Mephitica Alkalina*, a testimonial to its role in dissolving vesical calculi. The author cited twenty-eight patients and case histories. There was much testimony but little or no evidence of the medication's efficacy in freeing patients from disturbances caused by calculi in the urinary bladder. Franklin, it has been noted, found he was more comfortable in the presence of an alkaline urine, the likely explanation of the symptomatic success achieved by Falconer and his followers with his remedy.[90]

Some Famous Patients

Many celebrated men have been afflicted with vesical stone. Chief Justice Marshall of the United States Supreme Court was operated upon by Philip Syng Physick, who removed 800 to 1,000 calculi by perineal lithotomy in 1831. Polk, later president of the United States, was lithotomized successfully at age seventeen (1812) by McDowell, the founder of ovariotomy and also a skilled lithotomist.[91]

The diarist Samuel Pepys was cut for stone at Mrs. Turner's in Salisbury Court in 1658 by the surgeon Thomas Hollier of St. Thomas's Hospital. Pepys observed the anniversary annually in a festive manner. Marin Marais, a distinguished Parisian composer and violist, underwent lithotomy for vesical calculi about 1720. He later set to music the emotions which he experienced during the ordeal. The score is entitled "Tableau de l'operation de la taille."[92]

Robert Walpole first Earl of Orford, suffered long from renal and vesical stone but refused operation; the disorder eventually cost him his life. He was treated with James Jurin's *lixivium lithontripticum*. Over a period of seven weeks during his final illness, the patient took thirty-six ounces of the remedy, which Jurin said was at least four times stronger than the strongest capital lye soap.[93]

One of the most famous victims of vesical calculus was Napoleon III, who was suffering from stone when France declared war on Germany in 1870. It is puzzling that an ill emperor and his ministers, who were acquainted with his condition, would invite war with a powerful enemy when France was badly prepared. Perhaps the decision can be explained as the poor judgment of a very sick monarch.

After the defeat of France Louis Napoleon escaped to England. As a gay young blade he had early contracted a Neisserian posturethral stricture, which hampered the passage of a catheter. Early in 1873 Sir Henry Thompson, who had been successful in relieving King Leopold I of Belgium of a bladder calculus by lithrotrity in 1863, tried unsuccessfully to crush the bladder stone in Louis Napoleon. A few days later the emperor died. At autopsy, fragments of a calculus were found in the bladder. The left kidney had been destroyed by pyelonephritis. The patient undoubtedly had suffered episodes of uremia.[94]

Summary

The facility and agility with which experienced perineal lithotomists two centuries ago removed vesical calculi, often with astoundingly low mortality, neither equaled nor surpassed with the arrival of anesthesia and antisepsis, is an unending source of wonderment. A quarter-century elapsed following Lister's first publication (1867) on antiseptic surgical principles before the record of the great eighteenth-century perineal lithotomists was attained by modern lithotomists who resorted to the simpler suprapubic operation.

Three features stand out prominently in the story of perineal lithotomy: (1) Entry into the bladder was gained by a complicationless urethrovesical incision that did not extend into the confines of the prostatic capsule, containing a rich plexus of blood vessels. The anatomic explanation of the need to avoid incising the prostatic fascia came only with Pattison's demonstration (1820) of the significance of the prostatic capsule and fascia for lithotomy. (2) Open management of the wound as employed by Franco, which provided for the free escape of urine and served to irrigate the wound, was a telling factor in the achievement of acceptable mortality records. (3) The two-stage perineal lithotomy accentuated the importance of open wound management. Even at the hands of the less practiced it was attended with a very low operative mortality for its time, an accomplishment intelligible now in Billroth's demonstration of the virtual immunity of the granulating wound to infection by ordinary pyogenic organisms.

Franco emerges as the great innovator in the lithotomy story. Stellar surgical artists of the eighteenth century like Cheselden, Le Cat, Hoin, Pouteau, Maret, and Saucerotte achieved a success rate with perineal lithotomy that is truly astounding. By the mid-nineteenth century the mortality rate for perineal lithotomy in the hands of a few American surgeons also was impressive.

Patients and their surgeons of the late nineteenth century were spared the trying and painful ordeals of the preanesthetic era. Suprapubic lithotomy replaced the perineal approach for removal of vesical calculi as prophylactic surgical antisepsis found acceptance. Lithotrity and litholapaxy gradually lessened the need for operative lithotomy. Perineal lithotomy for stone, useful in its time, has disappeared. Moreover, vesical stones, once frequent in most countries of Western culture, for whatever reason, are rarely seen in these areas today.

(For notes, see pp. 600–607.)

CHAPTER 5

Prostatic Obstruction

PROSTATIC OBSTRUCTION is an affliction of the aging male before "he goeth to his long home."[1] It is occasionally observed in men in their fifties, but symptoms of frequency, urgency, and urinary retention suggesting need for surgical relief are common in the seventies and eighties, involving probably 30 percent or more of this age group.

Direct surgical attack upon the site of obstruction was a late development. Before the 1880s, save for a few isolated efforts directed at ameliorating the situation by an incision in the prostatic urethra, the patient was committed to a "catheter life." In 1884 the distinguished London urologist Henry Thompson had only one suggestion beyond use of the catheter — galvanism applied to the bladder.[2] Yet just a few years after this defeatist pronouncement surgeons in America and England came forward with recitals of successes that promised hope and relief to sufferers from prostatism. The delay seems particularly surprising in that more than a century earlier Pouteau and other surgeons had records of proud accomplishment in the removal of large vesical calculi by perineal lithotomy that often demanded incision of the prostatic urethra and the underlying gland. Moreover, several talented investigators had taken an interest in this geriatric problem, including the Italian Giovanni Battista Morgagni, the first distinguished gross pathologist, and John Hunter.

The normal prostate in the young adult is a small glandular and muscular structure, weighing approximately 20 grams, composed of two fairly large lateral lobes, a small middle lobe between the openings of the ejaculatory ducts into the prostatic urethra, and a small posterior lobe.[3] The contour of the prostate has been likened to the ace of hearts on a playing card.[4] Hypertrophy between the sixth and ninth decades of life concerns primarily the two lateral lobes and the middle lobe.

Morgagni, in 1761, was probably the first to recognize that there was no actual stricture in the urethra in prostatic hypertrophy; on the contrary, he concluded that urinary obstruction was occasioned by compression of the urethra from enlargement of the lateral prostatic lobes. For the majority of prostatic obstructions, he was right. He missed the significance of the mid-prostatic lobe, to which Everard Home lent emphasis forty-two years later.

Morgagni recounted the case of a seventy-year-old man who experienced considerable difficulty in voiding; a lithotomist was unable to procure an exit for the urine by catheter. At postmortem, the muscles of the urinary bladder were found to have increased in size to resemble the strong muscle bundles of the heart. The prostate gland, "in the form of a pear," left scarcely any passage and was "affected with an inflammation in the lower part; from the continual impetus of the catheter." Morgagni related another similar instance.[5]

Amussat (1840) agreed with Morgagni that the prostatic urethra never contracted as the organ enlarged. In fact, Amussat found he was able to thrust his middle finger into the prostatic urethra in many specimens at postmortem.[6]

Home (1811) probably published the first surgical monograph on diseases of the prostate gland, incorporating a lecture he had given before the Royal Society in 1806. Home asserted that he was the first to detect the presence of a mid-prostatic lobe, that it had escaped the attention of Morgagni and his own mentor and brother-in-law, John Hunter. Home's suggestion for management was the soft gum elastic catheter, which, when not in use, he suspended upon a metal stylet to preserve the desired curve. When reasonably cold, the catheter maintained the curve of the stylet. Home passed these catheters with and without the stylet and left them in place for variable periods of time, thus reducing, he said, the spasticity of the urethra at the vesicourethral juncture.[7]

In his treatise on *Animal Oeconomy* John Hunter in 1786 described the normal descent of the testes. He remarked that the secondary sex organs, such as the prostate, the seminal vesicles, and the penis, are dependent upon the testes for maturation. Hunter related that in the "land-mouse" and the mole the seminal vesicles are scarcely discernible in winter but very large in summer and that the vesicles vary in size according to the size of the testes. Hunter experimented with castrated young male animals, noting that as they grew older the prostate did not enlarge. However, he did not attempt castration of patients in the hope of diminishing urinary obstruction from prostatic hypertrophy.

In management of clinical aspects of the problem Hunter began by passing a catheter. Occasionally he left a bougie, without a lumen, in situ in the urethra for a few days, urine draining alongside it. When he encountered great difficulty in catheterizing a patient's bladder in the presence of urethral stricture or prostatic hypertrophy, he resorted to passing a trochar through the rectum into the bladder, allowing it to remain in place from twenty-four hours to a few days. After temporary drainage of the bladder via the rectum, Hunter observed it was often easier to catheterize the patient and obtain flow through the urethra. Whereas Hunter debated directing his attack upon the prostate causing urinary retention, he refrained from doing so [8]

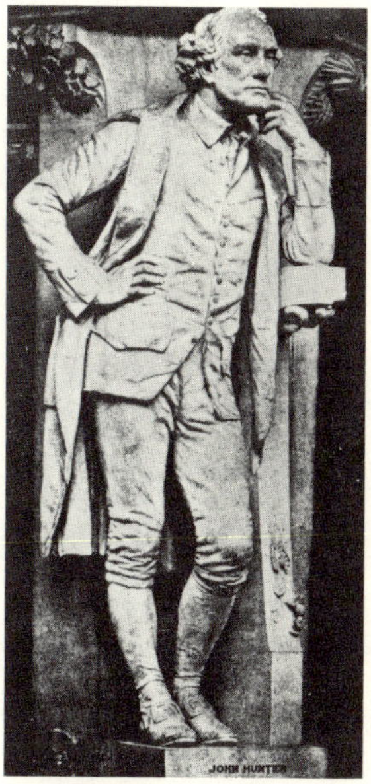

5.1 John Hunter (1728–93) introduced science into surgery, founded a great school of surgeons bearing his name, and developed the world's finest museum of surgical pathology. Statue at Royal College of Surgeons, England.

A century after Hunter, Joseph Griffiths of Edinburgh alluded (1890) to his observation that when a young bull was castrated, the prostate gland remained small. Griffith's extended Hunter's inquiry to the dog and cat, also studying the histologic changes attending castration. In a three-year-old dog castrated at the age of two years, Griffiths found the prostate small, firm, tough, and fibrous, unlike the large soft glandular organ of the normal male dog. A very similar situation followed castration of male cats, especially when done at three weeks of age.[9]

Robert A. Moore (1936) reported the autopsy findings of a man aged thirty-nine who had undergone castration at thirty-four in the hope of escaping the social stigma of being a homosexual. The prostate was considerably smaller than normal for his age, and the "seminal vesicles were exceedingly small."[10] There are few if any other published accounts of the study of the prostate some years after castration in adult men. The effects of castration in prepubertal boys, however, in delimiting growth of the prostate and the seminal vesicles have been recognized since ancient times and are described in early records.

That eunuchs castrated as very young boys retain preadolescent soprano voices, have beardless faces, with maintenance of the prepubertal status of the secondary sex organs, including prostate, seminal vesicles, and penis, has long been common knowledge. That eunuchs are free from enlargement of the prostate, common in aging men, too has long been recognized.

Eunuchs were known in China eleven centuries before Christ and were highly prized as servants in households and government in the Orient and the Eastern Mediterranean countries.[11] Oriental princes placed eunuchs in charge of the bedchamber and in the seraglios of their harems. Eunuchs are mentioned in both the Old and New Testament. Matthew writes that some eunuchs are born so, some eunuchs are made so by man, and "some made themselves eunuchs for the Kingdome of Heaven's sake." That eunuchs rose to important positions is reported in Acts 8:27, where there is reference to "a man of Ethiopia, a eunuch of great authority under Candace, Queen of the Ethiopians, who had the charge of all her treasure."

Emasculation of young slave boys was not uncommon, for they commanded a considerably higher price than did others in the slave market. They were sold as eunuchs for Moslem harems into the twentieth century. Tivadar Duka, who first brought the name of Semmelweis to the attention of Lister, spent some time in the British Bengal army in East India. He wrote (1866) it was the practice of "gangs" of eunuchs there to emasculate young boys purchased illegally from impoverished Hindu parents. On maturity they were hired out as entertainers. A "clean sweep" operation was done of scrotum, testes, and penis. Duka said the mortality of the procedure was approximately 50 percent, primarily from hemorrhage.[12]

Edmund Andrews of Northwestern University, a well-known contributor to surgical literature, wrote that at the end of the nineteenth century Coptic priests in Egypt castrated Nubian and Abyssinian slaves at about eight years of age and sold them into the Turkish market. The priests usually performed the complete operation, cutting away the entire scrotum, testes, and penis, which deplorable practice commanded a formidable mortality. Andrews adds that whereas the Church frowned upon the barbarity of castration eunuchs were employed in the Vatican choir of Rome well into the nineteenth century.[13]

Nineteenth-Century Conservative Therapy of Prostatism

In his monograph on the urinary bladder, the prostate gland, and the urethra in 1855, Gross, Nestor of American surgery, said that despite "the numerous attempts that have been made from time to time to place it [treatment of prostatic hypertrophy] upon a scientific basis, it must be confessed, however humiliating the acknowledgement may be, that it is eminently empirical, tentative, and unsatisfactory." Gross conceded that the only direct attack upon the problem was the catheter. Beyond that he recommended "a full bleeding." He added that introduction of the catheter is "the most important operation that a practitioner is obliged to perform."[14]

Although Gross's treatment was not imaginative, at least his frankness was provocative in a century when many eminent surgeons, including Charles Bell and Velpeau, avoided discussing therapeutic aspects of prostatic obstruction altogether in their texts. The distinguished London surgeon Benjamin Brodie, in a monograph of 1842 on diseases of the urinary organs, could only suggest use of the catheter. The Heidelberg surgeon Chelius in 1844 advised bleeding, application of leeches to the area around the rectum, baths, and enemas. When these procedures failed, Chelius resorted to the catheter. As late as 1884, Frederick Gant of London called prostatic hypertrophy incurable and said that the patient should be taught to catheterize himself, preferably with a gum elastic catheter.[15]

Prior to prostatectomy, the catheter life was inescapable for the patient suffering urinary retention from enlargement of the prostate. Many an aging man carried a catheter on his person and used it to obtain relief from distention. It was even possible to conceal the catheter in available walking sticks or umbrella handles. The hazard of inducing infection of the upper urinary tract through catheterization, with resultant pyelonephritis and uremia, was widely recognized. Paget (1875) believed that conservative methods were preferable, when possible, and warned against introducing the patient to the catheter until urinary retention supervened.[16]

Origins of the Catheter

Metal sounds were used from ancient times to encourage the passage of urine. Celsus wrote of a bronze tube, slightly curved and 9, 12, or 15 fingerbreadths in length, applicable, he said, when the passage had collapsed in an old man. Bronze sounds were found among other surgical instruments in the ruins of Pompeii. Later silver and sometimes gold were favored materials, being far more flexible, resisting encrustation by urine.

Albucasis described a silver sound to "draw off the urine." It was "slender and smooth and hollow like the quill of a bird's feather; as slender as a probe; about a span and a half in length;

and with a tiny funnel at the end." The sound in his illustration is straight. Curved sounds were generally more popular because they followed the normal curvature of the male urethra beneath the pubis. The anatomist Vidius (1508–69) applied mouth suction to an inlying catheter. G. A. Della Croce (1573) constructed catheters and sounds of gold, silver, lead, tin, leather, and the skins of fish and birds.[17]

Paré understood the functional anatomy of the prostate but failed to recognize hypertrophy of the prostate as a cause of obstruction to the outflow of urine. His catheters were used largely to detect vesical calculi. In his treatise on lithotomy Fabricius wrote of catheters to explore for stone in the bladder and to relieve urinary retention. He preferred flexible silver sounds and remarked that a large instrument frequently succeeded when a smaller one failed. He advised pulling the penis upward toward the umbilicus during catheterization, thus eliminating some of the urethral curve. The Belgian Joannes van Helmont recommended catheters of thin hide, but these proved impractical because when wet they softened.[18]

Many attempts were made to produce flexible catheters, including weaving silk thread about a thin cylinder of silver. Macquer was apparently among the first to conceive of fabricating flexible sounds from gum elastic, imported from the New World shortly after the discovery of America. Bernard, a Paris goldsmith who made surgical instruments, liquefied gum elastic in ether and placed several layers of the liquefied material upon molds of wax. When dry, he plunged the preparation into boiling water, thus liquefying the wax mold, which was discarded. Bernard eliminated the metal in the flexible sound and began with a tissue of silk which was then dipped in liquefied gum elastic. These catheters could remain in the urethra for a week to ten days without producing much irritation or becoming rough or in any degree dissolved, wrote John Syng Dorsey of Philadelphia. He found Bernard's product superior to any other then on the market.[19]

First Operations Involving Prostatic Incision

In a postmortem study Guthrie (1834) first described obstruction of the vesical neck by a bar of tissue in the prostatic urethra. Moreover, he devised a concealed knife, activated by a spring to be passed in a curved metal cannula through the urethra. When the instrument entered the vesical neck, the surgeon released the spring that controlled the knife, which cut into the prostatic urethra posteriorly and also as it was withdrawn. The knife disappeared into the cannula on withdrawal. Guthrie reports its use in two cases. Several years later L.-Auguste Mercier of Paris described and illustrated in a number of publications (1839–56) incision and excision of small obstructing bars at the vesical outlet by a knifelike punch passed through the urethra. The procedure, which fostered spontaneous evacuation of the bladder and also facilitated catheterization, had a few imitators in France but encountered no evidence of acceptance in Britain and little in America until implemented by Hugh H. Young of The Hopkins in 1912, complemented with a visual aid, as will be discussed later. In 1885 the New York surgeon John Gouley found Mercier's method useful, chiefly because the patient could catheterize himself quite readily following the removal of the obstruction. Gouley reported that Mercier had used his urethral knife on more than four hundred patients with considerable success.[20]

The distinguished Paris pathological anatomist Jean Cruveilhier cites an interesting episode of prolonged relief of prostatic obstruction following a novel maneuver at the hands of Georges La Faye, a Paris surgeon. La Faye encountered difficulty in catheterizing Jean Astruc, the famous eighteenth-century Paris physician. On digital examination of the rectum La Faye felt a tumor near the neck of the bladder. When the tumor was perforated with a sharp urethral sound, a catheter could be introduced and was left in place for fifteen days. Astruc's urinary retention was eventually overcome, freeing him from dependence upon a catheter for the remaining ten years of his life.[21] La Faye's technique obviously lacked the sophistication of Guthrie's and Mercier's, yet his success with Astruc antedated their more substantial achievement.

In an operation which he described as a prostatotomy (1884), Reginald Harrison of Liverpool made a perineal urethrotomy and incised the prostatic urethra in the midline posteriorly, extending the incision into the substance of the prostate. The urethrovesical orifice was then dilated with the finger or a large bougie. Thomas Annandale (1888) employed either a suprapubic indwelling catheter or a perineal cystostomy to relieve urinary retention from enlargement of the prostate. He found that the latter technique provided better drainage.[22]

In 1874 Enrico Bottini of Italy devised an intraurethral galvanocautery, a lithotrite-like instrument for destroying obstructive prostatic tissue. In later models (1877) he incorporated a water-cooling device to prevent overheating of the instrument.[23]

Before prostatectomy found general acceptance, perineal cystostomy with an indwelling catheter, as employed by Gouley, Harrison, and others, provided the best continuing relief for sufferers from prostatism. Prostatectomy was a great boon for such patients, relieving them of dependence upon manipulation of catheters for a comfortable existence at a period in their lives when the hand often loses its cunning and vision dims.

Retaining the Inlying Urethral Catheter

To avoid the problem of repeated catheterization in chronic urinary retention, surgeons were faced with the task of improvising techniques to keep the catheter snugly in place. Adhesive tape strapping over the hairless penis usually sufficed. Another adjuvant measure was to pass a threaded needle through the superficial surface of the rubber catheter and fasten such threads to hairless areas adjacent to the urethra. Techniques were even described in which threads tied to the pubic hair achieved the objective.[24]

Frederic Foley's self-retaining latex urinary catheter, far less irritating than rubber, incorporated a balloon near its tip, inflatable with air or water, which resolved the problem of catheter anchorage. The instrument has proved very serviceable and has become the prototype of other balloon-tipped catheters, including the Fogarty blood vessel catheter.[25]

In a discussion pertaining to care of the bladder in paraplegic patients, Cushing (ca. 1906) indicated that male patients so afflicted were much better off with a suprapubic cystostomy than with an indwelling urethral catheter. The availability of antibiotics has enhanced the protection of paraplegic patients from ascending pyelonephritis attending division of the spinal cord.[26]

V. H. K. Moorhouse of the University of Manitoba stressed the ability of some dogs with complete severance of the thoracic spinal cord to support their weight on their hind legs. This surgeon saw one of these dogs in 1932 carrying his hindquarters in a little buggy attached to a harness. The animal was in good health and had coped with the handicap for several months. His automatic bladder responded readily to the Credé maneuver.[27]

Hazard of Rapid Emptying of the Chronically Distended Bladder

In the third edition of a monograph on the prostate (1868) Thompson recounts the hazard of sudden complete emptying of an obstructed distended urinary bladder, describing an instance in which an "old man was placed upright against a wall, the catheter introduced, and six pints of urine were withdrawn in full stream; but the water had no sooner ceased to flow than the patient fell, dead, at the surgeon's feet." Obviously postural hypotension and consequent syncope played the important role in the patient's quick demise. Gant said that rapid complete evacuation of the overdistended bladder had "the effect of shock to the system." Warnings of this danger continued to be heard periodically through the 1930s, but the exact reason was not known. As a precautionary measure Cornelius Van Zwalenburg of Riverside, California, employed a urethral catheter drainage system in which the urine was drained into a receptacle several inches higher than the bed; the receptacle was gradually lowered as the patient improved.[28]

C. D. Creevy of the University of Minnesota was among the first, in 1932, to resolve the issue by pointing out that chronic retention was a potent factor in increasing the urinary tract's susceptibility to infection. Moreover, indwelling catheters, before access to specific antibacterial agents, readily invited infection. Elek in 1956 definitely established that foreign bodies in wounds enhance greatly the chances of infection, a situation that applies also to inlying catheters in blood vessels and the urinary tract.[29]

Even today, with emphasis upon sterility of the procedure, and use of less irritating instruments than the conventional red rubber catheter of forty years ago, transient bacteremia not uncommonly attends the prolonged use of indwelling urethral catheters. Withdrawal of the catheter or the administration of a sulfanilamide or an antibiotic quite consistently and quickly overcomes the threat of spreading infection.

Prostatectomy

William Belfield of Chicago had nothing to say about prostatic hypertrophy or its surgical relief in his monograph of 1884 entitled *Diseases of the Urinary and Male Sexual Organs*.[30] Within a few years he was to become an important contributor to the field. Almost simultaneously a number of other surgeons in the United States and in Britain introduced excisional techniques for prostatic hypertrophy. Among them were A. F. McGill of Leeds, Eugene Fuller of New York, and Peter Freyer of London. Obstructing prostatic tissue was excised with knife and scissors or was enucleated with the index finger.

McGill in 1887 described suprapubic prostatectomy in which

he enucleated the obstructing prostatic lobe. He prefaced a subsequent account of the procedure by saying that the orthodox treatment of an enlarged prostate was: "Teach the patient how to pass a soft catheter for himself, and let him pass it once or twice daily. When this treatment is successful nothing more is required." At the time of his report McGill's operative experience was limited to three patients, all of whom apparently did well. McGill had been preceded by Belfield by less than a year. In a brief presentation of a few lines Belfield (1887) described how he had evulsed the mid-lobe of the prostate by the suprapubic route.[31] *Garrison-Morton* (1970) credits Fuller with priority for the innovation of near total prostatectomy in 1895, although subsequent examinations of excised specimens did demonstrate that one of McGill's excisions included the lateral lobes as well as the mid-prostatic lobe.[32]

Freyer augmented a 1901 report in a subsequent monograph in 1906. He believed, with Velpeau, that enlargement of the prostate is analogous to fibroid disease of the uterus. John Hunter had contended that enlargement of the prostate was essentially inflammatory in origin. Freyer described the prostate as being like two halves of an orange surrounding the urethra, readily enucleated with the finger. When the tissue to be removed peeled away more like the skin of an apple than of a tangerine, one needed a knife or scissors to complete the operation.

The illustrations published by Fuller and especially those by Freyer indicate that the middle and lateral lobes of the prostate could be completely removed in this manner. The operations were carried out through a suprapubic incision, with a hospital mortality rate of approximately 13 percent. When successful, this operation brought considerable relief to the patient and terminated catheter dependency for a host of aging males throughout the world.

In many instances, said Freyer, he could remove each half of the prostate on either side of the urethra, leaving the urethra intact. When the dissection was difficult, the prostatic urethra came away with the segment of the prostate. Freyer related in 1906 that he had performed 312 prostatectomies with 22 deaths, a mortality rate of 7 percent, certainly very good for that day.[33] Freyer had nothing to say about two-stage prostatectomy, which was very popular through the second and third decades of this century.

Terence Millin (1945) of Dublin initiated retropubic prostatectomy in which the vesicourethral neck of the bladder is exposed with excision of the prostate, uniting the membranous urethra to the vesical neck.[34] This is a somewhat more complete removal than achieved by the usual transvesical suprapubic prostatectomy. Millin's contribution came at a time when emphasis was no longer upon completeness but rather upon provision for an adequate urinary outlet in which only obstructing prostatic tissue is removed by the popular transurethral resection; this development made a firm specialty of urology, for general surgeons obviously would not assign the much needed time to master the intricate technique of excision of prostatic tissue with the electric knife.

Several surgeons performed vasectomy in the false belief that shrinkage in size of the prostate would follow. Today vasectomy in the operation of prostatectomy is reserved solely to preclude occurrence of epidydimitis from an indwelling urethral catheter.

Visual Aids

In his first attack upon the problem (1909), Young opened the urinary bladder suprapubically and excised prostatic tissue obstructing the vesicourethral orifice. The operation was a failure and the patient succumbed. Young then devised an illuminated punch of two cylinders passed through the urethra. Under direct vision, the obstructing prostatic tissue was seen and when the internal cutting cylinder was pushed home the obstructing tissue engaged in the punch came away on withdrawal of the instrument. Young's first operation by this method was performed as an office procedure. In his report of more than a hundred cases in 1912, Young advised it be done as a hospital procedure. He expressed satisfaction with the accomplishment for median-bar obstruction and for hypertrophy of the middle lobe of the prostate. In the hands of William Braasch of the Mayo Clinic the method became widely used.[35]

Maximilian Stern (1926) of Chicago and Joseph McCarthy (1931) of New York launched transurethral resection, slicing away bits of prostatic tissue with an electric cutting current, thus widening the tunnel of the prostatic urethra.[36] This is certainly the most favored operation today, especially in America; usually only a few grams of obstructing prostatic tissue are removed in the procedure.

Today urologists in the United States adept and practiced in transurethral prostatic resection are able to remove obstructing prostatic tissue with surprisingly low mortality rates and with satisfaction to both patient and surgeon.[37] Proponents of transurethral resection content themselves with providing an adequate tunnel through the prostatic urethra and the underlying prostatic tissue. A few perform the operation through a perineal cystostomy, thus increasing the maneuverability of the resectoscope. Advocates of either the transvesical or the retropubic approach continue to emphasize the completeness of the procedure, which is apparently no longer the major problem.

Castration for Prostatic Hypertrophy

In a succession of papers (1893–1904) J. William White of Philadelphia advocated excision of the testes as a solution for urinary retention occasioned by an enlarged prostate, a suggestion debated vigorously at the time. Arthur T. Cabot of Boston remained a skeptic. The mortality rate was surprisingly high, varying from 13 to 18 percent in the hands of advocates, probably a reflection of application in terminal cases. Perhaps a third of White's patients upon whom orchiectomy was performed suffered from cancer of the prostate.[38] Strangely enough, neither White nor any of his successors followed up with an account relating the nature of the histology of prostatic tissue removed in the orchiectomies.

White's innovation preceded that of George T. Beatson (1896) of Glasgow, who performed excision of the ovaries in females for advanced cancer of the breast, an operation that has been revived in recent decades and found to be an effective palliative hormonal attack upon the problem of late breast cancer.[39] Over the past three decades orchiectomy has been endorsed by Charles Huggins (1941) as a therapeutic measure for cancer of the prostate.[40] Whether castration will cause regression of benign prostatic hypertrophy in older men and animals is not definitely known.

There appears to be no general agreement among urologists and oncologists on the best treatment for prostatic cancer. A few favor Young's total perineal prostatectomy for early cases. Most apparently advise orchiectomy or administration of agents to suppress plasma testosterone. A few reserve treatment for the appearance of metastases causing symptoms.[41]

Prostatectomy was a surgical triumph for the prostatic patient, but why was it so long in coming?[42] It will strike the reader who has perused the preceding chapter on perineal lithotomy as strange that a direct surgical attack upon the prostate was essentially a development of the late 1880s, during the early days of elective surgery. Perineal lithotomy by the mid-1700s was already a relatively safe and effective operation in many hands. The delay is all the more remarkable in that the London surgeon-sanitarian John Simon created a ureterorectal anastomosis in 1851 in a thirteen-year-old boy with congenital absence of the anterior wall of the bladder. The intact ureters were brought in juxtaposition to the rectal wall and a necrosing ligature between ureters and rectum was employed to establish a ureterorectal fistula, draining the major portion of the urine into the rectum. Only implantation of the ureters into the rectum or an end-to-end anastomosis of the divided ureters to the rectum could have succeeded in diverting all the urine. Simon's patient survived this heroic operation for almost a year.[43] An additional thirty-six years intervened before surgeons in America and Britain began their excision and enucleation techniques upon the enlarged prostate, a far simpler operation than that undertaken by Simon in 1851.

Summary

Whereas extraction of vesical calculi via perineal lithotomy was a well-developed and successful operation by the middle of the eighteenth century, the prostatic patient with urinary retention was usually treated by an indwelling urethral catheter into the last decade of the nineteenth century. Morgagni (1761) recognized that urinary retention in the aging male was usually occasioned by hypertrophy of the lateral lobes of the prostate. John Hunter (1786) demonstrated the dependency of prostatic hypertrophy upon the testes; when these were excised in young animals, the prostate gland remained prepubertal in size. Hunter's brother-in-law Home (1811) established the role of the median prostatic lobe in causing urinary retention.

Endovesical means of alleviating urinary retention occasioned by median-bar enlargement of the prostate were developed by Guthrie (1834), Mercier (1839), and others, but relief for prostatic hypertrophy causing urinary retention came only in the closing years of the nineteenth century, when operative removal of the obstructing prostatic tissue brought relief to many patients with prostatic hypertrophy and urinary retention. In a succession of papers in the 1890s White observed the dependence of prostatic hypertrophy upon the testes, an extension of Hunter's observations a century earlier. White, however, failed to recognize and establish definitely that improvement attending removal of the testes was confined to patients with prostatic malignancy, an observation made by Huggins in 1941.

(For notes, see pp. 607–11.)

CHAPTER 6

Intestinal Obstructions

THE MODERN TREATMENT of intestinal obstruction began with Frederick Treves of the London Hospital, who, in his revised monograph of 1899, said, "It is less dangerous to leap from the Clifton Suspension Bridge than to suffer from acute intestinal obstruction and decline operation." Treves had grown in stature and boldness in the fifteen-year interval since his first presentation on the subject in 1883, for which he had been awarded the Jacksonian Prize of the Royal College of Surgeons of England.[1]

Every innovator has to contend with the past. It is difficult to swim upstream against established opinion. Treves could not ignore completely the orthodox practice of the day. In publishing his revised monograph, therefore, he still included such conventional procrastinating treatments as posture, opium, purgation, metallic mercury, electricity, enemas, and inflation of the bowel with water, air, and other gases. He listed, without endorsement, puncture of the bowel with a fine needle or trochar, and he mentioned, too, the more dangerous procedure of enterocentesis, in which the trochar or needle is left in the bowel for varying periods of time for temporary decompression or with the hope of establishing an external fistula.

Early Conservative Management

The inverted *posture* was long a therapeutic device in the management of acute obstruction, especially for the reduction of intussusception, as advocated by Jonathan Hutchinson, a prominent London surgeon, in 1878. It was used in the Middle Ages at Salerno in reduction or surgical repair of abdominal hernias. Patients undergoing herniorrhaphy in head-down positions are pictured with explanatory verses in Caspar Stromayr's manuscript of 1559. Said Pott (1771): "The nearer the posture approaches to what is commonly called standing on the head, the better, as it causes the whole packet of small intestines to hang, as it were, by the strangulated portion, and may thereby disengage it."[2] Astley Cooper (1804) suspended patients with strangulated hernia in an upside-down position over the shoulders of a strong ward attendant when taxis failed to achieve reduction, but he never found it a satisfactory answer.

As late as 1926, S. Monrad at the Queen Louise Hospital in Copenhagen used manipulative *taxis* through the abdominal wall under chloroform anesthesia in cases of intussusception, a measure superseded by the hydrostatic pressure devices of C. P. B. Clubbe and P. L. Hipsley of Australia, who employed a column of water and a rectal tube to chase the intussusceptum back. Yngve Olsson and Gustaf Pallin replaced water pressure with a column of barium, permitting fluoroscopic confirmation of the completeness of the reduction.[3]

The great London physician Thomas Sydenham (1624–89) is widely quoted for his views on the management of intestinal obstruction with *opium*. With its use he reports abatement of symptoms attending "bilious colic." He also recommended rest, as well as horseback riding, to lend repetitive succussion to the distended coils of the intestine, hoping thus to encourage evacuation. He ascribed considerable benefit from keeping a warm kitten on the patient's naked belly in cases of ileus.[4]

Two centuries later, in 1879, we find Hugh Owen Thomas of Liverpool even more enthusiastic than Sydenham over opium for intestinal obstruction. Thomas pointed out that the latter depended on adjunct measures which he did not advocate, but he extolled Sydenham's employment of rest and opium and recognition of the potential harm of enemas in intestinal obstruction. Thomas obviously did not appreciate fully the significance and hazards of mechanical obstruction. He was fearful of surgical entry into the peritoneal cavity and entertained the notion that many obstructions were functional in nature.[5] Moreover, he was supported in the knowledge that operations were attended by high mortality rates.

Many astute clinicians of the mid-nineteenth century regarded mechanical obstructions with an attitude of hopelessness, feeling it their duty to ease the patient's transit into oblivion. Said the London physician William Brinton in 1867, "Certainly nothing in the whole action of remedies can surpass the comparative painlessness into which I have seen an agonizing intussusception converted [by belladonna with opium] during the many days that have intervened before its unavoidable termination in death."[6]

Treves remarked that employment of *metallic mercury* in large doses was of "very ancient date" in treating obstruction.[7] Its use as a favorite remedy for intestinal obstruction dates back at least to Marianus Sanctus of the sixteenth century, who gave as much as 3 pounds and then rolled the patient, hoping that the heavy mobile metal would work its way through the occluding lesion and be evacuated in the stool. Lead shot had previously been employed for the same purpose.[8] Many pounds of mercury were often given by physicians in their anxiety to avoid an operation. This archaic practice continued until the general acceptance of operative management.[9]

A cecostomy by Pillore of Rouen in 1776 for obstruction of the colon eventuated in death twenty-eight days after the innovative operation because of preoperative oral administration of 2 pounds of metallic mercury over a period of a month. Postmortem examination disclosed that loops of the small intestine had sunk into the pelvis; the patient redistended, and the mercury failed to pass.[10]

Electrical stimulation too had its vogue, promoted by Leroy-d'Étiolles in 1826. The most famous recipient of this heroic treatment was the French actor François Talma (1763–1826), one of Napoleon's favorites, whose slow demise, "assisted" by an ever increasing number of Paris consultants, was as agonizing a final act as any in the great tragedian's career. Talma had suffered periodic bouts of obstruction since 1809. By 1825 these became more frequent and disabling, yet he continued to fill his demanding roles on tour and at the Comédie-Française before enthralled audiences. On June 3, 1826 the sixty-three-year-old actor made his last appearance, playing the dying Charles VI with heartbreaking realism. For four months, as Talma's condition worsened, with episodes of epigastric pain, distention, vomiting, and distress, the popular remedies of the era were prescribed by many renowned consultants, including François Broussais, Bégin, and Dupuytren. Purges, enemas, diets, ice packs, baths, douches, visits to spas, rests in the country, and numerous applications of leeches, as many as thirty to the abdomen or anus, were all given trial.

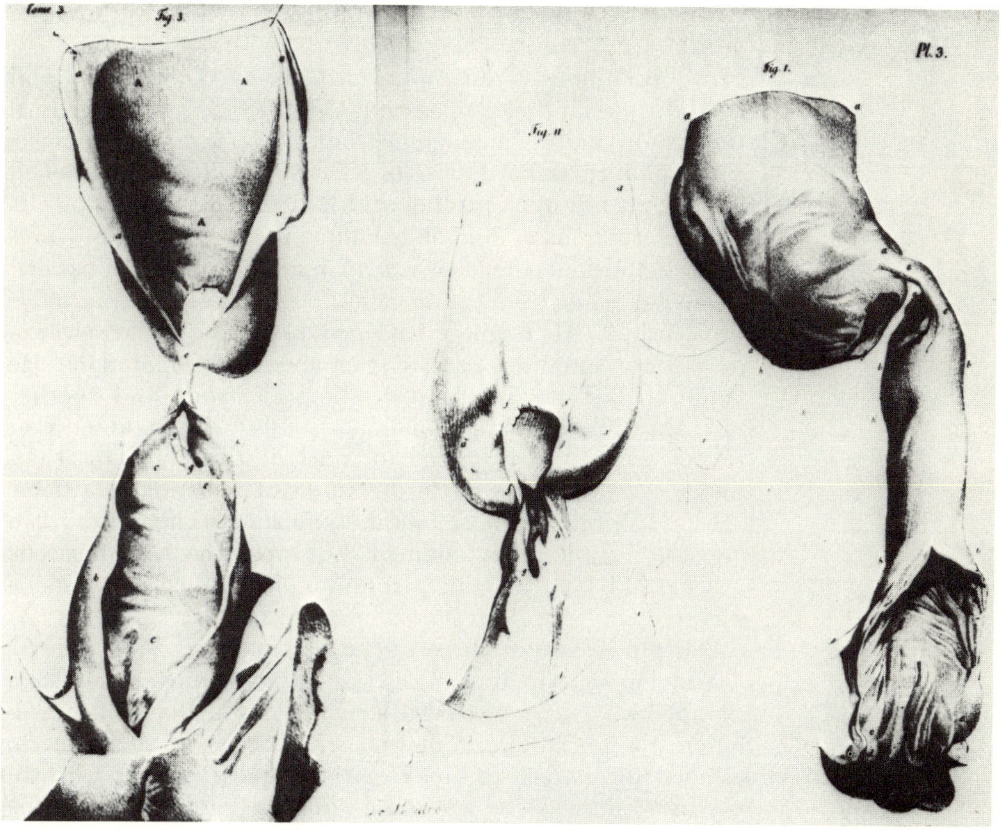

6.1 Talma's recurrent volvulus. He died without colostomy. From L. Biett, "Histoire de la maladie de Talma," *Report. gén. d'anat. et physiol. path.* (1827), 3:118.

Dupuytren made a rectal examination with an esophageal sound, detecting an impassable obstacle at a distance of 6 to 7 inches from the anus, and diagnosed an organic narrowing of the intestine. A colostomy would undoubtedly have been lifesaving, but operation was apparently never considered. As a final resort electric currents were twice applied during the week of Talma's death in October. At necropsy, a benign stricture was encountered in the upper rectum, owing undoubtedly to recurrent volvulus with ballooning of the proximal bowel and perforation.[11]

The eminent French neurologist Guillaume Duchenne in 1855 reported a few successes with use of the faradic current in intestinal obstruction. Ordinarily, one of the electrodes was placed in the rectum, the other on the patient's abdomen. Occasionally one of the electrodes was introduced into the stomach with the aid of a tube.[12]

Several editions of an American book by G. M. Beard and A. D. Rockwell on electrotherapy (1871–78) featured electrical stimulation in the management of constipation and bowel obstruction. In his Paris thesis of 1880 J.-B. Ballouhey continued to praise the role of electrotherapy for intestinal obstruction.[13] Its virtue, if any, was undoubtedly limited to the possible enhancement of intestinal peristaltic activity in some instances of paralytic ileus.

Recently A. M. Bilgutay has encouraged the use of electrotherapy for intestinal paresis after abdominal operations. He employed an intraduodenal dwelling electrode and another upon the abdomen to stimulate peristalsis.[14] In the absence of controls it would be difficult to conclude that the clinical improvement noted was solely the result of increased peristaltic activity accruing from electrical stimulation. Theoretically, in any case, faradic stimulation of the upper reaches of paretic bowel could help to initiate resumption of normal peristaltic activity.

Adolph Kussmaul introduced *gastric lavage* for pyloric obstruction in 1869. By 1884 he was enthusiastic over its use as a therapeutic device for bowel obstruction on the thesis that washing out the toxic bowel content, regurgitated into the stomach, lessened the hazard to life. Heinrich Curschmann, a German internist, said its value was second only to that of opium in the management of bowel obstruction. Although the method was warmly endorsed by many clinicians, too often the success was temporary and followed by death. As late as 1891 Edward Martin and H. A. Hare of Philadelphia continued to extol the virtues of gastric lavage in coping with the problem of acute intestinal obstruction.[15]

A conventional treatment for strangulated hernia was to *puncture* the distended intestine percutaneously with a needle. permitting trapped gas or fluid to escape, thus facilitating reduction of the hernia by taxis. F. D. W. Mensching, in a Rostock thesis of 1756, commended intestinal puncture for ileus. Otto Leichtenstern (1876) believed that the procedure when carefully performed "was quite without danger." Notable, if not commendable, was the persistence of the Boston clinicians John G. Blake and Bigelow (1876), who treated a patient over a period of eighteen weeks by periodic, frequent punctures of the abdominal wall, employing a Potain aspirator to remove gas and fluid. Frequent enemas and liberal administration of opium were adjuvant measures. In commenting upon the situation, Bigelow indicated that the patient had learned to call for the needle and aspirator, select the site, and perform the puncture himself, using a small needle a third of a millimeter in diameter. In the end starvation and obstruction took its toll, suggesting definitely that reluctance to operate could be overdone. Blake also added in a footnote that cases of successful operation by "gastrotomy" had come to his attention in the British literature.[16] Surgeons of that day obviously knew little or nothing of the courage of French surgeons of more than a century before.

When John W. Ogle summarized the literature of intestinal puncture in 1888, including the opinions of surgeons then active in London hospitals, he favored its use despite its hazards. He had nothing to say concerning operation for bowel obstruction. In 1891 Martin and Hare were still advocating percutaneous intestinal puncture as a therapeutic device of distinct value.[17]

It is also of interest that surgeons of that day protested abdominal section for bullet wounds of the abdomen. In fact, at the start of World War I, contestants on both sides of the conflict were still advising nonoperative management.[18]

Early Surgery for Intestinal Obstruction

Persistent vomiting accompanied by pain and abdominal distention should be treated, according to Hippocratic writings, "with enemas and inflation of the rectum by means of a bladder attached to a pipe."[19] Surgery in the Hippocratic writings is discussed under the caption, "The Physician's Repository"; obviously, therefore, surgery was not often regarded as a primary indication in the management of disease.[20]

Probably the earliest reasonably authentic report of operation for intestinal obstruction is that of Praxagoras of Cos, who was born about 340 B.C. In extreme cases of "iliac passion" he made an incision over the swelling of a strangulated hernia in the inguinal area, freed the gut, and cut into the bowel to establish an artificial anus.[21]

In the fifth-century texts of *Sushruta Samhita*, strangulated hernia was considered incurable. Application of the cautery over the swelling was advised to encourage cicatrization and to prevent recurrent hernia.[22]

Saliceto in the thirteenth century was among the first Italian surgeons to restore use of the knife in surgery; the cautery had been favored by the Arabs. He operated for strangulated hernia and employed animal bowel as an internal splint or stent over which continuity was reesetablished by resuture of the proximal and distal ends of the divided bowel. Lanfranc, a pupil of Saliceto, used animal trachea as the internal splint over which to approximate the divided bowel segments after excision of the devitalized segments, a procedure the "Four Masters" had recommended.[23]

Franco (1556) is to be regarded as the real originator of the planned direct attack upon strangulated hernia. He gave a careful account of his technique. He made an incision over the swelling and divided the constricting band, inserted a cannula the size of a goose quill into the distended bowel, and returned it to the peritoneal cavity. Nicaise suggests that Paré's description (1575) of the operation was borrowed from Franco and that Paré did not actually perform it. Paré advocated long periods of recumbency and trusses for hernia.[24] Franco too wrestled with the problem of scrotal hernia. After returning the abnormal scrotal content to the abdomen, Franco, and subsequently others, strove to preclude recurrence of the hernial descent by tightening up the fascial structures of the inguinal area in various ways. The most widely used was cautery, which caused contraction of the inguinal fascias.In other instances Franco ran a sharp curved needle, armed with an unabsorbable suture, beneath the spermatic cord, tying it tightly, thus occluding the hernial sac and incorporating the spermatic cord with the adjacent fascial structures; sometimes the testis was removed by incision. Franco stated that he had employed these diverse methods for ten years in Bern. Woodall (1655) treated the iliac passion by glisters (enemas) and such remedies as ingestion of horse dung in wine, perhaps a reflection of the superstition that like cures like.[25]

Pierre Pigray of Rouen, Paré's pupil, in 1615 described how he operated for strangulated hernia: the incision was made over the swelling, the peritoneum was deliberately opened, and a finger was inserted into the wound as a guide in the division of the constricting band occluding the intestine. It was Pigray's practice to smear his finger with fresh butter or oil of sweet almonds to facilitate its introduction into the wound. If the strangulated intestine was not readily released from the constricting band, he advised tapping the distended bowel with a needle to permit escape of gas. An intestinal wound, he concluded, heals like any wound of the abdominal wall.[26]

More than a half century later Paul Barbette of Amsterdam advised surgery for intussusception, asking, "Would it not be better to make an incision and draw out the strangulated intestine with fingers, than to leave the patient in danger of his life?"

There is no testimony, however, that he followed his own suggestion. The usual reaction in such cases was probably that of Rau. Heister relates that he and his teacher Rau encountered dead bowel when operating upon a patient for strangulating hernia in 1707. Rau informed the patient he would die, gathered up his instruments, and left, declining to excise the strangulated segment.[27]

In 1692 the Dutch anatomist Antonj Nuck supervised a successful operation performed by a young surgeon for volvulus employing the suggestion of Barbette.[28] Theophilus Bonet, in discussing *dolore iliaco*, relates a similar instance in which an army surgeon operated so successfully upon a baroness for volvulus that she endowed him with a life pension.[29]

The Royal Academy and Renaissance of Surgery in France

La Peyronie, with Mareschal, founded the French Royal Academy of Surgery in 1731, an innovation that is responsible in large measure for Paris being regarded as the world's leading surgical center for a century.[30] The discussions of that body revived interest and hope among surgeons in dealing with intestinal obstruction and strangulated hernia, concerning which the literature of surgery had been relatively silent since Pigray.

Mery operated upon a young woman for strangulated hernia with advanced gangrene at the Hôtel-Dieu in Paris in 1701. He excised several feet of gangrenous bowel and established an artificial anus. The patient recovered and was dismissed two months after operation.[31] In 1723 La Peyronie opened the peritoneal cavity of a thirty-five-year-old man with intestinal obstruction; he excised the devitalized bowel, bringing the adjacent loops into the wound as an artificial anus. By making traction upon a suture placed through the mesentery between the adjacent loops, he was able to hurry the union; the fistula closed spontaneously. Results exceeded expectations; within a month evacuation followed the normal pathway. In 1743 La Peyronie performed a similar operation.[32]

Surgeons early learned that a suture placed through the antimesenteric borders of the two adjacent loops was effective in eliminating the spur for which Dupuytren (1828) devised an enterotome, not unlike Mikulicz's version many decades later.[33] Velpeau (1851) mentioned instances in which the abdominal swelling of pregnancy hastened closure of an artificial anus.[34]

Antoine Louis, the perpetual secretary of the Academy, provided that august assembly and posterity with two long treatises

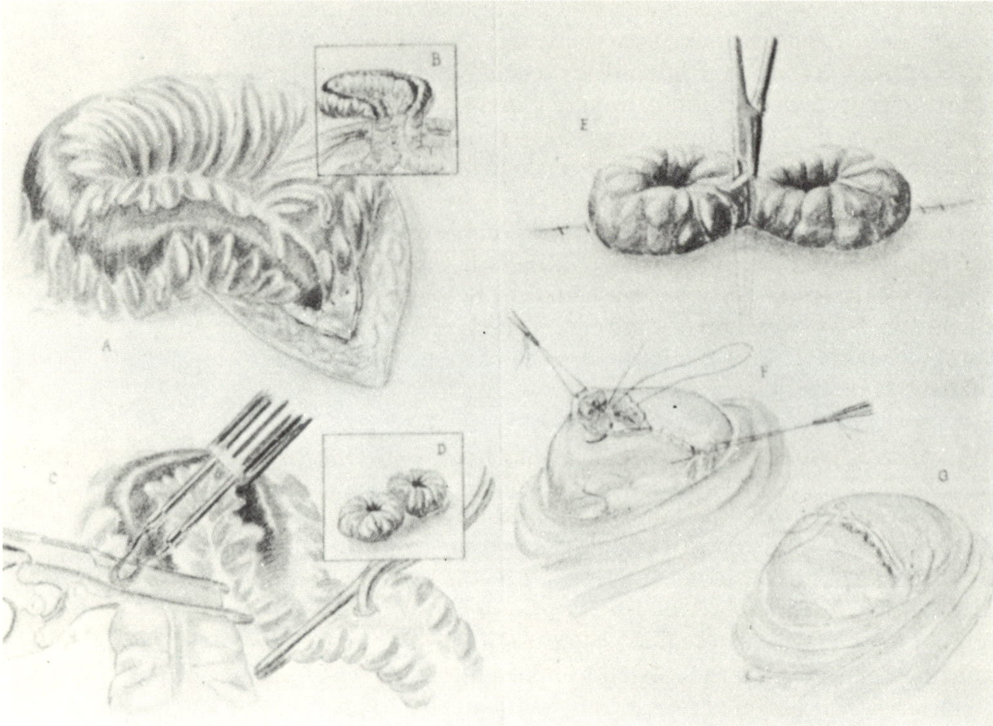

6.2 Adaptation of Dupuytren's enterotome to divide spur in colostomy. From O. H. Wangensteen, *Intestinal obstructions*, 3d ed. (Springfield, Ill.: Charles C Thomas, 1955).

on strangulated hernia (1757, 1768), summarizing a number of reports and practices of the period. A veritable rash of papers in the memoirs of the Academy accompanied his second presentation. The elder Pipelet, a director of the Academy, reported the case of a fifty-six-year-old woman upon whom he had operated in 1740. He excised several inches of dead bowel, creating an artificial anus. Four months later, following vigorous catharsis, feces were expelled via the rectum and within fifteen days the wound was healed. The patient survived twenty-six years, Pipelet tells us, dying at age eighty-two of causes unrelated to the obstruction.[35]

A few years later Regnauld recounted a most extraordinary case. He had operated upon a twenty-five-year-old man in 1772 for a strangulated inguinal hernia, finding it necessary to excise 6 to 7 inches of gangrenous bowel. He left the adjacent ends of the healthy bowel in the wound. Fifteen days after operation, following administration of cathartics and a vermifuge, feces were extruded via the rectum. With repetitive and vigorous employment of purges, most of the feces, by the twenty-sixth day after operation, were evacuated normally. Soon thereafter the wound healed completely and the patient was dismissed. A month later, the patient reappeared with signs of intestinal obstruction. After the patient had vomited for twelve hours and showed no improvement, Regnauld reopened the wound and the bowel with a bistoury and recovered prune stones and skins of baked potato. The bowel was left open in the wound; twelve days later, there was a large stool. By the twenty-eighth day the wound was healed and the patient remained well. Regnauld indicated that the incentive for the operation came from Louis's presentation of 1768, which admission and achievement prompted the Academy to award its gold medal to Regnauld. He was also given a civil honor in Rome for the accomplishment.[36]

It is fitting to conclude the account of this period of French surgery by alluding to the posthumous treatise of Petit, who devised the tourniquet (1718). Petit apparently operated with unusual success for strangulated hernia. Among a small group of eleven patients, he had seven definite survivors. In only one instance, however, was frank gangrene present, necessitating an artificial anus.[37]

Unfortunately, the successes of Mery (1701), La Peyronie (1723), Pipelet (1740), and Regnauld (1787) failed to make a durable impress upon surgeons of that day, just as the earlier successes of Franco (1556) and Pigray (1615) had failed to stimulate imitators. Half a century was to elapse before a young Paris surgeon illumined the subject with a bold paper.

In 1819 L. J. Maunoury wrote a significant and magnificent thesis, for its time, on strangulated intestinal obstruction, in which he was outspoken in his criticism concerning the timidity of the contemporary surgeons of the Hôtel-Dieu. He recounted several instances in which Dupuytren and Joseph Récamier were less than aggressive in operating for strangulated hernia. They delayed operation in the face of obvious and compelling indications. In several instances Dupuytren had failed to divide the constricting band completely; in others he had not recognized or dealt with the devitalized intestine in a manner that would have ensured recovery of the patient. In one instance Dupuytren, employing his finger as a dissector, made several superficial cuts in his finger without releasing the strangulated bowel from the constricting band. Surgeons were still debating whether the peritoneal sac should be opened when operating for strangulated hernia. Maunoury indicated that Dupuytren was not alone in these defections and that Le Dran and other writers had recorded similar difficulties. When patients did poorly, it was Dupuytren's practice to apply sixty to eighty leeches to the lower abdomen and about the anal canal.

Maunoury felt strongly that abdominal section should be done earlier and more often and that excision of dead bowel with establishment of an artificial anus was in order.[38] That an observing young surgical house officer's critique exhibited a sophistication and a forward look exceeding that of his superiors should suffice to admonish all teachers of surgery to be attentive and alert to suggestions of juniors. More time had to elapse on the surgical scene before his suggestions came to be implemented regularly in cases of strangulated hernia. Maunoury obviously deserved well at the hands of his superiors. However, we have no indication that his frank and wise appraisal was rewarded by a fitting academic opportunity in Paris. Many years later he was Chief of Surgery at the Hôtel Dieu in Chartres.

The English School of Surgery

Across the English Channel a brilliant group of British surgeons, represented by Cheselden, Pott, John Hunter, and Hunter's distinguished pupil, Astley Cooper, were making surgical history. Yet Hunter dismissed the subject of intestinal obstruction with allusion to two cases of intussusception and mere mention of hernia. Pott's experience in operating for strangulated hernia was meager.[39]

Cooper, who wrote a superb and well-illustrated text on hernia (1804–7), certainly does not appear to have been aggressive in attacking strangulated hernia. Charles Jones, who audited and reproduced many of Cooper's lectures, related that he leaned heavily on the use of tobacco enemas: "It is a most unpardonable neglect in the practitioner not to use tobacco in strangulated hernia, which ought to be impressed on the mind of every surgeon." Cooper also recommended bleeding the patient 20 to 22 ounces.[40]

Jones noted that Cooper was very pessimistic in his lectures over the outlook in strangulated hernia when mortification of the bowel was present: "It is seldom patients are strong enough to get through this process, 19 in 20 dying before; nature, however, sometimes succeeds but the instances are few."[41] From Cooper's own recorded observations it is clear that in some instances at least the bowel was allowed to slough without any attempt being made to excise the devitalized intestine. When

Cooper operated for strangulated hernia and encountered devitalized bowel, he incised that segment and left it in the wound.[42] French surgeons seventy-five years earlier had routinely excised such segments, establishing an artificial anus which, in the hands of a few surgeons like Mery, La Peyronie, Pipelet, and Regnauld, closed spontaneously or by simple revision of the wound.

A century after Cooper's operation in 1821 on King George IV for removal of a wen from the royal head, John Bland-Sutton wrote, "His anxiety lest erysipelas supervene seems scarcely compensated by the baronetcy which the King bestowed upon him as a reward for the successful issue of the operation."[43] This statement tells much of the surgery of that day and of Cooper. But modern surgeons should reserve their censure. Perusal of Aston Key's 1844 edition of Cooper's *Anatomy and Surgical Treatment of Abdominal Hernia*, which appeared three years after Cooper's death, serves to indicate that his operations for strangulated hernia met with greater success than those of other surgeons of his time. Among 33 operations for strangulated hernia, he lost 14 patients, or 42.4 percent. Of 31 operations collected by Cooper from other English surgeons and reported in the same monograph, 17 patients died, or 54.8 percent.[44]

The French surgeons had reported isolated cases. Several surgeons of other countries had written monographs on hernia, including Pott (1756), Richter (1778–79), Camper (1801), Scarpa (1809), and Cooper's pupil, Benjamin Travers (1812). In none of these is to be found a factual account of the experience of the author. William Hey (1803) related that when he operated early for strangulated hernia, 2 in 9 died (22.2 percent); in the later cases, 3 in 5 (60 percent). Travers put the situation well in discussing a death from strangulation: "If by good fortune a barber surgeon . . . had pushed his lancet into the swelling, the patient . . . would have recovered."[45]

The end effect of strangulation of the bowel of that day was more commonly looked upon as inflammation than as devitalization. The reliance by many present-day investigators and surgeons on antibiotics for strangulating obstructions reflects the prevalent opinion of 150 years ago, viz., that strangulation is essentially inflammatory in nature.

Early Techniques of Intestinal Anastomosis

Allusion has already been made to the use of animal trachea by the "Four Masters" of the thirteenth century in reestablishing intestinal continuity after excision of gangrenous bowel. The French military surgeon Duverger in 1747 excised several inches of gangrenous small intestine and its mesentery and reunited the ends with a few sutures over a piece of animal trachea, returning the bowel to the peritoneal cavity. The trachea was expelled in the stool on the twenty-first postoperative day and the patient convalesced satisfactorily. In canine experiments (1804) Cooper employed isinglass successfully in suturing divided intestine. He related that Thomson of Edinburgh in canine experiments had placed four inner sutures and four external sutures approximating divided intestine, cutting the sutures on the knot. On sacrificing the dogs on the tenth postoperative day, Thomson observed that the sutures were being discharged into the lumen. Lancelot Haire, formerly surgeon to the Haslar Naval Hospital, described cutting on the knot after amputation in 1786, a suggestion he attributed to an unidentified surgeon friend of "great abilities." Haire said that the stumps healed in ten days and that the ligature, with little pain to the patient, was soon discharged.[46]

Ramdohr, a German surgeon, in 1727 excised two feet of gangrenous small bowel and its mesentery, invaginating the proximal end of the bowel into the lumen of the distal segment and fixing it with a few sutures. Jobert (de Lamballe) (1824) effected an end-to-side anastomosis employing this technique in both dogs and cats. He employed a continuous waxed suture which was left untied with one end protruding through the wound. On the fifth postoperative day the suture was withdrawn by gentle traction. Dogs operated upon in this manner recovered and maintained functional intestinal continuity.[47]

Antoine Lembert described a technique of intestinal suture in 1826 which is still in vogue and which bears his name. He reviewed prior techniques of intestinal anastomoses and the experimental work of Cooper and Travers. His experiments were on the dog. He described employing interrupted sutures that pierced the entire thickness of the bowel wall except the mucosa, placed 6 to 8 mm. apart. No sutures were tied until all had been placed. The manner of placement of the sutures provided for serosal inversion. Lembert observed that such sutures were extruded into the lumen of the bowel, a circumstance suggesting that in practice his sutures actually did include the mucosa as well.[48]

Halsted (1887), in a few beautifully executed experiments, rightfully pointed out that such is not good practice, that sutures penetrating the intestinal lumen produce bending or kinking of the intestine accompanied by serosal adhesions, perhaps indicating a leak through the needle tract to the peritoneal surface. Halsted and others have observed that sutures extending into the lumen of the bowel are extruded into the bowel. On the contrary, Halsted noted in his experiments, when the suture needle includes the submucosa but does not enter the bowel lumen, the sutures remain in place and are not extruded either to the peritoneal surface or into the lumen of the bowel. Inasmuch as the mucosal blood vessels lie in the submucosa, surgeons have used pallor of the serosal bowel surface over the needle point as a determinant that the suture needle had included the submucosa; the increased tissue resistance to the needle provided additional evidence thereof.

Lembert stated that his method was applicable to any manner of uniting segments of intestine and could also be used on the stomach. His suture is in fact a good description of a one-layer anastomosis. Some of his protocols suggest that a lesser inversion of the intestinal wall would have eliminated the stomal obstruction occasionally observed.

Peter Olch, long an ardent student of Halsted and his important contributions to the literature, observed that the National Library of Medicine's copy of the monograph *Experimental and Critical Inquiry into the Nature and Treatment of Wounds of the Intestine* (1843) by Samuel D. Gross had a marginal notation in Halsted's handwriting on pages 4 and 5 which read "copy," obviously a note to his secretary.[49] Gross had pointed out that the submucosa is the strongest coat of the intestine; his publication ante-

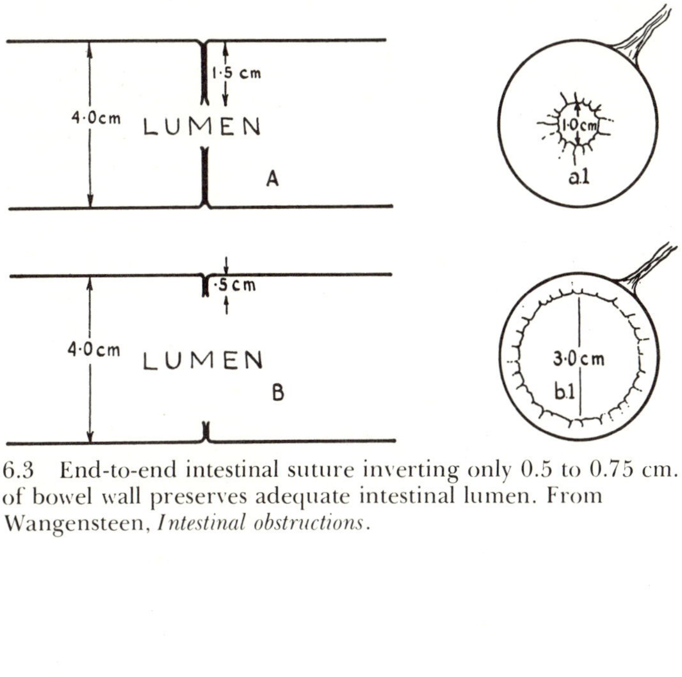

6.3 End-to-end intestinal suture inverting only 0.5 to 0.75 cm. of bowel wall preserves adequate intestinal lumen. From Wangensteen, *Intestinal obstructions*.

dated elective surgery by four decades. In his treatise of 1887 on intestinal suture, Halsted does not include a reference to Gross's observation; he does, however, allude to Lembert.

J. B. Murphy of Chicago introduced a button (1892) for quick intestinal anastomosis. The small circular metal button had two parts; each part was inserted into a segment of the two hollow viscera to be approximated with a purse-string suture of catgut. The two buttons, male and female, were then pushed home; a spring held them firmly in position. A continuous over-and-over catgut suture or interrupted silk suture sufficed to terminate the operation. The button passed spontaneously distally into the intestine and was ordinarily readily evacuated per rectum. In the repair of an incisional hernia in a patient operated upon fifteen years previously, in whom a scout roentgen film of the abdomen prior to operation had not been made, the silent button was found and removed, undoubtedly a rare occurrence.

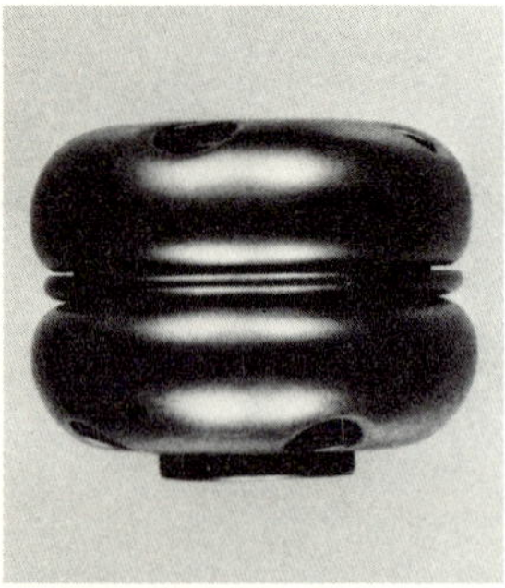

6.4 Murphy button for quick intestinal anastomosis. Gift from Charles E. Rea, St. Paul surgeon.

The Murphy button has disappeared from the current surgical scene but was widely used by many surgeons well into the third decade of this century. Several of the senior author's teachers used the device. In May 1928 he saw Hermann Küttner of Breslau, a very talented surgeon, perform a gastrojejunostomy employing such a button. Its sole advantage was the quickness with which the operation could be performed. One of Halsted's last papers concerned use of the Murphy button in resections of the lower colon.[50]

Colostomy and Enterostomy for Obstruction

Emphasis in the surgical management of intestinal obstruction until the mid-nineteenth century had been largely upon the strangulating types. Occlusions of the distal colon and upper rectum were exceptions. In 1710 Alexis Littre had suggested, without performing the procedure save on an infant after death, opening the colon in the lower left quadrant for imperforate anus, an operation which C. Duret of Brest performed successfully in 1793.[51] Pillore's temporary success (1776) with cecostomy for cancer of the lower bowel — an operation that ended disastrously because of the prior administration of 2 pounds of mercury — has been mentioned.

In 1798 Henric Callisen of Copenhagen suggested that the colostomy for imperforate anus be performed extraperitoneally in the lumbar area. Interest was renewed by Amussat's adoption of the procedure for cancer of the rectum and distal colon (1839). The operation maintained its popularity for almost fifty years, until Thomas Bryant of Guy's Hospital in 1885 and other surgeons reverted to the intraperitoneal maneuver of Pillore and Duret to achieve decompression of the distended and obstructed colon.[52]

As has already been indicated, French surgeons of the mid-eighteenth century, following the example of Mery and La Peyronie, excised segments of devitalized small intestine for strangulated hernia, drawing the orifices of the proximal and distal ends of the bowel into the wound, creating an artificial anus. By 1873 there were 80 instances of colostomy for obstruction in the literature, with a mortality of 32.5 percent.[53] Most of the patients had been operated upon before acceptance of antiseptic surgery, a noteworthy achievement.

Sometime in 1839–40 Auguste Nélaton of Paris attempted what was described as a simplification of Maunoury's 1819 suggestion. Nélaton, whose fame as operator and clinical lecturer would become internationally acclaimed, was probably at the time recognized only as a promising young surgeon who had worked as an undergraduate *externe* for the late Baron Dupuytren at the Hôtel-Dieu. Nélaton fixed a distended loop of bowel, proximal to the obstruction, in the wound by a number of sutures penetrating into the lumen, and concluded the procedure by incising the exposed bowel. The patient did not survive. In 1849 Nélaton was able to claim a success with the method. Another success, in 1852, concerned the son of a Hamburg merchant. Nélaton was by then Professor of Clinical Surgery at the Faculty of Medicine, and his wards were crowded with students from many countries. Armand Trousseau, who became Professor of Clinical Medicine at the Hôtel-Dieu that year, was also a consultant in the case. Trousseau telegraphed for permission for the operation and was advised to hold off until the parents arrived. Nevertheless, recognizing the seriousness of the situation, Nélaton proceeded at once. The patient survived and some months later Nélaton closed the enterostomy opening. Trousseau, known to us as a physician, similarly reported 5 enterostomies for obstruction of the small intestine with 2 recoveries.[54] Walter F. Atlee, one of Nélaton's American followers, reported that Nélaton had operated 8 times for strangulated hernia with 4 deaths during 1852–54. In 3 additional cases in which an artificial anus was established during operation for strangulated hernia, Atlee relates that Nélaton had 2 deaths. In 1867 Nélaton said he had had 4 successes in 9 attempts.[55]

It is of considerable interest for this discussion that the type of enterostomy described by Nélaton was depicted and employed by Kocher in 1911 and was also the type used by Victor Bonney in 1916.[56] The publications of Oscar Witzel of Bonn (1891, 1894) described an oblique enterostomy over a catheter which eliminated the difficulties, such as the development of a persistent fistula, presented by earlier types of enterostomy.[57]

Again, "Little Circumstances"

That operations of the magnitude described herein, undertaken with little or no apparent observance of late nineteenth-century principles of prophylactic antisepsis, had surprisingly good success in a few hands constitutes a fresh source for speculative wonderment. Observance of "little circumstances" and surgical cleanliness, as in amputation and perineal lithotomy, provide the likely answers. Nélaton has been praised for his postoperative care and use of sanitary measures. He was said to have developed a technique of avoiding unnecessary introduction of fingers and instruments into the peritoneal cavity and took care too that fecal matter did not leak into it.[58]

In the perusal of accounts of many authors, only twice have we noted wine or brandy used in operations for strangulated bowel. Barthélemi Saviard (1702) opened a strangulated hernial sac and poured warm wine and brandy over a somewhat discolored loop of bowel before returning it to the peritoneal cavity. The patient recovered. The recovery of Duverger's patient whose gangrenous bowel was excised and the proximal and distal ends resutured over animal trachea has already been mentioned. Duverger washed the gangrenous segment and the sac with fortified fomentations, probably brandy. The trachea, too, had been submerged in warm wine and in balsam of Peru and *Commandeur* (a strong alcoholic solution) before implantation.[59]

Debates over Whether and When to Operate

Long beyond the time that antisepsis in surgery began to encounter favor, surgeons and physicians were reluctant to advise surgical intervention for obstruction. Admittedly, excision of a large ovarian cyst, the first abdominal operation to find acceptance, did not entail replacement of distended intestinal coils and was therefore a far simpler procedure than operations for obstruction accompanied by great distention. Annandale (1870–71) and George Buchanan (1871) had each published reports of isolated operative successes in the British literature, suggesting that serious consideration be lent surgical exploration for bowel obstruction.[60] The conservative approach to intestinal obstruction had strong advocates among British surgeons in the later 1870s, as revealed in a lively discussion on the subject initiated at the annual meeting of the British Medical Association of 1878 at Bath. Hutchinson, a surgeon of the London Hospital, maintained that "exploratory operations for the relief of abdominal obstruction, the cause of which cannot be diagnosed, are not warrantable." He advocated manipulative measures for both diagnosis and treatment. However, he suggested with "some delicacy," as a surgeon speaking to a Medical Section of the Association, that cases of mechanical obstruction were surgical, not medical. He lamented the fact that usually by the time a surgeon is called "the stage at which abdominal taxis is most hopeful has passed."

The opposition to Hutchinson's views was most forcefully expressed at a later medical meeting by T. P. Teale of Leeds. He favored exploration of the abdomen in case of bowel obstruction on the grounds of theory and experience and described six apparently hopeless cases in which he felt operation had not jeopardized the patient's chance of recovery. The pros and cons were revealed in a number of articles in the *British Medical Journal* for at least a year after the original meeting.

Caught off guard and stimulated by Hutchinson's address, Allbutt had ventured a few remarks at Bath, suggesting that intussusception was best left without operation, indicating that he had only gone so far as to employ percutaneous intestinal puncture for the distention of obstruction. Later (1879) he published a retraction, still stressing the importance of opiates but ending with strong support of his fellow surgeons of Leeds, notwithstanding that among Teale's first six operative interventions, only one patient survived.[61]

In a subsequent meeting of the British Medical Association in 1883 the Liverpool surgeon Rushton Parker urged the extension of protracted palliative management of intestinal obstruction. In protest, Lawson Tait, the famous and controversial Birmingham gynecologist, remarked that an accurate diagnosis can only be made by exploration, which is better performed before than after death.[62]

It was the 1885 paper of E. H. Greves of Liverpool that gave operative intervention its first strong forward thrust in England. His patient had been completely obstructed for five days. Greves had employed abdominal taxis, as recommended by Hutchinson, enemas, and intestinal insufflation — all without success. A consultation was held, and R. N. Pughe, a local surgeon, performed abdominal section under antiseptic precautions. A loop of ileum near the cecum was found to have been obstructed. The band was divided and the patient recovered.[63]

In the discussion following the presentation, the majority favored nonoperative therapy. Among these was Thomas, who with his continued and ardent advocacy of opium management of intestinal obstruction undoubtedly did much to retard early surgical intervention throughout the British Isles. In discussing Greves's presentation, Thomas said that cases of acute intestinal obstruction "belonged to the department of medicine, the surgeon was a mere assistant. . . . An operation may be required in a few hours or it may not be required for weeks." Differential diagnosis he felt was of very little importance to the surgeon and still less to the physician. Shortly thereafter Thomas published a monograph entitled *The Collegian of 1666 and the Collegians of 1885*. This was a diatribe against surgical intervention and a comparison of his own views with those of Sydenham of two centuries before.[64]

In general, physicians continued to insist that the mortality of exploration was such that it was better to persist with nonoperative methods. Had not Sydenham and Brinton achieved good results with opium, percutaneous intestinal puncture, and conservative methods? Why change? The perseverance reported by Blake and Bigelow, previously alluded to, probably constitutes a record.

The Philadelphia surgeon John Ashhurst, who had been mildly enthusiastic over operation for acute intestinal obstruction in 1874, had a change of heart by 1886. Probably chastened by his own experience and encountering few suggestions of acceptance from his colleagues, he extolled the old remedies of bleeding, leeching, opium, and enemas.[65] At the 1887 German Surgical Congress Otto W. Madelung sounded a cautious note relative to operations for bowel obstruction, stating that he believed he had hurried a number of patients to their deaths thereby. Mikulicz agreed, adding that he had retreated from his formerly more aggressive surgical attitude; his experience had taught him that often laparotomy offered no hopeful prospect. In 1888, at the first Congress of American Physicians and Surgeons, Reginald Fitz of Boston maintained that even after the diagnosis of intestinal obstruction was made, conservative management should be continued for forty-eight to seventy-two hours before the patient was turned over to the surgeon. Nicholas Senn presented the view of surgeons and in general agreed with Fitz. In the ensuing discussion T. G. Morton, a Philadelphia surgeon, said that examination of the records of the Episcopal and Women's hospitals disclosed no instance of operative interference for intestinal obstruction and similarly that he had failed to find any record of such at the Pennsylvania Hospital in the preceding twenty-five years.[66] In his presentation Senn defended the ancient practice of rectal insufflation in the treatment of intestinal obstruction.[67]

The management of intestinal obstruction was a major topic for discussion at the German Congress of Internal Medicine in 1889.[68] Leichtenstern, one of the main reporters, avoided all discussion of operative treatment, concentrating on symptoms and effects of obstruction. He felt as he had in 1876 that stercoraceous vomiting had no significance in the determination of the site of obstruction, a thesis often since repeated by many observers. In fact, there are those who have insisted that feculent vomiting occurs only in obstruction of the colon.[69]

Paul Fürbringer's assessment probably reflected the general attitude: "The medical management of intestinal obstruction is not so bad, nor the results of surgery so good as to warrant calling in the surgeon." Curschmann, the other chief reporter, felt that surgeons should be consulted but stressed that all conservative medical measures should be tried before committing the patient to the surgeon.

It was against this background that Treves began to speak out for early operative intervention. Yet, in discussing the management of strangulating obstruction before the New York Academy of Medicine in 1863, in considering all the common conservative practices of the day, John O'Reilly concluded by condemning them all, saying, "Young surgeons are apt to follow the precepts of their Masters in all the details and will thus let slip by sometimes the favorable opportunity for saving the patient's life by a timely operation."[70] Sage advice indeed for its time, as it still is for our day.

Handicaps of the Surgeon in 1900

Treves and the surgeons of his era faced handicaps both of diagnosis and of fluid management. He mentions use of the stethoscope only once in his 1899 monograph. To make certain the colon was not obstructed, an enema was administered; if a fluid splash was heard with the stethoscope over the cecum, it was a reasonable inference that the colon was clear. X-rays were unavailable; Gottwald Schwarz of Vienna in 1911 was the first to point out the virtue of scout x-ray films in distinguishing which intestinal loops were distended. An important paper by Hans Kloiber of Germany in 1919 served to emphasize the importance of x-rays in localizing the level of obstruction. In 1920 J. T. Case of Battle Creek alluded to their value in the recognition of post-operative ileus.[71]

The problem of fluid administration was equally challenging. Treves depended solely upon proctoclysis. A decade later hypodermoclysis came into vogue with only sporadic mention of intravenous administration. It had been forgotten that O'Shaughnessy in 1831 had advocated and employed intravenous fluids containing both the Na and K ions lost in the severe diarrhea of cholera.[72] Two decades later (1850) Carl Schmidt again called attention to the loss of these ions in severe diarrhea as a significant factor in the fatal outcome. Ringer (1880–82), in experiments upon the frog's heart, established the importance of the K ion as a normal constituent of physiologic fluids. Rudolph Matas of New Orleans (1891) reported successes with intravenous fluid administration, but the method did not catch on widely for another quarter of a century.[73]

Demise of the Autointoxication Theory

The origin of the theory of autointoxication as the principal cause of death in bowel obstruction traces back to Amussat. He formulated this theory, according to his Parisian friends, after the death of his friend and patient, the famous French clinician Broussais, the keenest exponent of leeches and depletion for every trying medical situation. Broussais had a rectal hemorrhage and died after fulguration of a low-lying rectal cancer. In extenuation of the unfortunate outcome Amussat reported (1839) that death was caused by absorption of noxious materials from the colon,[74] a theory since invoked as solace by many a surgeon disappointed over his poor accomplishment in the management of bowel obstruction.

George Whipple and his associates in a series in the *Journal of Experimental Medicine* (1913–17) reported isolation of a toxic proteose from filtrates of intestinal content in obstructed intestinal loops, which lent renewed credence to the seventy-five-year-old theory of autointoxication. J. A. Hartwell and J. P. Hoguet's discovery (1912) that dogs could be kept alive for three weeks with high jejunal obstruction when given saline solution, however, cast glimmers of doubt upon the thesis. R. L. Haden and T. G. Orr (1923–24) subscribed to the Amussat theory, believing that saline solution rendered the toxin of bowel obstruction inert. Clarification of the mystery came when Gamble and his Harvard associates showed very nicely in 1925 that saline solution provided an excellent substitute for the fluid and electrolytes lost by vomiting.[75] Such, of course, was the therapeutic thesis of O'Shaughnessy and Schmidt for the severe diarrhea of cholera and dysentery. Gamble's significant observations initiated studies of the fluid and electrolyte requirements of surgical patients that have been a great boon to the surgeon in almost every sphere of his activity.

The almost miraculous resuscitative action of saline solution in high jejunal obstruction has no counterpart in low ileal obstruction, an observation which led to more than a decade (1928–39) of concentrated research by the senior author and a large number of his associates. Louis Sperling showed (1935) that intraluminal pressure maintained at the level of capillary blood pressure for twenty to twenty-eight hours resulted uniformly in patchy necrosis of the intestinal mucosa with loss of viability and transperitoneal migration of noxious substances from the bowel lumen into the peritoneal cavity. By dividing the cervical esophagus of dogs and inverting the aboral end Charles Rea (1939) adduced proof that the source of gaseous distention in bowel obstruction was swallowed air. Following this preparation dogs supported with saline-glucose solutions could survive for as long as eight weeks after complete obstruction of the ileum and only minimal quantities of fluid and gas were found accumulated proximal to the obstruction at postmortem.[76]

Significance of the blood loss factor in venous mesenteric occlusion emerged in experiments in dogs, revealing that when the venous return was obstructed to four feet of small intestine, death occurred in five hours and was owing primarily to hemorrhage (1932). Several years later (1956) John Perry and associates pointed out that the increased density of the bowel in venous mesenteric occlusions, observed previously, could be of practical use in the recognition of clinical venous mesenteric strangulations with the aid of pneumoradiography. In arterial mesenteric occlusions, however, blood loss is minimal. Horace Scott (1932) noted that dogs with occlusion of the terminal arteries to a segment of ileum four feet in length survive considerably longer, death being caused by transperitoneal migration of noxious substances from the bowel lumen.[77] Such occlusions, therefore, are not identifiable by pneumoradiography.

Distinguishing Symptoms of Small and Large Bowel Obstruction

Strangely, clinicians as late as the mid-1930s failed to distinguish between the behavior of obstruction of the small and large bowel. Feculent vomiting was considered characteristic of colic obstruction, obviously a hangover from the period antedating elective abdominal surgery when internists were the physicians of the body cavities and failed to correlate postmortem findings with antemortem symptoms. As a result, prevailing opinions were carried over into newer texts. Unable to distinguish fact from fiction, new authors, with older texts before them, copied what they noted therein into their compositions. The subtle but significant distinction of believing what one sees, rather than seeing what one believes, has importance in understanding this deception.

In 1929, a patient with enormous intestinal distention but without vomiting was observed in the senior author's clinic; exploration disclosed a cancer of the distal sigmoid colon with threatened perforation of the cecum, accounting for the tenderness noted in the right lower quadrant. Similar observations soon established that this was a regular occurrence in colic obstruction. Observation and experience also demonstrated that copious regurgitant, feculent vomiting is characteristic of obstruction of the small bowel. The lips of the ileocecal valve apparently are responsible for this strange behavior in colic obstruction, an occurrence known to Caspar Bauhin (1579) and to Richard Heschl (1880) — important observations which had been overlooked by clinicians.

Colic obstruction attended by enormous distention, limited to the colon, demands immediate surgical decompression. Peroral intestinal intubation cannot possibly overcome the distention in time to avert perforation of the cecum; a colostomy proximal to the obstructing agent is definitely in order. In most instances a diverting colostomy upon the transverse colon is performed, inasmuch as most colic obstructions are occasioned by malignancies of the distal reaches of the colon. Whereas cecostomy suffices to tap the distended segment, it is not as safe an operation in the presence of great distention of the colon as is colostomy; moreover, cecostomy provides only a vent and not an effective diversion of the fecal stream.

As a consequence of the work of competent investigators in many laboratories concerned with various facets of the problem of intestinal obstruction, the following have come to be recognized as the significant features in management: fluid and electrolyte therapy, replacement of blood loss, decompression and release of the obstruction, the earliest possible identification of strangulating obstructions, and excision of devitalized bowel.

The Mortality of Intestinal Obstruction, 1889–1929

After the Liverpool debates of 1885, the congresses of 1887 and 1889, and the appearance of Treves's book in 1899, one would reasonably have anticipated signs of improvement in the management of intestinal obstruction. The clinical literature of the first three decades of this century, however, reveals only here and there any suggestion of progress. As recently as 1929 C. Jeff Miller of New Orleans reported the mortality of bowel obstruction at the Charity Hospital for the preceding five years as 65 percent, a figure essentially that of forty years before, when physicians and surgeons were hesitant to operate in such cases. Miller indicated that surgery was undertaken as soon as the diagnosis was made, but he lamented the difficulty of achieving early diagnosis. He and his associates had failed to appreciate the significance of the pathognomonic sign of *intestinal colic* (borborygmi), readily audible with the stethoscope, along with recurrent gas pains. Scout x-ray films of the abdomen were not employed.[78]

A group of very competent New York surgeons of that era stressed the great hazards of enterostomy as a therapeutic device for acute obstruction, pointing out that the mortality of the enterostomy group was 90.9 percent for the 1916–19 period and 77.7 percent for the 1920–23 period, falling to 24.2 percent in the 1924–27 period. Kocher's (1911) and Moynihan's (1926) published illustrations indicate clearly that methods of enterostomy inviting trouble were employed by some of the keenest exponents of abdominal surgery during the first quarter of the twentieth century.[79] As the senior author has been at pains to point out for forty years, enterostomy must be accompanied without visible evidence of spillage. In the experience of his clinic over long years, the mortality of blind enterostomy for acute small bowel obstruction was approximately 10 percent.

Lessons of History

However contrite Astley Cooper was over his results with strangulated external hernia,[80] the success rate today is not strikingly better. Surgeons of Cooper's day had difficulty deciding on an operative course. Without anesthesia, antisepsis, asepsis, or rubber gloves, Cooper's reported achievement with strangulated external hernia and nonviable bowel is not far different from that of many large clinics today. Let us look briefly at this sobering record.

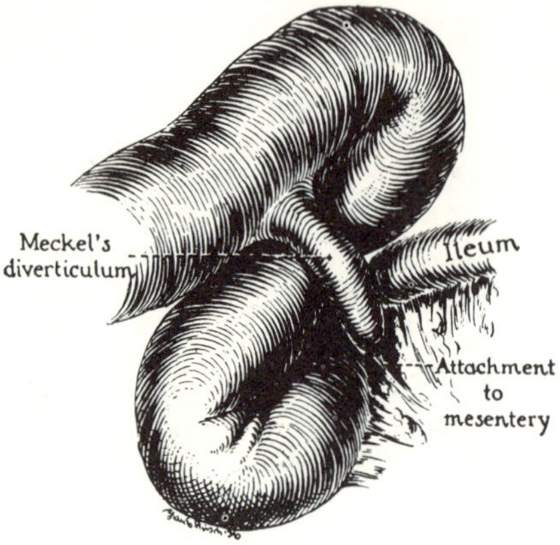

6.5 Strangulating obstruction caused by Meckel's diverticulum.

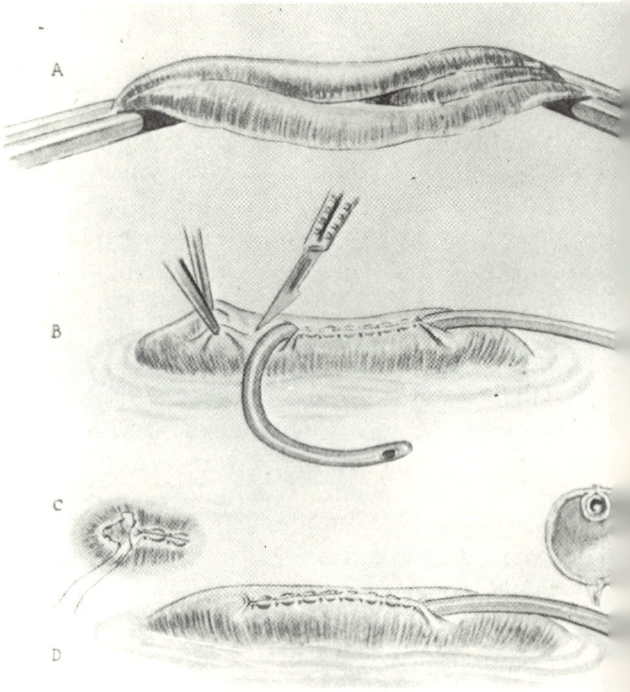

6.6 Adaptation of Witzel enterostomy.

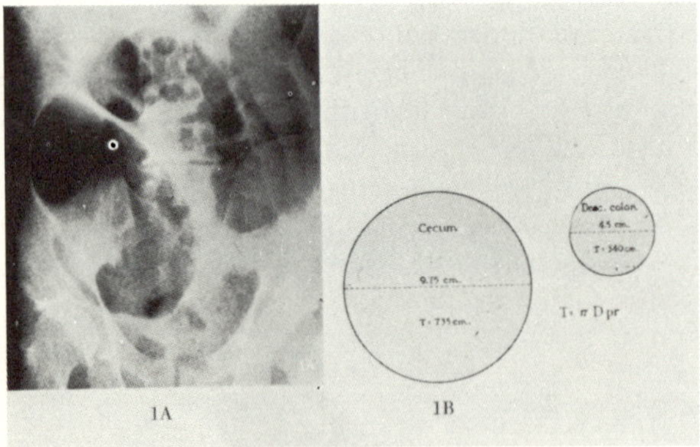

6.7 Differentiating large and small bowel obstructions.

From Wangensteen, *Intestinal obstructions*.

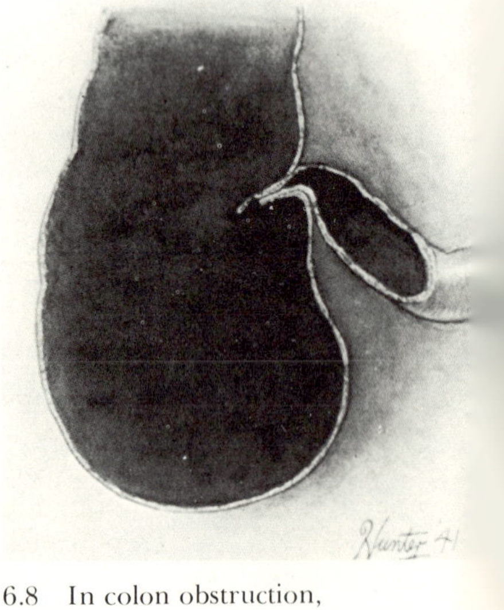

6.8 In colon obstruction, competent ileocecal valve and sphincter create a closed loop in colon.

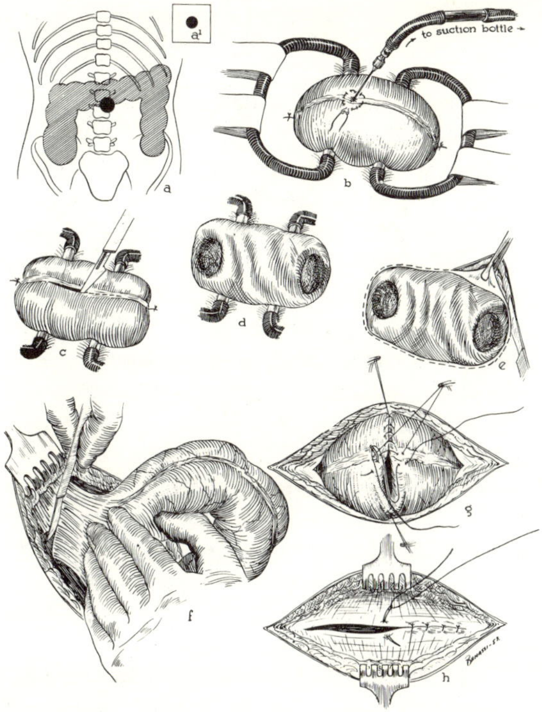

6.9 Technique of temporary colostomy on transverse colon and closure; resection is occasionally needed to reestablish functional continuity.

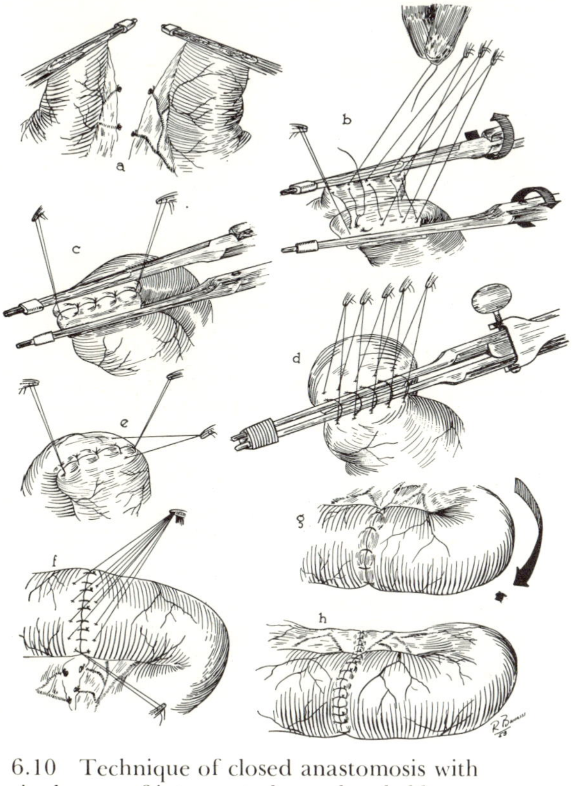

6.10 Technique of closed anastomosis with single row of interrupted nonabsorbable sutures.

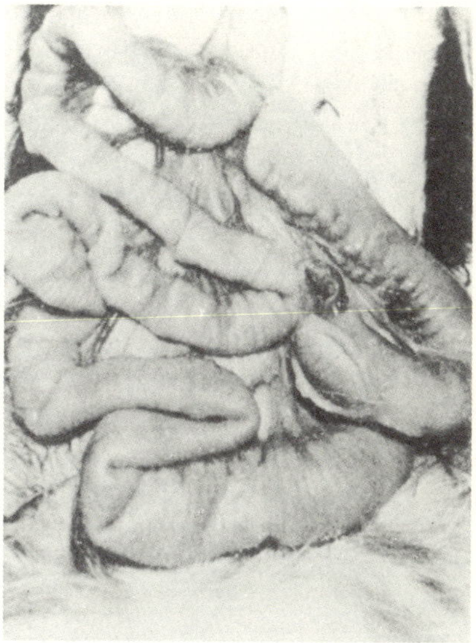

6.11 Cervical esophagostomy with closure of distal end of divided esophagus obviates intestinal distention when distal ileum is obstructed.

From Wangensteen, *Intestinal obstructions.*

In a study of the experience of the University of Pennsylvania Hospital (1940–50), Paul Nemir, Jr. (1952) observed a hospital mortality of 9.6 percent for strangulated hernia and 37.5 percent for patients with gangrene necessitating intestinal resection. Nemir stated that employment of antibiotics in the second five-year study carried no suggestion of improvement in the accomplishment. A more recent report from the same hospital (1962) by Jonathan Rhoads and his associates mentions a mortality of 35 percent for internal strangulations.[81]

J. P. Jarboe and J. H. Pratt from the Mayo Clinic (1947) reported a series of 26 patients with gangrenous femoral hernias demanding excision of bowel; the mortality was 73 percent. In an additional 78 patients in whom the bowel was viable and could be restored to the peritoneal cavity without resection, there were only 5 deaths, a mortality of 6.1 percent. In a small series of 7 strangulated hernias requiring resection, J. Y. Brown of St. Louis (1905) reported only 1 death, a mortality of 14.2 percent, very good indeed for that day. E. C. Saltzstein and colleagues (1962) from the Cook County Hospital in Chicago reported a series of 100 instances of strangulating obstruction necessitating resection. The overall mortality was 41 percent, essentially that of Astley Cooper. In 41 cases of strangulated external hernias, the mortality was 48.8 percent.[82]

The report (1948) of the Clinical Research Committee of the London County Council on patients admitted to several London hospitals for strangulated external hernias indicates that even of those operated upon within 6 hours of the onset of symptoms, 8 percent will require inversion of devitalized areas or intestinal resection. Of those operated upon within 12 hours of onset, 10 percent will need such additional surgery before intraperitoneal replacement of the bowel; within 24 hours, 13 percent; within 48 hours, 30 percent. Beyond 48 hours, 54 percent will require aggressive surgery. The overall mortality for the 336 strangulated hernias was 20.2 percent; for those requiring intestinal resection, 52 percent.[83]

Claude Frankau (1931) made a broad study of the problem of strangulated hernia in Great Britain. The overall mortality of 1,487 patients with strangulated hernia — inguinal, femoral, or umbilical — was 15.6 percent. Among the 99 patients requiring intestinal resection, the mortality was 41.4 percent. J. Englebert Dunphy (1940), in reporting the experience of the Peter Bent Brigham Hospital with strangulated femoral hernia, noted that of 31 patients with obstruction and viable bowel, all survived. Of 20 patients with gangrenous intestine, 50 percent died.[84]

Clarence Dennis and Richard L. Varco (1947) reported only a 10 percent mortality in a small series of operations for strangulated femoral hernia in which the afferent and efferent loops were divided through viable bowel, removing the strangulated segment with the surrounding peritoneal sac intact. This technique harks back to Pipelet's operation in 1740. He dealt successfully in a similar manner with bowel incarcerated below Poupart's ligament, completing the operation by establishing an artificial anus in the wound.[85]

Harbingers of Improved Accomplishment (1930–40)

The 1930s marked the beginning of a new era in the management of intestinal obstruction with the application of suction to indwelling gastroduodenal tubes. When intestinal decompression was achieved in this manner, the risk of peritoneal contamination was nil. The limitations of the method had to be learned. It could be persisted in too long or misapplied to a patient harboring strangulating obstruction.

Gradually the lessons of decompression came to be widely appreciated by the rank and file of surgeons and greatly improved results in acute intestinal obstruction were obtained. By 1940 Leland McKittrick and S. P. Sarris of the Massachusetts General Hospital were able to report a mortality of 20 percent, a third of that of C. L. Scudder from the same institution in 1908 (60 percent), half of that of E. P. Richardson in 1920 (41 percent), and considerably better than that of M. A. McIver in 1932 (44 percent).[86]

The improvement continues. Employing peroral intubation at operation, facilitated by a stylet and a tube containing a coiled spring embedded in its wall, Arnold Leonard and Edlich have been able to achieve a satisfactory decompression quite uniformly without enterostomy or enterotomy. When the bowel is viable and not perforated, the operative risk has been astonishingly low (1 death in 73 successive patients, or 1.4 percent). With the attachment of an inflatable directional fingerlike balloon at the very end of the tube and proximal to the more conventional balloon, Edlich and his colleagues (1967) have been able to intubate the duodenum under fluoroscopy prior to operation even in patients with great distention. When the tube has progressed beyond the duodenojejunal angle, inflation of the balloon attached to the intestinal tube encourages its descent. In this manner, patients with postoperative paralytic ileus have been decompressed without operation, and many with mechanical obstruction come to operation already remarkably well decompressed. Robert L. Goodale (1976) has employed the flexible gastroscope to advance the long intestinal tube through the pylorus and beyond with considerable success.[87]

Success with Congenital Intestinal Atresia

This is the era of the vascular surgeon, in which every surgeon cultivates the art of the jeweler. It is not surprising to hear daily of technical feats that would have been regarded as just short of miraculous a few decades ago. J. H. Louw of Capetown in 1967 reported a mortality of only 3 percent in operations for the correction of congenital atresia.[88]

These successes herald the beginnings of a new day in the management of obstruction of the newborn. Successively surgeons have learned to deal with the challenging problems of great distention and with the intricacies of small-caliber anastomoses. Now they must strive to solve the problem of strangulating obstruction, today's largest factor in the mortality of obstruction.

Role of Antibiotics in Strangulating Obstructions

Over the past twenty years the beneficial effect of antibiotics upon prolongation of life in experimental strangulating obstructions has been emphasized and extolled by a large number of competent investigators. Their writings have prepared the profession to anticipate equally as beneficial effects in patients. In fact, from the reports of Robert Zollinger (1964), Burke Syphax (1965), and their associates, it would appear that the employment of antibiotics has definitely improved the outlook for patients with strangulating obstructions.[89]

It is to be remembered, however, that the clinical situation is rarely, if ever, strictly comparable or analogous to experiments in which the antibiotic therapy can be initiated prior to obstruction and before the devastating effects of tissue devitalization are well in evidence. The patient with strangulation is seen usually after six to ten or more hours have intervened. The nonviable intestinal mucosa is no longer an effective barrier and becomes incapable of performing its normal function of restraining the migration of bacteria and toxic substances through a dead or dying wall into the peritoneal cavity. What is needed under these circumstances is the earliest possible identification of the true nature of the situation with prompt excision of the dead tissue.

Studies of inflammation, in which wounds of guinea pigs are contaminated with bacterial cultures, suggest very definitely that when more than three hours have intervened before systemic or local antibacterial administration is invoked, suppuration cannot be avoided. All studies of wound debridement too indicate that effective wound revision within four hours offers the patient a far better prospect than antibiotic therapy without wound debridement. Strangulating obstruction is essentially a problem of wound revision and debridement. Antibiotics are not to be withheld, but without excision of the devitalized bowel they are useless.

The commonly held view of Cooper's day that strangulation resulted in inflammation has long since been repudiated. In 1840 Malgaigne wrote a review and critique of the surgical management of strangulated hernia. He concluded by sounding a warning to recognize early that grave complication of strangulation, "inflammation."[90] The rise of histological anatomy under the influence of Henle, Rudolf Virchow, and others laid the ghost of that misnomer. Today we must take heed lest our therapy of strangulating obstruction fails to recognize that mucosal necrosis constitutes the fundamental problem and the real threat.

A shift in emphasis in the management of devitalized tissue in strangulating obstruction is, therefore, very much in order. Persistence of dead bowel is synonymous with the presence of a deadly foreign body. All the antibiotics in all the pharmacies of London, New York, and Paris cannot rival the accomplishment of early excision in such situations.

Current reports of experienced and competent surgeons indicate significantly that not only patients but members of our profession, too, are not fully alert to the inherent dangers of strangulated external hernias. One can be certain that the incidence of strangulated hernia with gangrene was greater in Cooper's day than now. His achievement of a hospital mortality of 42 percent compares not unfavorably, however, with current achievement for the late case. There were few if any early cases in Cooper's time: surgeons accepted the responsibility of operating only when it was obvious that death was otherwise inevitable. Progress has been made, in that larger numbers of patients with strangulated hernia now come to operation earlier. Yet, that mortalities not unlike those of Cooper's day continue to be reported in clinics of large experience indicates unequivocally that a new direction of emphasis is in order. Investigators need to bend their efforts to the definition and elaboration of techniques of recognizing internal strangulations within a few hours after hospital entry. For the continuing high mortality of strangulation in external hernias, there is only one explanation: neglect and failure to appreciate the potential seriousness of the situation.

In experiments on intraperitoneal autolysis of tissues in the senior author's laboratory forty years ago it was observed that bacteria-containing tissues like liver and intestine quickly killed the recipient dog, while equal weights of kidney and spleen were well tolerated. When Lester Dragstedt implanted liver from unfed newborn puppies, the autolysis was well borne.[91] That Morgagni in 1761 knew that intestine mortified more quickly than other tissues suffices to indicate what an astute observer he was.[92]

Antibiotics can retard bacterial growth, but it is very unlikely that their administration can significantly slow the death of tissue deprived of its blood supply. This is the vital question in strangulating obstructions. The only way to solve the problem directly is to remove the devitalized bowel as quickly as possible.

The Promising Future for the Treatment of Strangulating Obstructions

As indicated earlier, the increased density of the bowel in venous mesenteric occlusion enables the clinician to recognize this variety of strangulation by the employment of pneumoradiography — the density of the strangulated coils makes them appear as if barium-filled. Echograph techniques undoubtedly too would serve to identify the situation.

The real problem is recognition of arterial mesenteric occlusion in which there is little or no increase in the density of the bowel wall. Peritoneal tap advocated by H. D. Root and associates (1965) in the recognition of threatening situations attending abdominal trauma could prove helpful too in identifying the presence of a segment of gut deprived of its arterial blood supply. Root concluded that peritoneal cell counts in excess of 200 leucocytes per ml. on uncentrifuged specimens indicated a serious peritoneal insult.[93]

Ghanem and Goodale (1970) noted that when the arterial blood supply to short or long segments of gut in the dog, rat, or mouse is interrupted surprisingly high peritoneal leucocyte counts are observed in the peritoneal fluid within six to eight hours; on the contrary, leucocyte counts of the peripheral blood, both capillary and venous, exhibit only modest increases. This marked contrast between the high peritoneal leucocytosis and the fairly normal counts in the peripheral blood is virtually diagnostic of strangulating obstruction in the presence of intestinal colic. Conrad Jenson and Grafton Smith (1956) in the senior author's clinic had urged peritoneal tap for the recognition of internal strangulating obstructions. The studies of E. Amundsen (1963), W. O. Barnett (1958), Isidore Cohn (1961), C. E. Yale (1963), and many others suggest that collection of the intraperitoneal fluid in such instances may be adapted as a diagnostic tool by injections into the peritoneal cavities of mice.[94] The search for evidence of identifiable early radiographic changes in the mucosal pattern attending mesenteric arterial occlusions in dogs with Thiry fistulas also may prove helpful.

The management of acute intestinal obstruction is essentially a team-effort responsibility. Success with conservative decompression demands that the team have an enthusiastic and experienced intestinal intubator. In fact, the Minnesota experience showed that it was feasible to decompress many distended patients with virtually complete obstructions of the small intestine quite effectively prior to operation. One cannot know how the bowel is obstructed; in consequence, operation is necessary. At such operations, the bowel, in most instances, is found empty and quite well decompressed save for a few distended loops just proximal to the obstructing agent. Moreover, at operation, inlying catheters can invariably be quickly advanced to decompress completely any remaining distended coils, thus making it possible to deal directly with the obstructing agent.

Attending the performance of enterostomy for high-grade obstruction of the small intestine, measurements of fluid and gas escape demonstrated that, following the initial large output of both, the external drainage of gas and fluid often declined sharply, indicating that functional continuity of the intestinal stream had been reestablished. The persistence of large amounts of fluid drainage through the enterostomy catheter suggests definitely that the obstructing agency is still operative. These were the observations that led to the trial of suction applied to an inlying duodenal tube in the senior author's clinic (1931) in effecting decompression. It was the expertise of Leonard and Edlich in extending the techniques of intestinal intubation that made it possible to decompress the distended small bowel effectively prior to or at operation and without recourse to external drainage.

Plainly, the next step is an all-out attack on the discouraging problem of strangulating obstructions. Only early detection followed by immediate intervention can provide a satisfactory answer. The surgeon must constantly bear in mind that in grave abdominal emergencies the situation is comparable to that of a drowning man. He is brought to shore; it is not the proper time for a swimming lesson. In 1930 the death rate of intestinal obstruction per 100,000 population was 10; in 1951, 6; in 1972, 3.3, which figure also includes operations for hernia without obstruction. The gains represent a notable achievement; when, however, the public and our profession become fully alert to the urgent necessity of interfering surgically in all strangulating varieties of bowel obstruction, there is good reason to believe that the present mortality could be halved. We know what the problem is, and how to solve it, but we have to address ourselves with determination to resolve it.

Obstruction of the Vermiform Appendix

In 1812 John Parkinson of London reported perforation of the appendix distal to a fecalith in a postmortem examination on a boy of five years of age. Adolph Volz (1846), of a German village near Munich, observed perforation of the appendix, which he attributed to obstruction by a fecalith within the appendical lumen. Fitz (1886) described the entity as an inflammatory lesion, calling the sequence of events leading to perforation "appendicitis."[95]

In a monograph of 1930 Ludwig Aschoff of Freiburg stated that appendicitis was essentially an inflammatory lesion occasioned by the streptococcus type B of Gundel.[96] The senior author and associates, skeptical of such an explanation and favoring a mechanical origin, began a systematic study in a number of animals. It had been generally presumed that the appendix, attached to the cecum, was poised toward absorption of its fluid content rather than toward secretion.

Every premise must be tested to establish its validity. One of the first animals examined was the rabbit. When its vermiform appendix was ligated at the juncture with the cecum, nothing happened; when, however, the base of the vermiform appendix, very like its human counterpart, was ligated, perforation distal to the site of ligation occurred in 70 percent of instances within ten hours. A large number of animals, including monkeys and baboons, were tested without encountering anything like what happened in the rabbit, but when the base of the appendix was ligated in the chimpanzee the situation observed in the rabbit was duplicated, with observed intraluminal pressures exceeding diastolic blood pressure. In that era the conventional operation for cancer of the colon was the Bloch-Mikulicz exteriorization procedure, a circumstance that provided an opportunity to exteriorize the appendix also. In twenty-two such clinical situations, largely in elderly people, the appendix appeared grossly normal in fifteen. In all fifteen of these patients temporary ligature of the base of the appendix over a twenty-four-hour period of observation, followed by excision of the appendix, was attended by secretory pressures in excess of diastolic blood pressure; these observations elicited useful information and without harm to any patient. In rabbit, chimpanzee, and man, a polymorphonuclear exudate appeared in the lumen as well as in the appendical wall, very much like the histologic picture of spontaneous appendicitis in man.[97]

The distended appearance of the obstructed appendix with its accompanying thin wall, a constant finding in appendical perforation, attests to the circumstance that perforation is not primarily an inflammatory lesion but an obstructive lesion. In fact, the intraluminal pressures found in the presence of obstruction are the highest secretory pressures observed in man.

In 1736 Claudius Amyand, a surgeon at St. George's Hospital, operating for a scrotal hernia accompanied by a fecal fistula, found that the latter was owing to perforation of the appendix by a pin lodged in its lumen. He excised the appendix, repaired the hernia, and the patient recovered. This and F. F. Mestivier's postmortem account (1759) of an encrusted pin lodged in the appendix with perforation were probably responsible for the emphasis upon foreign bodies in the genesis of appendicitis by Fitz and others.[98]

In 1843 Willard Parker of New York City evacuated an appendical abscess successfully through the abdominal wall. He reported this and two additional cases, also with recovery, in 1866.[99] There is no indication that he removed the appendix in any instance.

Excision of the obstructed appendix as the primary operation did not become standard procedure until its advocacy by Charles McBurney of the Roosevelt Hospital in New York (1889). As late as 1902, just a few days before Treves operated upon Edward VII, who was awaiting coronation, Treves stated that there is no disease in the appendix until the peritoneum is involved and advised that operation be delayed five days after onset of the attack, except in "ultra-acute" cases. This was the practice he followed with King Edward, successfully draining an abscess following rupture of the appendix.[100]

In 1930 the death rate from appendicitis was in excess of 15 deaths per 100,000 population in the vital statistics of the United States. For several years now it has been 0.7, a truly remarkable achievement. The impressive reduction in the mortality rate for appendicitis since the preceding studies were undertaken four decades ago was occasioned obviously by the general acceptance of early operative intervention, advances in anesthesia, better trained surgeons, much improved postoperative care, and an awareness of the great hazards of an obstructed appendix.

In 1935 appendectomy ranked as the fifteenth most important cause of death in the United States, accounting for 16,142 deaths. Among policyholders of the Metropolitan Life Insurance Company, appendicitis was the ninth most frequent cause of death. In 1973, with a greatly increased population in our country, 1,066 deaths were reported from appendicitis. If surgeons followed the practice of obstetricians in New England, who examine carefully and critically every maternal death at delivery, the current mortality of appendicitis would also progressively decrease.[101]

In 1952 R. W. Toon observed that when antibiotics were administered to rabbits attending ligature of the base of the cecal appendage, neither the incidence of perforation nor the volume secreted was diminished, yet death from peritonitis was greatly decreased in the treated rabbits.[102]

Summary

The acceptance of operative management of acute intestinal obstruction traces back to Franco (1556), who, like the Greek surgeon Praxagoras (born about 340 B.C.), operated for strangulated hernia by establishing an external fistula at the site of the necrotic bowel. Throughout the eighteenth century a number of French surgeons operated successfully for internal strangulations, excising the dead bowel and establishing a temporary external fistula, restoring intestinal continuity secondarily by uniting the adjacent intestinal orifices. Despite these achievements operation for bowel obstruction actually did not catch on until near the end of the nineteenth century. Mortalities of 40 to 65 percent were usual through the first three decades of this century. Several observers reported that the diagnosis was difficult to establish, overlooking the circumstance that *intestinal colic* is a constant concomitant and pathognomonic occurrence in bowel obstruction. Additionally, differentiation between obstruction of the small and large bowel on the basis of symptoms had been badly confused, most holding the feculent vomiting was a sign of obstruction of the colon, unwilling to believe what they saw, but accepting what prior authorities had proclaimed.

With the elaboration of effective and safe operative techniques and the development of new nonoperative methods of decompressing the distended and obstructed bowel, the mortality of intestinal obstruction has diminished considerably. The mortality of congenital intestinal atresia, once almost uniformly fatal, in practiced hands today is in the area of 3 to 5 percent. Strangulating obstruction with loss of intestinal viability remains today the main challenge. Satisfactory methods for recognition of both venous and arterial mesenteric occlusion are available. A high level of clinical suspicion should evoke their use early enough to ensure favorable outcomes where failure has long been the rule.

Reliance upon antibiotics to control the threat of transperitoneal bacterial migration from dead and dying intestinal mucosa is irrational, a measure of delay that courts disaster. Excision is plainly indicated. When early recognition of strangulating obstruction is followed by immediate operation, the last barrier to improved accomplishment with the bowel problem will have been removed. In surgical clinics professing keen interest in the management of bowel obstruction, with acceptance of the responsibility as a team effort, the current overall mortality does not exceed 5 percent.

Obstruction of the lumen of the appendix by a fecalith is the usual cause of perforation or gangrene of the appendix. The extraordinary secretory capacity of the appendix in rabbit, chimpanzee, and man was demonstrated in the 1930s. Obstruction, not inflammation, is the responsible causative factor in perforation and mortality in appendicitis. A 97 percent reduction in its mortality has occurred over the past four decades in the United States; a residual annual mortality of approximately 1,400 lives still persists that can only be whittled down by continued critical adjudication of the cause of death in fatal cases. Such periodic assessments in local medical journals will create an atmosphere of alertness that is bound to affect the issue for the better.

(For notes, see pp. 611–20.)

CHAPTER 7

Gastric Surgery

The first operations performed upon the stomach concerned closure of penetrating injuries and the removal of accidentally swallowed sharp objects that threatened perforation of the gastric wall. Surgeons' efforts were not rewarded in elective surgery of the three body cavities — abdomen, thorax, and calvarium — until a prophylactic program of antisepsis was developed. Many have puzzled over McDowell's good fortune in achieving the first successful ovariotomy in 1809 and a succession of three favorable outcomes at the time of his publication (1817).[1] The first successful elective gastric operation was Billroth's partial resection for gastric cancer in February 1881.

Gastric Wounds

Toward the end of the sixteenth century Johann Schenck of Bohemia reported a recent instance of recovery from a gastric fistula caused by a spear in a hunting accident. The victim kept the fistula reasonably dry with linen cloth. Schenck described another case in which the wound finally closed spontaneously. Several similar lesions with fortunate outcomes were remarked by a succession of observers over the next two centuries.

In 1767 Nolleson *le fils* treated a Palatinate soldier whose stomach had been opened by a saber cut in the left hypochondrium. The patient was conveyed to a hospital in a "nearly hopeless state." The gastric wound was closed by suture, and the external wound was covered with wine dressings. The soldier was bled nine times in the next three days; even so, he recovered.[2]

Gastrotomy for Removal of Foreign Bodies

A peasant knife-swallower in Prague used to entertain his audiences by pulling a concealed knife from his gullet after quaffing a large stein of beer. His trick was to pass a nine-inch-long knife, handle first, down his gullet, withdrawing it by seizing the blade. During a performance in 1602 the knife descended into the lower reaches of the esophagus beyond the exhibitionist's grasp; when the beer was drunk, the knife slid into his stomach. There it remained for seven weeks until removed through an incision by the barber-surgeon Florian Matthis of Brandenburg. A complete report of the event, one of the first authenticated removals of a foreign body by gastrotomy, was made in 1609.[3]

A somewhat similar situation was reported in 1640 by Daniel Becker, professor of medicine in Königsberg. Andreas Grünheide, residing in a nearby town, awoke one morning feel-

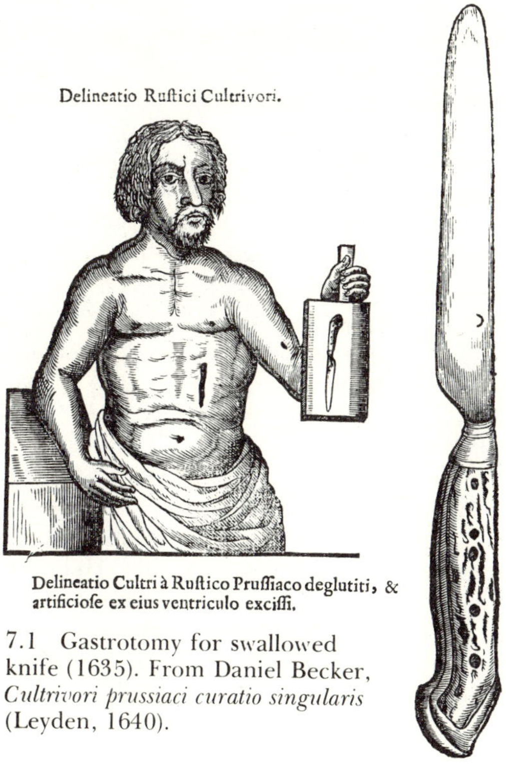

7.1 Gastrotomy for swallowed knife (1635). From Daniel Becker, *Cultrivori prussiaci curatio singularis* (Leyden, 1640).

ing nauseous. To provoke vomiting, he tickled his throat with the shaft of a long knife; the blade slipped from his fingers and the knife descended into the lower esophagus. Grünheide stood on his head but to no avail. To moisten his throat, he took a drink of beer, whereupon the knife slid into his stomach. Becker brought his patient to Königsberg for consultation with the entire Medical College. The decision to remove the knife by incision was agreed upon, and the operation was performed on July 9, 1635, by Daniel Schwabe, a wound and lithotomy surgeon, in the presence of Becker and other local physicians. The patient was bound to a board and the site selected for the incision over the palpable point of the swallowed knife was marked with charcoal. On its withdrawal, Grünheide joyfully announced it was his knife. The gastric wound was closed and the patient recovered completely, returning to his farm work; he married in 1641.[4]

A previously unpublished account of an 1819 gastrotomy was reported by Pierre Huard and M.-J. Imbault-Huart in 1971. It concerned a twenty-four-year-old French woman who inserted a silver fork into her throat to induce vomiting. The fork escaped her fingers and slid into her stomach. For five months she was asymptomatic, then periodic distress developed and a tender abdominal mass could be felt. The well-known Montpellier surgeon Delpech was summoned and advised gastrotomy. The abdomen was opened by Cayroche of Monde on May 1, 1819, while three servants restrained the patient. The prongs of the swallowed fork were embedded in the gastric wall. When disengaged, the fork came away readily and the patient recovered completely.[5]

In 1886 Benno Credé published an account of twenty-six foreign bodies removed from the stomach by gastrotomies, crediting the Becker account (1640) as the first authentic case. The other twenty-five instances occurred in the nineteenth century, and most of the patients were salvaged by operation.[6]

Gastrotomy Studies of Patients with Gastric Fistula

In 1803 Jacob Helm of Vienna studied gastric digestion in a patient, Mrs. Theresia Perzin, aged fifty-six, whose gastric perforation led to a persistent gastric fistula. Helm's observations confirmed Spallanzani's earlier experiments upon a number of animals in which he established the digestive power of gastric juice. Helm's investigations, the first such in a human being, contributed no new information.[7]

Beaumont's observations (1833) upon Alexis St. Martin rank

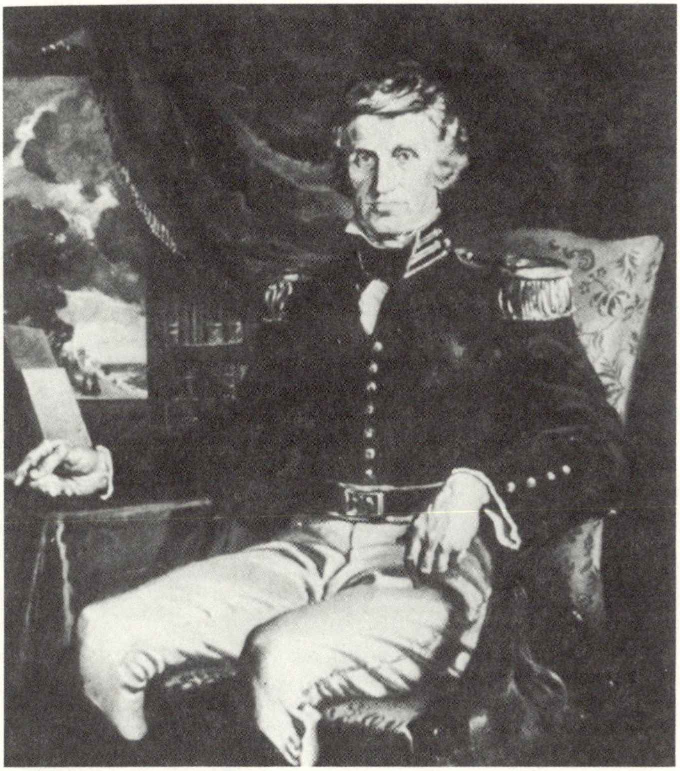

7.2 William Beaumont (1785–1853), pioneer American army surgeon in military outposts, conducted basic studies of gastric secretion in fistulous patient.

among America's finest contributions to medicine. The subject was a Canadian voyageur who suffered a persistent gastric fistula from a shotgun blast, June 6, 1822, on Mackinac Island, an American military outpost in the straits of Lake Huron. Most of Beaumont's studies on his patient were actually made after 1825 when stationed at Fort Crawford in Prairie du Chien, Wisconsin. He correctly concluded that the gastric juice in St. Martin's stomach contained a "chemical principle" other than hydrochloric acid (conclusion #24). Equally important was Beaumont's observation that the empty stomach was achlorhydric; it needed the stimulus of food to elicit secretion of gastric juice (conclusion #25), an observation not appreciated by clinicians until well into the twentieth century.[8]

On reading Beaumont's 1833 historic monograph Johannes Müller and Theodor Schwann (1836) of Berlin boiled a sample of gastric juice and noted a loss of proteolytic quality, verifying

Beaumont's conclusion #24 that gastric juice contained a "chemical principle" other than hydrochloric acid. Schwann named the ferment "pepsin," recognizing that in the Hippocratic writings the term "pepsis" indicated the "cooking" activity of the stomach upon food.[9]

It is of more than passing interest that Dragstedt, who was certainly the greatest among surgical students of peptic ulcer, suggested (1936) deleting the qualifying adjective "peptic" in describing ulcer, indicating that the more proper designation should be "acid ulcer." Donald Ferguson (1950) showed that perfusion of the cat's esophagus with gastric juice obtained from patients with duodenal ulcer caused the cat's esophagus to perforate regularly within two hours and occasionally within twenty minutes. On the contrary, perfusion of the cat's esophagus with 0.10 normal hydrochloric acid caused only slight reddening. In 1958 it was shown by Root and associates that when the cat and the perfused gastric juice were cooled, the proteolytic effect of the warm gastric juice was missing.[10]

A number of investigators have studied gastric secretion upon fistulous subjects since Beaumont — notably Otto Gruenewaldt (1853), A. J. Carlson (1912–15) upon his subject Fred Vlcek, and Stewart G. Wolf and Harold G. Wolff upon Tom Little (1943) — studies well known to all students of gastric secretion.[11]

Gastrostomy

The operation gastrostomy was used to study gastric secretion in sheep by the Paris physiologist Pierre Flourens (1832), who opened the rumen, reticulum, and omasum in successive experiments. He was interested in the phenomenon of rumination of quadrupeds and noted forceful gastric contractions when he introduced his finger in the various pouches; these contractions were inhibited by vagotomy but not by division of the lower thoracic spinal cord.[12]

The surgeon Nicolas Blondlot of Nancy helped the physician Henri Braconnot (1835) recover gastric juice from dogs that had swallowed sponges with attached strings. Braconnot correctly concluded the the juice contained hydrochloric acid. Eight years later Blondlot made gastric fistulas in dogs and found that the gastric acid was phosphoric.[13] He obviously failed to observe the advice of Beaumont that the gastric mucosa needed the stimulus of food to secrete. Today clinicians are aware that the presence of free hydrochloric acid with a low pH in a fasting stomach suggests that the patient may have a duodenal ulcer.

The Russian physiologist Wassili Bassow (1843) made gastrostomies upon dogs to explore the clinical promise of the operation. In making a canine gastrostomy H. Adolf Bardeleben (1849) of Berlin divided the cervical esophagus to prevent swallowed saliva from entering the stomach. His observations made no contribution to the physiology of gastric secretion. At a meeting of the Christiania (now Oslo) Medical Society on May 8, 1837, the Norwegian surgeon C. A. Egeberg made the suggestion of performing gastrostomy upon a patient having difficulty in swallowing. Sédillot of Strasbourg (1849) was the first to perform gastrostomy upon a human being. The operation was done to relieve a patient with increasing difficulty in swallowing — for the past three months he had been able to take only liquids and was declining rapidly. The patient survived the operation less than twenty-four hours; the lesion was described as epithelial cancer of the esophagus at autopsy.[14] The first successful gastrostomy was made by Aristide Verneuil (1876) in a boy of seventeen with a lye stricture of the esophagus. The Paris physiologist Charles Richet (1878) used Verneuil's patient for studies of gastric secretion. K. G. Lennander (1908) reported a successful gastrostomy in the management of acute gastric dilatation accompanying perforation of peptic ulcer.[15]

Gastric Cancer

Billroth (1829–94), the founder of gastric surgery, was the most innovative visceral surgeon of his day. Son of a German father and a Swedish mother, he was born on the Baltic island of Rügen. Following education in Berlin, Billroth became an assistant in Langenbeck's clinic, then professor of surgery in Zürich in 1860. He declined professorships in Rostock and Heidelberg, but in 1867 he received an invitation to the professorship in Vienna, a professional opportunity he could not refuse. Billroth was, at forty-one, already an international figure in surgery. The surgical school which he built in Vienna continued, with creative and productive pupils, until Hitler's destructive invasion. Billroth was certainly the greatest surgical teacher of the nineteenth century and ranks among the finest ever. His love of music, his friendship with Brahms, and his other cultural interests revealed in his prolific correspondence show how happily he was attuned to the life of Vienna in its heyday.[16]

A keen surgical pathologist and microscopist and a self-taught microbiologist, Billroth did not capitulate completely to the germ theory of disease until after Koch's publications on the life

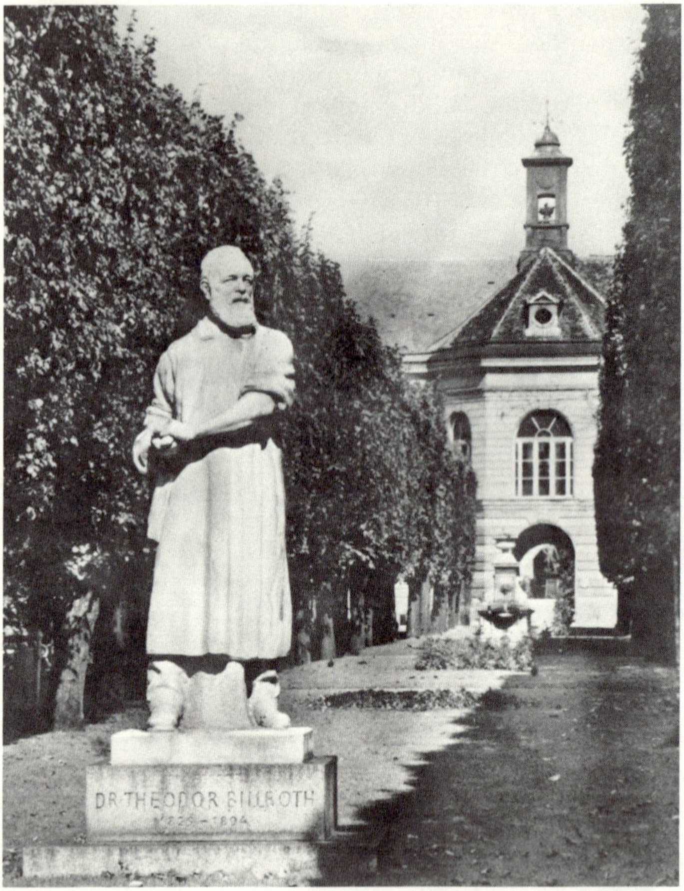

7.3 Theodor Billroth (1829–94), famous Vienna surgeon, first to operate successfully for gastric cancer (1881). Statue in garden, Allgemeines Krankenhaus, Vienna.

story of anthrax (1876) and the pathogenicity of bacteria (1878). After sending his pupils Anton Wölfler and, subsequently, Mikulicz to Lister's clinics in Edinburgh and London, Billroth was persuaded to give Lister's practices a try. In his early Vienna period he and Vincenz Czerny had worked out on dogs techniques for resection of the cervical esophagus and excision of the larynx. In 1874 Carl Gussenbauer and Alexander Winiwarter in Billroth's laboratory devised a technique for gastric resection. By 1876 they had developed what has come to be known as the Billroth I distal gastric resection with a gastroduodenal anastomosis. Two of their seven dogs survived for a long period of time. When sacrificed eight months after operation, one of these had anastomotic neostomal ulcers; two of the seven died of suture leakage.[17]

Billroth, now a convert to Listerian practices, save for omission of the carbolic spray, was ready for a surgical attack upon gastric cancer. He knew that J. E. Péan of Paris (1879) and Ludwik Rydygier (1880) of Culm had made such attempts unsuccessfully, their patients dying of suture leakage. Billroth's historic operation was performed on January 29, 1881, and was announced in print six days later in a letter addressed to the editor of *Wiener medizinische Wochenschrift*.[18] Billroth obviously appreciated the importance of the achievement, but his patient, Therese Heller, died of residual cancer in less than four months. Herbert Ziegler (1939), who studied the hospital record, found that an hour was consumed preoperatively in washing out the patient's stomach until the contents returned clear. Chloroform anesthesia was administered by a surgical assistant.

Billroth made a high transverse incision, 11 cm. in length; in subsequent gastrectomies he usually employed a vertical incision. The patient's abdominal wall was very thin. A few metastatic lymph nodes were encountered, one of which on section revealed the presence of medullary cancer. The duodenum was divided 1.5 cm. distal to the tumor through normal tissue, and so similarly proximally on the gastric side. Billroth closed the lower segment of the divided stomach with carbolized silk sutures, effecting a gastroduodenal anastomosis at the lesser curvature. The sutures included the entire gastric wall except the mucosa. He made a serosal approximation, tying the interrupted sutures only after the approximated wound edges were inverted; twenty-one sutures approximated the edges of the gastric wound not employed in the anastomosis; thirty-three sutures were used to effect the anastomosis. Frau Heller had a hurried pulse, accompanied by fever of 102° F, but by the third postoperative day she was doing extremely well and eating. The wound showed no reaction on the sixth day and the cutaneous sutures were removed; the patient left the hospital twenty-two days after operation. Following Heller's death on May 24, 1881, Heschl, a pupil of Carl Rokitansky, performed the autopsy, apparently in the house where the patient died, and removed the residual stomach.

Within eleven months following Billroth's first operation, according to Ziegler, twenty-one such operations had been done, and by 1890 there had been forty-one gastric resections in the Billroth clinic with nineteen operative successes. Two years after Billroth's death Hans Haberkant of Danzig (1896) re-

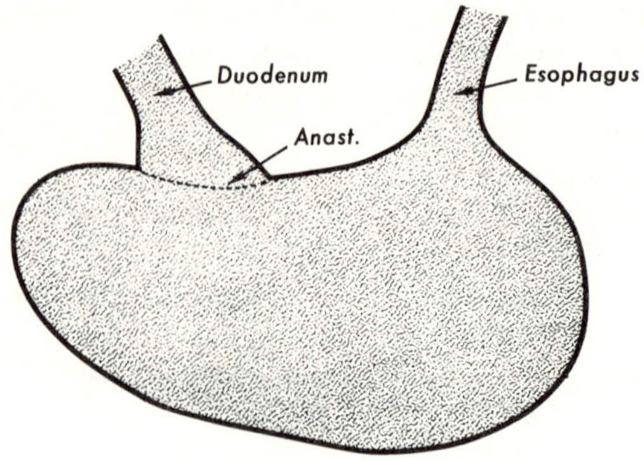

7.4 Therese Heller's residual stomach at autopsy, four months after operation. Redrawn from Herbert Ziegler, "Billroths erste Magenresektion," *Krebsarzt* (1949), 4:49–59.

ported that a total of 257 resections had been performed for gastric cancer with an operative mortality of 54.4 percent.[19]

The first successful total excision of the stomach for cancer was performed by the Swiss surgeon Carl Schlatter (1897), who anastomosed the divided esophagus end-to-side to the jejunum. C. B. Brigham (1898) did the first successful total gastrectomy in America. The patient survived more than eighteen years, dying of unrelated causes, a circumstance that throws considerable doubt on the completeness of the excision, for it is well documented that survival of more than three years following total gastrectomy, before the availability of vitamin B_{12}, was, indeed, most unusual.[20]

In 1810 Daniel Merrem, a staff surgeon in the Westphalian Army Corps, published a Latin account of three pylorectomies upon dogs. He apparently removed the pyloric sphincter and a very short segment of duodenum and stomach on either side. In the anastomosis Merrem employed very few sutures, making a substantial inversion of tissue. Two of the dogs survived the operation for different periods of time.

Merrem ascribed earlier attempts at experimental pylorectomy to a "very distinguished teacher" in Philadelphia who had performed such operations unsuccessfully on dogs and a rabbit two years before Merrem's exploit. Merrem does not name the professor but states that he was once "first physician to the Hessian auxiliaries." In a Hunterian Lecture at the Royal College of Surgeons in 1927, J. M. T. Finney mentioned Merrem's publication of 1810 and pursued the inquiry concerning the identity of

Merrem's famous American professor. After studying with great care the record of John Jones during his term as professor of surgery at King's College, New York, Finney concluded that Jones, a Philadelphian, was the unknown from whom Merrem obtained the suggestion that pylorectomy was feasible. Owsei Temkin, who translated the experimental data in Merrem's Latin thesis of 1810, concluded (1960) that Merrem's incentive came from Christian Friedrich Michaelis, professor of surgery at the University of Marburg, who had been in Philadelphia with the Hessian troops.[21]

William H. Welch in 1885 wrote very discouragingly of surgery for gastric cancer, indicating that there were no reported cures, even though Billroth's surgical success had "made a great sensation in the medical world."[22] One of the real problems, obviously, was late diagnosis. Theodor Storm, a German poet who died of gastric cancer in 1888, wrote of his difficulty in a poem entitled "Beginn des Endes." The three stanzas of four lines each may be summarized in a few words: "It is a prick; it is nothing; it is too late."

Observations with incomplete excision suggest that the silent interval for gastric cancer, before reassertion of symptoms, is in the area of two years. W. C. Roentgen's great discovery was first announced in 1895, but clinical application of x-rays for diagnosis of gastric lesions did not come until about 1910. Walter B. Cannon's physiologic studies upon the upper alimentary tract appeared at the turn of the century.[23] Surgeons of the first five decades of this century spent their professional lives on the wrong side of the gastric cancer woodpile. Fresh cases were pouring in daily, but only late symptomatic cases were recognized. Expert roentgenologists readily detected polypoid and infiltrative lesions that caused a defect in the gastric wall, but they only rarely recognized mucosal gastric cancers. The Japanese development of more precise techniques of gastroradiography accompanied by gastroscopy changed all this for the better.

Over the past three decades there has been a great decline in incidence of observed gastric cancer in the United States and in Scandinavia, but not in Japan, Chile, or Iceland. Approximately 25 percent of patients operated upon in gastric surgical clinics in Japan have mucosal gastric cancer. Instead of filling the patient's stomach with barium as their American counterparts were accustomed to do, the Japanese radiologists give the patient to swallow not more than 2 ounces of barium, with a sticking quality promoting ready adherence to the mucosal folds; 200 ml. of air is injected into the stomach through a nasal tube before the examination begins. All patients with the slightest suggestion of a suspicious lesion are subjected to gastroscopy. A five-year survival rate of 25 percent is commonplace in Japanese clinics. The best the senior author's clinic was able to achieve was a 17 percent survival of all gastric cancer patients, 604 cases, observed over a nine-year interval (1950–58), a modest accomplishment that certainly could be greatly improved upon with today's tools.[24]

Early Experimental Vagotomy Studies

In 1814 Brodie noticed that the mucosa of the empty stomach was dry a few hours after bilateral vagal section. F. H. Bidder and Carl Schmidt (1852) observed that sight and smell of food excited gastric secretion. Moritz Schiff (1867) found that dogs remained in good health and nutrition after bilateral subdiaphragmatic vagal section.[25]

Rudolf Heidenhain of Breslau was the first experimentalist to employ Listerian principles in canine surgery. His isolated denervated gastric pouches initiated scientific experimental studies of gastric secretion.[26] A dozen years later Ivan Pavlov, Heidenhain's great Russian pupil, made innervated gastric pouches upon which Pavlov and his colleagues Mme. E. Schumova-Simanovskaja (1889) and N. P. Jurgens (1892) assessed the effect of truncal vagotomy; Pavlov recognized cephalic, gastric, and intestinal phases of gastric secretion. The work of the Pavlov School, for which Pavlov was awarded the Nobel Prize in 1904, is the finest in the literature of the subject.[27]

Before the dawn of the twentieth century there was a well-established rationale for the performance of vagotomy for peptic ulcer. Karl Schwarz (1910) said "no acid, no ulcer," an expression that became dogma for clinicians;[28] however, as already pointed out, the digestive power of gastric juice is completely dependent upon pepsin, a digestive enzyme with great proteolytic power.

Early Clinical Trials with Vagotomy

By the second decade of this century European surgeons had begun invoking division of the vagal trunks above as well as below the diaphragm for a variety of conditions with gastric symptoms. Eugen Bircher (1920) of Aarau, Switzerland, performed incomplete subdiaphragmatic vagotomy for twenty such patients; in 1931 he reported that most of them remained well.

In a small monograph (1925) he pictured and described selective vagotomy of the gastric fundus, a procedure revived in recent years and currently performed as the vagal interruption of choice in many clinics.[29]

André Latarjet of Lyons (1922, 1923) performed truncal vagotomy either above or below the diaphragm; of twenty-four vagotomized patients, six had duodenal ulcer. Noting that division of both vagal trunks interfered with gastric emptying, Latarjet added gastrojejunostomy to correct the situation.[30]

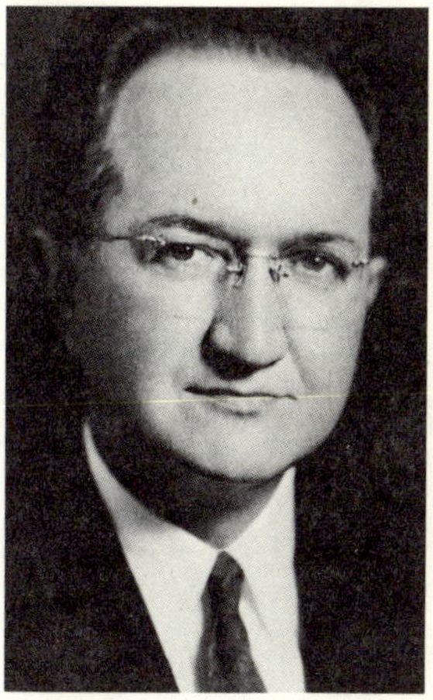

7.5 Lester R. Dragstedt (1893–1975) reinvoked vagotomy for duodenal ulcer (1943).

Twenty-five years later Dragstedt and Frederick M. Owens (1943) reported supradiaphragmatic vagotomy for duodenal ulcer, noting, as did Latarjet, that vagal division occasioned gastric retention; Dragstedt reverted to the abdominal approach, adding a complemental gastrojejunostomy.[31] Dragstedt, trained as a physiologist, has left a very durable impress upon the role of vagotomy in the surgery of peptic ulcer.

Strangely enough, gastric resection for duodenal ulcer had by the 1940s found such wide acceptance universally that it was not to be readily pushed aside. A committee of the American Gastroenterological Association (1952) had divided opinions on the merits of vagotomy for duodenal ulcer. It was A. V. Pollock (1952) of Leeds who saved the day for vagotomy. In a careful follow-up study of 589 patients operated upon for peptic ulcer in the Yorkshire area, he observed an incidence of neostomal ulcer in only 3 percent of the cases, a study that lent vagotomy a much needed lift.[32]

Well-controlled clinical trials are necessary to reaffirm suggestions pointed up by experimental laboratory data. Duodenal ulcer remains the physician's as well as the surgeon's greatest challenge in control of the peptic ulcer diathesis. Today most gastric surgeons invoke vagotomy as an integral part of their operations for duodenal ulcer.

John C. Goligher, D. Johnston, and their Leeds colleagues have recently reported upon twenty-one patients who underwent highly selective vagotomy for duodenal ulcer over a variable period extending up to six and a half years; periodically all were subjected to insulin testing. All responded negatively shortly after operation; a year later 62 percent of responses to insulin stimulation were positive, with a demonstrable slight increase in acid secretion; 90 percent eventually responded positively, but recurrent ulcer was observed in only one of the patients (4.76 percent), a recurrence rate that compares favorably with results in truncal vagotomy.[33]

Some surgeons favor vagotomy and antral excision; many

electing highly selective vagotomy of the gastric fundus find it unnecessary to perform a drainage operation. Over the past decade truncal vagotomy and pyloroplasty have been the most popular combination of operative procedures for duodenal ulcer. Alton Ochsner (1970) of New Orleans and Leslie Wise and Walter F. Ballinger (1974) of St. Louis are among a few continuing to advise extended gastrectomy for duodenal ulcer, the operation of choice three decades ago.[34]

Gastric Ulcer

No discussion of chronic gastric ulcer is complete without considering the possibility that the defect may be cancerous. For high-lying defects on the lesser curvature, some surgeons elect to perform the Madlener operation, resecting the stomach distal to the defect, reasoning that such is the logic of gastric resection for duodenal ulcer. Those partial to the Madlener operation for high-lying gastric ulcer have not infrequently discovered to their sorrow that the defect later proved to be malignant. With adequate exposure it is not technically difficult to excise a paraesophageal-lying gastric ulcer; the excision and anastomosis produce a gooseneck-like but very functional esophagogastric juncture. The entire acid peptic area of the stomach in such instances should be sacrificed to thwart the occurrence of acid-peptic esophagitis.[35]

Gastrojejunostomy and Pyloroplasty for Duodenal Ulcer

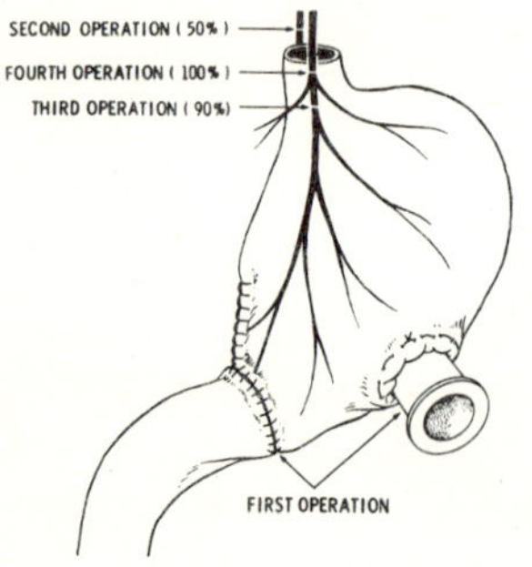

7.6 Kemp's canine experiments evaluating completeness of vagotomy. From Donald R. Kemp, "Effect of progressive vagal section on the stimulated output of gastric juice," *Austral. & N. Z. J. Surg.* (1973), 43:295.

Once very popular in America and Britain for duodenal ulcer, gastrojejunostomy and pyloroplasty were outmoded in the late 1920s. Richard Lewisohn (1925) of Mount Sinai Hospital, New York, reported that the observed incidence of neostomal ulcer following gastrojejunostomy for duodenal ulcer was 34 percent. Moynihan (1932) was still defending the procedure toward the end of his professional career, indicating that among 1,000 such operations for duodenal ulcer he had lost only one patient; the incidence of neostomal ulcer was 1.8 percent. Moynihan obviously used up much luck![36] Patient follow-ups are more thorough today.

H. Schmilinsky (1918) undertook to effect total intragastric regurgitation of the content of the proximal duodenojejunal loop, describing the procedure as an internal pharmacy. The operation proved to be a complete failure in that it provoked a continuous stimulus for the gastric phase of gastric secretion, attended by a very high incidence of neostomal ulcer.[37]

Billroth Resections for Duodenal Ulcer

Hans Haberer, a professor of surgery at Cologne, long the keenest exponent of the Billroth I resection (gastroduodenostomy), gave it up in 1939 because of the high incidence of neostomal ulcer. The lesson had to be relearned several years later. N. B. Ordahl and associates at two Boston Veterans Hospitals (1955) announced an 18 percent incidence of neostomal ulcer; Goligher's observed incidence was 17 percent, and Sten Wallensten of Ørebro, Sweden, reported neostomal ulcer in 11 percent of patients undergoing a Billroth I resection for duodenal ulcer. A complemental vagotomy has rectified this situation to the end that the incidence of neostomal ulcer after Billroth I and II operations is much the same.[38]

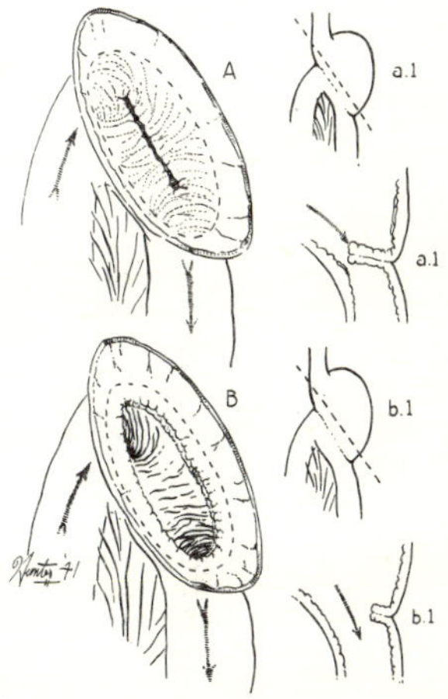

7.7 Technique for preserving patulous gastric stoma in gastric operations. From Wangensteen, *Intestinal obstructions*.

A significant paper by D. H. Stern and J. H. Walsh (1973) provided a cogent explanation for the greater liability of Billroth I resections for duodenal ulcer to provoke neostomal ulcer. They observed after antral excision in Billroth I resections that ingested food entering the duodenum stimulated gastrin release, not observed in the Billroth II operation in which food bypasses the duodenum and enters the jejunum directly. From this occurrence the authors infer that the proximal reaches of the duodenum also secrete gastrin.[39]

Before the employment of complemental vagotomy the Billroth II procedure continued to be the operative choice of most gastric surgeons, the majority favoring the Hofmeister partial gastrojejunal anastomosis over the Reichel-Pólya anastomosis of the jejunum to the entire length of the residual proximal stomach. H. W. Scott, Jr. (1965) reported an incidence of neostomal ulcer in 24 percent of patients undergoing Billroth II resections without complemental vagotomy at the Vanderbilt clinic, an incidence considerably higher than observed by other gastric surgeons. Even so, most agree that a complemental vagotomy does minimize the possibility of neostomal ulcer after Billroth II resections for duodenal ulcer.[40]

Segmental Gastric Resection

Mikulicz (1850–1905) initiated segmental resection in 1897. He was born in Czernowitz, Czechoslovakia. His father had suggested that young Johann become an orientalist. He decided in favor of medicine, which he studied in Vienna, beginning in 1875. He became an assistant in the Billroth clinic in 1879. After brief periods as professor in Cracow and in Königsberg, Mikulicz settled for the remainder of his short professional life in Breslau, where he had a distinguished career. Mikulicz and Anton Eiselsberg were among Billroth's finest pupils. Both developed eminent surgical schools of their own. Peptic ulcer of the lesser curvature was Mikulicz's special indication for segmental gastric resection. Bernard Riedel of Jena and Erwin Payr of Leipzig wrote of their experiences with segmental resection in 1909. Thereafter little was heard of the procedure. In 1948, the senior author adopted the operation for difficult duodenal ulcers perforated into the hepatoduodenal ligament — an experience demonstrating the reason the procedure failed in the hands of European surgeons was that transverse division of the proximal antrum interfered with gastric emptying. The addition of a complemental pyloroplasty (1952) resolved the matter.[41]

Segmental gastrectomy has proved an ideal operation for chronic gastric ulcer of the mid-lesser curvature and is to be preferred to sacrifice of the antrum as performed in the Billroth operations. For duodenal ulcer segmental resection has not been as successful, being accompanied by recurrence of symptoms in 8 percent of cases, half of which required reoperation; unfortunately, complemental vagotomy does not appear to lessen the incidence of this complication as it does in the Billroth operations. In performance of the operation the antrum is vagotomized; it was the senior author's practice initially to excise most of the lesser curvature of the residual fundic pouch, a maneuver that undoubtedly sacrificed additional vagal fibers.

Tetsuo Maki (1967) of Japan performed a glorified segmental gastrectomy, leaving only 1.5 cm. of antrum proximal to the pylorus and removing the remainder of the antrum. Interestingly, at this level of transverse antral section, a complemental pyloroplasty is not needed, a view that Maki and associates have reaffirmed in a more recent study (1975).[42]

Management of Peptic Ulcer Perforation

The first successful *closure* of a perforated gastric ulcer was reported by Hermann Kriege (1892) of Barmen, Germany; twenty hours intervened between perforation and the operation by Kriege's superior, Ludwig Heusner, not because of failure to recognize the nature of the emergency but because Heusner was otherwise occupied. H. P. Dean of London (1894) is credited with the first successful closure of a perforated duodenal ulcer, but a complete reading of the case record reveals that the patient died postoperatively in the hospital of an adhesive band obstruction.[43]

Haberer was an early advocate of gastric *resection* for perforated peptic ulcer and, in fact, reported two successes in 1919. In 1927 Axel Odelberg of Stockholm reported twenty such operations with one death. Other early advocates of gastric resection for acute peptic ulcer perforation were Serge Yudin, an accomplished innovative Russian surgeon (1929–39),[44] and Michael E. DeBakey (1940) of Houston. DeBakey and G. L. Jordan, Jr., suggested (1969) that primary resection be done only in patients with a history of peptic ulcer.[45] Recurrent ulcer attends mere closure of the perforation in approximately one-third of cases. For acute emergencies, theoretically, the simplest operation should be the best.

That the empty stomach of a dog could be perforated with little risk was demonstrated in the early 1930s. On the contrary, perforation of the full canine stomach commanded a formidable mortality, even with early surgical closure of the perforation.[46] These circumstances suggested that *nonoperative therapy*, using suction applied to an indwelling duodenal tube, would suffice to keep the stomach empty, permitting the perforation to close. The procedure was carried out successfully in 1932 on a medical student; a few years previously a perforated duodenal ulcer had been closed for him by suture. Between 1932 and 1935 an additional six patients with perforation were treated similarly with success. An eighth patient with a huge pneumoperitoneum succumbed; the total experience was published in 1935, but this mode of attack was then abandoned — unfortunately it was not then realized that a large pneumoperitoneum was synonymous with a large perforation. In fact, at autopsy the fatal case presented a free duodenal perforation almost 2 cm. in diameter, obviously demanding immediate surgical closure; so much gastric juice had leaked through the perforation that a large hole had been digested in the right diaphragm. Several years later Hermon Taylor (1946, 1957) of the London Hospital adopted the procedure, as did the American Army surgeon Colonel Sam F. Seeley (1956).[47] The method is rarely used today, but in patients with a small pneumoperitoneum who for some reason are not good operative risks the procedure should be considered.

Antral Exclusion

Eiselsberg (1860–1939) was a migratory Austrian medical student who studied successively in Vienna, Würzburg, Zürich, and Paris. He was trained in surgery under Billroth in Vienna (1884–87) and later became a member of his surgical staff. At age thirty-three Eiselsberg accepted a professorship at Utrecht (1893), where he remained until 1896, when he moved on to Königsberg; five years later (1901) he became chairman of the first surgical division at the University of Vienna, a post he held until a year before his death. Eiselsberg was a handsome, soft-spoken individual with a genial personality. He attracted a large number of pupils who later were to distinguish themselves in surgery. He was recognized as a great teacher at both graduate and undergraduate levels.

Like most European surgeons of his generation Eiselsberg was a general surgeon of diverse interests, concentrating primarily upon the gastrointestinal tract. He (1895) devised the operation of antral exclusion primarily for cancers of the stomach, which he regarded as irremovable. He divided the stomach proximal to the lesion and closed the distal segment, anastomosing the jejunum to the upper normal gastric pouch. Of the sixteen patients in his report two had peptic ulcer; the chief indication for performance of the operation for a few years, until the procedure was abandoned, was the difficult duodenal ulcer. Haberer (1913), a pupil of Eiselsberg, expressed misgivings over the acceptability of antral exclusion and by 1921 had abandoned it altogether, saying that the incidence of neostomal ulcer attending its performance for duodenal ulcer warranted its discontinuance. Hans Smidt (1924) of Jena observed that gastric secretory responses in dogs given meat were increased 82 percent after performance of the antral exclusion operation, a finding confirmed by Eugen Enderlen and L. Zukschwerdt (1931) of Heidelberg. Dragstedt and his associates (1951) provided significant confirmation of this occurrence.[48]

The work of W. Heneage Ogilvie of London with Billroth II resections (1936, 1938), with and without antral exclusion, served to persuade surgeons of the ulcerogenic influence of the procedure. Excision of the mucosa in the antral pouch, Richard Wilmanns (1926) found, eliminated the neostomal ulcer-provoking quality of the operation. W. R. Waddell and M. K. Bartlett (1957) attempted to resurrect the procedure, combining it with truncal vagotomy. The work of L. R. Sauvage and Henry N. Harkins (1953) and William D. Kelly (1954) has provided convincing evidence that complementing antral exclusion with vagotomy fails to protect against neostomal ulcer.[49] Edward Mason and his colleagues at the University of Iowa have demonstrated through their operations for obesity that when 95 percent of the stomach is excluded, followed up by a Roux Y type of anastomosis, the incidence of neostomal ulcer is only slightly more than 1 percent, a surprising occurrence in the light of the high incidence of neostomal ulcer attending exclusion of smaller segments of the stomach as performed by Eiselsberg and by Hugh Devine of Australia. Moreover, Mason does not add a complemental vagotomy.[50]

Vital Statistics

In the vital statistics of the United States for 1930 there were 6 deaths per 100,000 population from peptic ulcer, 15.6 from appendicitis, and 10 from bowel obstruction. In the vital statistics for 1972 there were 3.8 deaths from ulcer, 0.6 from appendicitis, and 3.3 from intestinal obstruction (a figure which also included deaths from unobstructed hernias). There was a 36.7 percent reduction over these forty-two years in the mortality of peptic ulcer, 97.2 percent in appendicitis, and 67 percent in intestinal obstruction; obviously the reduction would have been even greater if deaths from unobstructed hernias were excluded. Hemorrhage, the most serious threat, is largely accountable for the situation in peptic ulcer. In 1950 the mortality figure for peptic ulcer was essentially what it had been in 1930. Over the last quarter century there has been definite improvement, but a more critical appraisal of how to deal with the problem is sorely needed; an effective antipeptic agent should be of immense help. Cimetidine appears to offer promise on this score. Stress ulcer figures prominently in the persistent mortality from hemorrhage in peptic ulcer. Meredith P. Smith (1977) has assessed the incidence of duodenal ulcer perforation in Seattle hospitals and operations for the relief of chronic duodenal ulcer; he concluded that the incidence of duodenal ulcer in the area had declined by 35 percent over the past ten years.[51]

There are effective methods available to deal with the serious threat of hemorrhage from peptic ulcer states, but none unfortunately is consistently successful. The problem obviously needs critical evaluation by our most talented clinicians. The brilliant investigator Pasteur always had in mind the need to relate the significance of his discoveries to the practical art and the public interest.

Zollinger-Ellison Syndrome

In 1955 Zollinger and E. H. Ellison of Ohio State University described a syndrome of hypersecretion of gastric juice, an entity that had long gone begging for recognition. The authors described a severe peptic ulcer affliction in two patients, characterized by atypically located peptic ulcers, not responding to conventional surgery for duodenal ulcer. It is probably the most severe of all peptic ulcer diatheses. A twelve-hour nocturnal secretion without stimulation may approximate 3 liters of gastric juice with high potential digestive power containing as much as 300 mEq. of hydrochloric acid, contrasting with a normal value of 18 mEq. Diarrhea is frequently an associated symptom. Patients who have undergone several gastric resections with persistent symptoms and recurrent neostomal ulcers should be suspect. Hemorrhage, perforation, and obstruction are not uncommon sequelae of the disorder.

Following description of the syndrome by Zollinger and Ellison, most gastric surgeons of experience could readily recall a patient or two in whom repetitive gastric resections had failed to control what they had then regarded as instances of duodenal ulcer. R. A. Strøm of Norway (1952) had in fact described a patient who had undergone three prior gastric resections and in whom later excision of an 8-gram tumor from the tail of the pancreas had given complete relief. Strøm described the tumor as a pancreatic insuloma containing "atypical beta cells," indicating their likely relationship to an increased acid-peptic activity. F. Forty and G. M. Barrett (1952) of England related the occurrence of peptic ulceration in the distal duodenum in a fifty-five-year-old woman presenting an islet cell adenoma of the pancreas. R. A. Gregory and associates extracted a gastrinlike substance from a pancreatic tumor in a case of Zollinger-Ellison syndrome.[52]

Many of these pancreatic tumors are malignant, accompanied by hepatic metastases. Stanley R. Friesen of the University of Kansas (1967) has demonstrated that attending total gastrectomy the metastases may occasionally disappear. Such tumors in the pancreas are often multiple. For the occasional single pancreatic tumor, its excision is indicated; for multiple tumors, complete gastrectomy.[53]

There are well authenticated instances of like tumors or hyperplasia in other endocrine organs that may account for the syndrome. Multiendocrine tumors of the pituitary and/or parathyroid glands may also account for development of the series of events observed in the more frequent Zollinger-Ellison syndrome. A symposium on gastrointestinal hormones was convened in Galveston in 1974. From discussions there it would appear that the stomach, duodenum, and upper jejunum are emerging as an endocrine organ, secreting hormones that influence gastric digestion. Several of these have been described and chemically identified.[54]

In October 1977 the Nobel Prize Committee announced its award to three distinguished American scientists working in the neuroendocrine field: to Rosalyn Yalow for telling immunoassay studies on gastrin; to Roger Guillemin and Andrew Schally for demonstration of the presence of neuroendocrine cells scattered widely over the surface of the cerebral cortex, as well as in the duodenojejunal mucosa, cells responsible for the secretion of neuroendocrine hormones previously believed to be found only in the hypophysis and hypothalamus.

Total Gastrectomy for Polycythemia Vera: Justifiable Procedure?

Polycythemia vera, a disease of obscure etiology, has no completely satisfactory treatment. Phlebotomy and drug therapy to suppress regeneration of red blood cells from the bone marrow have been the usual modes of management. Thirty years ago a patient was seen frequently in consultation over a period of three years in the hematologic clinic of the Department of Medicine at Minnesota. The patient, a carpenter by trade, had been a railroad employee until he lost a leg in an accident. A diagnosis of polycythemia had been firmly established. Complete blood studies were carried out on a number of occasions. The hemoglobin was usually in the range of 17.5 grams, with red cells in the 6,400,000 range, the hematocrit approximately 52 percent, and leucocytes usually in the 15,000 range. Preoperative blood volume studies revealed 9.6 liters, certainly a grossly increased volume for a man of fifty-two years, of slight build, weighing 150 pounds. (Some months after total gastrectomy the blood volume was reduced to 4.8 liters, a reduction of 50 percent.) Gastric analysis on a fasting stomach showed consistently small volumes of acid with free hydrochloric acid of 31 mEq. with total acid of 60 mEq., an observation suggesting the presence of an acid-peptic diathesis. The patient had been treated over the three-year interval by repeated phlebotomies in which 800 to 1,000 ml. of blood were removed and by x-ray irradiation of long bones and spleen. He constantly had occult blood in the stool and periodic bouts of vomiting heavily tinged with blood followed by melena and constant abdominal pain. There had been psychotic episodes; fatigue and weakness were prominent complaints. The phlebotomies effected a temporary reduction in the hematocrit and the hemoglobin, but on hospital revisits within a month's time the usual high values had returned. Sternal bone marrow aspiration revealed the red cells to have a mean corpuscular diameter of 7 micra; 44 percent of the leucocytes were lymphocytes; the erythropoiesis was normoblastic; normoblasts and megakaryocytes were increased in number; no evidence of leukemia. Two years after gastrectomy sternal biopsy showed hyperplasia of the bone marrow. Numerous megakaryocytes were still in evidence as were marrow platelets.

The senior author, having seen the patient frequently during his hospital admissions and outpatient visits, timidly suggested total gastrectomy. The suggestion met with no enthusiasm by our competent hematologists and internists, nor by other leaders in the field, nor could we find any precedent for such a procedure. Because of the constant abdominal pain, the episodes of bleeding from hyperrugated mucosal gastric folds (identified by both roentgen and gastroscopic examinations), and the lack of durable success attending phlebotomy and x-ray treatment, it was finally agreed to submit the patient to total gastrectomy, an expedient he welcomed. The procedure was carried out by our surgical colleagues David State, Ivan Baronofsky, and David Gaviser on May 3, 1947. The operative specimen included several centimeters of the lower esophagus exhibiting squamous mucosa, and the distal end of the resection included a few centimeters of duodenal mucosa. Apart from evidences of erosive gastritis and hyperrugation of mucosal folds, the stomach specimen was not remarkable.

Interestingly, no phlebotomies were found necessary after the operation. Bleeding from the digestive canal disappeared as did the abdominal pain. The patient's health improved despite weight loss and continued fatigue. With dietary advice and frequent small meals, his weight stabilized at 132 pounds, somewhat below his preoperative weight. The Sippy regimen was no longer necessary. He was not able to sustain a full day's work schedule, but his health was considerably better than the preoperative status.[55] He survived the total gastrectomy for sixteen years and four months in fairly good health on vitamin B_{12} injections and ingestion of frequent small meals. He succumbed to a squamous cell cancer of the upper thoracic esophagus on July 29, 1963. On encountering increasing difficulty in swallowing, the patient returned to the University Hospitals but too late to undergo excision of the esophagus; tracheal involvement at its bifurcation was already in evidence.

No similar instance has been reported in the medical or surgical literature over this long interval of time. It would appear, therefore, to be an approach to a problem which at present is not well controlled or managed and which warrants further exploration. Total gastrectomy for gastric cancer in the senior author's hands has been a satisfying experience, followed by long-term survivals, with ready availability of vitamin B_{12} and supervised feeding. One patient continues well and active after twenty-seven years. Survival for twenty years is not uncommon. Loss of weight and fatigue are frequent but not incapacitating. The long survival in reasonably good health for more than sixteen years would suggest a trial of gastrectomy in other patients with polycythemia vera not well controlled on medical management.

Congenital Hypertrophic Pyloric Stenosis

An extramucosal pylorotomy for congenital hypertrophic pyloric stenosis was performed by W. Conrad Ramstedt of Münster on August 23, 1911, and again on June 18, 1912; both operations were successes. Before this W. Weber (1910) of Dresden had two successful operations upon infants in which he drew the adjacent serosa over the divided pyloric muscle. In 1908 Henri Dufour and Pierre Fredet of France reported successful instances of extramucosal myotomy in which the longitudinal incision was closed transversely.[56] In consequence, the operation is often termed the Fredet-Ramstedt procedure.

The important role of two American pediatric surgeons in performing the operation has been unique. In 1937 E. J. Donovan of New York reported 243 operations with a single hospital death (0.41 percent); Robert E. Gross (1953) indicated that the mortality at the Boston Children's Hospital since 1940 had been under 1 percent.[57] In many German surgical clinics in the 1927–28 period there still remained traces of a preference for gastrojejunostomy.

Gunshot Wounds of the Abdomen

The American gynecologist Sims advised early routine operative intervention for gunshot wounds in a series of papers in the *British Medical Journal* in late 1881 and early 1882.[58] Interest was stimulated by the unfortunate sequence of events following the attempt on President Garfield's life in July 1881. The president was fired upon from behind with a .42-caliber revolver at a distance of six or eight feet. He lingered for several weeks and finally succumbed from rupture of a mycotic aneurysm of the splenic artery. The advice of the day was to remove lodged bullets or other foreign bodies. Examination of the clinical records discloses that the wound was probed by "socially clean" hands seventeen different times.[59] Had a strip of sterile adhesive plaster been applied over the point of entry of the bullet to the right of the president's spine, and all probing of the bullet tract with nonsterile fingers and probes been avoided, Garfield probably would have survived to run for reelection.

In a subsequent study of bullet wounds of abdominal hollow viscera Charles T. Parkes (1884) of Chicago shot into the abdomen of anesthetized dogs that had been draped with sterile precautions for operation. Spillage of intestinal content was an almost uniform finding, and the operative mortality was high.[60]

When George H. Makins returned from the Boer War (1899–1900) in South Africa, he wrote a monograph on his experiences. It is to be remembered it was an itinerant type of warfare, not permitting establishment of bases for emergency operations. Makins concluded that nonoperative management of abdominal bullet wounds was the wisest scheme, attended with a mortality of 33 percent. Senn's (1900) inference at the siege of Santiago in the Spanish-American War was the same.[61] Be it said to the credit of American surgeons at Buffalo that when President McKinley was felled by an assassin's bullet (September 1901) at the Pan American Exposition, the attending surgeons operated immediately. The president was on the operating table within seventy-five minutes of the shooting, a record rarely achieved in our finest hospitals today. Roswell Park, Buffalo's outstanding surgeon of that period, was away at a consultation in Niagara Falls, some miles distant. A special train was dispatched to return him to Buffalo, but by the time he reached the Exposition Building, Matthew Mann, a well-known local gynecologist, had almost completed the operation. The points of entry and exit of the bullet through the stomach were closed. The bullet had penetrated the pancreas, but Mann failed to find it.

The president's convalescence in the beginning was smooth, but he died about a week later of an anaerobic infection of the retroperitoneal area, a challenging therapeutic prospect even today. Harvey R. Gaylord, the accomplished goiter pathologist, spent seven hours doing the postmortem but failed to find the bullet; the president was a large man.[62]

Shortly after the outbreak of World War I the London surgeon P. Lockhart Mummery wrote (November 1914), "I should like to reiterate the view, which I hold most firmly, that wounds involving the bowel should not be treated by immediate operation, even if proper facilities are available." Mummery's therapeutic reliance was upon complete rest, no food, and morphine. Not long thereafter (July 1915) Enderlen and Sauerbruch, well-known German surgeons of the Axis, concluded that early operation for all gunshot wounds of the abdomen was definitely in order. When patients with wounds of the intestine were treated conservatively, 94 percent died; when subjected to operation, the recovery rate was 44.4 percent.[63]

Frederick F. Cartwright, well-known London anesthesiologist and author of several informative historical monographs, has pointed out that in the Russo-Japanese War (1904–5) Princess Vera Ignatievna Gedroitz, a Russian surgeon, brought a well-equipped ambulance train close to the front and was "enabled to operate upon battle casualties in good conditions and within a short time of wounding. She adopted a policy of operating for early penetrating wounds of the abdomen and her results were better than any that had yet been attained. Further back at the base hospitals results were still poor; the point to be noted is that Princess Gedroitz, by means of her ambulance train, was able to operate upon her patients within a very short time of wounding."[64]

Gerald W. Shaftan (1960) has recently shown that under careful hospital supervision penetrating wounds of the abdomen, both stab wounds and small-caliber bullet wounds of the intestine, may be treated conservatively and with surprising success; in fact, it would appear that the mortality actually is less than in an operative series.[65] Shaftan's mortality in 125 consecutive cases treated nonoperatively was 0.8 percent; in those with visceral injuries operated upon the mortality was 20 percent. Shaftan has justified this regimen with adequate supporting data in subsequent papers in 1966 and 1969. It is very unlikely, however, that nonoperative management on a wide scale could be carried out under conditions of warfare.

Summary

The earliest recorded operations upon the stomach dealt with knife wounds and the removal of sharp swallowed objects. Several such accounts are to be found in the literature of the sixteenth and seventeenth centuries.

Gastric fistulas in man permitted several nineteenth-century observers to study gastric secretion. The observations of Beaumont (1833) upon St. Martin remain a classic. Beaumont established the presence of a "chemical principle" in gastric juice other than hydrochloric acid. He also recognized that the normal empty stomach needs the stimulus of food to provoke secretion. Müller and Schwann (1836) boiled canine gastric juice and noted loss of the digestive power of Beaumont's gastric ferment, which Schwann called pepsin.

Flourens (1832) performed gastrostomy on sheep to study secretion, and Blondlot (1843) made a similar study on dogs. The studies of Heidenhain (1878) and his brilliant pupil Pavlov (1892) on canine gastric fistulas and isolated pouches are the finest in the literature. Pavlov established definitely the significant role of the vagus in gastric secretion. Heidenhain in morphologic and secretory studies identified correctly the acid-peptic secreting antral segment of the stomach, which areas surgeons and the physiologist Gregory have shown to have great influence in stimulating and eliciting acid-peptic secretion from the fundic area.

Present-day operations for peptic ulcer received their thrust from the work of gastric physiologists. Duodenal ulcer and the Zollinger-Ellison syndrome (1955) are manifestations of the peptic ulcer diathesis most difficult to control, the latter requiring total gastrectomy if the causative pancreatic tumor cannot be found and excised.

Chronic gastric ulcer yields readily to segmental gastric resection. Excision to eliminate the possibility of cancer is an important consideration.

Obstruction, perforation, and hemorrhage are frequent complications of peptic ulcer, remediable by surgery. Mortality from hemorrhage constitutes today the most important challenge to the profession. Better ways to control hemorrhage need to be evolved.

Over the past two decades there has been a general retreat in the management of duodenal ulcer away from extensive gastric resections and away from truncal vagotomy to highly selective vagotomy of the gastric fundus and corpus, an operation that does not mandate pyloroplasty. Both patients and physicians find these conservative operations more acceptable than extensive gastric resection. Some type of vagal section of which Dragstedt was a vigorous proponent has become an integral part of surgery for duodenal ulcer. Recent studies suggest that effective conservative antacid and antipeptic drug therapy may be available; if extended trials confirm these observations operation for duodenal ulcer will obviously become less frequent.

Billroth (1881) at the Allgemeines Krankenhaus in Vienna had the first operative success with gastric cancer; the patient survived the operation but succumbed to cancer four months later. The outlook has continued poor, owing primarily to late diagnosis. Over the last decade Japanese radiographers and gastroscopists have very definitely improved the situation. Employing air-contrast media followed by gastroscopic examination, Japanese clinicians have been able to identify mucosal lesions with fairly consistent regularity, a circumstance that has heightened the survival rate after operation considerably. Unfortunately, the silent, asymptomatic interval for gastric and most visceral cancers is in the area of two years. For some obscure reason, there appears to have been a very definite decrease in the incidence of gastric cancer in many Western countries, including the United States. A similar decrease in incidence has not been observed in Hungary, Iceland, Japan, or Peru. These occurrences suggest the possibility of extrinsic environmental factors in the genesis of gastric cancer.

Observations on the Zollinger-Ellison syndrome have invoked intense investigation into the mechanism of gastrin release. It would appear that the antral, duodenal, and upper jejunal mucosa actually constitute an endocrine organ, a conclusion that the Galveston symposium (1974) did much to reaffirm.

The case history of a patient with polycythemia vera who survived total gastrectomy sixteen years and four months before dying of cancer of the cervical esophagus is cited. This occurrence suggests that gastrectomy may constitute an additional approach to a baffling problem not yet well controlled.

Acceptance of the need to close bullet wounds of the abdomen emerged in the midst of World War I. Before this, it had been thought the patient stood a better chance of recovery if treated conservatively, primarily with morphine. Wounds of the abdomen, whether by bullet or knife, are likely to penetrate the gut. In civil practice Shaftan and others have shown that the recovery rate accompanying conservative management in selective cases is good, but such management is of little usefulness in military surgery.

(For notes, see pp. 620–25.)

CHAPTER 8

Tracheostomy and Respiratory Obstruction

ON DECEMBER 14, 1799, a deeply concerned family physician and two consultants at Mount Vernon, Virginia, conferred over the worsening condition of their sixty-seven-year-old patient. George Washington was struggling for breath with a septic sore throat. All the timely measures such as copious bleeding, laxatives, emetics, blisters, and poultices had been tried. The youngest member of the trio, Elisha C. Dick, graduate of the new Medical School of Pennsylvania, advanced a daring alternative — tracheostomy. The proposal was considered but vetoed by his orthodox Edinburgh-trained elders, although Dick offered to take full personal responsibility for a failure.

Earlier remedies were continued and the former president was dead before morning, probably from suffocation and depletion, after fourteen hours of illness.[1] A tracheostomy might well have been life-saving, but it was too radical a suggestion for the year 1799 and for so eminent a patient. Nearly a quarter century passed before the consultant's proposal would be justified.

The First Tracheostomies

Tracheostomy is, in fact, an old operation, but it was not used frequently until after Pierre Bretonneau's adoption of it in 1825 to relieve an obstructive diphtheritic membrane of the larynx.[2] Asclepiades (ca. 124–40 B.C.) of Bithynia, who spent most of his professional life in Rome, is said to have first performed tracheostomy.[3] The performance is credited to him by Galen and Caelius Aurelianus (fifth century), neither of whom practiced it. Aurelianus called the operation Asclepiades' "futile and irresponsible idea." The Greek surgeon Antyllus (second century) suggested that the third or fourth tracheal rings should be divided to provide an airway in the operation.[4]

Albucasis was called to treat a slave girl who had tried to commit suicide by cutting her throat with a knife and had severed part of her trachea. He sewed up the tracheal wound and the girl recovered, demonstrating that the trachea would heal following incision,[5] an important observation for subsequent attempts to open the windpipe.

Although earlier authorities had described the operation, the first account of a successful tracheostomy apparently was that published in 1546 by Antonio Brasavola, an Italian physician. He opened the trachea of a patient who was on the point of death from respiratory obstruction caused by an abscess in juxtaposition to the windpipe. The patient recovered.[6]

The writings of Hieronymus Fabricius ab Aquapendente (1537–1619), great surgeon and anatomist of Padua, and his pupil Julius Casserius (ca. 1561–1616) provided good descriptions of the technique of tracheostomy, an operation which neither of them ever performed. Fabricius was not enthusiastic over opening the trachea for respiratory obstruction but did approve of it as a last resort. He sketched the history of the operation, tracing back to early Greek and Arab physicians. Fabricius insisted on a median-vertical incision, directly over the midpoint of the cervical trachea. He described a tracheal cannula with provision for fastening at the back of the neck with tapes. The cannula was to be placed between cartilaginous rings and kept in place for a few days. Fabricius' concept of tracheostomy approximated current practices.[7]

In 1620 the Paris surgeon Nicolas Habicot (1550–1624) published a book listing four successful cases of an operation entitled "bronchotomy commonly called laryngotomy," reviving interest in opening the trachea for respiratory obstruction. He also devised a cannula which he inserted between two tracheal cartilages. Habicot's equipment for the operation reflects evidences of a modern design, save that he employed only a single tracheal cannula.[8] After Habicot's report twenty-three other successful tracheostomies were recorded over the next two hundred years.[9]

George Martine of St. Andrews, the earliest British tracheostomist on record, was apparently the first (1730) to recommend a double tracheostomy tube, an inch in length, with the obvious advantage that the inner tube could be removed and cleaned several times a day without disturbing the patient. He said the idea had been suggested by "one of our Ministers here."[10] Removal of a single tube for cleaning was not only inconvenient but painful. Early surgeons usually employed a knife or lancet to make the tracheal opening. Some passed the cannula over a sharp pointed instrument; most, however, passed it alongside the lancet or after the tracheostomy opening was made.

Desault recommended that laryngotomy be made above the cricoid cartilage, as distinguished from tracheostomy performed below it.[11] In general, openings into the trachea above the second cartilaginous tracheal ring are to be avoided because of the risk of provoking chondritis of the cricoid cartilage, a troublesome source of subsequent tracheal stenosis.

William Lawrence, a distinguished English surgeon of the early nineteenth century, advised (1815) making a small slit in the tracheal ring beneath the site of insertion of the tracheal tube to provide a salvaging air vent should the tracheal tube become obstructed. He was apparently the first to excise slips of tracheal cartilages in performing tracheostomy.[12] Johann Dieffenbach of the University of Berlin later supported Lawrence's idea.[13]

Bretonneau (1778–1862), a Tours physician, described diphtheria as a special entity in a monograph of 1826, in which he reported his first successful tracheostomy for laryngeal obstruction. His two previous attempts, both on children, had been last resort measures and had failed, although one child, who had stopped breathing before the surgery, was revived and lived twelve more hours.[14] Meanwhile Bretonneau continued to do research on dogs and cadavers — his celebrated pupil Velpeau has related how adept he was at procuring the latter, even though it meant nocturnal visits to the cemetery.[15]

In June 1825 the four-year-old daughter of the Count of Puysegur was brought ten leagues (about twenty-five miles) to Tours by her father, who suspected that she had what was called malignant angina. The count, who had lost three young sons in recent years with the disease, had followed Bretonneau's studies and hoped he might be able to avert a fourth tragedy in the family. The child had been ill four days; her condition rapidly deteriorated. By the seventh day Bretonneau determined once again that tracheostomy offered the only chance of salvation. Profiting by experience, he prepared carefully for the operation, adapting a single silver tube as a cannula instead of the rubber sound that had proved unsuitable in his earlier cases. The little girl had a difficult time. The tube, which was used for eleven days, became detached or had to be removed for cleaning almost daily and was sometimes replaced with great difficulty, but the patient had regained her health and normal voice three weeks postoperatively.[16]

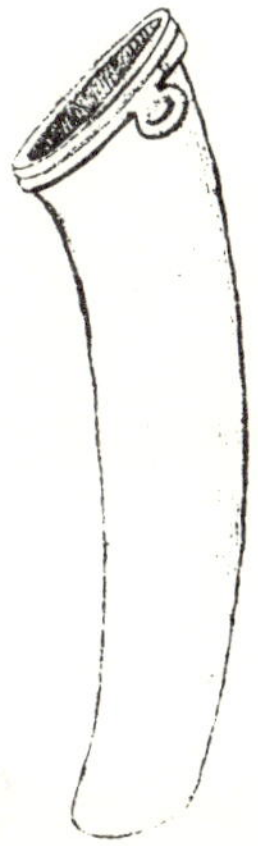

8.1 Pierre Bretonneau's tracheostomy tube. From Bretonneau, *De la diphthérite* (Paris, 1826).

Thereafter Bretonneau urged opening the trachea in the presence of a laryngeal diphtheritic membrane obstructing respiration; to this thesis his other famous pupil, Trousseau, also lent considerable momentum. Trousseau originated a dilator to spread the tracheal opening while the tracheal cannula was being inserted. Bretonneau and Trousseau used a midline incision of both skin and tracheal cartilages.[17] They accepted the term "tracheotomy" and it was so known for almost a century.[18] In the last two decades, however, the term "tracheostomy" has supplanted "tracheotomy," as "colostomy" did "colotomy" at an earlier date to designate a skin stoma rather than a mere opening of the colon.

Tracheostomy and the Hangman's Noose

Antoine Louis (1784) tells of a Londoner who led a double existence as butcher and highwayman and was ultimately detected in his thievery and condemned to be hanged. A young surgeon who had performed successful tracheostomies on dogs bribed his way into the prison and persuaded the condemned man to permit him to perform a tracheostomy the night before the execution, leaving a small tube in the trachea. The next morning the prisoner was duly hung. When cut down he was still alive, but he survived only a few minutes.[19] An open airway failed to protect the victim from the damage occasioned by occlusion of the arterial flow to the brain and injury to the spinal cord.

The official hangman's noose is a slipknot placed posteriorly at the level of the upper cervical spine. The weight of the victim and the height of the trap are important factors in the extent of the resultant havoc; a drop of two to four meters is usual. Venous occlusion of blood returning from the head and obstruction to arterial inflow are obvious consequences; fracture of the hyoid bone and thyroid cartilage are not uncommon. Less apparent but consistent accompaniments are rupture of the upper spinous ligaments with frequent dislocation of the second or third vertebral bodies occasioning irreparable damage to the spinal cord. Fracture or fissure of the lens has been observed.[20] Prior tracheostomy is unlikely to make resuscitation possible in a body suspended for several minutes, attending this ordeal.[21]

Persons who commit suicide by hanging rarely adjust the knot of the noose to the posterior midline of the neck. Ernest W. White (1884) reported the instance of a woman who hanged herself with portions of her clothing and, when found some minutes later, was apparently dead — unconscious and apneic. A physician revived her by artificial respiration and she survived. In a famous case in 1740 the body of a young man hanged for rape came to life when laid out for dissection in the Barber-Surgeons' Hall, London. He fully recovered and was reprieved from the death sentence.[22]

Nineteenth-Century Tracheostomy Mortality

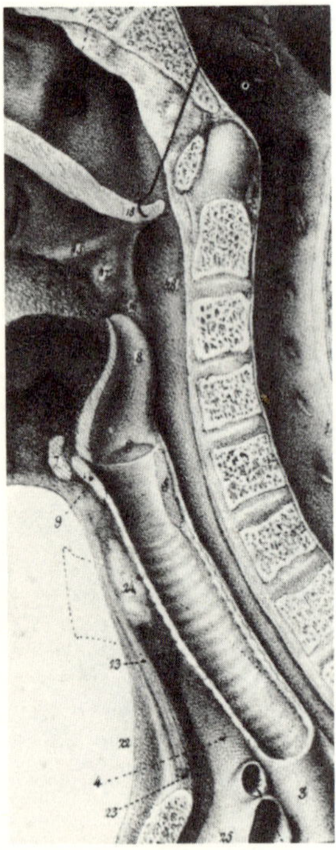

8.2 Relationship of trachea, esophagus, and vertebra. Location of Bretonneau's tube shown by dotted lines. From Bretonneau, *De la diphthérite*.

Throughout the nineteenth century tracheostomy was most often done for diphtheritic obstruction of the larynx or for croupous pharyngitis and laryngitis. The death rate of the operation was high.

Trousseau wrote in 1835 that he had saved 9 children among 36 submitted to tracheostomy (75 percent mortality). By 1847, according to Velpeau, Trousseau had 20 successes in 60 cases, and Bretonneau 5 or 6 cures out of 18 or 20. Velpeau said that he himself had lost the 4 children upon whom he had attempted tracheostomy for croup and that it had been ineffectual in a large number of patients at hôpital des Enfans.[23] There, under the leadership of Trousseau (1849–58), 466 tracheostomies were performed with 126 successes, a mortality rate of approximately 73 percent — "very satisfying," said the reporter. Tables reveal that the mortality of patients with diphtheria subjected to tracheostomy in Paris hospitals in the 1870s was usually around 75 percent. Universally, there obviously had been little, if any, improvement in the outcome of tracheostomy performed for diphtheria. From 1862 to 1869 the Langenbeck clinic in Berlin admitted 221 patients with diphtheria; tracheostomy was not performed on any of them.[24]

In describing the numerous techniques devised and the fatal complications frequently encountered with all methods, C. Hardy (1858) of Paris portrayed the miserable experience with tracheostomy by the mid-nineteenth century, although he maintained it was often the only expedient. His pessimism was reaffirmed by W. E. Steavenson's summary of results in 1873–82 with children treated in St. Bartholomew's Hospital and the Great Ormond Street Hospital for Sick Children. Fistulous openings above the larynx were dilated with catheters and sounds in attempts to create a breathing space. Persistence of the obstruction offered little hope of recovery. Steavenson occasionally sat up all night with his patient, ready to replace the tracheal tube should it be extruded.[25]

Billroth reported upon his experience from 1860 to 1876 of 22 tracheostomies of which only 6 patients survived (72.2 percent mortality). In almost all instances, said Billroth, there was considerable easing of respiration, but the patient died a few days later. In general, apart from mucus in small bronchi of the lungs, postmortem examinations were usually negative.[26] The salvage rate undoubtedly was better than in the time of Fabricius ab Aquapendente, but the persistently high death rate reflected the use of tracheostomy in diphtheria and croupous laryngitis and its performance as a last resort.

When the Paris surgeon Charles M. Maingault made a special plea for early performance of tracheostomy at a meeting of the Royal Academy of Medicine in 1832, Velpeau raised an objection on the grounds that the measure might not be necessary. Nevertheless, a year later Maingault reiterated his insistence on the importance of doing tracheostomy in good time if the measure was to succeed. The need for relieving tracheal obstruction when symptoms are first presented, rather than as an antemortem operation, is today generally conceded.[27]

In 1893 Emil Behring announced the treatment of diphtheria with diphtheria antiserum; in 1913 he was able to report an effective toxin-antitoxin in its management.[28] Public health programs employing toxin-antitoxin immunization have gradually eliminated the serious threat of diphtheria.

Tracheostomy Technique

The preferred skin incision for elective tracheostomy is transverse, midway between the thyroid cartilage and the suprasternal notch. This is accompanied by a vertical incision in the trachea excising short segments of the third and fourth cartilaginous tracheal rings, permitting easy insertion of the airway cannula.

Division of the cricothyroid membrane, a high type of tracheostomy, in a penknife kind of life-saving measure. It is justifiable only as an emergency procedure in acute respiratory obstruction, when neither time nor equipment permits performance of conventional tracheostomy. It does allow ready entry into the acutely obstructed respiratory channel, but often needs to be revised within twenty-four to thirty-six hours if glottic edema persists. A cannula left in the divided cricothyroid membrane except very temporarily invites stenosis from injury of the cricoid cartilage.

Indications for Tracheostomy

The chief reasons for performing tracheostomy are (1) mechanical respiratory obstruction and (2) obstruction occasioned by accumulations of secretions not readily removed. Obviously a combination of these factors may coexist, multiplying the hazards. One of the advantages of tracheostomy in the presence of fluid secretion in the bronchi is that it shortens the respiratory channel, reducing the ventilatory dead air space. Unconscious patients and those suffering head or chest injury are especially prone to accumulation of respiratory secretions, most readily removed by bronchial aspiration through a tracheostomy cannula.

Prophylactic Tracheostomy

With more frequent performance of tracheostomy for a variety of conditions, its value in relief of respiratory obstruction has

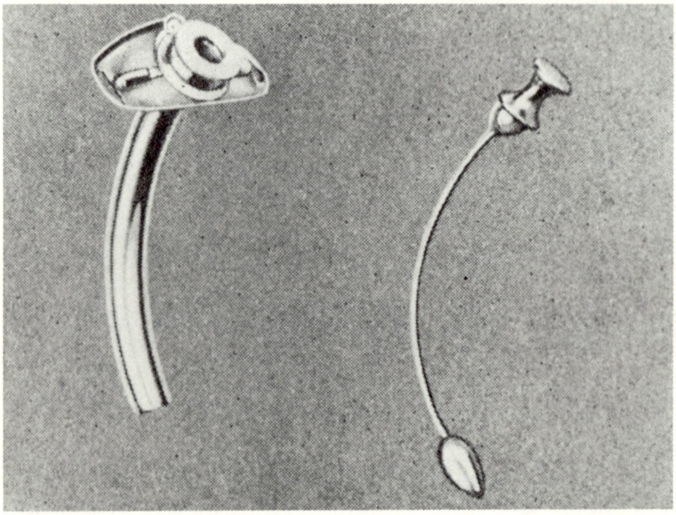

8.3 Modern tracheostomy tube illustrated by Chevalier L. Jackson.

definitely been proven. A quarter of a century ago the senior author employed prophylactic tracheostomy to lessen the risk in extensive surgery for excision of cancers of the alimentary tract in the elderly patient with low pulmonary reserve and a wet tracheobronchial tree who could not readily clear the respiratory tract by cough and expectoration. The bronchopulmonary tree could be kept relatively dry by this "instant bronchoscopic aspiration." Several challenges were met in this manner and the range of operation was extended to a number of patients who otherwise would not have tolerated major abdominal surgery.[29]

Every experienced surgeon has seen many instances in which, after successful aggressive operation for malignancy, including prophylactic tracheostomy, there appeared to be no way of caring for the patient when he was ready to leave hospital. Young surgical proteges have been known to remark, "the best thing for you to do is to take the patient home with you." Children's loss of interest in an aging parent is not unusual. Someone once remarked that a parent can support ten children, but ten children often find it difficult to support a needy parent. Loneliness among elderly patients, particularly men, is commonplace. Upon recovery after operation, if the spouse is gone, the patient often feels left alone in the world. An effective solution is to find, with the help of a trained social worker, a companion checker, bridge, or domino player to come to the hospital to encourage the patient, then join him or her for games at their living quarters. This simple device often rekindles interest in life, replacing desire for an early demise. The social aspects of a patient's care must not be neglected by the thoughtful surgeon. Praise be to those voluntary samaritans who help uplift the flagging spirits of the neglected and lonely aged.

Another bizarre behavior of ungrateful children that undoubtedly has been observed by many other surgeons has come to this surgeon's notice twice. The first concerned an elderly man in his mid-seventies with an extensive gastric cancer requiring total excision of the stomach. Expecting only a short survival, on the advice of his physician and attorney, he deeded all his property to two sons, who carried on an important business enterprise developed by the father. Five years went by and the patient was getting on very well, but was without resources. One of the two sons refused to participate in a plan providing the father an adequate annual income. The patient survived an additional seven years. The other case concerned a man in his mid-forties. He had a malignant melanoma over the left shoulder with axillary metastases and a nodule in the lung. On similar advice from his physician and attorney, he too consigned the business he had developed to two sons. The lesion in the lung proved to be a fibroma. Following excision of the local lesion and axillary metastases, he was active and well and wished to reenter his profitable food supply concern. One of the sons refused, indicating that half the property had been deeded to him. It can indeed be a strange and merciless world!

Gastric Reflux into Trachea during Sleep

It is conventional today to place balloons on tracheal and endotracheal tubes to prevent fluids from the mouth draining into the lower reaches of the trachea during operation. Stuart Arhelger (1951) demonstrated a quarter of a century ago the ease of regurgitation from an empty stomach into the trachea. In the evening before the patient went to sleep congo red was placed in his stomach by means of a duodenal tube, which was immediately withdrawn. The next morning tracheal aspiration was performed by a catheter passed through the nose or through a prior tracheostomy. The frequency with which the dye was aspirated from the trachea was surprising.[30]

The Mortality of Tracheostomy

Virtual disappearance of diphtheria and poliomyelitis has eliminated a frequent former indication for tracheostomy. Even so, the mortality of conditions necessitating tracheostomy remains high, in effect a reflection of the potential hazard of the illness compelling its performance. When used as an elective procedure to facilitate anesthesia for various types of operations, the risk to the patient is not augmented. Inasmuch as many of the situations for which tracheostomy is invoked present high-risk conditions, reduction of the mortality to negligible levels perhaps can never be regularly achieved.

A critical review of published papers on tracheostomy indicates clearly that there is a tendency to separate deaths owing to the operation from deaths owing to the disease for which the operation is performed. Nils Toremalm of Lund (1960) reported a zero mortality among 25 tracheotomized infants and children. When, however, the 6 deaths attending tracheostomy performed for "ventilatory insufficiency" are included, the overall mortality is 24 percent. Obviously, these cases constitute a high-risk group, yet, if one is to glean the value of the accomplishment in all patients to whom tracheostomy is applied, none should be eliminated. Similarly J. McK. Watts (1963) of the Alfred Hospital in Melbourne, Australia, reporting a mortality of 1.4 percent among 212 tracheostomies (1953–60), admitted that "there are other less dramatic complications which often contribute to death, but their responsibility is difficult to evaluate."[31]

Peter Oliver and associates of Boston reported upon 294 tracheostomies performed during 1950–59 in children under eighteen years with a mortality of 3.4 percent attributable to tracheostomy and its complications. The overall mortality, however, was 20.1 percent, highest when tracheostomy was invoked in diseases of the central nervous system (54.3 percent) and for congenital anomalies (26.6 percent). Interestingly, the mortality was only 5.3 percent when tracheostomy was done for infections causing respiratory embarrassment.[32]

Thomas G. Nelson (1958) reported an overall mortality rate of 38 percent in 300 patients undergoing tracheostomy. In the 160 patients for whom tracheostomy was performed to relieve respiratory embarrassment from accumulations of tracheal and other fluids, the mortality rate was 57 percent; in the 140 patients with mechanical ventilatory obstruction, a still somewhat formidable rate of 16 percent occurred. R. M. A. McClelland (1965) of Cardiff reported upon 389 tracheostomies carried out in the United Oxford Hospitals over a ten-year interval (1950–59) with an apparent mortality rate from the operation of 3.4 percent. Actually, however, 46 percent of the patients failed to survive.[33] Unrealistic evaluations, strangely enough, are not uncommon in this area of surgery in which significant advances have been made in recent decades.

Anesthesia for Tracheostomy

When general anesthesia was first used to facilitate tracheostomy, many patients died under anesthesia. When cocaine was made available in 1884, Chevalier Jackson of Philadelphia became an early strong advocate of its use in elective tracheostomy.[34] Several modern students of the problem have returned to use of general anesthesia in elective tracheostomy, especially when operating upon struggling children. Elective tracheostomy in adults is best performed under local procaine infiltration anesthesia. The isthmus of the thyroid gland, overlying the trachea, is divided, if in the way, for the making of an adequate tracheal window. Many emergency tracheostomies need to be performed without anesthesia.

It is of more than passing interest that over a century ago Trendelenburg (1871) invoked use of tracheostomy in inhalation anesthesia, employing an inflatable rubber cuff. He employed tracheostomy particularly for jaw resections and other extensive operations in the neck in which bleeding into the mouth or pharynx could occur. He coated the rubber balloon with flannel onto which chloroform was dripped.[35]

Endotracheal Intubation

Victor Ver Meulen and Herbert Birck (1968) believe nasotracheal intubation, despite a fairly high complication rate, commands a lesser mortality than tracheostomy. That injury of the upper respiratory tract attends such prolonged intubation is well known, including necrotizing tracheitis, glottic ulceration, and subglottic tracheal stenosis. Blair Fearon and associates (1966) from the Toronto Hospital for Sick Children reported that, out of 72 infants and children subjected to nasotracheal intubation for respiratory distress, 45 (62.5 percent) failed to survive, a measure, obviously, of the severity of the illnesses treated.[36]

Carl Lindholm (1969) of Uppsala has written an extremely knowledgeable evaluation of tracheostomy and nasotracheal intubation. He presents a table listing deaths "attributable to tracheostomy" varying between 0.0 and 7.9 percent. Unfortunately, the reader finds no report of the overall patient mortality. One learns that 10 deaths occurred among a total of between 1,200 and 1,300 children as a complication of prolonged intratracheal intubation.[37] Ignoring the overall mortality obviously attaches a complexion to the situation that does not portray the actual accomplishment. Faithful and reliable reporting of actual results attending treatment are essential to the progress of surgery. In chapter 19 of this book we allude to James Paget's (1862) differentiation between operative mortality and deaths after operation for which he believed the surgeon was not responsible. When prophylactic surgical antisepsis found acceptance, these mysterious, unaccounted for operative deaths largely disappeared.[38]

Whereas anesthesiologists are likely to prefer endotracheal intubation, otolaryngologists continue to find tracheostomy "the safest procedure for both short and long term relief of respiratory obstruction."[39] William John Glover of London, anesthetist (1972), favors, when practical, endotracheal intubation over tracheostomy, carried out as an elective procedure under general anesthesia in children; a nasotracheal tube is passed and the operation is performed without the patient struggling.[40]

Assisted respiration with a pressure-controlled mechanical ventilator is a very helpful device in conditions such as a flail chest wall, attending fracture of multiple ribs and the sternum, until normal ventilation has been reestablished.

Sterilization of plastic tracheal and endotracheal tubes demands special consideration. Conventional steam sterilization, as applied to metal instruments, is out of order. Current techniques include sterilization by gas, ionized radiation, and liquid disinfectants. No standard technique has yet been agreed upon; methods of achieving acceptable sterility are continually being reassessed.

Laryngeal Foreign Bodies

Raphaël Sabatier in 1810 described incision of the cricothyroid membrane for removal of lodged foreign bodies in the larynx. Sabatier found it to be a thick ligamentous membrane, 30 mm. in length and 9 mm. in width. He referred to the earlier work of Vicq-d'Azyr, who had performed division of this membrane on dogs with complete success, remarking upon its ease of access and that it was a simpler operation than tracheostomy.[41]

Lodgment of a piece of meat in the larynx has snuffed out many a life. Persons with upper dental plates miss the sensitivity of the soft palate in helping to direct swallowed food into the esophagus. In such emergencies, whether in the home or restaurant, use of the inverted posture and a thrust against the lower rib margin often succeeds in dislodging the obstruction. In fact, a sudden thrust to the epigastrium from behind by the locked hands of the operator will often suffice to eject a foreign body lodged in the larynx.[42] A finger introduced into the throat, encouraging the cough reflex, also is helpful.

Laryngeal Tumors

The father of laryngology in America, Horace Green of New York, wrote an interesting small monograph in 1852 on the surgical treatment of polyps of the larynx and edema of the glottis. He suggested that the nature of laryngeal polyps was not appreciated until the middle of the eighteenth century. Green cited several instances in which patients died from acute asphyxia, occasionally having had prior episodes of suffocation.

In removing polyps of the larynx, Green seated the patient on a stool with head directed backward. He stood behind with good light while an assistant depressed the patient's tongue. Green urged the patient to cough; if there was a pedicled polyp in the pharynx it would be extruded. Such a polyp could be aspirated into the larynx on inspiration and cause suffocation. Green's enthusiasm for peroral application of silver nitrate to laryngeal lesions occasioned him to overuse the method.[43]

The Laryngoscope

The Spanish singing master Manuel Garcia (1854–55) made a significant contribution to laryngology by demonstrating that the larynx could be inspected by aid of a small mirror attached to a long handle; with the patient facing the sun and the examiner standing behind the patient and pushing the mirror gently against the soft palate and the uvula, the movements of the vocal cords, responsible for voice phonations, could readily be inspected. Garcia's important work was done in London. He lived to be 102 and became an international celebrity, recognized for his contribution to the development of laryngoscopy.[44]

Cancer of the Larynx

At one period tracheostomy alone was used to treat cancer of the larynx when it became obstructive. Billroth's first laryngofissure was performed in 1870 upon a patient with tuberculosis of the larynx. The thyroid cartilage was divided in the midline, providing direct access to the larynx, permitting excision of an involved vocal cord. The patient succumbed two months later of pulmonary tuberculosis. Billroth then did a succession of laryngofissures for malignancies, followed in some instances, because of recurrence, by laryngectomy (total). Billroth's experience, first with laryngofissure, then with partial laryngectomy, and finally with a group of operations entailing total laryngectomy was indeed very disappointing, with no long-term survivals.[45]

Gurdon Buck of New York Hospital related the instance of a woman of fifty-three upon whom he performed laryngofissure in 1851 for intralaryngeal tumor, the patient surviving for approximately a year beyond the first of three operations. She died of asphyxia when, on withdrawal of the cannula for cleaning, neither she nor her daughter could replace it.[46]

On April 9, 1886, Bernhard Fränkel of Berlin read a paper at the German Surgical Congress entitled "First cure of laryngeal cancer through extirpation by the natural way." The patient concerned was Professor Julius Wiggers, who came to Fränkel from Rostock on the recommendation of Virchow in September 1881 with a bean-sized tumor of the right vocal cord. Fränkel seized the tumor with forceps and excised a portion of the right vocal cord, which he then cauterized with galvanocautery. A year later, in September 1882, he repeated the procedure. A third recurrence was removed in February 1884. At Fränkel's request, Professor Madelung, a general surgeon, then performed a neck dissection, removing several involved lymph nodes; no mention is made of laryngofissure at this time. In June 1884 Fränkel for the fifth time removed the tumor intralaryngeally. After that, apparently, the patient did well. Fränkel found the larynx normal on laryngoscopic examination in October 1885, and the patient wrote him on April 2, 1886, that he seemed completely well and that his voice was reasonably good.[47]

The account of this first successful intralaryngeal extirpation of a malignant growth was published by Fränkel in 1887, the year that marked the beginnings of an international controversy over the management of a lesion in the larynx of Crown Prince Frederick, son of William I, Emperor of Germany.[48] William had been a successful monarch and Frederick, a warm patron of the arts and sciences, was a great favorite among the German people. On the occasion of his father's ninetieth birthday, March 18, 1887, the crown prince, then fifty-six, made a speech in which a very noticeable hoarseness was obvious to all who heard him. The prince had consulted Carl Gerhardt of the University Faculty in Berlin, who had diagnosed a small growth on the posterior part of the left vocal cord. Gerhardt strove to remove it with the aid of a laryngeal mirror, but failed; he then cauterized the lesion a number of times. Although the growth seemed to disappear, hoarseness and discomfort remained. Frederick's wife, Crown Princess Victoria, the eldest child of Queen Victoria, alerted her mother in a letter of April 29, 1887, that all was not well with her husband. Again on May 7 the crown princess wrote her mother that Professor Bergmann was contemplating making an external approach from the neck (laryngofissure) to the lesion, in light of the circumstance that its removal through the larynx had been unsuccessful.

At this juncture Bismarck[49] entered the picture and convened a consultation, attended by Gerhardt, Bergmann, and a number of other consultants. All expressed approval of Bergmann's suggestion. Despite absence of microscopic proof of malignancy, a firm clinical diagnosis of cancer of the left vocal cord had been established by Gerhardt and confirmed by Professor Adelbert Tobold. In fact, Bergmann had planned to do the operation on Sunday, May 21, and had sent all the necessary instruments to Potsdam and made the nursing arrangements. Meanwhile exchanges between the crown princess and Queen Victoria urged postponement of the procedure until Morell Mackenzie, England's foremost laryngologist, had an opportunity to assess the situation.

Mackenzie arrived from London and saw Frederick on May 20. He was unwilling to approve the operation proposed by Bergmann until a microscopic diagnosis of cancer was produced. When three biopsies failed to reveal microscopic cancer, the operation was postponed indefinitely.

The summer of 1887 witnessed celebration of Queen Victoria's Golden Jubilee, the fiftieth anniversary of her ascent to the throne. Frederick and the crown princess spent considerable time in London, providing Mackenzie additional opportunities to examine the royal patient and to cauterize his laryngeal lesion. It was then recommended to the prince that he spend the winter in San Remo, Italy, where he would be attended by Fritz Bramann, Bergmann's assistant, and by Mark Hovell, Mackenzie's assistant. When Mackenzie visited Frederick in Italy on February 8, 1888, he found Frederick's condition distinctly worse. It was obvious that a tracheostomy was in order because of the patient's dyspnea. Bramann wished to wait until Bergmann came from Berlin, but the situation dictated immediate performance of the operation and it was carried out by Bramann on the afternoon of February 9. Mackenzie had declared he would assume no responsibility unless the tracheostomy was done at once.

A month later, March 9, 1888, Emperor William I of Germany died. His son, despite the inclement weather, returned at once to Berlin. Frederick III was emperor ninety-nine days and was obviously a very ill man over that entire period. He bore the tracheostomy reasonably well. Toward the end the cannula had to be replaced and a false passage was made by Bergmann. No effort was ever made to extirpate the lesion. Had the proposed laryngofissure been carried out when Bergmann first saw him, Frederick undoubtedly would have continued in reasonably good health for a period of time. However, it must be admitted, achievement with cancer of the larynx at that date was meager.

The autopsy was performed June 16, 1888, directly after the emperor's death. A translation of the memorandum signed by (among others) Mackenzie, Bergmann, Virchow, and Heinrich Waldeyer, a famous anatomist, appeared in the *British Medical Journal* on July 21, 1888. It read in part: "Cancerous destruction of the larynx, with secondary disease of a rather large lymphatic gland at the lower part of the left side of the neck, and a cutaneous nodule on the right side near the wound. Oesophagus, unaffected. Inflammatory destruction of the upper portion of the windpipe and the neighbouring parts. Numerous bronchiectases, with putrid contents. Near these, bronchopneumonic suppurating gangrenous patches." In a separate report on the same page Virchow and Waldeyer confirmed the microscopic diagnosis of cancer.

The mismanagement of Frederick's laryngeal cancer caused international repercussions of great moment. Despite his signature attesting the gross presence of cancer of the larynx on the occasion of the autopsy, Mackenzie actually did not capitulate completely to this thesis. He never fully recovered from the damage done his reputation by his hesitant indecision and died four years later, a greatly disappointed man.

In an attempt to "present both sides of this memorable case" the *British Medical Journal* (October 13, 1888) published summaries of the German attack on Mackenzie and of the latter's defense. Mackenzie was severely criticized by the German authorities for his interference and mismanagement and for his insistence on a positive microscopic diagnosis before surgery was undertaken. Mackenzie made the tragic error of ignoring all clinical signs. Despite the absence of histologic diagnosis any seasoned clinician would have agreed with Bergmann. What could be seen through a laryngoscope indeed manifested a myopic view of the situation. Bergmann pointed out that microscopic evidence was particularly unreliable in this instance because it "was hardly possible to reach the portion of the tumour containing characteristic elements."

Mackenzie defended his stand against surgery in part on the poor results achieved by laryngofissure and even by laryngectomy, saying that of 22 published instances of laryngofissure, only 2 were successful; of 35 cases of partial excision of the larynx, only 1; and in 138 of total extirpation, only 8. Certain it is that the results of the management of laryngeal cancer at that date were poor. Yet to ignore the presence of advancing cancer and to delay performance of tracheostomy for relief of respiratory obstruction until near death on any patient, let alone a crown prince about to succeed his father as Emperor of Germany, was obviously a serious error in judgment.[50] Mackenzie's insistence on a positive microscopic diagnosis of cancer on excised biopsy specimens was of course his great mistake, which could be repeated today if the decision demanded a positive microscopic diagnosis in all instances. Certainly the surgery that Bergmann proposed on the basis of clinical findings was fully justifiable. Clinical findings must be considered in a diagnosis.

Similarly, microscopists in earlier decades had difficulty in recognizing the potential malignancy of small polypoid lesions in the urinary bladder. In fact, there are instances in which a lesion was diagnosed as benign by the pathologist in the presence of its observed clinical spread. Until very recently many pathologists continued to insist that most adenomatous polyps of the rectum and colon were benign. Basil Morson of St. Mark's Hospital for Rectal Diseases in London, through long pursuit of the problem and careful histologic studies, has succeeded in alerting the profession to the circumstance that these "benign lesions" are actually a frequent source of cancer of the colon and rectum.[51]

Another tragic neglect of a laryngeal cancer winding up with an emergency tracheostomy concerned the famous painter Sir John Millais. Treves was called by a fellow practitioner, George H. Hames, after midnight in May 1896 to the home of Millais, where he found Millais breathing with great difficulty, his face livid and his lips black. The patient had apparently been suffering from hoarseness periodically since October 1892.

A kneeling housemaid held a lamp so that Treves, also on his knees, could perform the tracheostomy. Hames attempted to anesthetize the patient with chloroform, but the anesthetic assembly fell apart. Treves opened the trachea when Millais appeared virtually dead. Artificial respiration was started by Hames, and the patient responded. The tracheostomy tube was fastened in position. Tracheostomy wearers cannot speak, of course, unless there is provision for air to enter the larynx through an aperture on the convex upper curve of the cannula.[52] Millais squeezed Treves' hand firmly as he left, a gesture that Treves said fully repaid him for all the difficulties of the emergency.[53]

These are, indeed, two tragic occurrences emphasizing indecision and acceptance of tracheostomy only as a last resort in the relief of dyspnea caused by cancer of the larynx. Today, such postponement would be regarded as malpractice. Cancer of the larynx can be treated quite satisfactorily by laryngofissure in very early stages and by total laryngectomy when the lesion extends beyond the vocal cord. X-ray radiation is sometimes used instead of laryngofissure. It has the advantage over surgery in avoiding persistent hoarseness from loss of a vocal cord. Combinations of radiation with surgery are also being tried out in many clinics; a definitive plan has yet to be evolved.

At the German Roentgen Congress in 1968, radiotherapy of cancer of the throat and larynx was broadly discussed. A report indicated that among 243 patients proved to have cancer of the larynx, in 24 cases (10 percent) the diagnosis had only been established by laryngofissure,[54] the procedure Bergmann had proposed for Crown Prince Frederick.

C. L. Jackson and C. M. Norris (1963) reported a five-year survival rate of 91 percent with early lesions of the vocal cords treated by irradiation. This figure compares favorably with somewhat more advanced cases treated by partial laryngectomy, in which they obtained a five-year survival of 87.6 percent, increased to 91.9 percent by reoperation for residual cancer in 15 instances.[55]

Today, for extensive lesions, complete laryngectomy followed by radical neck dissection is a generally accepted procedure. As in most cancers the ultimate outcome is dependent upon early diagnosis. Certainly hoarseness lasting more than a week without obvious cause is an indication for laryngoscopic examination.

Rehabilitation of the laryngectomized patient has received great attention in recent years. The artificial larynx has been largely discarded and the most promising devices appear to be electronic, employing a pulsating diaphragm that transmits vibrations from the side of the neck to the larynx and oral cavity during speech.

Summary

Relief of respiratory obstruction in the larynx and upper reaches of the trachea by tracheostomy traces back to antiquity, when it was usually performed only as a last antemortem resort. The need to perform such operations early has finally become generally recognized. A double-lumen tracheostomy tube introduced approximately two and a half centuries ago has greatly facilitated maintaining an open breathing space; the inner tube is merely removed and cleaned periodically. Laryngeal obstruction by diphtheritic membrane, a frequent indication for tracheostomy in the nineteenth century, has disappeared since the introduction of antidiphtheritic measures early in this century. Inasmuch as the indications for tracheostomy are usually life-threatening, the mortality attending the operation still remains high. Peroral endotracheal intubation for edematous temporary tracheal obstruction is often preferred to tracheostomy.

That laryngeal biopsy cannot always be depended upon to give histologic proof of malignancy was well established ninety years ago in the international controversy over the management of Germany's Crown Prince Frederick's hoarseness. Even today in 10 percent of instances the diagnosis still has to be made by laryngofissure.

(For notes, see pp. 626–31.)

CHAPTER 9

Empyema

BARON DUPUYTREN, threatened with death by empyema, said he would rather die by the hand of God than by that of surgeons. And well he might have made such a decision, for the chance of death from the operation in 1835 was exceedingly high, in the area of 60 percent. Dupuytren had weighed the possibilities for some time and selected his assistant Sanson to do the surgery, but at the last moment he rejected the measure as futile. He died twelve days after the diagnosis.[1] Empyema took the life of Maria Theresa, Empress of Austria, in 1780. She was bled twice for an axillary abscess and given a powerful emetic. The abscess ruptured into the pleura because of the delay in opening it; the ensuant empyema caused her death.[2]

Shortly after Dupuytren's death several sessions of the French Royal Academy of Medicine were devoted to a discussion of the management of empyema, in which a number of well-known Paris physicians and surgeons participated. Larrey recommended pulling the skin of the lower thorax upward, followed by a short incision with a bistoury at the upper border of the rib of an intercostal space. When the upward traction on the skin was released, the opening into the pleural sac was automatically sealed over, avoiding an open pneumothorax. Some suggested puncture of the pleural collection, but just how this was to be achieved was not described. There was no agreement on the advisability of removing all or only a portion of the exudate. A few insisted that a bilateral open pneumothorax was well tolerated by healthy dogs; others contended it was uniformly lethal.

No guiding principle emerged from the prolonged debating. No discussant had an experience beyond a case or two. Opinions were freely expressed. The physician Pierre Louis, who had already rejected overused phlebotomy in 1835 for most illnesses, in this discussion of 1836 reported 150 cases of "pleurisy" at La Pitié in which one or more bleedings were performed by lancet, including also leeches; "all 150 patients were cured," said Louis.[3]

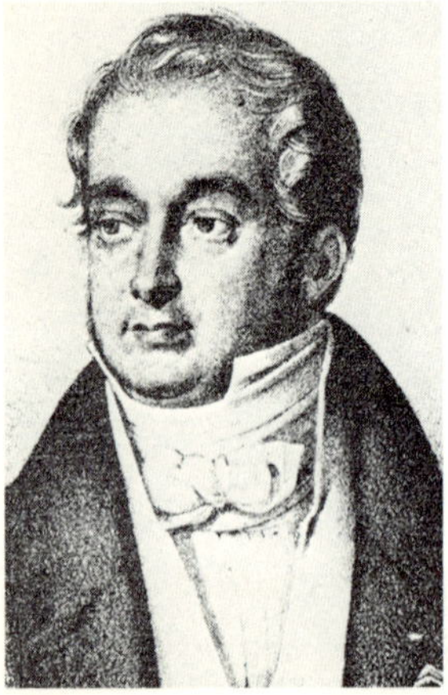

9.1 Dupuytren chose to die of empyema by the hand of God (1835).

Six years after Dupuytren's death, Sédillot (1841), a senior surgeon and professor at the military hospital of Val-de-Grâce in Paris, wrote a comprehensive report on operation for empyema in a *concours* thesis, saying that such surgery had fallen into discredit because it was misunderstood and badly executed.[4] Including experiences of his own, he alluded to forty-three instances of empyema, widely scattered in time, beginning in the seventeenth century. Sédillot spoke of the Hippocratic rule that evacuation of an empyema should not be undertaken until about the fifteenth day after the onset of symptoms, when the pleural exudate would have acquired detectable density. This observation of Hippocratic medicine was amply confirmed by experience with the management of empyema in the influenza epidemic during World War I.

Sédillot named four manners of treating empyema surgically: (1) incision, (2) cauterization, (3) intercostal aspiration, and (4) rib resection. He said that Hippocrates urged opening the thoracic cavity in the third costal interspace, counting ribs from below. Sédillot apparently rediscovered the Hippocratic views on the management of empyema, which recognized the importance of delaying open chest drainage until the exudate was no longer serous and found that dependent drainage was optimal when instituted at the lowest margin of the pleural cavity. Émile Littré, an eminent historian and philologist and an ardent student of Hippocrates and his school, was also aware of the Hippocratic doctrine on the treatment of empyema, a thesis Littré developed in his ten-volume series on Hippocrates (1851). Guido Majno (1975) has more recently alluded to the conservative views of Hippocrates in dealing with empyema. C. D. O'Malley (1964) stated that Vesalius (1547), resurrected operative management of empyema, which had long been neglected.[5]

Needle Aspiration

In 1843 Trousseau performed thoracentesis on a seventeen-year-old girl who was seemingly near death from acute pleurisy. Making a small incision with a lancet at the upper border of the ninth left rib, he pulled the skin up so that the incision corresponded with the eighth costal interspace. Trousseau plunged a hydrocele trocar into the pleural cavity and aspirated an amber fluid that flowed readily. When he removed the cannula, the skin wound closed spontaneously. The patient began to breathe easily, the pleurisy ameliorated, and within sixteen days she was well on the way to complete recovery. The next year (1844) Trousseau described a second successful case, as well as a third patient with puerperal fever, peritonitis, and pleurisy who died after three punctures. Trousseau was the "prophet of the future," but his instrument was so heavy it was better fitted "for the side of a barrel than for the human chest," remarked Henry Bowditch. H. M. Hughes and Edward Cock of Guy's Hospital reported (1844) upon 25 patients treated with paracentesis thoracis by them and other members of the staff over the years 1833–44. Repetitive aspiration of the pleura by trocar was employed. The mortality in the 25 cases was 36 percent.[6]

Several other names are identified with needle aspiration and/or intercostal siphonage of pleural exudates. These include Bowditch (1852), Georges Dieulafoy (1870),[7] F. C. Hewett (1876), Pierre Potain (1886), and G. Bülau (1891), all well known to students of the problem.[8] Bowditch credits Morrill Wyman of Boston (1850) with the innovation in America. It is related that Wyman removed the pleural exudate from a patient with a large exploring needlelike trocar attached to a suction pump on February 23, 1850, and repeated the aspiration a few days later. Bowditch asked Wyman to perform the procedure on one of his own patients April 17, 1850. Bowditch later announced to the medical world that the innovation belonged to Wyman, who rarely published.[9]

William Osler in 1879 was appointed physician to the Montreal General Hospital, an institution he knew well from undergraduate days at McGill and as a volunteer in the autopsy room and wards after his return from two years of study abroad. By the time the thirty-five-year-old Canadian left Montreal to become professor of clinical medicine at the University of Pennsylvania (1884), he had attracted a following of students and had started his great collection of specimens, rare books, and clinical notes. It was from the last that he no doubt drew his description of three recent cases of empyema treated successfully at Montreal General Hospital, adding, "These three cases of empyema stand out very distinctly in my memory, inasmuch as they are among the few instances in which I have seen good recoveries in this disease."[10] The practice was to employ aspiration followed by dependent open intercostal drainage, a procedure that anticipated the lessons of management of empyema during World War I.

In 1886, when Rickman J. Godlee, Lister's nephew and biographer, reported on treatment of empyema, aspiration was his conventional mode of therapy. In a few instances rib resection also was done. Godlee strangely concluded that the drainage vent should not be at the lowest segment of the chest, for, he said, this portion of the cavity closes first owing to the rise of the diaphragm. Godlee preferred to excise a short segment of the rib, followed by exploration of the pleural cavity with the finger. In children Godlee often removed the drainage tube at the end of two weeks. If the tube had been withdrawn and fever recurred, he urged immediate dilatation of the sinus tract.

Godlee wrote of patients treated in two London hospitals, a group of 30 children from one to ten years old, at the North-Eastern Hospital for Children and a second group of 20 patients varying in age from five and one-half years to forty-nine years at the Brompton Hospital. There was one death (3.3 percent mortality) at the Children's Hospital and three in the second group (14 percent mortality). The overall mortality rate was 8 percent.[11]

Controversy over Open Drainage

At the 1890 meeting of the German Congress of Internal Medicine held in Vienna there was a long discussion on the management of empyema, in which both physicians and surgeons, including Billroth, participated. Karl Immermann, professor of medicine in Basel, introduced the subject. He reported the use of aspiration in a series of 74 patients, some of whom he deleted from the account because of tuberculosis, septicemia, or puerperal fever, leaving 57 patients with what he regarded as conventional empyema. Of these 57 patients, 3 died (5.26 percent mortality). Immermann said he disagreed with the Berlin surgeon Ernst Küster,[12] who believed that continuous aspiration lengthened the healing period. Immermann concluded that repetitive aspiration provided the greatest protection for the patient.

The second paper in the series was given by Max Schede, professor of surgery at Hamburg. Schede said that Jacob Estlander (1879) did not do extensive rib resection, that he resected only 4 to 6 cm. of three or four ribs. In other words, Estlander's operation provided only very adequate drainage of the empyema cavity.[13] On the contrary, Schede resected long segments of as many as nine ribs in adults with chronic empyema. In fact, says Schede, in 1878 he had come to the belief that not only the ribs but the thickened pleura also should be excised, thereby bringing an extensive musculocutaneous flap in contact with the visceral surface of the lung, obliterating the empyema cavity.

The discussion following the presentations by Immermann and Schede was begun by the physician Oscar Fraentzel of Berlin, who said he favored Bülau siphonage drainage over open rib resection. Curschmann, a Leipzig internist, preferred aspiration to surgery and found little difference in the healing periods of aspiration and open operation. In the main, physicians participating in the discussion favored aspiration, while most of the surgeons advised preliminary aspiration followed by rib resection.

Emanuel Aufrecht, a physician of Magdeburg, wrote in 1894 that, contrary to the opinion of most other physicians, he favored rib resection. He tried to sterilize the empyema cavity with a 2 percent solution of carbolic acid, in the presence of a large drain, a method popular in France forty years earlier using iodine compounds.[14] Aufrecht reported that among 36 patients subjected to rib resection, there was only one death, a patient who on entry had a tracheal rattle in the throat and died following evacuation of 3 liters of foul stinking pus, which to a surgeon portends the likely presence of gangrenous lung.[15]

One might reasonably have expected that acceptance of prophylactic surgical antisepsis, which found general recognition about 1885, would lower the mortality of empyema considerably. In individual reports of the period no significant difference is readily discernible.[16] However, on summarizing the mortality in twelve reports in the international literature between 1802 and 1876, the authors found the overall mortality for 98 patients was 26.5 percent. In ten reports employing conventional antiseptic practices, dating from 1875 to 1896, among 236 patients treated for empyema the overall mortality was 14.8 percent; obviously, a very definite advantage had accrued from employment of antiseptic practices.

Experiences of World War I

In the influenza epidemic that swept the Western world during World War I, streptococcal cellulitic pneumonia followed by empyema was pandemic among civilians of all ages as well as in the military forces of the Allies and the Central Powers. The mortality in treated cases of empyema among both civilian and military personnel was astonishingly great, occasioned in large measure by failure to appreciate the danger of establishing open pneumothorax in the presence of a serous exudate. Most of the empyemas in that period were streptococcal in nature, accompanied by a serous exudate containing little fibrin; fibrinous sticky exudates are far more likely to accompany pneumococcal empyemas, reflected also by the uniform presence of fibrin in the pulmonary alveoli. When open drainage was undertaken early in streptococcal empyema, the lung collapsed completely and it was exceedingly difficult to reexpand it. Moreover, the admission of atmospheric pressure into the pleural cavity on one side brought about a mediastinal shift, with consequent displacement of the contralateral lung, diminishing the patient's vital capacity.

Graham and Bell, representing the Empyema Commission of the United States Army, came to the conclusion (1918) that it was wise to tap the pleural cavity in patients with empyema either by a needle or an intercostal catheter. In this procedure a negative pressure could be maintained within the thorax by suction. Open drainage was performed only when tap by intercostal tube proved inadequate. The research was done in the Hunterian Laboratory of W. G. MacCallum at The Hopkins with dogs as the experimental animals. The study showed that the mediastinum was mobile and not fixed as some previous writers had suggested.

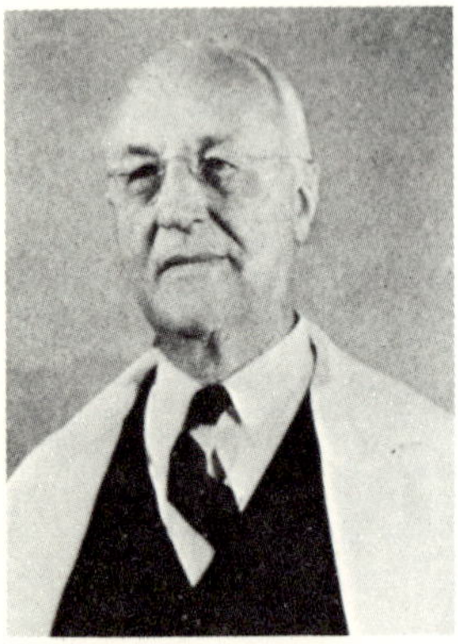

9.2 Graham confirmed value of closed drainage for serous streptococcal empyema in World War I (1918).

The same journal in which Graham and Bell gave their report contained an editorial statement from the Surgeon General's Office declaring that the "evacuation of the pleural exudate by operation early in the disease involves greater risks, without compensating benefits, than removal by aspiration. Much of the relief offered by operation without its attendant dangers can be offered by aspiration, repeated according to indications." Irrigation of the empyema cavity with Dakin's solution (hypochlorite) was advocated in all instances in which a bronchopleural fistula was not present. Other recommendations were expansion of the lung by blowing against resistance, the use of negative pressure and gentle suction devices, and properly controlled respiratory exercises.[17]

The experiences of World War I with the surgical management of empyema reenforced the importance of the Hippocratic rule of not being too hasty in establishing open pleural drainage. In the 1920s the surgeon often made it regular practice to place on the wall at the head of the patient's bed a series of small sealed glass tubes of aspirated exudate. Only when more than 50 percent of the exudate was cellular debris was recourse made to open chest drainage. Meanwhile, from the beginning of the empyema, the pleural cavity was aspirated frequently at a low point posteriorly, permitting small quantities of air to enter the cavity to aid in the displacement and removal of the exudate.

That not all physicians immediately utilized the lessons of World War I in the management of empyema is reflected in the following experience. In the fall of 1925 the University of Minnesota acquired a full-time professor of medicine, Hilding Berglund of Sweden, who came directly from the laboratory of Otto Folin at Harvard. On a crisp October morning the senior author noted the professor leaving his house and stopped to offer him a ride to the hospital in my Model-T Ford, introducing myself as the current senior surgical resident. The professor said "You are just the person I need to see." He then related a situation which concerned a young patient, a student with empyema, for whom he had recommended open rib resection. Said the professor, "The physicians in the Health Service know nothing of the therapy of empyema and have never heard of Hippocrates, who insisted that wherever pus is present, it must be completely evacuated." It was also clear that the professor too was not familiar with Hippocrates' reservations concerning the need for cautious delay in opening the pleural cavity to drain a serous pleural purulent collection.

What began as a friendly discussion of the surgical management of empyema had become a controversy of some proportions by the time we reached the hospital doors. I politely suggested that the professor read what Evarts Graham had said upon the matter. The mention of Graham's name occasioned the professor to exclaim, "I see for the first time a dim light on your mental horizon." Thereupon I wrote out two recent references by Graham and handed them to the professor.

Within the hour I was visited by our distinguished professor of pharmacology, Arthur D. Hirshfelder, who said, "Owen, you must go to the professor at once and apologize." I replied, "I find it difficult to do so, for I am certain that my stand in the matter is sound." Said my faculty friend, "It makes no difference. You are only beginning to scale the academic ladder. Don't make the mistake of contending with a professor." The matter had also reached the attention of Dean E. P. Lyon, whose appointee I was, as well as of my teacher, Arthur Strachauer, professor of surgery, neither of whom had any advice to offer.

All of this occurred on a Friday morning. Late the next Tuesday afternoon, while I was washing my hands following some dressing changes, Professor Berglund, who had just returned from presenting a clinic concerning the patient in question, said, "Doctor, those references you gave me were not bad, in fact, not half bad," a rather generous concession for a professor to make to a young surgical house officer. Thereafter, we became fast friends and often discussed medical-surgical interphase problems.

Adequacy of Aspiration

It must be understood that closed aspiration of empyema collections in the thorax with rigid walls is not as efficacious as suction applied to a hollow viscus like the stomach, with contractile walls from which the entire contents of the viscus can be quickly aspirated if the tube is properly placed. Not so in the thorax. No matter how great the negative pressure suction, the pleural collection cannot be completely evacuated unless the lung expands concomitantly. This shortcoming of the closed aspiration method can be overcome in part by periodic admission of air, with the patient in the sitting position, thus permitting greater evacuation of the collection. Similarly, irrigation with saline solution will dilute the purulent collection, thereby enhancing the efficiency of closed aspiration. It is to be admitted, however, that the last drop of exudate in a pleural cavity is rarely removed by closed aspiration.

If, however, rib resection is done at the most dependent posterior segment of the collection when the pleural exudate has become thick, open drainage is more likely to provide a dry pleural cavity. The empyema is cured only when the lung is completely reexpanded. Delay in initiating adequate drainage of an empyema is, therefore, a deterrent to ready expansion of the lung.

Assessment of Methods in 1932

George Heuer, one of Halsted's most versatile trainees, writing on acute empyema in 1932, alluded to the great variation in the mortality rate of empyema, pointing out that the mortality of pneumonia, from which empyema stems, also varies considerably. He stated that before World War I the preferred method of treatment was open rib resection but that the studies of Graham and Bell and others had focused on its hazards in streptococcal empyemas.

Heuer related that in a series of 425 patients with empyema at The Hopkins from 1889 to 1921, treated almost exclusively by rib resection and drainage, the mortality in all acute empyemas in which no other lesion was present was less than 6 percent; in children between the ages of five and ten, the mortality was zero. At the Cincinnati General Hospital during the period 1922–30, when Heuer was professor of surgery, in a series of 158 cases in which no other lesion was present the mortality of closed aspiration drainage was 1.4 percent. Yet in the patients treated at the same hospital in 1927, the mortality had been 50 percent. The point is, there is a mortality of disease as well as of treatment; the virulence of the disease can vary greatly.

Heuer recommended Dakin's solution as an irrigant in the management of empyema, believing it acted as a solvent for fibrin and necrotic tissue. The force of Fleming's statement of 1919, that most antiseptic agents introduced into wounds did more harm to tissues than to bacteria, had not yet been fully appreciated by surgeons. The average healing period in most empyemas in Heuer's series was thirty-nine days from institution of treatment until closure of the empyema cavity. In one instance it was ten days. Joseph Danna of New Orleans (1931) wrote of aspiration attended by air replacement without external open drainage; among thirty-five patients treated in this manner there were two deaths (5.7 percent mortality).[18]

Reexpansion of the Lung

Some of the difficulty with the management of empyema just before and during World War I was occasioned by failure to evacuate all the exudate from the pleural cavity. This obviously was in a period antedating the availability of antibiotics. It is now standard practice to use needle aspiration followed by drainage with an intercostal catheter placed posteriorly, because ill patients lie on their backs; this is followed in turn by rib resection when the pleural exudate is fairly thick.

Young surgeons today have had little experience with acute suppurative empyema, because the administration of sulfonamides or penicillin for pneumonia has usually precluded the development of empyema. Osler characterized pneumonia as the old man's friend,[19] and still it is, unfortunately, for viral varieties of the illness rarely respond favorably to available chemotherapeutic or antibiotic management; there is no current effective treatment.

Today's surgeon is more likely to encounter empyema as a

complication of a hemorrhagic collection in the thorax, following trauma or an operation in which the pleural hemostasis was imperfect. In World War II surgeons recognized the importance of mobilizing the lung by incising the slight thickening of the visceral pleura directly overlying the lung, permitting it to expand.

After World War I our civil hospitals had many patients whose empyemas had been drained by open pneumothorax far too early; in consequence, the lung had receded from the chest wall, so that Schede's multiple rib resection type of thoracoplasty was required to bring the chest wall to the lung.

When the lung does not reexpand quickly attending drainage of the empyema, thumb-nail thickening of the visceral pleura in empyema binds the lung down. On the contrary, the parietal pleura in chronic empyema becomes very thick, frequently an inch or more. The cause of this disparity in behavior of visceral and parietal pleura is not well understood. It may be a matter of the lymphatic drainage of the pleural cavity in the presence of infection, undoubtedly greater to the parietes of the chest wall. Effective drainage of the pleural cavity accompanied by respiratory exercises and forced expiration in which the patient blows water from one bottle into another, without the aid of gravity, is a useful expedient in encouraging lung expansion. Most of all, early evacuation and effective drainage are the significant factors in achieving early and complete reexpansion of the lung to obliterate an empyema cavity. When the pleural surfaces are healthy, healing occurs as it does in any wound by creeping proliferation of fibroblasts that gradually approximate the collapsed lung to the chest wall, obliterating the cavity.

A teaching model demonstrating the techniques of achieving lung expansion in empyema can be a useful method to instruct nurses, students, and ward personnel. A balloon with an attached tube is passed through a cork into a glass bottle attached to a mercury thermometer; the bottle also has an outlet for suction. It becomes quite evident that when the tube leading to the balloon is occluded, no amount of suction can expand it; when, however the outlet to the atmosphere is open to permit suction the balloon distends completely and fills most of the space within the glass walls of the container. This model serves to demonstrate the futility of attempting quick obliteration of an empyema cavity with closed suction drainage unless the lung expanded directly.[20]

It is very unlikely that antiseptic solutions injected into the pleural cavity have a useful influence in sterilizing the empyema cavity or in effecting expansion of the lung. Moreover, because of the toxicity of antiseptic agents when retained within the pleural cavity, their use can be dangerous to the patient.

The Origin of Pulmonary Decortication

Delorme, the well-known French military surgeon, in 1894 recognized the need to remove the slightly thickened visceral pleura overlying the lung and devised an operative procedure to liberate the lung, permitting it to expand. The exact origin of the procedure, which came to be known as pulmonary decortication, is somewhat difficult to place. A. H. Ferguson of Chicago (1897), who reported upon a successful partial visceral pleurectomy after an extensive Schede rib resection, stated that George Fowler of Brooklyn had reported a case earlier than Delorme. It concerned a residual empyema cavity of long standing, complicated by a bronchopleural fistula; by mobilizing and freeing the lung from the parietal pleura near the diaphragm, Fowler had succeeded in gaining partial expansion of the lung. Paul Reclus of La Pitié, Paris, stated that Delorme reported a brilliant result attending such an operation four days after its performance but that on the fifth postoperative day the patient was in syncope. Reclus condemned the operation.[21]

In the performance of pleural visceral decortication, the surgeon must strive to peel off the slightly thickened pleura as one would peel an orange. If the pleura comes off as when one peels an apple, the surgeon can be in difficulty owing to pulmonary seepage and the creation of many small bronchial fistulas.[22]

Carl Eggers of New York (1923) described a radical operation for chronic empyema, illustrated with excision of six to eight ribs, including intercostal muscle bundles and thickened parietal pleura. The operation differed only slightly from the Schede (1890) operation, Eggers's approach being posterolateral in contrast to Schede's, which was anterolateral. Schede's approach produced far greater deformity of the chest wall than Eggers's posterior approach.

The force of such wide excision brings the musculocutaneous tissues of the chest wall to the lung, obliterating the empyema cavity. Eggers's illustrations would suggest that mobilization of the lung in his operation played a very minor role in obliterating the empyema cavity.[23] The extensive rib removal and concomitant excision of intercostal muscle bundles including vessels and nerves is inevitably followed by a huge hernia of the upper abdomen on the same side. In order to avoid this unwarranted complication of the Schede type of chest wall collapse, it is possible to convert the intercostal muscle bundles into intercostal muscle ribbons.[24] In the presence of greatly thickened parietal pleura, however, it is not always easy to preserve intact every intercostal artery, which is, of course, necessary for the survival of each intercostal ribbon. This technique of dealing with greatly thickened parietal pleura in chronic empyema may therefore be only a partial success.

Gunshot Injuries of the Lung

Surgical management of gunshot wounds of the lung was an outgrowth of World War I. The French military surgeon Pierre Duval (1918) said that wounds of the chest had been considered trivial, based on experiences with small-caliber bullet wounds. Such wounds were comparatively benign unless a large vessel was injured. In World War I, however, shell wounds with dangerous sequelae were encountered.

Duval estimated that 24.2 percent of missile wounds of the lung were from small-caliber bullets, entailing a mortality of 2 percent; 75.8 percent were high-caliber shell wounds commanding a mortality of 28.2 percent. Contrary to accepted opinion of the day, he believed that surgery upon the lung was feasible, that hazards of open pneumothorax were negligible, and that it was safe to open the thorax, examine the lungs, remove foreign bodies, and suture the damaged lung surfaces. Duval believed that approximately 70 percent of patients with lung injuries could be saved by early operation. In a subsequent symposial discussion on war wounds of the lung at the Clinical Congress of the American College of Surgeons, Duval expressed similar views, urging early surgery and deemphasizing the risks of opening the thorax.[25]

In the mid-1930s four small children were brought into the wards at Minnesota's University Hospital, each shot through the thorax with a .38-caliber revolver by their father, who was despondent because the mother of the children was dying from a cancer of the cervix; the father then hanged himself in the farm silo. All the children recovered without incident, responding favorably to intercostal suction drainage. The air-containing lung, the least dense of all body tissues, floats on water. Life-threatening situations regularly attend wounds of the heart, the great vessels, and bullet wounds that fracture ribs, which then become secondary missiles.

Summary

The streptococcal empyemas with a thin serous exudate accompanying the pneumonias of the worldwide influenza epidemic of 1917–18 commanded a formidable mortality. The lessons in the management of empyema have been long and painful. Hippocrates recognized the importance of delayed aspiration of serous exudate and opposed draining the empyema collection prior to fifteen days after its onset; drainage was established by incision along the superior border of the rib adjoining the intercostal space chosen for the drainage site or by trocar inserted into the space. Whereas Sédillot (1841) wrote of intercostal trocar drainage, it did not catch on in France until Trousseau's papers of 1843–44 or in America until Bowditch advocated needle aspiration in 1852.

It took the disastrous experiences of World War I with open external drainage to reestablish firmly the Hippocratic principles of therapy. Graham and Bell (1918) rediscovered the truth of the Hippocratic observations, which Sédillot (1841) clearly reaffirmed. The noted German thoracic surgeon Sauerbruch (1929) stated that the mortality of open drainage treatment for streptococcal empyema during the influenza epidemic of 1918–19 was 90 percent.[26] It is astounding how significant lessons of the past have to be relearned.

With the availability of sulfonamides and antibiotics (1934–45) empyema and its antecedent, bacterial pneumonia, no longer constitute a dangerous threat, relieving surgeons of a serious responsibility that often necessitated formidable operations for the management of chronic empyema. This and similar occurrences reaffirm the role of research and how the activity of surgeons is changed thereby.

(For notes, see pp. 632–34.)

CHAPTER 10

Cesarean Section

DELIVERY OF AN INFANT through an incision in the dead mother's abdomen got its name ostensibly from the belief that Julius Caesar entered the world in this manner. However, as Friedrich Osiander, a well-known nineteenth-century Göttingen obstetrician, has pointed out, Caesar's mother Aurelia was still alive when Caesar was forty-eight years old, in an era when such operations were performed only after death of the mother in Western countries.[1] Nevertheless, the legend of Caesar's birth was often recalled in early surgical treatises, including that of Guy de Chauliac, and was a popular subject in Renaissance illustrations.[2]

Cesarean Section on Dead Mothers

Guy, in a brief passage on childbirth in his 1363 *Grande chirurgie*, refers to the necessity of removing the infant before burying the dead mother, saying it was forbidden to do otherwise by the king's ordinance. He advised cutting the woman with a razor the length of her left side, avoiding the liver on the right, and taking the child out with the fingers. He said that when ordinary maneuvers failed to extract a dead baby from a living mother it should be pulled out by hooks, "entier ou en pieces."[3]

Guillemeau, writing in 1609 of the *Happy Deliverie of Women*, tells of Caesar being "rip't out of his Mothers wombe, at the verie instant she died,"[4] adding, "Lawiers iudge them worthy of death, who shall burie a great bellyed-woman that is dead, before the child be taken foorth." Although he speaks of the need for haste to save the baby, Guillemeau says that the surgeon must first be assured the mother is dead and that "her kinsfolkes, friends, and others that are present, do all affirme and confesse, that her Soule is departed." Despite the likely delay in obtaining such a consensus, Guillemeau names two women from whom on their deaths he extracted live babies, "Monsier Paraeus [Paré], and the Curate of St. Andrew, being present."

Guillemeau said he had twice performed cesarean section on living mothers in the presence of Paré and had witnessed three others done by three skillful Paris surgeons. All the women died. Adds the author, although successes with cesarean section on living mothers are alleged, "*One Swallow makes not a Spring*."[5]

Paré put great emphasis on the urgency for doing cesarean section as soon as the mother died, saying that a surgeon should be in readiness for the task. He said such ancient practices as keeping the dead woman's mouth or other orifices open would not bring air to a child in the womb.[6] He also discussed in graphic detail the ways to remove a dead child from a living woman, dismemberment being one expedient. When the limbs were off and only the head remained, he tried to engage a hook, known as a crochet, in the infant's mouth, eye, or beneath the chin to facilitate extraction.

Records of living infants from thirty-six cesarean sections performed after the mothers' deaths have been tabulated from the world literature of the nineteenth century; by the mid-twentieth century over eighty more such cases had been reported. Assessments before 1700 are difficult to appraise, for accounts of living babies rescued from the uteri of dead mothers, some of whom, Lazarus-like, had been buried for days, place great strain upon twentieth-century credulity.[7]

Cesarean Section on the Living

Paré said nothing could persuade him that a live baby could be cut from the belly of a woman without her dying from the great wound, and he marveled at the "insolency of those that affirme that they have seene women whose bellies and wombe have bin more than once cut, and the infant taken out." A reply to Paré's repudiation soon appeared in *Hysterotomotokie*, a remarkable little book published in Paris in 1581.[8] The author, Rousset (1535?–90), was physician to the Duke of Savoy and later practiced as a surgeon in Paris.

Rousset reported that fifteen successful cesarean sections with living offspring had been accomplished in the preceding eighty years, six of these on the same woman. From this account it can be inferred that the maternal mortality in the sixteenth century was no worse than that reported for the last decades of the nineteenth century. Rousset divided his case histories into two categories: reports from persons he believed reliable, and "histoires oculaires," cases in which he had personally counseled the patient or obtained the testimony of the surgeon, husband, or other witnesses "who were present in goodly number." He himself did none of the operations. The patients and surgeons, often barber-surgeons, are named, as well as the French villages concerned, and details are given of the deliveries.[9]

A year later Rousset's text was put into Latin by Bauhin. In an appendix Bauhin reported several other cesarean sections from the sixteenth century in which both infant and mother survived, operations which he had neither performed nor observed, but which were recounted by persons whose veracity he apparently did not question.[10] Bauhin credited the 1500 story of Jacob Nuffer, a pig-gelder of Sigerhausen, Switzerland. When thirteen midwives and several lithotomists had been unable to effect the delivery of his wife, Elizabeth Alsbach, Nuffer expelled them from the room and responded to his wife's pleading to go ahead with the operation. After securing permission of the local governor, Nuffer laid his wife on the table, opened her abdomen, and extracted the infant without injury. The wound "was sewed up after the fashion of a veterinarian"[11] and healed nicely. Bauhin adds that in subsequent pregnancies the mother was delivered of four children in the normal manner and that the cesarean child lived to the age of seventy-seven. Several students of cesarean section doubt the authenticity of the Nuffer account. Some are skeptical inasmuch as the woman later had several normal labors.[12] However, there are so many instances of normal delivery in pregnancies after cesarean sections that this circumstance need not invalidate the report.

In 1933 Walter Oswald published an account of a pamphlet found in the library of the city archives of Frankfurt am Main. It recorded the performance of 7 cesarean sections by a midwife before the year 1411, with a fortunate outcome for mother and child in each instance, antedating Rousset's cases by a century. The pamphlet carries the title *Gefangene und Irre* [Prisoners and the Insane] and contains a long letter written in old German, ending with the signature of Jost von Pern. The dubious account obviously concerns illicit relations between patients and supervisors in the mental institution and prison where the pregnancies occurred; the midwife was probably a friend of Pern. It is indeed odd that the achievement did not find its way into the literature of an earlier day. Existence of the pamphlet, however, is bona fide.[13]

It seems strange that many historians are skeptical of the success with cesarean section upon living women in the sixteenth and seventeenth centuries, for it apparently had long been a last resort among primitive African women. During travels in Central Africa in 1879 R. W. Felkin, a medical student, witnessed a cesarean section in Uganda. The operation, he said, was customarily performed by men in the hope of saving mother and child when midwives were unable to accomplish delivery. The parturient was about twenty years old. She had been "liberally supplied with banana wine, and was in a state of semi-intoxication." She was fastened naked to the bed by ropes of bark. The operator stood at her left side, holding a knife aloft with his right hand, "muttering an incantation," following which he washed his hands and the patient's abdomen, first with banana wine and then with water. A bold incision extending from the pubis to the umbilicus severed the abdominal wall and entered the uterus; in fact, the infant also sustained a wound in the right shoulder. A red-hot iron was used to stop the bleeding points. When Felkin left the area eleven days later, both mother and baby were doing well.[14]

A British consul, writing of *Travels in Abyssinia and the Galla Country* (1848–60), related that a *waggayra*, a native Galla surgeon, had recently performed a cesarean section before many spectators. The author's informant, who had been present at the ordeal, said that the scene was horrible and that "all hid their eyes from a sight so startling."[15]

Acceptance of Cesarean Section on the Living

Apparently the first authentic cesarean section verified by medical witnesses was performed in Wittenberg on April 21, 1610, by Jeremiah Trautman, a local surgeon. The event was reported by Daniel Sennert, a professor in the Academy of Medicine at Wittenberg and a consultant in the case. He was among several other professional observers. The patient, Ursula, wife of Martin Opitz, had received a blow to the abdomen, rupturing muscular structures in the abdominal wall. A large hernia resulted on her left side, which was found to contain a gravid uterus. Sennert and his Academy colleagues were consulted well before labor began. They reasoned that natural delivery would probably be impossible and decided upon cesarean section when the time came for delivery. After extraction of the infant, the uterine wound was left open; the uterus apparently could not be returned to the abdominal cavity. The patient died, undoubtedly of sepsis, twenty-five days later; her infant survived for nine years.[16] The operation was therefore only a partial success and not the landmark in surgical history acclaimed by some authors.

In a monograph of 1596 Geronimo Mercurio, an Italian, described the technique of cesarean section, advocating its use upon pregnant women with rachitic contracted pelves. The operation was performed in the patient's bed; four assistants restrained her and three women assisted the surgeon. The abdomen was opened through a paramedian vertical incision, the uterus by a transverse incision. Hemostasis was achieved with hot moist packs to which wine and the juice of red roses were added. To sustain the patient during and after the ordeal, a drink of white wine, egg yolk, sugar, butter, and cinnamon was provided.[17]

When called in 1689 to deliver a woman of about thirty-three who had been in labor for five days, the French surgeon Jean Ruleau summoned a conference of professional confreres and demonstrated that the narrow outlet of the patient's rachitic pelvis made normal delivery impossible. He then proceeded to execute a successful cesarean section "with order and diligence." In publishing this experience in 1704, Ruleau said it showed that cesarean section should be done when needed to save the lives of both mother and child. He enumerated the materials needed for the performance, including two razors, needles, small sponges (well washed and dried), linen dressings, *baume d'Arcæus*, oil of roses, egg white, and aromatic wine.[18]

By 1700 published reports of cesarean deliveries became more frequent, particularly in Europe. Among them should be included the "cattle horn" cesareans — instances in which pregnant women were gored in the abdomen by a bull or cow — occupational hazards of a pastoral society, which are scarcely to be counted as triumphs of surgery. In some cases a physician was called to conclude the cesarean section; in others the animal's horn had penetrated the uterus, provoking spontaneous delivery of the infant. "It used to be a byword in Scotland that the operation was never successful unless it was performed by a cow," said Tait in 1890.[19]

Meanwhile, the high mortality of cesarean section, as well as theological questions concerning the propriety of the procedure,

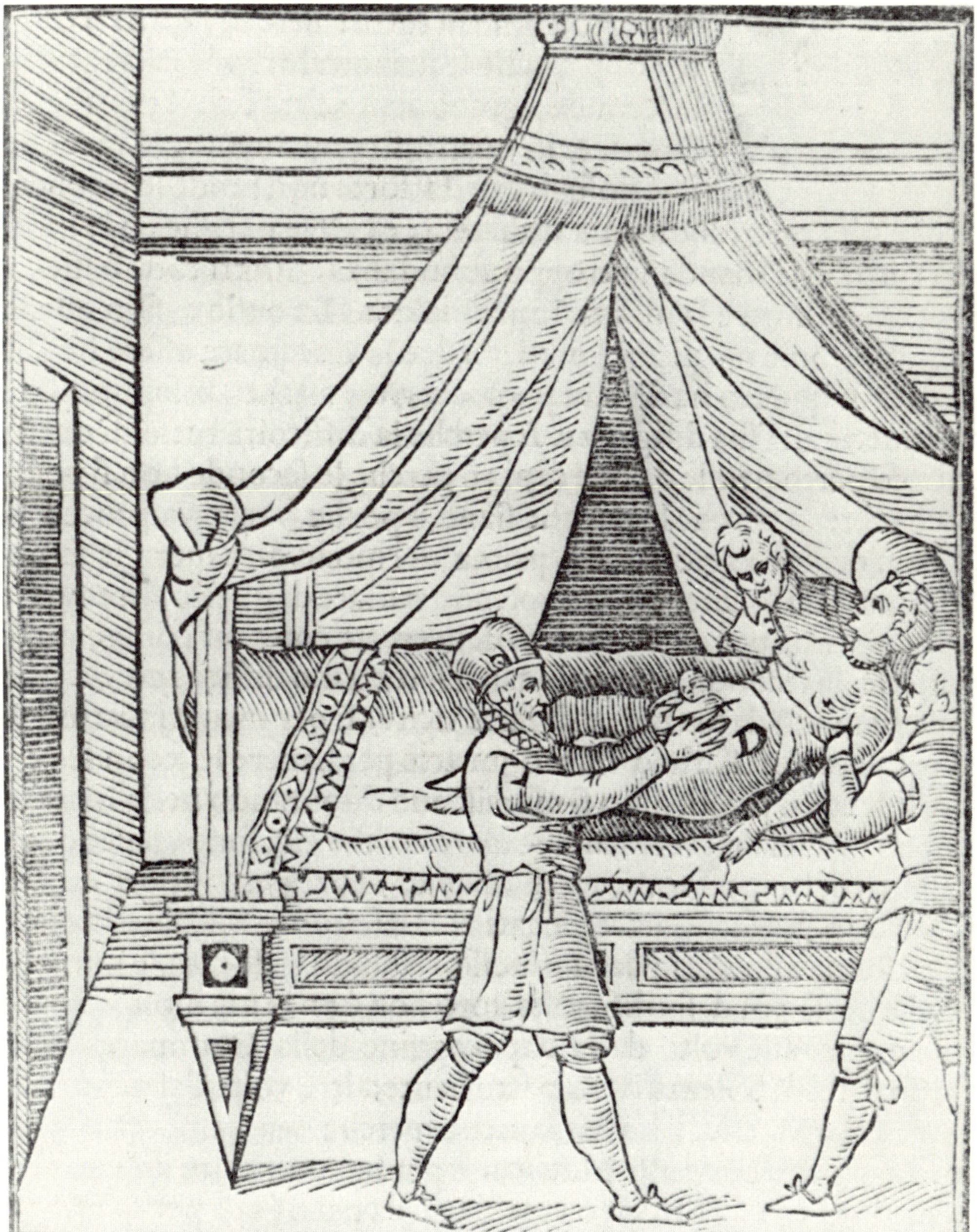

10.1 Cesarean section. from Geronimo Scipione Mercurio, *La commare o riccoglitrice* (Venice, 1621). Courtesy National Library of Medicine.

caused much debate. Dionis, who published his work on midwifery in 1718, insisted that cesarean section should not be done unless the mother was dead, adding that those who ventured to perform such surgery on living women deserved to be punished.[20]

Most early surgeons and accoucheurs in Britain were extremely skeptical of the value of the operation, which succeeded in many countries before it did in England. Percival Willughby, a mid-seventeenth century physician who practiced midwifery in London and Derby, said that cesarean section was not used in England, having "proved unfortunate to severall, under whose hands the women have perished," and that Primrose had called it a "rash piece of work . . . a practice to bee abhorred."[21]

Apparently the first successful cesarean in the British Isles was performed by an Irish midwife, Mary Donally, in about 1738. The patient, as reported by a surgeon in County Tyrone, Ireland, was about thirty-three years old — Mrs. Alice O'Neal, the mother of several children. She had been in labor for twelve days, attended by women who failed in efforts to terminate the delivery. Donally, "eminent among the common People for extracting dead Births, being then called, tried also to deliver her in the common Way: And her Attempts not succeeding, performed the *Caesarean Operation*," opening the abdominal wall and the uterus with a razor. She took out the dead child and secundines and closed the incision. Having no suture material available, Donally held the parts together "till one went a Mile and returned with Silk and the common Needles which Taylors use." Apart from a hernia, the patient did very well and in four weeks was able to walk a mile.[22]

John Hull of Manchester, a member of the Corporation of Surgeons of London and other distinguished societies, published his *Defence of the Cesarean Operation*, in the form of a letter to a critic in 1799. He had had some experience with the procedure and preferred a midline incision in the linea alba. Hull exhorted members of the profession to be more sympathetic toward acceptance of the operation which, he said, had saved many lives. His enthusiasm seems a little extreme, for he could find only two women who had survived among seventeen cesarean sections in the British Isles, and both their babies had died. Only eight children had lived. His own record in two cases was one living child.[23]

In 1801 Hull published a translation of two memoirs by the French champion of cesarean section, J.-L. Baudelocque. These constitute a brilliant summation of the merits of the procedure, particularly in cases of distorted pelvis. The first memoir, presented in 1798 to the Society of Medicine in Paris, won that body's unanimous opinion that it was a physician's duty to resort to cesarean section in "cases determined by the Art."[24]

Results in France by 1834 were considerably better than those reported for Britain. The disparity was owing in part to the circumstance that the British frequently practiced craniotomy and resorted to the cesarean procedure only in desperate situations, said Paul Dubois, a distinguished French surgeon and accoucheur. He quoted figures from 1801 to 1832 disclosing 110 cases of cesarean section with 48 surviving mothers and 63 living children.[25] Edward W. Murphy of University College, London, in 1852, wrote that the mortality of cesarean section among British surgeons was nearly 75 percent, whereas Continental surgeons recorded a maternal mortality of 41.2 percent, 152 of 369 women dying following the operation. Of the combined British and Continental experience, Murphy observed a maternal mortality among 409 patients of 44.2 percent. Joseph Späth, an experienced Vienna obstetrician and gynecologist, said the overall mortality of cesarean section in 1878 was about 60 percent; although the achievement was improving somewhat, he believed this figure was probably an understatement inasmuch as favorable outcomes were more likely to be reported. Septicemia and peritonitis were the common causes of death.[26]

Cesarean section in 1822 was called one of the most dangerous operations in surgery; the indication for it was prolonged labor with no sign of progress. Yet Osiander relates the readiness of dying women to accept the ordeal of cesarean section, with one of his patients saying, "In God's name, if only my child can live!" Another mother approaching death urged Osiander to get on with the section, "so she could sense the child lying upon her abdomen."[27]

Autocesarean Section

Instances in which desperate women have resorted to performance of cesarean section upon themselves are well known in medical literature. One account repeated by several writers concerns a Negro slave in Jamaica who in 1769 performed a cesarean section upon herself, using a butcher's broken knife with a blade about two and a half inches long. The incision in the linea alba of the abdomen was made with such force that she opened her abdomen and uterus, also cutting into the child's right thigh, "three lines deep, and two and a half inches long." A Negro midwife was summoned; she cut the navel cord and replaced the protruding intestines. Later the plantation surgeon opened the abdominal wound, washed the intestines, extracted the placenta, and sutured the abdominal wound; at this period it was not customary to stitch the uterine wound. The mother recovered; the infant died of tetanus six days later.[28]

In another account (1960) a young Yugoslavian farm wife, six or seven months pregnant, expecting her husband home after a year's work in America, performed cesarean section upon herself, apparently in a wooded area of their farm. She incised her abdomen above the pubis, opening the uterus, and extracted the fetus, which she threw into the bushes; then she sutured up the skin and walked half a kilometer home. She was in bed ten days and was finally taken to a local hospital where she died of sepsis; a portion of the infected placenta remained. The author stated he knew of two similar instances in the area.[29] The story depicts very obviously a state of desperation, verging on insanity, in an unfortunate guilt-ridden woman.

Craniotomy

In the nineteenth century there were frequent debates over whether craniotomy should be done in protracted difficult labors exhibiting no progress or whether an attempt should be made to deliver the baby by cesarean section, which posed even greater risks for the mother.

After Charles D. Meigs of Philadelphia had twice (1831, 1833) performed craniotomy on a dwarfed woman, "Mrs. R.," she again became pregnant. Meigs refused to perform a third craniotomy, and the patient was placed in the care of William Gibson, professor of surgery at the University of Pennsylvania. In the presence of a number of the city's leading surgeons and physicians, Gibson succeeded (1835) in saving both infant and mother by cesarean section. The onset of labor was awaited before the operation was scheduled, and some two hours more were spent in obtaining the patient's consent. Several of the spectators assisted manually in the performance. Two years later Gibson and Meigs repeated the operation on the same patient with similar success. The list of consultants and attendants for the procedures was a veritable "Who's Who" of the Philadelphia medical hierarchy. The mother was still alive in 1879, as were her two children and six grandchildren.[30]

Early induced labor was sometimes employed to obviate cesarean section or craniotomy in cases of contracted pelvis. As late as 1922 Herbert Spencer of University College Hospital, London, used induced premature labor three and a half times as often as cesarean section, which, he said, was performed too frequently in England and America.[31]

Uterine Suture

Acceptance of the use of sutures to close the uterine wound came relatively late in the history of cesarean section. Apparently Rousset (1581) had considered it but had dismissed the idea, believing that contraction of the uterus following removal of the infant would suffice. Lebas, a master surgeon of Mouilleron, France, is credited with the first application of sutures when in 1769 he was called to a neighboring town where a young surgeon was unable to deliver a thirty-year-old parturient who had been in labor for four days. The child was dead, a protruding arm had been amputated, and the cervical os had closed on the stump of the arm. Lebas decided that cesarean section was imperative and proceeded rapidly to operate with a razor. The child and the placenta were extracted through a transverse incision below the umbilicus. Lebas placed three sutures in the uterus to arrest bleeding, a most extraordinary procedure, said the physician who reported the incident. The patient recovered fully in about ten days without special therapy. There were no complications, although at one time gangrene of the wound was feared.[32]

By the mid-nineteenth century only a few other uses of uterine suture in cesarean section had been described, but thereafter the reports became more frequent, particularly from pioneer American surgeons (1852–80). The Sänger operation of 1882, which included deep and superficial suture of the uterine peritoneum, was rapidly accepted in Germany and more slowly in Great Britain. In reporting his technique Max Sänger listed sixteen cesarean sections in which silver sutures had been used on the American frontier, with a maternal mortality of 50 percent.[33]

Low Transverse Uterotomy

Sänger credits F. A. Kehrer (1882) with the low transverse opening in the cervical uterine segment. However, Théodore E. Lauverjat had made such a uterotomy in 1788.[34] Fritz Frank (1907) of Cologne described a peritoneal exclusion cesarean in which he deliberately opened the peritoneum through a transverse incision, attaching it by suture to the visceral peritoneum behind the uterus. He reported thirteen consecutive successful operations using this procedure.[35]

Extraperitoneal Cesarean Section

Extraperitoneal cesarean section on a living patient was performed by the German obstetrician F. A. Ritgen on October 1, 1821. The child lived, but the mother died.[36]

Physick of Philadelphia was among the first to take note of the anatomic advantage of performing a cesarean extraperitoneally and suggested that the peritoneum be separated by gentle blunt dissection from the posterior surface of the bladder and the anterior surface of the uterus. Physick's "proposition," described in a letter by his anatomist colleague William Horner, appeared in William Dewees's *Compendious System of Midwifery* (1824), the first American obstetrical monograph. There is no evidence that either Physick or Dewees followed up on the suggestion, which Physick had frequently discussed with Horner.[37] Absence of the posterior rectus sheath in the lower half of the vertical rectus abdominis muscle greatly facilitates this maneuver.

Surgeons had long been aware that extraperitoneal operations are better withstood than those necessitating entry of the peritoneal cavity. The same may be said of the extrapleural approach to the trachea and esophagus in the upper mediastinum. Before urology became a firm specialty upon the advent of transurethral prostatic resection in the 1930 era, the senior author removed stones impacted in the lower ureter in juxtaposition to the bladder through a midline extraperitoneal exposure, readily achieved by gently pushing aside the peritoneum.

A flood of reports upon extraperitoneal cesarean section began to appear in the literature after 1870. The first American success with the method for both mother and child came in the hands of A. J. C. Skene of New York in 1875. T. Gaillard Thomas of Philadelphia had been an ardent advocate of the operation since 1870 but had to wait until 1878 to report his first success. The maternal mortality in these early efforts was approximately 75 percent.[38]

In 1879 Robert P. Harris stated that cesarean section was a dangerous operation but not the most dangerous in surgery, as had been alleged. He alluded to operative mortalities varying between 22 and 87 percent. Two years later he observed that if cesarean section was performed within "a few hours after the commencement of labor" the mortality would not exceed 25 percent. His meticulous statistical publications, emphasizing the importance of earlier operation, attracted attention abroad, although the attention was not always favorable. Tait dubbed him a "library surgeon."[39]

These additions — retroperitoneal approach, transverse opening of the lower uterine segment, and suture of the uterine wound — added much to the safety of the operation, as did prophylactic antisepsis and improvement in surgical technique. Edoardo Porro's (1876) suggestion of complementary hysterectomy when serious intrauterine infection threatened patients in prolonged labor also was a significant contribution.[40] Current practice appears to favor complete hysterectomy over the supracervical, when indicated.

Present-Day Aspects

Unlike prostatectomy, which emerged suddenly in the late 1880s, cesarean section has a long history, extending back for centuries. It was first employed to save the infant upon death of the mother, then in desperate situations it was used upon dying mothers after prolonged and unsuccessful labors, attended with inordinately high maternal mortalities. Finally, in the last two decades of the nineteenth century, it was invoked in more favorable situations, and with a gradual but pronounced drop in the mortality rate in recent decades.[41] In fact, today many clinics throughout the world have reported large series of successive cesarean sections without a maternal death.

J. A. O'Leary and C. M. Steer report that in the ten-year period 1952–61, among 40,888 deliveries at the Sloane Hospital for Women, Columbia-Presbyterian Medical Center, New York, 3,412 cesarean sections were performed, 165 of which were complemented by simultaneous hysterectomy. There were no maternal deaths in the cesarean deliveries, truly an astounding achievement. However, the morbidity rate in the cases with hysterectomy (30 percent) was considerably above that of a control group of cesarean operations with tubal ligation (16 percent). Serious complications in the former included perforation of the bladder (2 percent), vesicovaginal fistula (2 percent), and febrile states of undetermined etiology (5 percent).[42] It would appear, therefore, that hysterectomy should complement cesarean section only on positive indication.

In 1963 the incidence of cesarean section was 3.3 percent among 36,277 deliveries at the Bronx-Lebanon Hospital Center,

New York, and an affiliate voluntary hospital, as reported by M. D. Klein and associates. The incidence of primary cesarean section in multiparas was 0.51 percent.[43]

The 1971 edition of *Williams Obstetrics* cites a series of 3,285 elective repeated cesareans completed without maternal mortality.[44] Several factors have contributed to this fine accomplishment. Performance of the operation before the onset of labor has eliminated the sequel of complications attending prolonged and difficult labor, and the long-prevailing attitude that cesarean section should be done only as a last resort in otherwise hopeless situations has finally disappeared. In addition, the rachitic or deformed pelvis, the primary reason for cesarean section during many years after Mercurio's 1596 report, is rarely a current indication in Western countries. Early separation of the placenta with uterine hemorrhage, preeclampsia states, and persistent breech presentation now constitute the chief indications. As an elective procedure the classical cesarean has been virtually replaced by the extraperitoneal.

This achievement augurs well for future liberalization of the indications for cesarean section, such as abnormal birth presentations entailing risk to both child and mother. As applications widen, we may anticipate fewer birth injuries, relegating congenital spastics from cranial birth trauma to the past. Undoubtedly antibiotics have lessened the mortality, yet in the main, without any new facts or discoveries, the acceptance of elective early cesarean section before labor commences has produced extraordinary results, validating the thesis that the craft and art of medicine, implemented by knowledgeable and experienced representatives of a clinical discipline, can indeed complement significantly the accomplishments of scientific surgery.

Summary

It would appear unlikely that Julius Caesar was "rip't out of his Mothers wombe." She apparently was still alive when Caesar was forty-eight years of age. Authentic instances of living babies delivered by abdominal section from uteri of dead as well as living mothers are recorded in the literature of the late sixteenth and early seventeenth centuries.

The mortality of cesarean section remained inordinately high throughout most of the nineteenth century; in fact, it was not much lower than it had been before the acceptance of prophylactic surgical antisepsis. The problem was that the operative procedure was invoked only after protracted, difficult labor of several days had failed, by which time necrosis of the uterine mucosa and sepsis were already under way. During the past quarter century there has been a sharp reversal of indications for performance of cesarean section: a fetal intrauterine position portending protracted labor or a contracted osseous maternal pelvic outlet constitutes acceptable bona fide indication for the operation. In the recent literature from several clinics, where the latter indications prevailed, there are abundant reports of several thousand successive cesarean sections without maternal mortality. This is truly one of the great achievements of modern-day surgery, deserving the attention and emulation of the profession and pointing the way toward careful readjudication of the significant role of the time factor for operative intervention in many surgical disorders.

(For notes, see pp. 634–38.)

CHAPTER 11

Ectopic Pregnancy

WHEREAS CESAREAN SECTION has a long history, tracing back to antiquity, surgical relief of ectopic gestation was not accepted until late in the nineteenth century. It may surprise and probably shock the modern-day student to learn that from the 1850s into the late 1880s it was common practice to terminate such a pregnancy by destroying the fetus. The fetal sac was aspirated with a cannula or needle, or the fetus was killed with morphine injections or by an electric current delivered through needles.

Before this, ectopic pregnancy was usually fatal for both fetus and mother. The mother's survival was contingent on the dead fetus becoming an encysted lithopedion or being extruded through a paraumbilical abscess in the abdominal wall or via a rectal fistula. Such instances, sometimes verified at the mother's autopsy many years later, are to be found in the literature as early as the sixteenth century.

Far more frequent than abdominal pregnancy or an encysted lithopedion is tubal gestation with the threat of tubal rupture and life-menacing hemorrhage. Current achievement in management of these serious situations is truly remarkable, reflecting the importance of experience in the progress of surgery. A combination of early diagnosis with speedy recourse to operation and availability of blood for transfusion account for the startling reduction in mortality.

Abdominal Pregnancy

Albucasis, the distinguished tenth-century Arab surgeon living in Spain, was among the first to write of ectopic pregnancy.

According to his account, he was asked to treat "a woman who had become pregnant and the foetus had then died *in utero*; then again she conceived and the second foetus also died; and after a long while she got a swelling in the umbilicus which grew and eventually it opened and began to produce pus." When small bones were extruded from the wound, Albucasis, "mightly astonished," realized he was dealing with an abdominal pregnancy and a dead fetus. The patient recovered, but the sinus continued to discharge pus intermittently, suggesting that remnants of the fetus remained within the abdomen.[1]

An amazing occurrence is reported by the Dutch surgeon Abraham Cyprian. In 1694 he was called to attend a woman of thirty-two, who allegedly had been pregnant for twenty-one months. It was her third pregnancy. Cyprian was told that after nine months fetal movements stopped; she had no milk in her breasts, and her menses had started again. The fetus lay in her abdomen like a dead weight; there was pain in the area of the umbilicus, where a "fungous ulcer" appeared. Using a probe, Cyprian dilated the tract of the ulcer enough to admit his little finger and thereby felt a cranial bone.

When warned that she would die otherwise, the patient consented to an operation, and Cyprian made an incision in her left side, exposing a large fetus. By restraining extrusion of the patient's intestines with his left hand, he succeeded in extracting

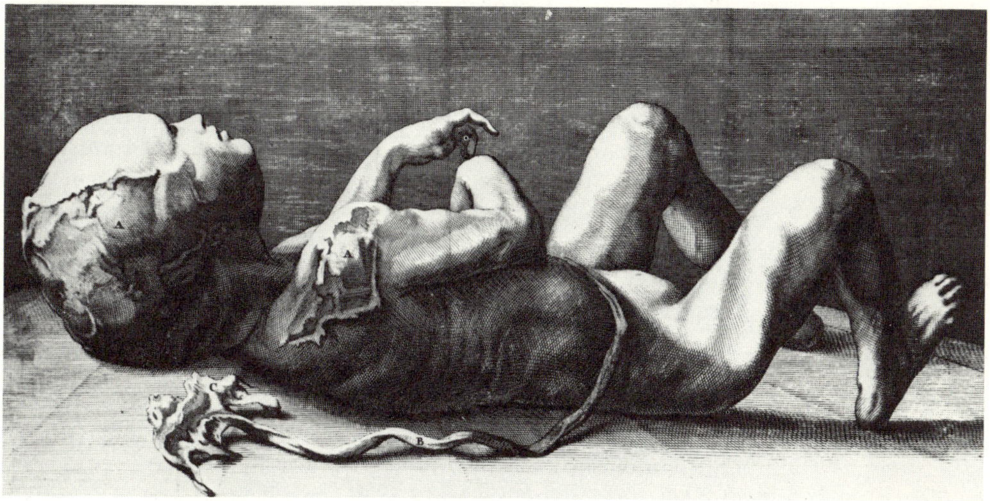

11.1 Abdominal lithopedion delivered by Abraham Cyprian (1694). From Cyprian, *Epistola historiam foetus humani post xxi menses ex uteri tuba* (Leyden, 1700).

the entire fetus with his right. It was completely intact save for some erosion over the right side of the infant's skull and shoulder. He closed the abdominal wound with four interrupted waxed through-and-through sutures, reinforced by a girdlelike dressing incorporating thin strips of wood. The mother recovered completely and subsequently had another child and then twins.[2]

A number of such curious reports of ectopic pregnancy appear in early medical publications, especially in the pages of the *Philosophical Transactions* of the Royal Society of London.[3] No typical case can be selected among these bizarre accounts, but the following cases were substantiated by postmortem reports, occasionally accompanied by illustrations of the lithopedion.

A Swabian woman in the area of Augsburg, Germany, aged forty-eight, supposedly pregnant, experienced the usual labor pains but failed to deliver. Later she had two normal confinements with healthy children. After she died in 1720 at the age of ninety-four, her abdomen was incised as she had requested. A large hard mass which was opened "with a blow of a Hatchet" confirmed her opinion that she had been carrying a dead fetus for forty-six years.[4]

Robert Houstoun, a Glasgow surgeon practicing in London in 1717, recognized the tumor of an abdominal pregnancy at term in a woman who had been delivered of eight children normally. He made the diagnosis on finding a small uterus and a hard cervix — the latter an astute observation, now a recognized sign of ectopic gestation. Despite pain and other symptoms for the next five years, the patient refused to let Houstoun open the abdomen to remove the fetus. In 1723, five months before she died, feces and fetal parts, including osseous segments, were discharged through a fistulous communication between bowel and fetal sac. The remainder of the child's skeleton was removed after death. Houstoun's report of the case before the Royal Society met with considerable opposition and was even attacked as fraudulent, although he presented an autopsy specimen. It was perhaps the first diagnosis at term of an ectopic pregnancy. Houstoun already had the distinction of successfully draining an ovarian tumor.[5]

Autopsy on a woman at Guy's Hospital in 1747 disclosed a hardened fetus, accounting for a pregnancy sixteen years before in which the patient could not deliver. An abdominal pregnancy had been diagnosed at the time, but it was considered "beyond the Reach of human Art to relieve her." In the meantime she had had four normal pregnancies and deliveries.[6]

As the defeatist attitude was gradually replaced by a more aggressive approach, a few successful cases were reported. A woman with a combined intra- and extrauterine ectopic pregnancy was treated by the New York surgeon John Bard in 1759. The patient, about twenty-eight years of age, had failed to deliver a child after nine months of apparent pregnancy. Shortly thereafter she again became pregnant and delivered a healthy child at term, but a tumor persisted on the right side of her abdomen. After nine weeks, fluctuation was perceived in the tumor. Bard then made an incision in the most prominent part of the tumor over the right rectus muscle, at the level of the navel. Fetid matter escaped, together with a phalanx of a child's finger. Additional bones were extracted, including those of the skull; there was a large quantity of pus. After ten weeks the wound was completely healed. The mother recovered good health and her milk supply was adequate for suckling the new infant.[7]

Ernst Heim, a popular Berlin doctor, reported an operation performed in 1813 at term upon a woman aged thirty-two, pregnant for the third time, upon whom he had made a diagnosis of abdominal pregnancy some months earlier. When labor pains began, Heim assembled ten of the most knowledgeable medical men in obstetrics in the area to advise with him. Debates among the doctors delayed the operation for four days; it was eventually done by a local surgeon. The mother died following the operation, but the infant boy, named MacDuff, was alive and well five years later.[8]

A mid-nineteenth century operation in the home, with a fortunate outcome for both mother and child, has been described by the Hamburg practitioner Johann Zwanck. The parturient was a large powerful woman of thirty-six years who had had two normal deliveries, the last thirteen years earlier. A diagnosis of extrauterine abdominal pregnancy was made. The operation was performed on September 16, 1837, in the patient's house at Altenwärder, an island in the Elbe River near Hamburg. Zwanck was aided by two assistants; when the hand of one of them became bloody, it was dried by an onlooker. No anesthetic was administered, but the patient did not complain of pain until closure of the abdomen. A large "over-term" boy was delivered intact, followed by spontaneous extrusion of half the placenta; the remainder came away with a gentle tug. The mother was bled 12 ounces on completion of the operation. In convalescence, twenty leeches were twice applied near the wound. A small milk secretion appeared in the patient's breasts two days after operation. When Zwanck, who was the child's godfather, visited the family a year later, he found the boy sitting in a chair dunking a piece of bread in a cup of milk and coffee.[9]

Lactation

The complex question of lactation in extrauterine pregnancy raised by Cyprian and others a few centuries ago is still of great interest to enquiring scientists. Lack of milk in the mammaries was one of the most reliable signs of abdominal pregnancy, wrote André Levret in 1750. By 1770 this experienced French accoucheur had amended his statement to say that there was no milk in the breasts unless the placenta had an intrauterine attachment. John S. Parry of the Philadelphia Hospital (1876) declared that secretion of milk did accompany abdominal pregnancy; John W. Taylor of Birmingham, England (1899), said that the breasts temporarily filled with milk when an extrauterine pregnancy went to term and the fetus died.[10]

In a 1975 appraisal Willard M. Allen commended the astute observation of eighteenth-century obstetricians. The placental relationship to lactation has been an important concern of his over many years. With reference to the question of lactation in abdominal pregnancy at term, Allen had the following to say: delivery of fetus and placenta induces lactation; delivery of fetus only produces prompt loss of estrogen, but does not induce lactation; death of the fetus near term frequently induces lactation; continued production of progesterone by the intraabdominal placenta is probably responsible for failure of lactation in these patients.[11] Whereas the problem is not completely solved, Allen, the keenest current-day student of the subject, does confirm the observations of early obstetricians.

Diagnosis

Before hormonal tests of pregnancy became available, early recognition of ectopic gestation was often difficult and uncertain. Tubal rupture with attendant severe hemorrhage and shock, as noted by Tait in a patient upon whom he failed to operate in 1881, was often the warning signal to both patient and physician.

The common symptoms of ectopic pregnancy are abdominal pain, irregular menstrual bleeding or amenorrhea, and a miscellany of other disturbances. Shoulder pain in these circumstances occasioned by irritation of the diaphragm is a symptom of bleeding into the peritoneal cavity.

Abdominal and pelvic tenderness, accompanied by a palpable

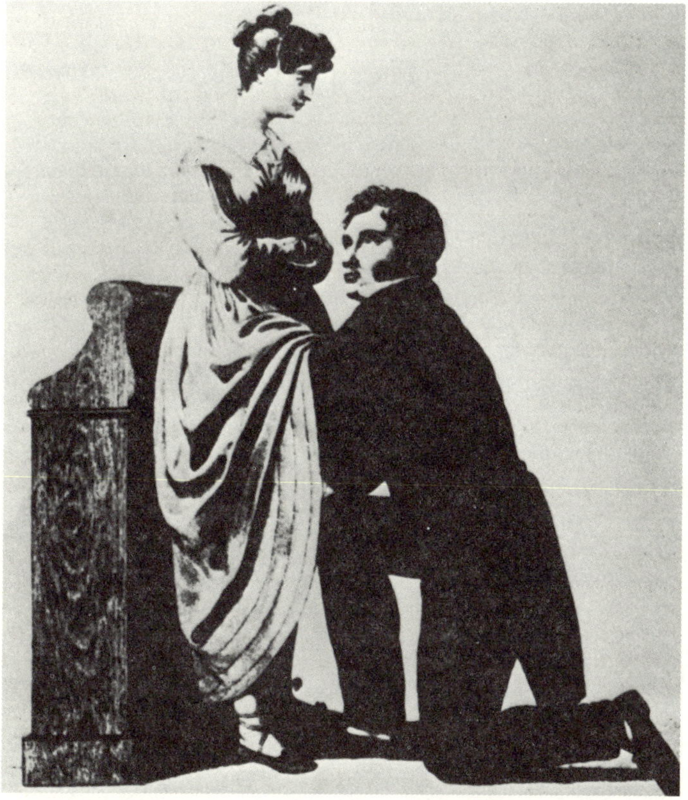

11.2 Conventional method of diagnosing pregnancy (1822). From J.-P. Maygrier, *Nouvelles demonstrations d'accouchemens* (Paris, 1822).

abdominal or pelvic mass, are the usual clinical findings in ectopic pregnancy.[12] Even at term, the cervix is not soft as in intrauterine pregnancy.[13] A positive reaction to the Friedman test confirms the diagnosis. Blood recovered from the pelvis by needle aspiration (culdocentesis) that does not clot, owing to the absence of fibrinogen, very definitely suggests ectopic gestation.[14]

Destruction of the Fetus

Until the mid-nineteenth century the literature on therapy of ectopic gestation was characterized by prolonged silence, the condition being regarded as nonremediable. Then a number of papers appeared extolling various means of destroying the fetus to save the mother, expedients that not infrequently sacrificed the mother too.[15]

Paulin Cazeaux (1850), a highly esteemed professor in the Faculty of Medicine in Paris, advised copious bleedings in the early stages of extrauterine gestation, saying that the "unfavorable influence on the child's life is not to be dreaded, since its death is the most fortunate event that could occur." He also suggested that an electric current might be used to destroy the fetus.[16]

Odoardo Bacchetti of Pisa in 1853 was the first to shock and kill a fetus by an electric current, which was passed through needles inserted into the cyst. The fetus gradually shrank in size following the application; menstruation recurred two months later. Variants of the method were soon put to trial, especially in America. In 1888 Abram Brothers of New York collected 43 instances in which ectopic pregnancy had been terminated "successfully" by electricity. Both galvanic and faradic currents had been employed. The number of electrolysis sessions varied from 1 to 24; the mean seems to have been between 8 and 10. Brothers believed that the method had a "brilliant future," although he did mention, in a footnote, that Tait had recently had 33 successes among 35 patients operated upon for removal of an ectopic fetus.[17]

Termination of an extrauterine pregnancy by perforating the sac with a trocar and evacuating amniotic fluid was an ill-advised inspiration accredited to several authorities, including Baudelocque, Basedow, and Franz Kiwisch of Prague. Its disastrous application by Simpson of Edinburgh in 1863 on a woman who was six months pregnant showed its dangers as well as its futility. The mother died three days after the puncture, and "the foetal heart could be heard almost up to the last."[18]

In 1863 J. D. Joulin of Paris proposed injecting atropine or strychnine into the fetal sac to destroy the fetus. Shortly thereafter, N. F. Friedreich of Heidelberg reported two instances in which repeated injections of morphine into a fetal prominence through the vagina or the abdominal wall terminated fetal movement, a method that enlisted a professional following in the endeavor to destroy the fetus and convert it into a "silent lithopedion."[19]

Friedreich's first patient was a twenty-year-old servant. On March 1, 1863, leeches were applied to the area of abdominal pain and reapplied ten days later. Friedreich finally concluded, by a process of exclusion, that the patient was harboring an extrauterine pregnancy, probably tubal in nature. Using a Pravaz syringe with a 6-inch needle, he injected the fetus through the vagina with 1/10th grain (6 mg.) of morphine acetate on March 15. The next day, employing the same approach, 1/7th grain (approximately 10 mg.) of morphine was injected, and on March 18, 1/6th grain (approximately 11 mg.). By March 19 a decrease in the size of the tumor was noticeable to palpation. The mother had a rather stormy convalescence but was discharged from hospital completely well on May 20.

Anyone inclined to favor "injecting poisons into the gestation sac" should read Case 4 in *St. Bartholomew's Hospital Reports*, 1883 (p. 35), wrote John Strahan (1889). In this "ghastly case," as Tait termed it, a woman five months pregnant was treated by electricity, injections of morphine — a "great dose" of 2 grains (130 mg.) by mistake — aspiration of amniotic fluid, and galvanopuncture in succession and occasionally repeated, over a four-week period, until fetal beats were finally no longer audible. The poor woman succumbed two days later.[20] O. Rennert and many others continued to use injections of morphine or electrolysis to destroy the fetus.[21]

Until the late 1880s, therefore, in England, France, Germany, Italy, and the United States, a conspiracy was prevalent among obstetricians to destroy the unborn child in extrauterine pregnancies, in the belief that it offered the mother the best chance for survival, although it was recognized that a "quiescent lithopedion" was a rare occurrence.[22]

Operative Management

In a study of the literature G. E. Herman of the London Hospital (1887) found twelve instances in which extrauterine pregnancies near term were resolved by posterior vaginal colpotomy. Five mothers survived, and two of their infants were alive at delivery. No effort was made in any of these five cases to remove the placenta, as was attempted in several of the maternal deaths. In early extrauterine pregnancy, Herman regarded delivery through the posterior vaginal cul-de-sac as dangerous.[23]

After debating the pros and cons of operation for ectopic pregnancy, Parry (1876) wrote, "Primary gastrotomy [laparotomy] for the relief of extra-uterine pregnancy is an unjustifiable operation . . . instead of diminishing, it increases the dangers of the mother." He based this view on comparative maternal mortalities, both obviously excessive at that period. Parry found secondary operations for evacuation of a dead fetus, on appearance of an abscess, more justifiable.[24]

When Tait addressed himself to the problem of operation for ectopic pregnancy, he had already had some experience with ovariotomy, not at that time attended with striking success. Perhaps this experience tempered his approach when, in the summer of 1881, he was called in consultation to see a woman, "blanched and collapsed," who had arrived in Birmingham by train. The diagnosis of hemorrhage into the peritoneal cavity from a ruptured tubal pregnancy was agreed upon, but Tait was "staggered" when the physician suggested he open the abdomen and remove the ruptured tube. Tait twice declined to operate; the patient died. The postmortem findings convinced Tait that surgery would have been feasible and probably lifesaving.

When the next such opportunity presented, in 1883, Tait at once advised abdominal section. However, as he later explained, he blundered by consuming time separating the adhesions instead of going first to the source of the bleeding and tying the vessels in the broad ligament. The patient died shortly after surgery. Finally, nearly three months later, on March 1, 1883, Tait could announce the first successful operation for ruptured tubal pregnancy. By 1884 he had done 5 such operations, and the only fatality was the first patient operated upon. A few years thereafter Tait (1888) had very obviously acquired an unusually favorable experience with the management of ectopic pregnancy. He could report 42 cases with only 2 deaths.

In 1884 Tait had declared that operation should always be done as soon as the diagnosis of extrauterine pregnancy was made; in 1886 he called treatment by electrolysis "nonsensical." He (1888) based his objections to such practices on two points: first, it was neither moral nor legal for a physician to destroy a viable unborn infant; second, the mother's interests were not best served by destroying the fetus. Tait labeled proponents of this method "abortion-mongers and reckless craniotomists." He said there is "no appeal against the decision to cut down and tie the bleeding point."[25] In fact, it can be said that it was he who led the way to the adoption of early operation for ectopic pregnancy.[26]

Progress in Management

A. Wiegand reviewed 210 operations performed at the Women's Clinic in Magdeburg, Germany, for extrauterine pregnancy during the thirteen-year period between October 1906 and September 1919. The mean age of the patients was slightly more than thirty-one years. Eight of the women died, a maternal mortality of 3.8 percent. Six of these deaths (75 percent) were owing to blood loss — this was a time before adequate blood storage was available for transfusion and concerned also the long years of World War I.[27] The achievement, although excelling only slightly Tait's 1888 performance with a 4.7 percent mortality, does represent an important advance over the accomplishment prior to Tait's advocacy of early operation for extrauterine gestation.

Over the years 1813 to 1907, H. Hudnall Ware, Jr., of Richmond, Virginia (1948), found 240 cases of full-term extrauterine pregnancy with living fetuses reported in the literature and an additional 61 cases in the interval 1907 to 1923. In an analysis of 236 abdominal pregnancies between 1919 and 1932, a maternal mortality of 14.3 percent was noted; this series included some instances of early ectopic pregnancy.

Among 249 cases (1933–46) of extrauterine pregnancy of seven months or more in duration, Ware reported that 37 mothers died, a mortality of 14.8 percent. Eleven of these left living babies. Of 251 babies in this segment of Ware's study, including two sets of twins, only 60 lived (24 percent). The overall infant mortality was 75.6 percent. Ware insisted that the placenta be left in situ and the abdomen be closed without drainage in late cases of ectopic gestation and that removal of the placenta should be reserved for instances in which its blood supply can be easily interrupted. If the placenta is attached to a vital organ, such as the intestine, efforts at removal are likely to provoke uncontrollable hemorrhage. Tubal rupture in early ectopic pregnancies is often accompanied by severe hemorrhage necessitating transfusion and is the primary cause of maternal death.[28]

Operation Only When Pregnancy Is Established

Jørgen Lund of Roskilde, Denmark, wrote in 1950 of early ectopic gestation. The study embraced essentially patients suspected of harboring an ectopic gestation who were hospitalized and treated expectantly until their pregnancy was confirmed. If a patient had a positive reaction to the Friedman test, satisfying the hormonal criterion of pregnancy, operation was undertaken immediately to remove the fetus and protect the mother against the likely sequel of tubal rupture and life-threatening hemorrhage. Proceeding in this manner, Lund stated, he succeeded in avoiding operation in 55 percent of these patients; the remaining 45 percent required operative intervention.[29]

Combined Intrauterine and Extrauterine Pregnancy

A. E. Winer and associates reviewed the 71 cases of combined intrauterine and extrauterine pregnancy in the world literature from 1948 through 1954, including 3 cases of their own at Cook County Hospital in Chicago. Of the intrauterine infants, 73 in number, 43.8 percent survived; of the extrauterine infants, also 73 in number, 5.4 percent survived.

Survival of the mother and the fetus depends to a great degree in such instances upon the treatment of the extrauterine component. If the cervix is dilated in a parturient near term, evacuation of the uterus is in order. Treatment of the ectopic pregnancy is surgical, whenever recognized, regardless of the presence of concomitant intrauterine pregnancy, except in cases near viability, when salvage might be a consideration.

The authors noted that the prior mortality of 14 to 19 percent, as of 1940, was in 1957 approximately only 1 percent. The one maternal death in the present series, said the authors, was nonobstetrical. Maternal morbidity remained high, especially when ectopic pregnancy had been overlooked.[30]

Recent Mortality Accounts

J. T. Armstrong and associates wrote of operations for ectopic pregnancy from 1951 through 1956 in two Houston hospitals, a review of 481 patients, among whom were 4 hospital deaths, a mortality of 0.83 percent. Among 9 abdominal ectopic pregnancies in the group, there were 3 living babies. Of the 4 deaths, 3 occurred in tubal pregnancies, the other in abdominal pregnancy. There were 11 repeat ectopic pregnancies in the group (2.2 percent); in 2 instances simultaneous intrauterine and extrauterine pregnancies were observed (0.41 percent). The peak incidence for ectopic gestation was among patients of twenty-seven and twenty-eight years. These authors regarded culdocentesis, needle puncture of the cul-de-sac between the uterus and rectum, as an indispensable diagnostic procedure. Incisional colpotomy was far less frequently performed; both procedures were helpful diagnostically. Shock was present in patients who bled profusely.[31]

A seventeen-year review (1947–63) of ectopic pregnancies at the Tulane Unit of Obstetrics and Gynecology in the New Orleans Charity Hospital revealed 699 instances of tubal or interstitial pregnancy. There was only one death in the series, a patient who was moribund on arrival at the outpatient clinic and was not operated upon, report Herman D. Webster, Jr., David L. Barclay, and Charles K. Fischer. Thomas W. McElin of Northwestern University notes (1977) that the current mortality of ectopic pregnancy is 1 in 800 (0.12 percent). Some series are being reported with no deaths, denoting the progress made over the past seventy-five years when management of ectopic gestation held out little promise of survival for the mother.[32]

Two series of abdominal pregnancies at the Charity Hospital in New Orleans were reviewed by W. D. Beacham and associates (1962). In the earlier series, July 1937 to July 1945, there were 22 patients, of whom 2 died; of 43 patients in the July 1945 to January 1962 series, 2 died. The overall maternal mortality for the 65 patients in both series was 4.6 percent, a commendable achievement in this, the most challenging of all types of extrauterine pregnancy. The authors stated that operation should be done as soon as the diagnosis is made and lent renewed emphasis to removing the placenta only when its blood supply could easily be cut off.

In the discussion following Beacham's presentation Allen said he had been able to carry several patients with extrauterine abdominal pregnancy to term, delivering the fetus by abdominal section. Allen left the placenta in situ, removing it at a later date, because efforts directed at its removal invariably would provoke serious hemorrhage.[33]

J. M. Rosenblum and his associates reported from Western Reserve University, Cleveland, upon 107 patients (1955–58) who underwent operation for tubal pregnancy without a maternal death. In about half the cases the involved fallopian tube was excised; in the others it was retained after extrusion of the fetus, in the hope of preserving a patulous lumen. Patency was tested by a salpingogram a few weeks after the operation. In the latter group, there were, in fact, 8 patients who subsequently had 9 intrauterine pregnancies, an incidence of 18 percent.[34]

In a sixteen-year survey of 905 cases of ectopic pregnancy, among 31,865 gynecologic admissions to New York's Harlem Hospital between the years 1942 and 1957, M. L. Bobrow and H. G. Bell (1962) noted a 1.4 percent maternal mortality. Culdocentesis was carried out as a routine diagnostic procedure. Culdoscopy, visual examination of the cul-de-sac, was done only in atypical cases; colpotomy was not used. It was the authors' practice not to transfuse the patient until the abdomen was opened and bleeding controlled, in the belief that transfusion before adequate hemostasis encourages bleeding.

In 61 percent the usual operative procedure was unilateral salpingectomy; less frequently, salpingo-oophorectomy (28 percent) was performed, with cornual excision of a segment of the uterus at the site of attachment of the fallopian tube. In the remaining 11 percent, a miscellany of operations, including hysterectomy, myomectomy, bilateral salpingectomy, and in a few instances even appendectomy, were done. There was a 23 percent incidence of subsequent normal pregnancies.[35]

Summary

The tenth-century Arab surgeon Albucasis recognized the presence of an abdominal ectopic pregnancy when fetal bones were discharged from an abdominal wall abscess in a pregnant woman; she survived the ordeal. Lack of milk in the maternal mammaries was recognized as a reliable sign of abdominal pregnancy by astute eighteenth-century accoucheurs. In 1770 Levret amended his earlier (1750) statement to suggest that if the placenta in abdominal pregnancies had an intrauterine attachment normal lactation could occur, an observation confirmed recently by Allen, a keen student of the problem of lactation in abdominal pregnancy.

It is startling to learn that until the mid-1880s the conventional management of ectopic gestation was to destroy the fetus by electrolysis or intrafetal injection of lethal doses of morphine or other deadly drugs, a procedure also hazardous for the mother.

Tait of Birmingham, England, introduced early surgical intervention to thwart lethal hemorrhage from rupture of a fallopian tube in ectopic pregnancy in 1884, reporting a maternal mortality of 4.7 percent in 42 patients. Maternal mortalities of less than 1 percent in large series of cases are now recorded, a remarkable advance.

(For notes, see pp. 638–41.)

CHAPTER 12

Ovariotomy (Excision of Ovarian Cyst)

One of the more interesting chapters in American surgery relates to the history of ovariotomy. When most surgeons around the world looked upon invasion of the peritoneal cavity for elective surgery as an unwarranted procedure, Ephraim McDowell in 1809 in America's hinterland of Danville, Kentucky, performed the first successful complete excision of an enormous ovarian cyst.[1]

McDowell began his medical studies with Alexander Humphreys of Staunton, Virginia, a graduate of the University of Edinburgh. After he had "read from two to three years" with Humphreys, McDowell went to Edinburgh and registered for medical classes in the sessions of 1793–94. The institution was then at the very zenith of renown, attracting students from all parts of the world and overshadowing in its appeal all the medical schools of Britain and Europe.

During his second year McDowell "took a ticket to the private course of the celebrated Mr. John Bell." A teacher with great charm, Bell stimulated his pupils to learn and inspired their ambitions; "many worshipped him; not a few idolized him." Bell apparently discussed the possibility of ovariotomy in his lectures[2] but had not mustered the courage to perform the operation. McDowell returned to Kentucky in 1795 to begin his professional career.

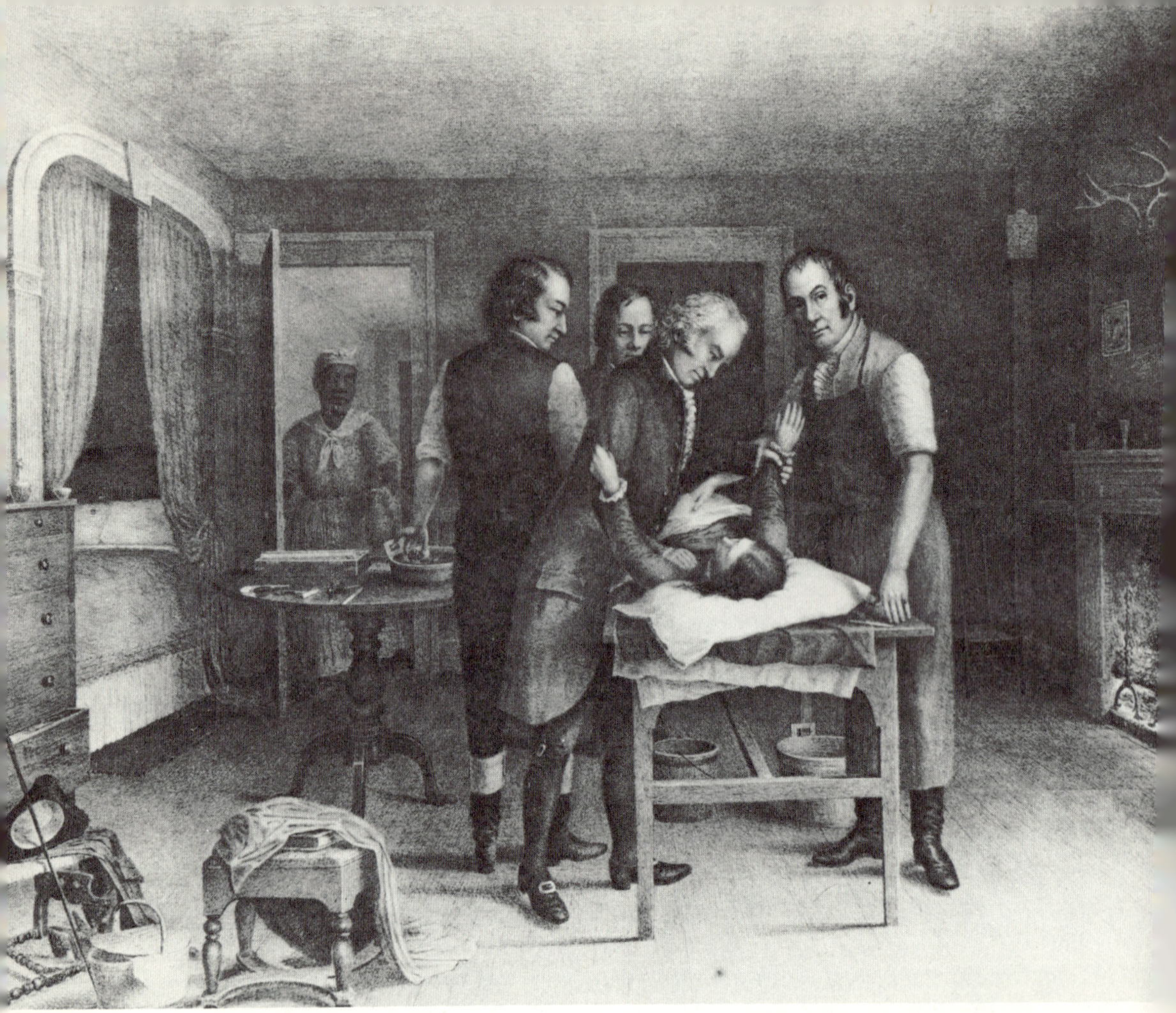

12.1 McDowell of Danville, Kentucky, performed the first successful ovariotomy Christmas Day on Jane Crawford (1809). Courtesy National Library of Medicine.

McDowell's 1809 Ovariotomy

In December 1809 Jane Crawford traveled sixty miles across the Kentucky mountain trails on horseback to Danville, bracing her large tumor against the saddle horn. McDowell had earlier examined the patient in her home, explaining that the only possible relief would be surgery, a novel and dangerous procedure. The operation, which was done on Christmas Day in the surgeon's house, took twenty-five minutes.[3]

Anesthesia was, of course, not then available, but opium had long been in general use for dulling the pain sense. In subsequent years McDowell wrote of giving his postoperative patients "cherry bounce," a fairly strong alcoholic concoction, and laudanum.[4] These agents may have been given to Mrs. Crawford. The family memoirs indicated that "she occupied herself repeating the Psalms" throughout the ordeal.[5] McDowell tied the ovarian pedicle with a long silk ligature brought out through the lower portion of the wound and closed it with interrupted through-and-through sutures of silk. He applied adhesive tape to coapt the skin edges between the sutures.

McDowell waited several years before venturing to announce his achievement, and he could then report two additional successful excisions of large ovarian cysts; both these patients were black women. He reportedly sent a copy of his report in care of his nephew William McDowell to Physick, America's most prominent surgeon. This dignitary apparently took no note of the article, probably incredulous that an unknown surgeon in Kentucky could have achieved what no one else in the world had yet succeeded in doing. The nephew then took the account to Thomas C. James, professor of midwifery at the University of Pennsylvania, who recognized its merit, read it to his class, and published it in 1817 in the *Eclectic Repertory*.

In 1819 McDowell reported two more ovariotomies, both in black patients, with one death. Despite making a 9-inch-long incision, McDowell's usual procedure was to incise and tap the cyst before removing its capsule, thus facilitating exposure and ligature of the ovarian pedicle and vessels. This practice may have caused the death of the fifth patient, from whose cyst 16 quarts of gelatinous fluid escaped, considerable of it into the peritoneal cavity. She died on the third postoperative day and necropsy disclosed the presence of peritonitis.[6]

McDowell had mailed a copy of his first report to his former teacher, but Bell was ill and away in Italy, where he died (1820). The copy came into the hands of an Edinburgh surgeon, John Lizars, who acknowledged McDowell's achievement in 1824, reporting an operation of his own in which no ovarian tumor was found. The next year Lizars reported three ovariotomies recently performed by himself, with two patients surviving. His writings brought McDowell's account to a wide audience and focused attention on ovariotomy as a feasible operation. Lizars said (1824) that there was "little danger to apprehend, in laying open the abdominal cavity" and that to delay in cases of diseased ovarium was "more dangerous than the operation."[7]

Repercussions of McDowell's Announcement

McDowell's report met with considerable skepticism. Among the unbelievers was James Johnson of London, who published his doubts in the *London Medico-Chirurgical Review* (January 1825), of which he was editor: "Dr. Mac visited the patient *at the end of five days*, though she had come to his own residence to have the operation performed!![8] He found her engaged in making her bed! she soon returned to her native place quite well [McDowell said in twenty-five days]. *Credat Judaeus non ego*." Johnson subsequently withdrew his criticism and asked "pardon of God, and of Dr. Macdowel of Danville" for his mistrust.

It is not known exactly how many patients McDowell eventually operated upon for ovarian cyst; 13 is the usual estimate, of which 5 are said to have died, providing a mortality of 38.4 percent, certainly a better score than achieved by several famous ovariotomists during the next few decades. McDowell (1819) used the designation "excision" of diseased ovaria. The term "ovariotomy" apparently was first applied by Charles Clay in *Medical Times*, 1843–44. Clay said it had been suggested to him by Simpson of Edinburgh.[9]

Beginnings of Acceptance of Ovariotomy

Washington L. Atlee of Philadelphia, one of the chief early proponents of ovariotomy in America, reported on the status of the operation up to 1851 in a table comprising 222 cases.[10] The first case listed was that of J.-B. Laumonier of Rouen (ca. 1781); however, careful reading thereof suggests that Laumonier's patient had a postpartum tubo-ovarian abscess.[11] Atlee's chart indicated an overall mortality for the period of 52 percent. After some juggling of figures he arrived at a considerably better record; however, deaths adjudged by the number of patients operated upon substantiates the 52 percent figure. Of surgeons who had done more than 5 ovariotomies, McDowell came out the best in the chart, with 5 patients and 1 death (20 percent mortality). Atlee's own achievement was given as 6 deaths among 15 patients (40 percent).[12]

In England as in America the first successful excision of an ovarian cyst was accomplished in an isolated country town. William Jeaffreson, a skillful practitioner in Framlingham, Suffolk, did the operation in 1836. London surgeons were severely critical of the innovation.[13]

The tenacious and belligerent Clay (1801–93) of Manchester entered the controversy in September 1842, when he performed his first ovariotomy, successfully removing a 17-pound tumor through a 24-inch vertical incision. Before the year was out he had done four others; two were failures. Clay continued to favor the exposure of the long incision. He met great opposition, bearing, as he said (1865), "the brunt and contumely of all that was levelled against the operation for many years *unsupported and alone*." There were other exponents during this period, notably I. Baker Brown, but the results Clay announced in 1856 commanded attention — 71 cases, 24 deaths (33.8 percent mortality). Clay accepted anesthesia with reluctance. His abusive replies to critics who questioned both the integrity of his reports and the propriety of his operations were typical of the controversy that marred the era, when claims for priority and successes aroused petty rivalry among great surgeons.[14]

Excision of an ovary was a fairly simple operation and no novelty. As was often pointed out in discussions, women had been castrated to please the kings in ancient Lydia;[15] moreover, the operation was not infrequent in many a veterinarian's practice. A large cyst with adhesions presents a greater challenge but is not ordinarily a formidable task. Technical details, such as length of the incision, treatment of the pedicle, whether to empty the cyst before removal, and the most suitable temperature of the operating room, became the basis of lengthy arguments in surgical circles yet were of less importance than the competence of the operator and his observance of cleanliness. With the advent of anesthesia and mounting statistics of success, excision of large ovarian cysts was no longer an oddity and a number of accomplished ovariotomists appeared in Britain.

T. Spencer Wells (1818–97), a London surgeon who had distinguished himself in the Crimean War, was one of the first to recognize the importance to surgery of Pasteur's research. In a memorable address to the British Medical Association at Cambridge in August 1864, he alluded to seven of Pasteur's papers concerning spontaneous generation, fermentation, and putrefaction, pointing out that the work of Pasteur would have great practical significance.[16]

Wells performed his first ovariotomy, a success, in 1858. He published a series of reports, keeping a careful record of all his operations, listing both successes and failures. His thousandth ovariotomy, in 1880, was the occasion of congratulatory editorials in the British press. Wells was an advocate of surgical cleanliness and one of ovariotomy's strongest supporters over long years, yet he apparently never achieved a better than 25 percent mortality rate with the operation until his adoption of antiseptic techniques in 1878. His mortality rate in the final 100 of his 1,000 cases was 11 percent.[17]

In 1892 Wells told of witnessing an ovariotomy in a large London hospital. The operating surgeon asked him how long he thought the patient would live. Replied Wells, "Not three days." "Why?" asked the surgeon. "Because," said Wells, "you came straight from the anatomical theatre where you had been demonstrating for an hour, and were followed by a crowd of dissecting students." The patient did not live forty-eight hours, dying of peritonitis.[18]

Thomas Keith (1827–95), one of Scotland's early and great ovariotomists, a pupil of Syme, has been overlooked in many surgical histories. When Keith performed his first ovariotomy in 1862, guided by the counsels of the "old men in the profession" who were watching, he hastened to close the wound, leaving a large quantity of extravasated blood in the peritoneum. Three days later, when the patient became septic, Keith removed several sutures, releasing a great quantity of fetid serum.[19] The patient recovered. Thereafter Keith became an ardent advocate of absolute hemostasis and closed the wound only when oozing was controlled.

Keith had 17 deaths in his first 100 ovariotomies without antiseptic agents. Over the next three years (1869–71) he used Listerian techniques, but when his results did not improve he discarded the method, trusting to cleanliness alone. No one could attend his operations who had recently visited a person with an infectious disease or participated in a postmortem examination. In 1876, finding he was still losing patients from "rapid septicaemia," Keith returned to Listerian principles. He eventually was able to report two series of cases in which the mortality varied between 3.8 and 4.1 percent.[20] Keith attained this record despite ill health; he had suffered bouts of vesical calculi since early youth.

Finding that Keith cured a greater percentage of patients than did other surgeons, both before and after using antiseptic techniques, Sims decided that "there must be something besides antisepsis to account for this difference" and went to Edinburgh in 1879 to witness Keith's performance.[21] Keith's success, Sims concluded, was owing to his being "systematic in everything he does." Keith used Lister's carbolic acid spray and carried out Lister's precepts very carefully upon his hands, instruments, and sponges, all well carbolized. Sims noted Keith's meticulous hemostasis but was surprised that Keith had abandoned restriction on visitors or assistants who had attended cases of infectious disease or had done autopsies, apparently believing that antisepsis would protect his patients.[22] Keith preferred the cautery for the ovarian pedicle.

Ovariotomy did not find ready acceptance in France. In a protracted discussion on ovarian cysts at the Imperial Academy of Medicine (1856–57) only one participant, Cazeaux, spoke in defense of the operation, saying it should not be proscribed without further examination. Malgaigne believed it to be too radical; Velpeau characterized it as "frightful"; both Cruveilhier and Jobert (de Lamballe) withheld their approval. Most of the debating concerned iodine injections or puncture of ovarian cysts, measures favored by many.[23]

After watching several ovariotomies performed in London, J.-N. Demarquay (1862) said he hoped this "bold" operation could be introduced in France but wondered if the difference in French and English native constitutions would not affect the results.[24]

The celebrated French surgeon of the era, Nélaton, said he was taxed with barbarity when he proposed ovariotomy. His first patient (1862)[25] died of tetanus, brought on, he claimed, by a quarrel with her neighbor two weeks postoperatively, just after he had presented the case as a success at the Academy. By 1869 Nélaton was reported to have performed 16 ovariotomies with 7 deaths, not a remarkable achievement for so skillful an operator.[26]

Eugène Koeberlé of Strasbourg reported the best results in ovariotomy in France at this period. Analyzing the 54 ovariotomies with 32 deaths performed up to 1862 in France, he said that in Paris the cures had been 1 in 6; in the provinces half the operations were successful; and his own cases accounted for three-fourths of the recoveries. He felt therefore that the operation was now "one of the glories of our surgical epoch." Koeberlé attached great importance to cleanliness in operating.[27]

Hegar Introduced Semmelweis's Techniques

The gynecologist Hegar (1830–1914) of Freiburg was the first among surgeons to adopt Semmelweis's prophylactic antiseptic practices in elective operations. He explained his technique in a communication (1876–77) in which he reported 15 consecutive successful ovariotomies. This was a real achievement for that day when many experienced ovariotomists were recording mortalities of 60 percent or more. Hegar, Semmelweis's first biographer (1882), was born in Darmstadt, the son of a practicing physician. Young Hegar worked with Gustav Simon in Heidelberg. In 1864 he was made chairman and professor of obstetrics and gynecology at Freiburg, succeeding Otto Spiegelberg.

Hegar was nominated subsequently as chairman for professorships at Giessen (1867), Strasbourg (1882), and Breslau, but remained at Freiburg as chairman for forty years, retiring in 1904; he was highly honored throughout Germany.[28]

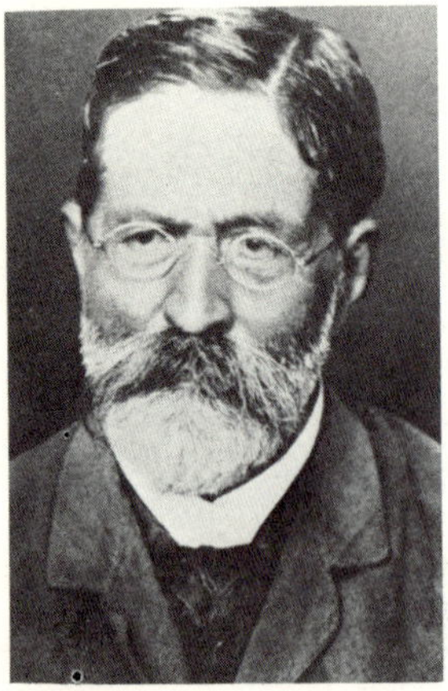

12.2 Hegar of Freiburg reported success with 15 consecutive ovariotomies (1876–77), following strictly the prophylactic surgical antisepsis of Semmelweis.

Hegar (1876–77) described his preparations for ovariotomy as follows: "The surgeon and his assistants remove their coats, elevate the sleeves of their shirts to the elbow, and wash their hands and forearms first with soap and water, followed by a wash in chlorine water prepared the day before. Before the incision is made, the abdominal wall is washed with chlorine water; similarly, the instruments are submerged in the same solution; the hands to be introduced into the peritoneal cavity are washed many times during the operation with chlorine water. The toilet of the abdomen is accomplished with sponges which have been treated with chlorine water. Silk sutures are similarly treated in the chlorine water."

The author goes on to say that spillage of small amounts of chlorine water in the peritoneal cavity is not injurious.[29] He stressed the importance of having the chlorine water freshly made. He believed it the best, even though the most expensive, disinfective agent. It had the advantage over phenol in that it irritated the tissues but little. Hegar could not commit himself to use of the phenol spray.

The author then continues, "We allow but six students to be present at operations and these must provide evidence that they have not been in a department of anatomy in the prior five or six days; that they have not attended any postmortems, nor been with patients who have an acute exanthem such as diphtheria, erysipelas, or pyemia."[30]

The Hegar paper obviously is an important document in the history of abdominal surgery, antedating by ten years Tait's (1886) significant contribution on ovariotomy. Hegar does not state exactly when he did his first ovariotomy. In a monograph of 1878 Hegar wrote of castration of women. He dealt with historical aspects of oophorectomy, indicating that he did his first bilateral excision of the ovaries on July 27, 1872. When Hegar and Rudolf Kaltenbach described the preparation of patients for gynecologic operations in 1874, they included many of the measures Hegar later developed in his ovariotomy routine. The rooms of patients to undergo such operations were disinfected with fumes of chlorine, as were the operating room and table. Instruments were placed in a strong solution of chlorine both before and after operation, and only a few students were permitted to examine the instruments; first they had to put aside their coats, roll up their sleeves, and wash their hands and forearms with soap and water, followed by a wash in a strong chlorine solution. Sponges were washed and placed in a chlorine solution prior to use. The vagina was routinely washed out with chlorine solution on completion of vaginal operations. Almost thirty years elapsed between Semmelweis's introduction of prophylactic surgical antisepsis (1847) for parturients and its innovation and adoption by Hegar, the first such use in the literature of surgery for elective abdominal surgery. Semmelweis (1861) had used his prophylactic surgical antisepsis with uniform success in the removal of uterine adenomatous polyps.[31]

Tait's Accomplishment

Tait, the greatest of the ovariotomists, began his work on ovariotomy in July 1868, in his twenty-fourth year, with a fatal case. He had performed 4 more ovariotomies, all successful, before he moved in 1870 from the little town of Wakefield to Birmingham. By 1878, among his first 50 ovariotomies there were 19 deaths (38 percent mortality), and he was "stung to the quick by the awful results." This was a "higher mortality than that of any British surgeon who has published his statistics," said Knowsley Thornton,[32] a lifelong antagonist.

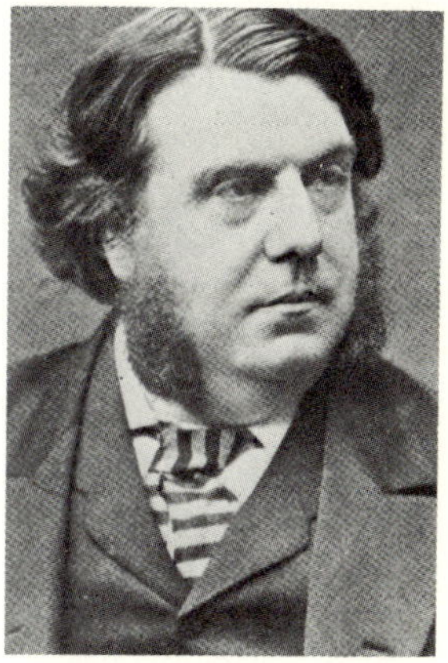

12.3 Tait of **Birmingham, England,** reported 139 consecutive successful ovariotomies without antisepsis (1886), observing only "high standards of surgical cleanliness."

Early in his surgical career Tait employed Listerian antiseptic practices. These he was to abandon, proclaiming his belief in "scrupulous attention to cleanliness of every kind and in all directions." Tait's practices have been described as the beginning of "aseptic as distinguished from antiseptic surgery," but one could not infer this from his own pronouncement: "My fear of germs has steadily diminished; so that, if I could get them in sufficiently large quantities, and found them dry, elastic, and absorbent, I would willingly stuff my pads with them instead of wool" — so wrote Tait in 1886 in reporting 139 consecutive ovariotomies (1884–85) without a death.[33] For one who disavowed the germ theory of infection, it was quite an accomplishment, especially before the days of rubber gloves, face masks, and steam sterilization.

Tait courted opposition and much of his professional life was spent in conflict. He and Spencer Wells, at one time intimate friends, parted ways quarreling over their results as well as over their techniques.[34] They differed concerning the management of the ovarian pedicle and other practical concerns of ovariotomy. Tait preferred the silk ligature. He washed out the peritoneal cavity with plain tap water, "full of germs," he said.[35]

In a monograph of 1884 in which he summarized 1,000 cases of abdominal section with a mortality of 9.3 percent, Tait said he had experimented with various anesthetic agents but finally had decided that a mixture of two parts of ether to one of chloroform was the safest and most practical anesthesia.[36]

The acme of Tait's career came in 1890 when he delivered the Address in Surgery at the annual meeting of the British Medical Association, in which he made a plea for the training of the surgeon as artist and craftsman, a proposal that was well received.[37]

The last five years of Tait's life were marked by more or less continuous invalidism. He was operated upon in London for stone and subsequently developed a renal infection. These and other factors prompted Tait to relinquish operative work, and he sought repose at his beautiful country house in the New Forest.[38]

The record of Tait (1886) has not been bettered, the only difference being that today with universal acceptance of prophylactic surgical antisepsis, uniformly good results are consistently achieved with excision of benign ovarian cysts. The designation "ovariotomy" in daily use among surgeons for more than a century too has disappeared, to be replaced by McDowell's choice, "excision."

McDowell's early success with ovariotomy was the prelude to the beginnings of abdominal surgery. French surgeons of the Royal Academy of Surgery (1731–92) had reported a number of good results in excision of strangulated bowel within the peritoneal cavity, yet these achievements did not lend the impetus to abdominal surgery that came from the favorable reports attending ovariotomy. Only, however, when prophylactic surgical antisepsis found general acceptance did abdominal surgery really catch on. Excision of an ovarian cyst does not involve the complicated techniques attending excision of segments of the alimentary canal — techniques acquired only through experience.

Summary

The first successful excision of an ovarian cyst compelling operation occurred outside academic halls in the Kentucky backwoods on December 25, 1809. The news was met by skepticism in this country and in England. Hegar of Freiburg (1876–77) presented a series of 15 successive ovariotomies without mortality, employing the prophylactic surgical antisepsis of Semmelweis (1847) in every detail and in each step of the operative procedure, an occurrence that marked the beginnings of elective abdominal surgery. A decade later Tait of Birmingham (1886), who rejected completely Listerian practices and belief in the germ theory of infection and relied solely on high standards of surgical cleanliness, reported 139 successive ovariotomies without mortality, an achievement that gave elective abdominal surgery a strong forward thrust.

(For notes, see pp. 641–44.)

CHAPTER 13

Vesicovaginal Fistula

A RENOWNED Berlin plastic surgeon has provided a dramatic account of unsuccessful attempts to close persistent vesicovaginal fistulas. Dieffenbach's (1836) description of the tortured existence confronting the woman with such a urinary lesion is as graphic as any found in the literature — excoriation of the thighs, furunculosis, the "revolting" smell of urine, contamination of clothing and mattresses, isolation and social rejection — all serve to indicate the severity of the handicap. Complete ostracism from society made many a sufferer hope for an early death. Yet urinary incontinence rarely endangered life.

No surgeon then could provide a list of successive operative cures in the repair of the vesicovaginal fistula. Dieffenbach (1792–1847) operated unsuccessfully upon several patients many times; one of these was a twenty-year-old Russian countess. When he removed the sutures some days after each surgical attempt, the urinary fistula was still invariably in evidence.[1]

The role of J. Marion Sims (1813–83) in devising what came to be known as the American operation for vesicovaginal fistula is indeed a fascinating story, constituting a significant contribution to the advance of surgery.[2] Born in a small South Carolina hamlet, Sims attended the state college in Columbia, where rudimentary chemistry seems to have been the only scientific offering. Subsequently he took a fourteen-week course of lectures at Charleston Medical College, and the next fall (1834) he entered Jefferson Medical College, receiving a diploma as "Physician and Surgeon" the following March.[3] During this five-month session

Sims occasionally assisted the professor of surgery in operations in a small clinic and did some dissecting; he stayed an extra month in Philadelphia to attend a series of private lectures by the well-known anatomist Pattison, recently back from England, Sims's favorite instructor.[4] So, without hospital training, postgraduate work, or foreign study, Sims came home to hang up his shingle (1835), probably no less adequately prepared for the profession than many other young men starting practice that year in rural America. After a short period of discouraging prospects, Sims moved to a town near Montgomery, Alabama. He survived several periods of ill health, fever, and persistent diarrhea, occasioned probably by contaminated drinking water,[5] an affliction that no longer plagued him after he subsequently went to New York in 1853.

Sims was urged by some of his fellow practitioners, as well as by plantation owners who operated large cotton fields with slave labor, to interest himself in the repair of vesicovaginal fistulas resulting from protracted tedious childbirth in young black women, probably because of rachitic pelves. Prolonged impaction of the fetal head was considered an indication for the application of forceps to quicken delivery. Sims consistently demurred, believing there was no cure for such complications of pregnancy.[6]

Sims's Innovations

While attending a large woman who had been thrown from her pony and thereby sustained a severe back injury, Sims found the uterus acutely retroverted. He recalled the advice of his teacher Thomas G. Prioleau of Charleston Medical College to place patients with this problem in the knee-chest position with forehead, palms of hands, and knees upon the table. When Sims did this, the inrush of air into the patient's vagina, with the force of atmospheric pressure (14.7 pounds per square inch), caused the uterus, almost spontaneously, to return to its normal position.

His enthusiasm kindled by this experience, Sims decided to have another look at the possibility of surgical correction of vesicovaginal fistula. He called back three black patients he had dismissed as inoperable; he added a story to the little private hospital he had built in his yard, contrived new instruments, and sought other cases in the countryside. In three months he was prepared and performed his first vesicovaginal surgery (1845) on Lucy, who bore the hour-long operation with courage. Anesthesia was not then available.[7] Sims freshened up the edges of the fistulous opening and closed the defect with a few sutures of fine silk. After some days, upon removal of the sutures, leakage of urine indicated that the fistula was still open.

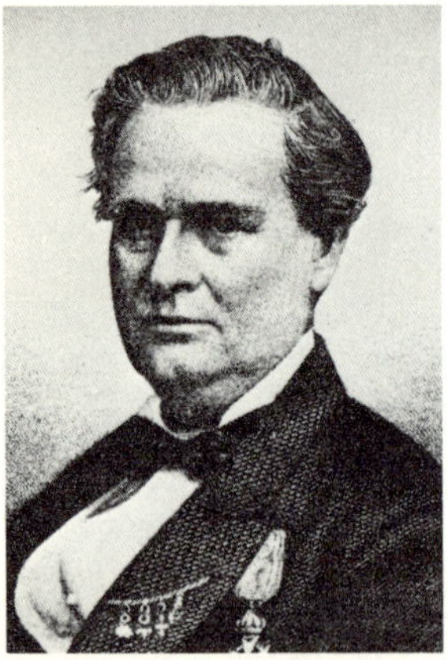

13.1 Sims of Montgomery, Alabama, defined criteria for success in closure of vesicovaginal fistula: adequate exposure, good illumination, knee-chest posture, fine silver sutures (1852).

Sims appreciated that a real handicap in the operation was tying the innermost suture in the vagina. His next innovation was placement of a perforated lead shot over the sutures, tightened down with a clamp. This operation was on Betsey. Again, when the sutures were removed, the leak persisted.[8] Sims's ultimate attack on the problem was to have a local jeweler prepare fine silver wire sutures of capillary thickness. In May or June 1849 he performed his thirtieth operation on Anarcha; four silver sutures were placed, accompanied by a catheter to keep the urinary bladder empty. A few days later Sims examined Anarcha and observed that the wire sutures were completely clean, without evidence of suppuration. When the wires were removed, no urinary leak occurred. After this success Sims promptly reoperated on Lucy and Betsey; both were cured within the space of a few weeks.[9]

In the beginning Sims employed a pewter spoon, but later an instrument maker provided him with a shiny retractor that reflected light, affording good exposure of the fistulous defect. Surgeons of that day operated largely with sunlight as the sole illumination, preferably with a northern exposure. Sims made a complete report of his technique in 1852,[10] including a few lucid schematic illustrations.

When the Civil War broke out in 1861, Sims was in New York; being a Southern sympathizer, he went abroad, where he spent much of the next few years. He was cordially welcomed by the leading surgeons in Ireland, his first stop, and demonstrated his operation successfully in Dublin. He was particularly impressed in Scotland by the skills of Syme and Keith.[11]

He apparently went next to Paris.[12] At this juncture Sims knew no French, but on his arrival at La Charité in October 1861 he was fortunate in meeting Edmond Souchon of New Orleans who was working in Velpeau's clinic there. Sims carried a letter from Mott of New York to Velpeau. The latter gave Sims an opportunity to repair a difficult vesicovaginal fistula, an operation Sims performed before a large assembly of distinguished Paris surgeons and with complete success. This brilliant occasion sufficed to provide Sims with many similar opportunities in Paris hospitals.

Thirty years later and a decade after Sims's death (1883) Souchon reported the circumstances surrounding the famous case of the French countess, a patient of Nélaton's, operated upon by Sims in the country in 1861. The patient was given chloroform and stopped breathing. Said Souchon, "It was then that Nélaton uttered the legendary cry 'head down.'" With complemental artificial respiration the patient was revived. Before the operation was completed, the patient had to be revived twice again. The patient survived and the operation was a success. It is obvious from this that the head-down position was already recognized by Nélaton as important for the revival of patients overanesthetized with chloroform,[13] antedating use of the posture by Trendelenburg and his assistant Willy Meyer by many years.[14]

Sims's great success with repair of a surgical lesion then generally regarded as incurable caused him to be lionized by Paris society. He was also warmly received by well-known surgeons in Britain, Brussels, and other important medical centers in Europe. The "American operation" rapidly won converts.[15]

As the Civil War drew to an end, Sims returned to New York. His success abroad had won him wide recognition, many honors, and helpful support from New York's affluent community. The famous Woman's Hospital came into being through the desire of friends to provide Sims an opportunity to continue his productive work.

Some years after his return from abroad, Sims fell on hard times in the hospital built for him. During his absence his trainees had prospered and won friends among the trustees, who, with staff approval, set a limit of fifteen observers at operations and asked that no patients with cancer of the uterus be admitted. There had been as many as seventy-three spectators in a small operating room when Sims operated; also, the stench occasioned by some of Sims's patients suffering from cancer of the uterus had been offensive to the hospital management.

Sims chose to ignore both regulations. In debates that followed he exhibited considerable irritation and threatened to resign, a defiance he confirmed in a letter. Unfortunately for all, his resignation was accepted January 18, 1874. Three years later, three of his erstwhile colleagues and friends addressed a pamphlet "To the Medical Profession," recounting the trustees' displeasure over Sims's ignoring the directives of the hospital board. They disclaimed any responsibility for Sims's expulsion from the staff. Sims was deeply hurt but responded with a dignified, factual account of the occurrence.[16] Thus ended in personal tragedy for Sims what has come to be recognized as an epic in medicine, correction of a defect attending protracted labor in childbirth abhorrent alike to victims and their intimate associates.[17]

Sims was not always a modest man. In 1857, five years after his first publication on the repair of vesicovaginal fistula, he delivered an address at the New York Academy of Medicine in which he expressed his conviction "that the use of silver as a suture is the great surgical achievement of the nineteenth century." Nevertheless, the final word on silver sutures is perhaps still to be heard. In an experimental study Ballinger and associates (1973) coated catgut, dacron and silk sutures contaminated with *Staph. aureus* and/or *Pseudomonas aeruginosa* organisms with 5 and 50 percent aqueous silver nitrate. The bacterial counts on short segments of such implanted sutures were significantly reduced (by approximately 90 percent).[18] Clinical trial is still awaited.

Sims's Predecessors in the Repair of Vesicovaginal Fistula

Sims had an important predecessor in the person of a London surgeon of note, Montague Gosset, a favorite pupil of Cooper, who in 1834 repaired a vesicovaginal fistula of eleven years' duration in a woman of forty-five years. Cooper had previously treated the patient without success. Gosset, too, placed his patient in the knee-chest position with knees and elbows resting on the operating table. He denuded the edges of the fistula and approximated them with three sutures of "gold wire, or, rather, silver-gilt wire." The first was removed on the ninth day after operation, the second after twelve days, and the third after three weeks. A urethral catheter was employed during the postoperative period to keep the bladder empty, and the patient was instructed to lie prone in bed. The fistula healed perfectly.

Gosset described the case in a letter to *Lancet* (1834), saying he had employed similar sutures for repair of cleft lip defects, in plastic operations on the eyelids, and to close fistulous openings. He found they did not induce ulceration with the rapidity of silk sutures.[19] Gosset's report did not find favor with the members of the profession, who were accustomed to operative failure in the repair of vesicovaginal fistulas. Why did not Gosset follow up on his advantage?[20] It was Sims's persistence and courage after a succession of failures that won him professional and public acclaim.

Sims said that the first operative cure of vesicovaginal fistula in America was reported by George Hayward (1839), a prominent Boston surgeon. He placed his patient in the lithotomy position, supine with knees acutely flexed, freshened the edges of the fistula, and closed the defect with a few interrupted sutures of "thread." A silver catheter was inserted to ensure an empty urinary bladder. By 1851 Hayward had operated twenty times on nine patients, three of whom were cured.[21]

John P. Mettauer, a country surgeon of Virginia, was the first American to have success with operative closure of vesicovaginal defects, having performed a repair in August 1838; however, the case remained unreported until 1840. Mettauer used wire sutures of lead, a procedure he amplified upon in a paper of 1847, and a retention catheter of silver.[22]

Other Techniques

There are a number of references to vesicovaginal fistula in the French literature of the early nineteenth century. Some of the patients were treated by caustics or cautery instead of suture. A few cures were reported.[23]

A. T. Vidal (de Cassis), a French surgeon, proposed obliteration of the vagina to close a vesicovaginal fistula and demonstrated his operation in public on a menopausal patient in 1832. The operation failed. In 1844 Auguste Bérard performed the Vidal operation for vesicovaginal fistula upon a thirty-year-old woman with an extraordinarily large defect. Initially the result was encouraging, but the patient succumbed from peritonitis seventeen days later. The operation raised "a tempest." Bérard was severely criticized by his colleagues for having caused the death of a woman too young to be submitted to so radical a procedure as obliteration of the vagina. In Vidal's technique, said Sims, "the bladder and vagina became a grand compound receptacle of urine and menstrual secretion."[24]

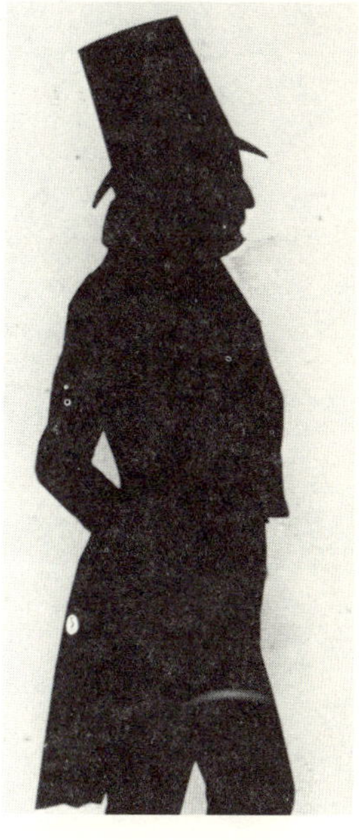

13.2 Mettauer of Virginia successfully closed a vesicovaginal fistula with sutures of lead (1838). Courtesy Richmond Academy of Medicine, silhouette collection.

Two names, said Sims, "stand out in bold relief" in the surgical repair of vesicovaginal fistula, Mettauer of Virginia and the French surgeon Jobert (de Lamballe). The latter, in a "sliding" procedure, mobilized a slip of skin from the vulva upon its own pedicled blood supply; the graft was rotated and attached by wire sutures over the defect, the raw surface facing the fistulous opening. This left the hairy portion of the pedicled graft within the vagina, a technique that did not find wide acceptance by the profession. Jobert never abandoned his technique. Reports of his cases continued to appear until 1862, shortly before his final illness. His total successes were said to have been 82 out of 137 operations.[25]

Gustav Simon (1868) introduced the suprapubic approach for repair of vesicovaginal fistula, a method subsequently advocated by Trendelenburg (1890), who added the feature of an extraperitoneal incision to open the urinary bladder. Trendelenburg closed the vesical fistulous opening with catgut and made no attempt to approximate the vaginal mucosa.[26] Three years later Leopold Dittel, a Viennese surgeon (1893), did the same operation transperitoneally. Maurice Collis (1861) modified the Sims procedure, separating vaginal and vesical walls of the fistula, closing the defect in two layers instead of in a single unit as done by Sims. He used thread sutures.[27]

J. C. Moir (1954) of Oxford University performed the Sims operation with the flap modification successfully in 130 consecutive cases; stress incontinence persisted in a few instances when complete reconstruction of the urethra was required. Naquib Mahfouz (1957) indicated that gynecologists preferred the "Sims-Sänger" operation, whereas urologists and general surgeons usually closed these fistulas transvesically above the pubis.[28]

Early Observations of Vesicovaginal Fistula

A large vesicovaginal fistula has been found in the mummified body of a Nubian woman named Henhenit buried near Thebes about 2050 B.C. She belonged to the harem of Mentuhotep II, a king of the Eleventh Dynasty in Egypt, and was about twenty-two years of age. She had an abnormal pelvis which would have impeded delivery of a fetal head. D. E. Derry, of the Cairo Egyptian University, who described the defect, believes it was a true vesicovaginal fistula resulting from protracted labor. The mummy, one of six examined by Derry (1935), was sent to him from the Metropolitan Museum collections, New York.[29]

Toward the end of the sixteenth century descriptions of vesicovaginal fistulas began to appear in the medical literature. The Dutchman Hendrik van Roonhuisen in 1663 recognized that such lesions are owing to pressure of the child's head upon the vesicovaginal septum. He regarded the situation as incurable. Even so, he related that in an attempt at operative correction he passed two catheters, one through the normal urinary meatus, the other through the fistula. He employed a speculum. The defect was closed by sutures, but details are not provided.[30] Whether Roonhuisen achieved any success is unreported and remains dubious.

Johannes Fatio, a surgeon in Basel, twice operated successfully (1675 and 1684) in cases of vesicovaginal fistula. With the patient in the lithotomy position and with the aid of a speculum, after freshening the margins of the fistula with fine scissors, he passed sharpened quills through the margins of the fistula and wound threads snugly about them, thus approximating the edges of the wound.[31]

Vesicovaginal fistula is rarely seen today because of the fairly consistent performance of early cesarean section in patients with breech presentations and other fetal positions portending difficult and protracted labor. Moreover, among peoples in geographic areas where diets are adequate, rachitic pelves are a rarity. The conquest of vesicovaginal fistula by Sims ranks as one of the great triumphs of nineteenth-century surgery.

Summary

Persistent vesicovaginal fistula, defying satisfactory surgical closure, had been a frequent sequel to prolonged labor in parturients through the first half of the nineteenth century. Many of its unfortunate victims prayed for an early death as the only acceptable resolution of their unhappiness.

In the nonacademic setting of Montgomery, Alabama, Sims (1852) evolved an operation for repair of this dreadful complication of prolonged labor that had condemned many unfortunate women of high and low station to isolation and social ostracism.

The innovation of cesarean section for intrauterine fetal positions and contracted maternal pelves portending prolonged labor has done away with the once much feared complication of vesicovaginal fistula and has immortalized the name of J. Marion Sims in the annals of medical history.

(For notes, see pp. 645–47.)

CHAPTER 14

Phlebotomy

BLOODLETTING as a mode of treatment for ills of various sorts is, indeed, an old practice. Why or how it started is difficult to ascertain definitely, yet it continued to be invoked through the final decades of the nineteenth century. The indications for venesection were never precise; in fact, healthy as well as sick people were often bled regularly twice a year, spring and fall, under the theory that "thinning the blood" promoted health. Surgeons abandoned phlebotomy before physicians were willing to discontinue its use.

Phlebotomy is mentioned in the Egyptian papyri and as treatment for pain and fever in the Hippocratic writings; Celsus at the time of Christ advocated and described its use, as did Galen more than a century later. Albucasis named thirty blood vessels suitable for the practice.[1] The great importance attached to bloodletting in the twelfth century is shown in the School of Salerno's popular *Regimen sanitatis* (Code of Health); the poem, intended primarily as a guide for the laity, passed through 240 editions. Several stanzas devoted to the subject of bleeding indicate how intent the public and the medical profession were on finding a universal remedy, or elixir, to ensure good health. Among the first publications after the invention of printing (1462) were calendars to predict by "judicial astrology" the proper times for bloodletting. Bleeding was often performed at the popular public baths by the bathkeeper, usually a barber-surgeon. The red and white barber pole became the symbol of his two historical functions, bleeding and bandaging.[2]

Phlebotomy — a Universal Remedy

During the next four centuries bloodletting continued to be used as a prophylactic and therapeutic measure, few doubting its efficacy or questioning its safety. Among the most ardent advocates was the sixteenth-century Italian Botallo, who practiced in Paris. He published a treatise in 1577 extolling venesection as therapy for practically every disease. Repeated bleeding to faintness was his recommendation.[3]

One of the chief functions of surgical interns in Paris hospitals was bleeding patients, both medical and surgical. This chore, which consumed an hour's time every afternoon, is said to have accounted for there being more surgical house officers than

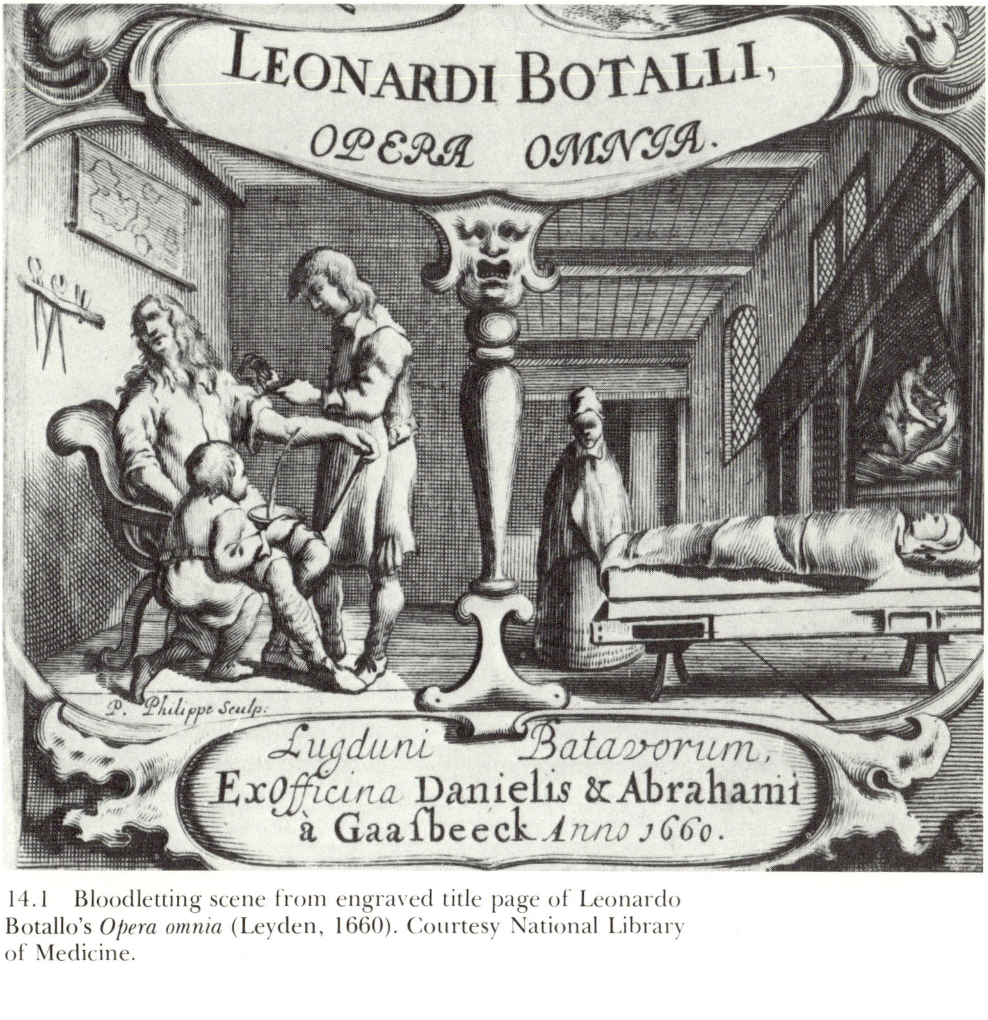

14.1 Bloodletting scene from engraved title page of Leonardo Botallo's *Opera omnia* (Leyden, 1660). Courtesy National Library of Medicine.

physician interns at the Hôtel-Dieu in the seventeenth century. The primary role of the physician house officers, remarked Charles Coury, "was to prescribe with dignity."[4]

Le Sage turned the abuse of bloodletting into fine satire in his *Adventures of Gil Blas* (1715–35). He told of a cleric who consulted a somewhat fictitious Dr. Sangrado for gout. The physician's two favorite remedies were copious bleeding and ingestion of huge quantities of warm water. "It is a mere vulgar error, that the blood is of any use in the system," said Sangrado. He instructed a surgeon to withdraw "six porringers of blood" and "as much more three hours hence" and then to repeat the process the next day. Within two days the cleric, at death's door, sent for a notary to make his will. The housekeeper, hoping for a legacy, kept everyone away until the notary had finished, saying, "you may bleed away when the will is done." Sangrado affirmed that the patient's speedy demise was "owing to their having been too lenient with the lance and too chary of their warm water."[5]

Three of the greatest figures in English medicine — William Harvey, Sydenham, and John Hunter — endorsed bleeding as a therapeutic measure. Harvey (1628) employed bloodletting in his study of the flow of blood in superficial veins. Sydenham never encouraged copious withdrawal of blood but used phlebotomy as first treatment for many disorders. Hunter advocated bloodletting for therapy of gunshot wounds and inflammation, although he warned against excessive bleeding. He advised application of leeches and punctures with a lancet in the inflamed area "to empty the vessels of the part to lessen the inflammation sooner, and, of course, to promote suppuration." Astley Cooper called phlebotomy the "most powerful constitutional means of relieving inflammation." He believed the beneficial effects came principally from its diminution of nervous power. "Sometimes the removal of a very small quantity of blood will occasion not only suspension of all the voluntary functions, but of the mental powers." He bled in amounts of 10 to 20 ounces.[6]

In the late eighteenth and early nineteenth centuries the plague of venesection was visited upon adult patients in most hospitals with no indication other than that they were there. In the early days of the Bristol Royal Infirmary, which opened its doors in 1737, venesection was imposed upon 73 percent of the admitted patients. As many as 32 were bled daily, 12 ounces constituting the average amount drawn at one sitting. The patient held the bleeding bowl to catch his own blood. In 1840 a student bled nearly 50 patients in one day there. When Syme was a young house surgeon at the Royal Infirmary in Edinburgh, he displayed a characteristic bit of independence by withholding venesection from a debilitated boy with compound fracture, directing that he be given porter and steak instead. The irate chief of surgery canceled Syme's order.[7] The illustrious British journal *Lancet* began publication in 1823 and probably chose its name to suggest the emphasis of that day upon the efficacy of bleeding to cure man's ills.[8]

Outside the hospital physicians often bled their own patients. There is no more telling example of the enthusiasm for phlebotomy than that of the Philadelphia physician Benjamin Rush. When ill, he himself willingly submitted to repeated bleedings, and critics have claimed that his sanguine faith in the practice so influenced his contemporaries as to make him indirectly responsible for the death of George Washington at Mount Vernon in 1799. Washington underwent four copious bleedings (about 80 ounces of blood) as treatment for his septic sore throat, probably a virulent streptococcal infection of the pharynx, that proved fatal in fourteen hours. A tracheostomy was urged by one consultant, Dick, but was rejected by the family physician and other consultants. Dick, and probably Mrs. Washington too, objected to the final bleedings. Washington himself favored the procedure and had even ordered his overseer, a veterinarian, to perform the first bleeding before the doctor arrived. In defense of the two physicians whose treatment unfortunately prevailed, they were following the orthodox measures endorsed by their Edinburgh schooling, the accepted practices of the day.[9] The famous Physick subjected himself to be bled 176 ounces during a bout of yellow fever in Philadelphia in 1797.[10]

Much the same therapy as Washington's was ordered a few years later (1838) when John Brown of Edinburgh, the physician author of *Rab and His Friends*, had a "virulent sore throat." He was treated first by six leeches and a mustard plaster applied to the painful area of his neck, then by twelve leeches behind his ear. When no relief from pain was obtained, Brown consented to withdrawal of 16 ounces of blood, with immediate and complete relief, a procedure repeated some time later, until he fainted, but again with satisfaction.[11]

Paul B. Beeson related that Daniel Drake (1785–1852), a roving professor between many medical schools of the Midwest and the architect of two encyclopedic volumes on *Diseases of the Interior Valley of North America*, was called in consultation by a Dr. Colby in 1837. The patient was Mrs. Salmon P. Chase who, two weeks after childbirth, was probably suffering from a low-grade puerperal fever. Upon the urging of Drake, she was bled 30 ounces. Then, over the protests of Colby she was bled another 20 ounces the next morning "to slow the pulse," following which the pulse accelerated and the patient expired, a sequence reminiscent of the bleeding purges of Sangrado.[12]

Use of depletion to treat illness was at its height in Europe in the early decades of the nineteenth century. Phlebotomy was complemented by purgation, measures to encourage perspiration, and emetics, cupping, and leeches, all in the belief that these exhausting remedies increased the patient's resistance. The primary advocates of such methods "to improve the patient's health" were the Paris physicians Broussais and his pupil J. B. Bouillaud who, said Garrison, "let even greater torrents of blood" than his teacher. Dupuytren also was an ardent devotee of phlebotomy for inflammation, even though he had seen a "clean" lancet provoke a dangerous phlegmon at the bleeding site. Oliver Wendell Holmes revealed from his visit to Paris in the 1830s that the dexterous surgeon Lisfranc, "when a phlebotomizing fit was on him," ordered a "wholesale bleeding of his patients, right and left, whatever might be the matter with them."[13]

Application of leeches to the operative site before as well as after operation was a favored practice of the period. The demand for leeches became so great that it outran the native supply in France and England. The total number of leeches imported into France in 1833 is often quoted as 41,500,000.[14] In 1832 the Manchester Royal Infirmary was spending 4.4 percent of its entire hospital budget on "that most singular and valuable reptile." Thereafter use of leeches decreased markedly. The number of leeches bought for St. Bartholomew's Hospital in 1908 had dropped to 400 from a total of 97,300 purchased in 1832. One of the earliest childhood recollections of Anna Dostoevsky, widow of the Russian novelist, was an illness at three years of age for which her doctor prescribed several leeches applied to her chest (ca. 1849). "How repulsive these writhing worms were . . . how they terrified me, and how I tried to tear them off," she wrote in her *Reminiscences*.[15]

Hazards of Phlebotomy

The dangers inherent in bloodletting, whether by lancet or leech, were mentioned by some early writers, but most forcefully by Van Helmont in the mid-seventeenth century. He condemned the practice entirely. Van Helmont's beliefs were invoked in 1791 by a Viennese veterinarian of distinction, Johann Wolstein, who published a twenty-year experimental study of bloodletting in animals and man. His findings repudiated venesection as treatment for all but a few conditions.[16]

Nathaniel Rumsey, a surgeon of Beaconsfield, England, reported in 1819 that fever was sometimes the effect of depletion by bleeding. A number of fatal cases of pyemia following phlebotomy in the records of the Royal Infirmary at Edinburgh were published by J. H. Balfour in 1833. Deaths from phlebitis ascribed to venesection appeared not infrequently in medical journals of that period.[17]

Bloodletting for diagnostic study is currently a significant cause of anemia and reticulocytosis in hospitalized patients in the United States, according to a 1973 study at Cornell Medical Center. The authors conclude that most adults hospitalized for three to four weeks have an average of 500 to 1,000 ml. of blood withdrawn for diagnostic purposes — 10 to 20 percent of their blood volume.[18]

The Final Era of Phlebotomy

The practice of bloodletting survived despite strong protests of the physicians Pierre Louis and Marshall Hall. Louis announced his study of the effects of venesection in 1828–35. He employed statistics to show that phlebotomy had little influence on the progress of pneumonia, yet in 1836 in a discussion of empyema Louis indicated that phlebotomy had been a primary factor in the healing of 150 cases of "acute pleurisy" that had come under his supervision (see chapter 9). Louis proclaimed the importance of experience over that of authority in medicine and was a great influence on many young Americans who came to study under him in Paris. The English physiologist Hall's emphasis (1830) was primarily on delineating rules, limiting the extent of bloodletting.[19]

In 1862 Stromeyer, a famous German military surgeon who still put faith in venesection, regretted that "young German surgeons glory in the fact that they have never ordered a bloodletting."[20] The tradition dies hard. In the first edition of his *Principles and Practice of Medicine* Osler (1892) remarked that "local depletion" was a good practice in inflammation and a lifesaving measure in pneumonia. Osler believed that in the first five decades of the nineteenth century bleeding was used too much and in more recent decades too little. When a healthy full-blooded man had high fever and a bounding pulse, Osler believed removal of 20 to 30 ounces of blood was almost uniformly beneficial, relieving pain and dyspnea. In the seventh and last edition of the textbook prepared by Osler alone (1909) he continued to advocate bleeding in pneumonia, advice that was retained through the sixteenth edition (1947) edited by H. A. Christian. In subsequent revisions of Osler's book there is no mention of phlebotomy for treatment of inflammation or pneumonia. Osler's thesis that the condition of patients with pneumonia is improved by phlebotomy appears to be finding support in the work of Harry LeVeen of the Bronx Veterans Administration Hospital in Brooklyn. LeVeen and his associates have observed (1978) that in patients with chronic pulmonary obstruction, by lowering the hematocrit from the 45 range to 25 by phlebotomy, patients breathe more readily, their color improves, and they regain their appetite. In other words, reducing the density of the blood improves tissue oxygenation and decreases the work load of a failing heart.[21]

Obviously, what was needed was a specific antibacterial agent, which only became available for clinical use with prontosil and sulfanilamide in 1935 and penicillin in the final years of World War II. Before this, surgeons had no remedial measures other than rest and elevation with which to combat infection and inflammation. In fact, the surgeon's role was essentially that of pus evacuator, opening and draining abscesses. When he did more, he usually did harm, especially in cellulitic phlegmons. There were proponents of both prophlogistic (heat and dependency, primarily) and antiphlogistic (cold and elevation) methods of combatting surgical infection.[22]

There is one indication for extended phlebotomy with good rationale that Physick employed at the very beginning of the nineteenth century, attended by syncope and profound muscle relaxation in the reduction of chronic dislocations, a matter to be discussed in chapter 16 on anesthesia.

Inflammation

Despite the broad application of phlebotomy to a great variety of conditions, its specific utilization for inflammation, especially of the soft parts, was widely recommended and practiced, even for visceral inflammation involving lungs and intraperitoneal infection. The rubor, calor, dolor, and tumor of inflammation were well known in antiquity and were discussed in the Hippocratic writings and notably by Celsus. It is not surprising, therefore, that bleeding was an old and honored measure to treat the local turgescence of inflammation.

John Hunter characterized inflammation as the reaction to injury or irritation. He did not know of the existence of bacteria. Today, we usually identify inflammation as the result of bacterial action. Whereas Leeuwenhoek had described protozoa and bacteria in a series of papers (1693–1718) many decades before Hunter, he did not recognize their pathogenicity. In fact, almost two centuries intervened before Koch (1876–78) established firmly the pathogenic character of bacteria.

Hyperemia, slowing of blood flow in inflamed areas, dilatation of venules and capillaries, stasis, exudation of fluid and leucocytes owing to increased penetrability of vessel walls — these are the sequels of bacterial injury and infection, responsible for the redness, heat, pain, and swelling of inflammation. Augustus Waller's demonstration in 1846 of the migration of leucocytes through capillary walls served as an important factor in shifting the emphasis from a humoral (fluid) to a cellular leucocytic influence in the defense against inflammation of bacterial origin.[23] Julius Cohnheim, one of the great pathologists of his time, established (1867–73) on a firm basis that pus resulting from a suppurative process was the result of migration of leucocytes through the endothelial lining of capillaries and venules in the area of inflammation, first the polymorphonuclear leucocytes, followed by the larger mononuclear leucocytes. Earlier it was generally believed that the cellular component of the exudate in the suppurating process originated from the local tissues, of which thesis Virchow, Cohnheim's teacher, had been an ardent advocate. Cohnheim's paper drew criticism from traditional pathologists. When Virchow studied Cohnheim's views, he capitulated to the latter's thesis of leucocytic migration through venular walls. Virchow elaborated upon the concept of the cell as the primary line of defense in inflammation. Current concepts of molecular biology continue to lend renewed emphasis to Virchow's views. L. J. Rather has written a brief but discerning account of Virchow's contributions to understanding the nature of the inflammatory process (1971).[24]

The important role of leucocytes in the phagocytosis of bacteria was illuminated by the famous Russian biologist Elie Metchnikoff (1884) and has survived the critical test of time. Lister (1890) was probably the first surgeon to appreciate the significance of Metchnikoff's theory of phagocytosis in the engulfment of bacteria and the role of leucocytes in delimiting the spread of bacteria and the extension of infection. Yet several pathologists, notably Ernst Ziegler of Germany (1889), persisted in the belief that engulfment of bacteria by leucocytes was a primary cause in the extension of infection.[25] The histiocytes of tissues and organs, the analogue of the vascular monocytes, also partake in the macrophage function of engulfing bacteria.

William Addison (1802–81), a British physician, dedicated many years to the study of leucocytic function. He concluded (1843) that there were two types of inflammatory process, one leading to suppuration and abscess formation and the other constituting a part of the normal healing process after injury.[26]

G. H. Brieger (1968) has written a full historical account of the development of knowledge relating to histologic and immunologic aspects of inflammation. The monograph of B. W. Zweifach and associates (1965) explored the limits of that day's knowledge and appreciation of the nature of the inflammation. J. V. Hurley's monograph on acute inflammation summarizes current views responsible for margination and attraction of leucocytes (chemotaxis) to the walls of venules in inflamed areas and factors that potentiate leucocytic emigration. Obviously, there is much yet to be learned of many aspects of inflammation.[27]

Summary

Phlebotomy survived as a frequently invoked therapeutic procedure for inflammation from antiquity into the nineteenth century. Harvey, Sydenham, and John Hunter endorsed its use. Astley Cooper believed phlebotomy to be the "most powerful constitutional means of relieving inflammation." When leeches and mustard plasters failed to relieve a painful sore throat, much testimony exists to indicate that copious bleeding did. In all the editions of his widely read book on *Principles and Practice of Medicine*, Osler, from the first (1892), and Christian through the sixteenth edition (1947) held to the thesis that extensive phlebotomy was a useful therapeutic remedy for pneumonia. Demonstration of migration of leucocytes through capillary walls shifted emphasis from a humoral to a leucocytic cellular influence as the important defense mechanism against inflammation of bacterial origin. Cohnheim (1867) established definitely that purulent accumulations resulted from migration of leucocytes through the endothelial lining of capillaries and venules. Metchnikoff (1884) elucidated the thesis that phagocytosis or engulfment of bacteria by leucocytes constituted an important factor in delimiting the spread of infection. The nature of inflammation continues to be a subject of earnest pursuit and study by microbiologists.

(For notes, see pp. 647–50.)

CHAPTER 15

Vascular Surgery

No chapter in surgery is more exciting than the control of hemorrhage. Galen alluded to accidental wounds of arteries made while trying to perform phlebotomy.[1] Use of the ligature to staunch hemorrhage is said to trace back to Celsus; it was reintroduced by Paré for amputation. Over the intervening years cautery had been the mainstay of surgeons in the control of hemorrhage; Guillemeau (1597), Paré's successor, reverted to its use. Petit (1718) made a significant contribution to hemostasis in surgery of the extremities with his screw compressor (tourniquet).[2]

Guillemeau and Dominique Anel (1710), Petit's pupil, are sometimes credited with proximal ligation for aneurysm many years before John Hunter's (1786) use of the method, yet the second-century Antyllus had preceded in boldness the great vascular surgeons of the eighteenth and nineteenth centuries; not only did he ligate both proximal and distal to aneurysms, but he also opened and obliterated the aneurysm, an operation that Matas (1888) elaborated upon many centuries later.[3]

Proximal or Distal Ligature?

Desault reintroduced Anel's method of proximal ligation for aneurysm in 1785, the year he became surgeon-in-chief at the Hôtel-Dieu. The patient survived only four days. When proximal ligature could not be done, Desault proposed and performed ligature immediately distal to the booming tumor; the blood could then reflux into the aneurysmal sac and leave via collateral vessels. This operation, he believed, was applicable to aneurysms of the external iliac and axillary arteries. After Desault died in 1795, his works were published by his devoted pupil Xavier Bichat (1801), giving the description of Desault's method and an account of the 1785 operation. Alexis Boyer (1818) wrote that Desault tied the femoral artery immediately proximal to a popliteal aneurysm in 1785. The aneurysm burst on the eighteenth day, and Desault apparently tied the artery distal to the aneurysm, preserving as many communicating branches as possible. The patient succumbed in eight months from caries of the tibia.[4]

Desault and Pierre Brasdor (1721–97) were contemporaries and both discussed ligature in Paris lectures. Brasdor did not perform the operation and apparently did not describe it in print; even so, through the years, his name has been linked with distal ligation for aneurysm.[5]

Bichat states that Deschamps of Paris employed Desault's operation in 1799. Deschamps convened a group of physicians to discuss treatment of an aneurysm nearly 17 inches in diameter of the upper thigh. Neither he nor several assistants who probed the wound at operation could find the artery distal to the aneurysm. Deschamps then made a mass suture of the area where the artery should be. The blood loss was negligible. On the fourth postoperative day, because the tumor was enlarging and the patient's condition worsening, Deschamps reoperated and opened the aneurysm with a large loss of blood, then effected proximal ligation. The patient died shortly thereafter.[6]

Guthrie also wrote of Desault, Anel, and Brasdor. At times, Guthrie seems confused, using the terms "below" and "above"; he obviously should have said "proximal" or "distal" to the aneurysm. Guthrie conceded that Deschamps was the first to improvise the suggestion of Desault. In London James Wardrop in 1825 reported an aneurysm of the carotid which he had successfully treated by tying the artery distal to the aneurysmal tumor.[7]

Hunter's proximal ligation for aneurysm was announced in print by his brother-in-law, Home (1786). Garrison earmarked Hunter's ligation of the femoral artery in the mid-thigh (Hunter's canal) for popliteal aneurysm as "his greatest innovation in surgery," a very ephemeral glory indeed if Hunter's renown were to rest upon that inadequate and long outmoded operation, which disregarded the important role of communicating arterial branches in perpetuating persistence of the aneurysm.[8]

Lancisi on Aneurysms

The seventeenth-century Italian surgeon Giovanni Lancisi, physician to Pope Clement XI and often regarded as the founder of cardiology, wrote a dissertation upon aneurysms which was first published in 1728, eight years after the author's death.[9] He related that a canon of the church, a man of fifty-five who was very fond of singing, had an aortic aneurysm presenting between the fourth and fifth ribs. Lancisi advised him to refrain from any exertion, including singing, that could compromise the status of the thoracic aneurysm. The patient asked a famous local surgeon of the day to provide a device to wear around his chest to restrain the thrust of the aneurysm and prevent it from breaking through the tissues of the chest wall. Said Lancisi, "The talented surgeon . . . made an iron belt with a spring, not unlike the spring truss" worn by patients with hernias, to retain the protrusion within the thorax. With this belt he "easily kept the projecting sac of the aneurysm by main force within the chest." The patient, encouraged and relieved, kept on singing, much to Lancisi's displeasure. Whenever the iron belt was removed, the thrust of the aneurysm against the tissues of the anterior thoracic chest wall was very evident. The canon died suddenly from rupture of the aneurysm in February 1699.

In his treatise, Lancisi alluded to "Gallic aneurysm," which he regarded as syphilitic; in fact, he was inclined to believe that most aneurysms, including the aortic and popliteal, were syphilitic in nature. From several patients Lancisi had extracted a story of inguinal buboes and a history of syphilis or gonorrhea. Lancisi, obviously an unusually competent history taker and observer, went into the background of his patients' illnesses in great detail, rationalizing symptoms to interpret their significance. In case reports he followed his patients to their deathbeds, relating their symptoms to the postmortem findings, and then set about striving to resolve how observations at postmortem accounted for the symptoms.[10]

Vascular Surgery in the Nineteenth Century

Astley Cooper was the keenest exponent of vascular surgery in the early decades of the nineteenth century. On November 1, 1805, he ligated the common carotid artery. Although the neck tumor disappeared, the patient died a week later, apparently of suppuration. A second effort on June 22, 1808, succeeded. The patient, aged fifty, was a porter whose job was to carry heavy bars of iron. In this endeavor Cooper ligated and divided the artery between the ligatures, following the example of another pupil of Hunter, John Abernethy (1764–1831) of St. Bartholomew's.[11] In 1796 Abernethy had dealt successfully with a high-lying aneurysm beneath Poupart's ligament, ligating and dividing the external iliac artery between ligatures an inch apart, a technique that established the superiority and greater safety of division of large arteries over simple ligature in the management of aneurysm.[12] This important departure from simple ligature of large arteries was unappreciated by other leading vascular surgeons of the nineteenth and twentieth centuries, including Britain's Guthrie and America's Mott and Halsted. In fact, the importance of Abernethy's practice remained unrecognized by surgeons for almost a century and a half, until Emile Holman of San Francisco showed experimentally the superiority and greater safety of division over single ligature of a large artery.[13]

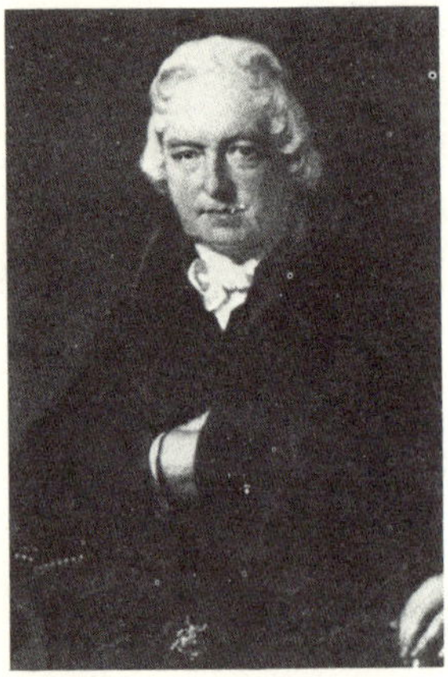

15.1 John Abernethy (1764–1831), pupil of John Hunter, demonstrated that division of large arteries is less likely than ligature to invite postoperative hemorrhage (1796).

Cooper pointed out that in ligating medium-sized and large arteries the ligature must be snug enough to rupture both the intima and the muscular layer of the arterial wall.[14] Herein lies the cause of subsequent hemorrhage at the site of ligation, fatal to all who underwent ligature of the aorta for aneurysm from Cooper's early case in 1818 down to Halsted's two patients with partial occlusion by aluminum bands.

In April 1817 Cooper ligated the abdominal aorta for aneurysm as a last resort for a patient with a continuing hemorrhage. Edward Osler, uncle of William Osler, was present as a student in Guy's Hospital surgical amphitheatre at the time. Cooper announced: "Gentlemen, I have the pleasure of informing you that the aorta is now hooked up on my finger." He tied the aorta with a single long ligature which was led to the external surface of the wound. The operation was performed on a Wednesday; the patient, a porter of thirty-eight years, died with cold extremities on Friday.[15] This operation was repeated twenty times over succeeding years, but almost uniformly failed.[16] In fact, successful operations on the aorta for aneurysms and occlusive disease came only in the 1950s with resection and homograft replacement of the excised segment.

Travers of St. Thomas's Hospital, in a cooperative effort with Cooper, wrote a historical account of the surgery of veins, including experiences of his own. A surprising revelation of this review was the frequency of suppuration and abscess attending ligature of varicose veins in the leg, occasionally attended by fatal pulmonary embolism.[17] In a Paris thesis J.-L. Jaillot (1857) advocated Anel's proposal of ligating the artery proximal to an area of suppuration to avoid hemorrhage. On the basis of experience Jaillot believed it to be a good technique, adding that the procedure had had wide application in the Crimean War.[18]

"The names of Scarpa and J. Bell, of Abernethy, Astley Cooper, and Mott, will long stand pre-eminent, as having improved our knowledge of the pathology of these diseases [aneurysms]," wrote Liston in 1838. He stated that aneurysm at the bend of the elbow was often occasioned by phlebotomy, the brachial artery being unintentionally pierced, and that such aneurysms were usually curable by the application of direct pressure.[19]

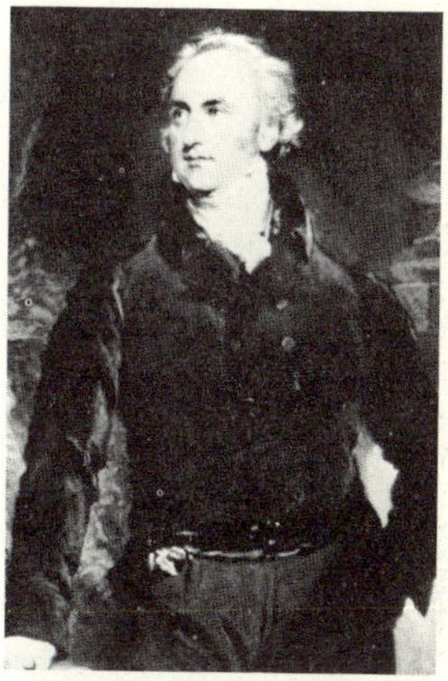

15.2 Astley Cooper (1768–1841), celebrated vascular surgeon, one of Hunter's most distinguished pupils. From a painting by Thomas Lawrence, Courtesy Royal College of Surgeons, England.

Commenting on ligating the carotid artery, Liston said, "The effects of disturbing the flow of blood to the brain was much dreaded in earlier times." He related that a case was described by J. Bell around 1807 in which "a poor woman was allowed to perish by hemorrhage from the sac, under the eyes of himself [Bell] and colleagues, a whole college of surgeons, at that particular period claiming to be surgeons to the Royal Infirmary of Edinburgh." Liston then went on to say that both carotids have been tied in the human subject with only brief periods of time intervening, and without any bad effects arising — a rather strange statement to come from so experienced a surgeon. However, that Liston did entertain misgivings over ligature of the carotid arteries is apparent in another statement: "I believe I have had fully as much experience in the management of tumours of the mouth and jaw, and of the face and neck, as any surgeon in this country and have never seen occasion to tie the carotid previous to, or during the operations for, their removal; and have never regretted omitting this supposed precautionary measure."[20] It would appear that Liston had altered his opinion relative to the harmlessness of ligating the carotid arteries.

America's first great vascular surgeon was Mott (1785–1865), long a distinguished member of the Bellevue Hospital staff in New York. He performed proximal ligature of the innominate artery for aneurysm in May 1818. The patient, a fifty-seven-year-old sailor, apparently tolerated total occlusion of this large artery very well but died of hemorrhage from the site of ligation twenty-six days later. In 1833 Mott reported the case of a twenty-one-year-old woman with a tumor of the right subclavian artery "as large as a hen's egg." He tied the artery within the scaleni muscles. Blood loss at operation was slight; morphine was given postoperatively. There were several episodes of bleeding and the patient died of a severe hemorrhage nineteen days after the operation. The ligature obviously had cut through the artery. For an aneurysm of the innominate artery involving the subclavian and the root of the carotid, Mott (1829) successfully dealt with the situation by tying the carotid artery. It concerned a tumor "the size of a pigeon's egg" above the clavicle in a farmer of fifty-one. Mott "considered it a proper case for the operation proposed by Brasdor, and . . . first successfully performed by the distinguished Wardrop." He tied the carotid artery "in the usual manner," and the patient recovered without complication. Mott (1831) also reported a case of diffuse femoral aneurysm for which he tied the external iliac artery. The patient, a boy of thirteen with a penknife penetration of the right thigh, recovered.[21]

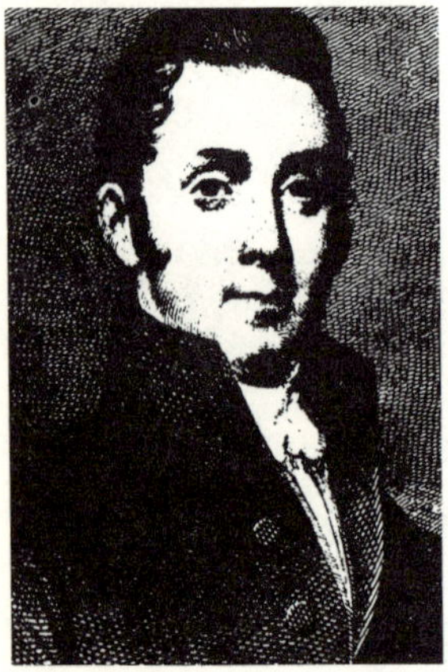

15.3 Valentine Mott (1785–1865), noted American vascular surgeon.

Mott had studied under Cooper in London and, according to a *Lancet* obituary notice (1865), "was the representative American surgeon and his name was a household word with British surgeons." The editorial commented that Mott had "tied the carotid forty-six times, the subclavian seven times — every one of them successfully; the iliac seven times — four successfully; and the femoral, fifty-two times; cut for stone one hundred sixty-five times, and amputated nearly one thousand limbs." Mott's success obviously was not that consistent.[22]

George W. Norris, a Philadelphia surgeon, made several historical analyses of mortality in operations for ligation of arteries. His statistics published in 1847 revealed 118 instances of ligature of the external iliac artery, the first by Abernethy in 1796, the last by J. G. Crosse, the well-known Norwich surgeon, in 1842. Of these, 85 patients survived; in some of these cases, amputation was necessary. There were 33 deaths, an overall mortality of 28 percent, a nice achievement for a period antedating anesthesia and prophylactic antiseptic surgery.

In a second paper in 1847 Norris reported similarly upon ligature of the carotid and the innominate artery; in 38 such operations for aneurysms of the carotid artery, there were 16 deaths, a mortality of 42.1 percent. The first operation reported was Cooper's in 1805; the last was G. White's in 1845. Cooper's first patient died; his second, in June 1808, survived.[23]

In 1845 Luigi Porta, professor of surgery at Pavia, published a series of experiments performed on 270 animals (mostly dogs, but also sheep, goats, and calves) between the years 1835 and 1844. Porta tried various types of ligature materials. He ligated the aorta of 60 animals, noting that paraplegia followed frequently; a few dogs survived the experiment. He also collected and summarized from the literature 600 instances in which large arteries had been tied; ligature of the aorta (4 patients) was fatal in all, as was ligature of the innominate artery (8 patients); lesser mortalities attended ligature of the common iliac and femoral arteries.[24]

A knowledgeable monograph of over 900 pages upon aneurysms and their treatment was written by Paul Broca (1856) when he was an *agrégé* of the Faculty of Medicine in Paris and surgeon to its hospitals. He recounted that manual and mechanical obliteration of the aneurysm by pressure proximal to, as well as distal to, the aneurysm had been practiced in antiquity and was described by Guy de Chauliac and others.[25]

Use of the galvanocautery for the control of aneurysms dates back to C.-G. Pravaz (1831) of Lyons and continued into the first decades of the twentieth century, the object being to try to coagulate the blood within the saccular aneurysm. Such aneurysms were stuffed with ligature material of varying sorts and also with fine wire through which an electric current was passed in the hope of hastening coagulation of blood and obliteration of the aneurysmal sac. Most of these methods, obviously, were dangerous and rarely succeeded.[26]

Halsted's Contributions to Vascular Surgery

In the first volume of Halsted's *Collected Papers,* 275 pages are devoted to surgery of the blood vessels, most of which concerns

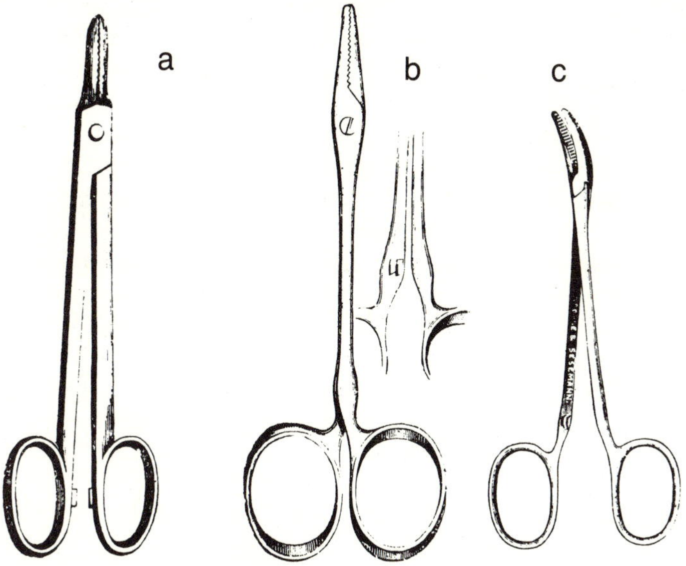

15.4 Spencer Wells's artery forceps: **c** is curved, facilitating ligature of divided vessels. From Thompson, *History of surgical instruments*.

aneurysms.[27] His first paper on the subject, presented before the Johns Hopkins Hospital Medical Society on May 23, 1892, was a brief account of a black man of fifty-two years, with premature white hair and beard, who had an aneurysm of the subclavian and axillary arteries. Halsted ligated the first portion of the subclavian artery and removed the aneurysm. The surgery was successful, certainly an aggressive and impressive operation. Halsted's next paper before the society, on March 20, 1905, was the report of an experimental study on the use of metal bands of silver and aluminum, successively tightened, in the belief that proper constriction would slow the blood flow and cause clotting within the aneurysm. The experiments concerned the aorta. One dog died from hemorrhage at the site of the proximal band, apparently the only instance of hemorrhage in the observations. Halsted performed approximately 90 experiments on 68 dogs, concluding "there may be a place in surgery for the partially occluding band." He reported two clinical cases: in one, an aluminum band was applied to the left common carotid artery; in the other, an attempt was made to place a band around the aortic arch; this patient died on the operating table before the band could be placed.[28]

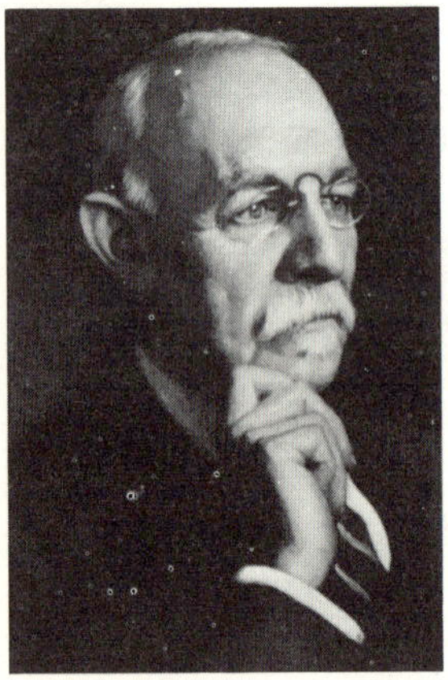

15.5 William S. Halsted (1852–1922), great vascular surgeon, developed a distinguished school of surgeons.

In his third paper Halsted suggested that partial occlusion of the aorta might succeed in curing an aneurysm, remarking that the most successful of such operations was performed by William W. Keen in 1899, the patient surviving forty-three days.[29] Keen (1837–1932), S. D. Gross's successor as professor of surgery at Jefferson Medical College, was the author and editor of several important medical texts. Halsted's fourth paper on ligature of major arteries was presented at the American Surgical Association meeting in June 1909. Herein he reported upon a physician with an abdominal aneurysm in whom he partially occluded the aorta between the superior mesenteric and the renal artery with an aluminum band. The patient survived forty-seven days, dying of an abscess at the site of application of the band, "the first [infection] in the annals of The Johns Hopkins Hospital in a clean abdominal case," said Halsted. The patient apparently survived four days longer than Keen's case in 1899. In a discussion of Matas's presentation before the American Surgical Association the following year (1910), Halsted said, "I regret that I have, as yet, no case to report of cure of an aortic aneurism, but I find great encouragement to further attempts from the result of the only case suitable for the application of a band to the abdominal aorta which it has been my fortune to treat."[30] Halsted's sixth paper concerned ligature of the common iliac artery, a paper also presented before the American Surgical Association (1912). Herein he related that in 1812 William Gibson, then the twenty-four-year-old professor of surgery at the University of Maryland, attempted unsuccessfully to ligate a left common iliac artery which had been pierced by a musket ball. Halsted goes on to describe an instance in which Mott tied the common iliac artery for aneurysm, using an aneurysm needle and a suture. Mott saw the patient several months after the operation and reported that the aneurysm had completely disappeared and that the patient remained well. Halsted presented a table listing thirty instances in which the common iliac artery was tied for aneurysm from 1880 to 1912.[31]

Halsted published several additional papers on partial occlusion of the aorta with a metal band, essentially experimental procedures. He then made a presentation before the German Surgical Congress in April 1914.[32]

Later Halsted studied dilatation of the subclavian artery distal to the site of impingement upon the artery by a cervical rib and enumerated similar cases going back to one of Herbert Mayo, published in the *London Medical and Physical Journal* in 1831.[33]

Of his numerous publications on vascular surgery, Halsted's most scholarly and interesting is that entitled "Ligations of the Left Subclavian Artery in Its First Portion," published in1921, one year before his death. It contains a good historical survey. In this article Halsted quoted at length from a paper of Osler, who had asked the Greek scholar R. W. Livingstone to translate Antyllus' account of aneurysms, preserved in the writings of the fourth-century Byzantine physician Oribasius. Antyllus tied the artery proximal to the aneurysm as well as beyond it with a double ligature of flax or gut. He then opened the aneurysm and evacuated its contents, an operation, said Antyllus, that could be effected without loss of blood — heroic surgery for that day.[34] Halsted quoted Broca, who stated that Antyllus not only created operative medicine but also the understanding of the pathology of aneurysms. Halsted then related that Aetius in the sixth century described the operation, subsequently attributed to Anel (1710), of ligating the brachial artery for an aneurysm at the bend of the elbow three or four fingerbreadths below the axilla, followed by opening of the sac.

Halsted concluded his informative paper by listing twenty-one aneurysms in which ligation of the first portion of the left subclavian artery was done.[35] The twenty-first case was his own and perhaps, said Halsted, the largest subclavian aneurysm ever operated upon. A good bibliography follows.

One notes these many contributions of Halsted on vascular surgery with increased admiration for a venturesome surgeon with scholarly instincts. Great student of the literature that Halsted was, it is strange that he had not employed Abernethy's (1796) division rather than simple ligation of large arteries in dealing with aneurysms; nor had he explored the use of vessel homografts of which Carrel had written (1908). Heparin was discovered at The Hopkins in 1916, but its use to preclude thrombosis came approximately fifteen years after Halsted's death.[36] Every student of surgery will applaud Halsted's thirty years of consecutive application to a surgical problem that had to await additional developments for signal achievement. His artistic and beautiful description of the effect of the ligature upon an aneurysm warrants repetition here: "The moment of tying the ligature is indeed a dramatic one. The monstrous, booming tumor is stilled by a tiny thread, the tempest silenced by the magic wand."[37]

Techniques of Blood Vessel Suture

Alexander Jassinowsky (1891) of Odessa experimented with arterial suture on dogs and calves in which he partially divided various arteries. He found complete division of arteries difficult to handle because of retraction of the divided vessel, whereas partial division with a bistoury could be sutured easily. Jassinowsky used the fine silk sutures employed by eye surgeons. He made sutures of the entire thickness of vessel walls and sutures sparing the intima in some and the adventitia in others. Partial divisions of the carotid arteries and the aorta were sutured with quite uniform success.

For clinical application, Jassinowsky recommended ligature of small vessels in which reanastomosis would prove difficult. For larger vessels the size of the axillary or popliteal, he favored attempts at suture. Attending complete division of arteries, he considered ligature adequate to effect hemostasis. He stressed the need to perform all such operative procedures under strict antisepsis.[38]

Julius Dörfler wrote of arterial suture (1899), reporting from Karl Garré's clinic in Rostock. He related several instances between 1894 and 1898 in which a number of clinical surgeons had repaired operative injuries of arteries successfully. He performed twenty arterial sutures in dogs employing essentially the method of Jassinowsky. He preferred the continuous suture over the interrupted suture. On reexamining anastomoses in which the full thickness of the vessel wall was employed in the arterial suture, he observed that the intimal suture within the arterial lumen was completely unchanged and without signs of inflammation or thrombus formation. In twelve consecutive suture repairs performed under strict antiseptic precautions, he had uniform success without complication or compromise of the vessel lumen. In approximating divided arteries he used either an interrupted mattress or running suture, approximating the intimal surfaces, or a suture which included only the adventitia and muscle layer of the vessel and did not penetrate the intima and the vessel lumen. He concluded that both modes of suture were about equally efficacious. He also reported upon J. B. Murphy's (1897) invagination of the proximal segment of a divided artery into the distal segment.

Dörfler began with the thesis that it was wise not to penetrate the intimal layer of divided vessels in the suture, but his own experiments demonstrated that a full-thickness suture of the vessel wall was satisfactory. He cited five clinical instances in which Lothar Heidenhain (1895) and F. Villar and Brachet (1895) used the entire thickness of the vessel wall for the suture with good results. The experiments of Villar and Brachet, however, were on the veins of dogs. Heidenhain had best results using running catgut sutures, intima to intima, in wounds of large arteries in both man and dog.[39]

In a series of papers between 1902 and 1908 Carrel, originally of Lyons, provided a clear description of vessel suture. He insisted on intima-to-intima coaptation in reapproximation of divided vessels. By placing three equidistant fine sutures on the divided vessel, he converted the lumens into equilateral triangles; and over-and-over continuous fine-silk suture effected a nice union. He carefully removed the adventitia from the vessel surfaces to be approximated.[40] Carrel's description was a refinement of the techniques of Jassinowsky and Dörfler, whom he neglected to cite. In two papers of 1907 and 1908 Carrel showed clearly that organ transplants were feasible, a possibility he predicted at the end of his 1902 Lyons presentation. He also recognized the greater tolerance of autografts over homografts and their increased chance for functional survival. It probably was chiefly for this segment of his work that Carrel was cited for the Nobel Prize in 1912, the first made for medical research performed in America.[41]

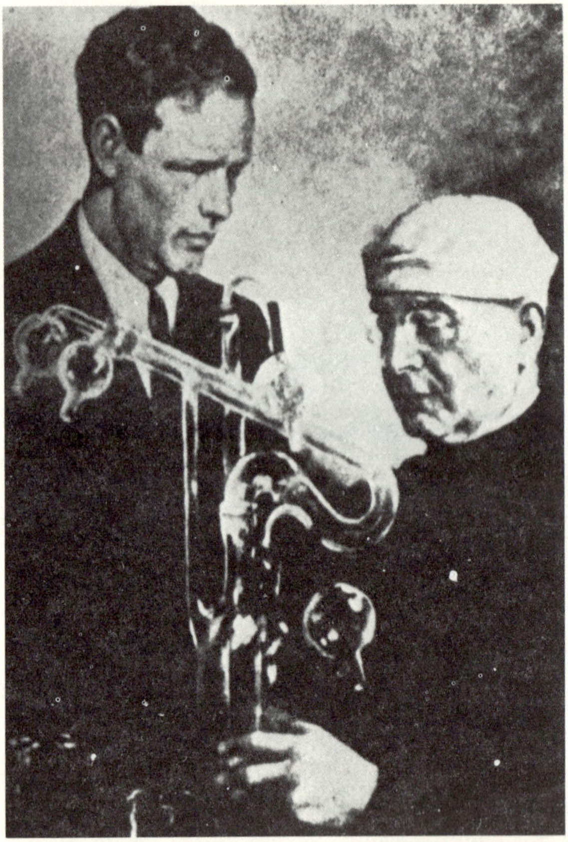

15.6 Alexis Carrel with Charles A. Lindbergh and their mechanical heart. Carrel (1873–1944), Nobel Laureate, was cited for contributions to vascular surgery.

Aids to Arterial Surgery

Perhaps in no other branch of surgery have there been as many important twentieth-century developments favorably affecting its technical procedures as in vascular surgery. Heparin and dicoumarin proved to be effective agents in the prevention of thromboses at sites of vascular suture. Perhaps equally important has been diagnostic arteriography in revealing the nature of arterial lesions needing the attention of the surgeon. Reynaldo dos Santos of Lisbon demonstrated in the late 1920s that percutaneous aortography could be achieved by injection of an opaque medium, allowing x-ray visualization of the aorta and peripheral arteries. Werner Forssmann described (1929) self-catheterization of the antecubital vein permitting x-ray visualization of the heart.[42]

Microsurgery, first adopted by the otologists, was subsequently invoked by many throughout greater surgery, including neuro- and vascular surgeons. A binocular microscope enables the surgeon to use suture materials and needles of very small caliber, permitting establishment of functional anastomoses in small vessels not achievable by conventional surgical means.

Jay McLean was a sophomore medical student at The Hopkins working with William H. Howell in physiology when he described (1916) an anticoagulant substance especially prevalent in the liver; the substance subsequently came to be known as heparin. The lung, too, was found to be relatively rich in heparin.[43] The work of the Toronto investigators A. F. Charles and D. A. Scott and the studies of J. Erik Jorpes of Stockohlm (1935), defining the chemical nature of heparin, made this anticoagulant practical for employment by surgeons. D. W. Gordon Murray and associates are credited with the first use of heparin for venous thrombosis (1937). Heparin has been a great boon to vascular surgeons. Whereas many of the techniques of operation upon arteries originated in the 1890s and early decades of this century, progress in vascular surgery was slow until anticoagulant agents became available. Jorpes stated (1950) that between 1942 and 1945 anticoagulant therapy of thrombosis became firmly established in Sweden. Before this the treatment had been conservative, with confinement of patients to bed until fever and acute symptoms subsided.[44]

Today anticoagulants are employed by surgeons to preclude thrombosis, usually for short periods of time. When long-term anticoagulant therapy is indicated, dicoumarin is the usual agent. It is less expensive and can be taken by mouth.

Extensions of Vascular Surgery

Modern-day vascular surgery permeates the entire surgical range, from relief of disability from varicose veins of the legs to the most intricate surgical procedures, such as those dealing with cerebral aneurysms, congenital and acquired arteriovenous fistulas, and portal hypertension. Holman (1924), one of Halsted's last protégés, by a series of careful studies, showed that in large arteriovenous communications the observed peripheral ischemic tissue changes are owing to lack of oxygen in the tissues beyond the abnormal arteriovenous communication, the blood returning preferentially to the area of lesser resistance in the vein, and that in large arteriovenous fistulas the consequent enlarged blood volume demands extra work by the heart, inviting cardiac failure. C. Walton Lillehei and associates (1950) demonstrated in canine experiments that large arteriovenous fistulas frequently provoke vegetative endocarditis.[45]

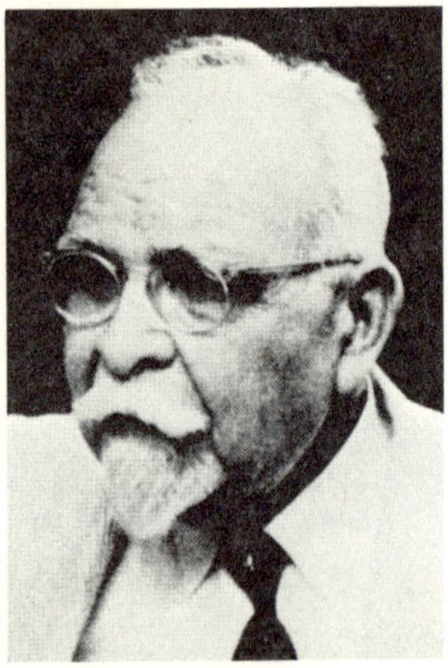

15.7 Rudolph Matas (1860–1957), well-known New Orleans vascular surgeon and scholar.

The Russian military surgeon Nikolai V. Eck (1877) performed the first successful experimental portacaval shunt, making a side-to-side anastomosis between the portal vein and the vena cava below the liver. The portal vein was tied above the anastomosis. This operation, devised to relieve portal hypertension and bleeding from esophageal varices, did not encounter clinical success until six decades later when Allen Whipple of Columbia-Presbyterian Hospital in New York (1945) established its feasibility. Many variations of the method are currently in use to achieve decompression of portal hypertension and relief of esophageal variceal bleeding owing to hepatic cirrhosis. An unwelcome common side effect of the portacaval anastomosis has been the appearance of encephalopathy (ammonia intoxication) occasioned by the portal blood entering the systemic venous circulation without being filtered and detoxified by the liver. Although the operation when successful does deal effectively with variceal hemorrhage and prolongs life, it is not an unmixed blessing. However, no acceptable substitute has appeared on the medical horizon to overcome the handicaps of hepatic cirrhosis other than abstention from alcohol, an addiction many of its victims find extremely difficult to relinquish. Varco's operation of excision of the esophagus does quell the bleeding from esophageal varices, especially in extrahepatic portal hypertension. The segments of jejunum employed in this operation for replacement of the esophagus tend to rebleed; nevertheless, the survival time has been impressive. These patients, however, in contrast to those with alcoholic cirrhosis, have normal hepatic function.[46]

Varicose Veins and Ulcers

Inasmuch as the veins of the body cavities have no valves, pressure of the column of blood from the level of the right cardiac atrium, in the erect quiet posture, is constantly testing competency of the venous valves below the inguinal ligament. Excision of the superficial saphenous veins ordinarily corrects the most frequent sequel of this situation. If, however, the deep veins of the leg too are involved, and especially if they have been the seat of thrombophlebitis, a potentially serious threat confronts the patient and his surgeon, viz., chronic venous stasis, not readily remedied. Ulceration of the lower leg and ankle area quite resistant to treatment is likely to ensue. Conservative management with snug bandages and frequent assumption of the horizontal posture to combat the force of gravity are among the more successful attacks upon the problem. Even so ulcers with a constantly wet surface may persist.

Schede (1877) and Trendelenburg (1890) employed excision of the superficial varicosities, including the saphenous vein. Strippers to remove that vein through short incisions were devised and are still in use. In successive papers dating from 1916 John Homans of Boston stressed the importance of the perforating leg veins that communicate with the deep venous system. He observed thrombophlebitis in refractory cases of varicose veins of the leg and in patients with chronic leg ulcers. In 1934 he alluded to the frequency of thromboembolism in such situations, a circumstance which Travers (1821) had recognized before the days of anesthesia. Homans (1941) urged "division of the superficial femoral vein, common femoral or even the common iliac vein" in instances of prior canalized thrombophlebitis.[47]

A fundamental requirement for healing in any wound is that it remain dry, free from exudate. Modes of dealing with chronic leg ulcers are legion. A group of six authors (1976) representing several disciplines from two Swedish university hospitals, Malmö and Uppsala, have come up with a very novel scheme of counteracting the customary wetness of these wounds. They employ a Swedish preparation known as Debrisan, porous hydrophilic spherical beads, 0.1 to 0.3 mm. in diameter when dry, capable of absorbing four times their weight in fluid and exudate. The authors report that chronic varicose ulcer wounds become dry when thus treated and quickly exhibit evidence of healing in about 75 percent of instances, permitting ready and successful application of skin grafts.[48] The principle is correct; time will tell whether it is a durable contribution.

Paracardiac Surgery

Wounds of the heart and large paracardiac vessels today can be sutured successfully if the patient reaches the operating suite in good time. Operation for relief of constrictive pericarditis was a twentieth-century surgical development featured first in Europe at the hands of Ludwig Rehn (1920) and Victor Schmieden (1923) of Frankfurt am Main and others, and in this country,

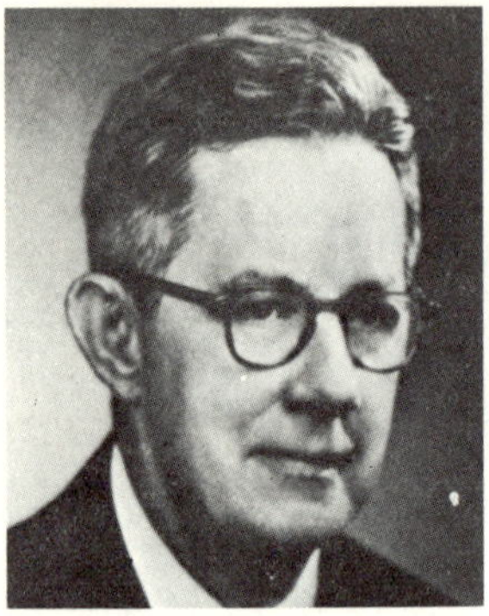

15.8 Alfred Blalock (1899–1964), creative vascular surgeon, famous for his blue baby operation.

notably, by Edward D. Churchill (1929) of Massachusetts General Hospital.[49] The development of paracardiac surgery was lent considerable impetus by Robert Gross of the Children's Hospital, Boston, in ligature of the patent ductus arteriosus (1939) and in its division (1944). A corrective operation for coarctation of the aorta by Gross and by Clarence Crafoord of Sweden came almost simultaneously in 1945. Division of vessels and bands surrounding and partially occluding the trachea or the esophagus by Gross (1945–46) was an additional significant milestone in the development of vascular surgery.[50]

Then came the Blalock-Taussig operation for blue babies (1945), in which the subclavian artery was anastomosed to the pulmonary, providing increased oxygenation of the blood. The procedure brought pink lips to cyanotic babies, a startling change that gave great hope to the profession and the public of the promise of vascular surgery.[51]

Mid-Twentiety-Century Innovations

The management of aortic aneurysms received new encouragement when Charles Dubost of Paris and associates (1951) excised a terminal sclerotic aorta (Leriche syndrome) and successfully inserted an arterial homograft. The possibilities of the procedure became immediately evident to many vascular surgeons. DeBakey and Denton Cooley of Houston, Henry Bahnson of Baltimore, and others promptly employed the method in the removal of aortic aneurysms, extending the surgery of great arteries. Presently synthetic materials of varying kinds replaced arterial homografts. The crimped dacron graft has proved especially useful in that flexion of the thighs does not cause acute obstructive angulation of the graft. Arterial and venous grafts trace back to Carrel's 1907 publication. Erich Lexer (1907, 1912) of Königsberg, too, substituted venous grafts successfully for diseased arteries.[52]

Pulmonary Embolism

It is to be remembered that during the mid-1920s and well into the late 1930s embolectomy was performed in many European surgical clinics and occasionally in the United States for pulmonary embolism. When a surgical patient was threatened with exitus from a pulmonary embolus, many a surgeon and his patient spent the night in the operating suite anticipating worsening of the condition and the need for an operation without anesthesia on an unconscious patient. Crafoord gained early international fame by this practice, attended with some successes. At the 1928 sessions of the German Surgical Congress, Martin Kirschner, then of Tübingen, presented his patient who in 1924 had undergone the first successful pulmonary embolectomy.[53]

Today one rarely hears of pulmonary embolectomy. Usually the situation can be resolved by the administration of anticoagulants, intravenous heparin, followed by a maintenance dose of oral dicoumarin for a temporary period while the hazard threatens. For repetitive episodes of clot migration, surgeons occasionally interrupt the vena cava below the renal veins by ligature, application of a clip, or insertion of a screen filter that precludes central movement of large clots. T. J. Fogarty and associates (1963) devised a catheter of the Foley variety which, when inflated, can assist the removal of a venous thrombus or an arterial embolus.[54]

Open Heart Surgery

John Gibbon of Philadelphia initiated studies in the 1930s directed at development of a pump oxygenator which would make it possible to do open cardiac operations. His first attack on the problem was to demonstrate that when the pump oxygenator was used, dogs could survive ligature of the primary pulmonary artery for relatively long periods of time. Gibbon's first clinical success with the pump oxygenator came on May 6, 1953, in the repair of an interatrial septal defect.[55]

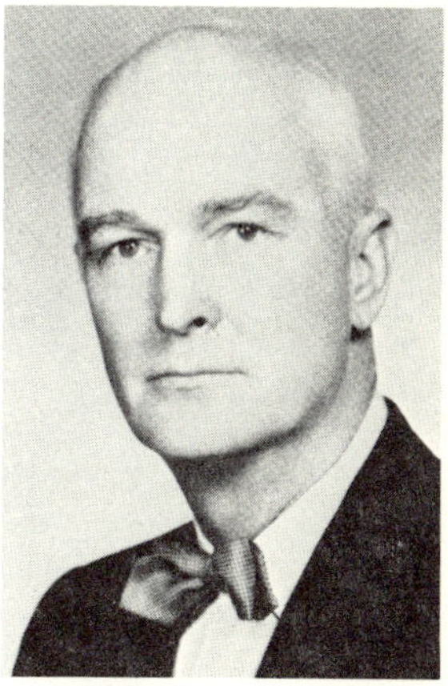

15.9 John H. Gibbon, Jr. (1903–73) initiated intracardiac surgery with development of pump oxygenator.

The Minnesota surgeon C. W. Lillehei and his coworkers Varco, Herbert Warden, Morley Cohen, and Raymond Read (1954), using a donor — often a parent — and cross circulation, were able to report successes in a variety of congenital cardiac defects. The same group then used gravity transfusion in a few infants and in young children (1954–55). In 1955 they reported several successes with the bubble oxygenator developed by Richard DeWall, marking a period in time when open cardiac surgery became a reality.[56] In fact, the world's first successful open heart operation on man was done by F. John Lewis in the University of Minnesota Hospitals on September 2, 1952. It concerned an interatrial septal defect which Lewis closed under hypothermia. The afferent inflow occlusion lasted seven minutes.[57] Dennis, also a pioneer Minnesota student of intracardiac surgery, had performed two unsuccessful open heart operations with a pump oxygenator before Gibbon's 1953 success.[58] Today corrective procedures have come to replace the palliative operation initiated by Alfred Blalock for congenital cardiac lesions. Moreover, replacement of calcified valves has become possible with synthetic or homograft valves.

The most commonly performed operation upon the heart currently appears to be vascular venous grafts from the aorta to the coronary arteries distal to demonstrated blocks in the lumen. Surgeons are far more enthusiastic over the procedure than physicians; nevertheless, the operation is catching on.

Cardiac transplantation came through the work of Christiaan Barnard (1967) of Cape Town, South Africa,[59] and Norman Shumway of Palo Alto, whose investigations on cardiac autoreimplantation date from 1960. Shumway (1976) indicated that the first three months after cardiac transplantation are the most challenging because of the threat of rejection; of patients who survive three months after transplant surgery 77 percent are alive at one year, 45 percent at two years, and 35 percent at three years — truly a laudable achievement when one recalls that these are hopeless cases not responsive to any form of conservative management. When immunosuppressive measures can be invoked that do not produce leucopenia and invite infection, the accomplishment will be greatly enhanced.[60] Several investigators in the United States and Russia believe that a substitute mechanical heart also affords great promise, if only the problem of hemolysis can be thwarted.

A close cooperative effort between the departments of surgery and physiology came into being at the University of Minnesota when Maurice Visscher returned as professor of physiology in 1936. A large number of talented and skilled surgeons spent from two to three years in the physiological laboratories under the tutelage of Visscher and his associates, acquiring an intimate knowledge of the circulation, a circumstance in large measure accounting for the progress in intracardiac surgery at the University of Minnesota in the 1950s. Today, innovative cardiac surgeons with expertise dot the geography of all continents. To open heart surgery, one of the most outstanding advances in twentieth-century surgery, an impressive worldwide group of surgeons have contributed significantly.

Summary

The bold operation of the second-century surgeon Antyllus for aneurysm has a modern twentieth-century ring. He employed both proximal and distal ligation, then opened the sac and obliterated the aneurysm. In the sixteenth century Paré reintroduced the ligature of Celsus in amputation. Petit's screw compressor (1718) promoted survival of the ligature in the control of hemorrhage in extremity surgery.

Abernethy of St. Bartholomew's, one of John Hunter's celebrated pupils, pointed out the advantage (1796) of dividing rather than occluding large arteries by ligature in dealing with aneurysm. As perusal of the record indicates, division is far less likely to be followed by hemorrhage, a lesson not generally appreciated by the most distinguished vascular surgeons of both England and America until experimental proof by Holman in 1942. Jassinowsky (1891) of Odessa and Dörfler (1899) of Rostock demonstrated the feasibility of arterial anastomoses prior to the work of Carrel (1902), whose technique of arterial suture was a refinement of their methods.

Anticoagulants have been a great boon for the advance of vascular surgery. McLean (1916), a Hopkins medical student, extracted the anticoagulant heparin from liver; two decades intervened before its use became practicable. Facets of vascular surgery concern virtually every segment of surgery. New twentieth-century developments have come about in many areas, including management of arteriovenous fistula, aneurysm, portal hypertension, and varicose veins.

Paracardiac surgery was represented by such operations as pericardiectomy, division of patent ductus arteriosus, correction of coarctation of the aorta, and removal of vascular bands about the great vessels and esophagus of the upper mediastinum. These were important first steps in launching cardiac surgery. Subclavian-pulmonary artery anastomosis, which brought pink cheeks and lips to blue babies with congenital heart disease, caught the public imagination, presaging great future development for intracardiac surgery.

An important innovation of the 1950s was excision of the terminal aorta by Dubost for arteriosclerotic disease, followed by insertion of an arterial homograft. The suggestion has been extended by DeBakey and other enterprising surgeons to include both abdominal and thoracic aneurysms. Crimped dacron grafts have come largely to supplant arterial homografts, and, for smaller vessels, venous grafts have proved extremely useful.

The outstanding contribution in this century to the advance of surgery has been intracardiac surgery. For centuries physicians dominated the therapy of cardiac disorders. The surgeon's role in extending effective therapy to congenital and acquired heart disease including coronary artery occlusion has been impressive. The application of the skill of another discipline to that of surgical talent was fundamental in the accomplishment, viz., knowledge of support of the circulation, a requirement that could only be supplied by students of cardiopulmonary function.

(For notes, see pp. 650–55.)

CHAPTER 16

Anesthesia

THERE WAS PROBABLY good cause in 1820 for Reverend Sydney Smith's scornful reproach: "In the four quarters of the globe, who reads an American book? . . . What does the world yet owe to American physicians or surgeons?" The voice of Ralph Waldo Emerson rang out clearly seventeen years later in reply to the British taunt, summoning his countrymen to cultivate their own intellectual leadership. Said Emerson: "Our day of dependence, our long apprenticeship to the learning of other lands, draws to a close. The millions that around us are rushing into life, cannot always be fed on the sere remains of foreign harvests." Although his dream was never fully realized, Emerson heralded the severance of American reliance upon foreign inspiration.[1] Perhaps nothing lent as much support to his prediction as did the American discovery of ether and nitrous oxide anesthesia.[2] The latter agent, once relegated to secondary consideration, has proved to be the more enduring innovation.

Discovery of Inhalation Anesthesia

Nine years after Emerson's historic speech ether was used in an operation at Massachusetts General Hospital. The story is familiar. William T. G. Morton, a dentist who had used ether in the extraction of teeth, called on the Harvard professor and surgeon John Collins Warren to suggest that his material could be administered to prevent pain in other operations; Warren, aged seventy, waited only for the first suitable case in which to make

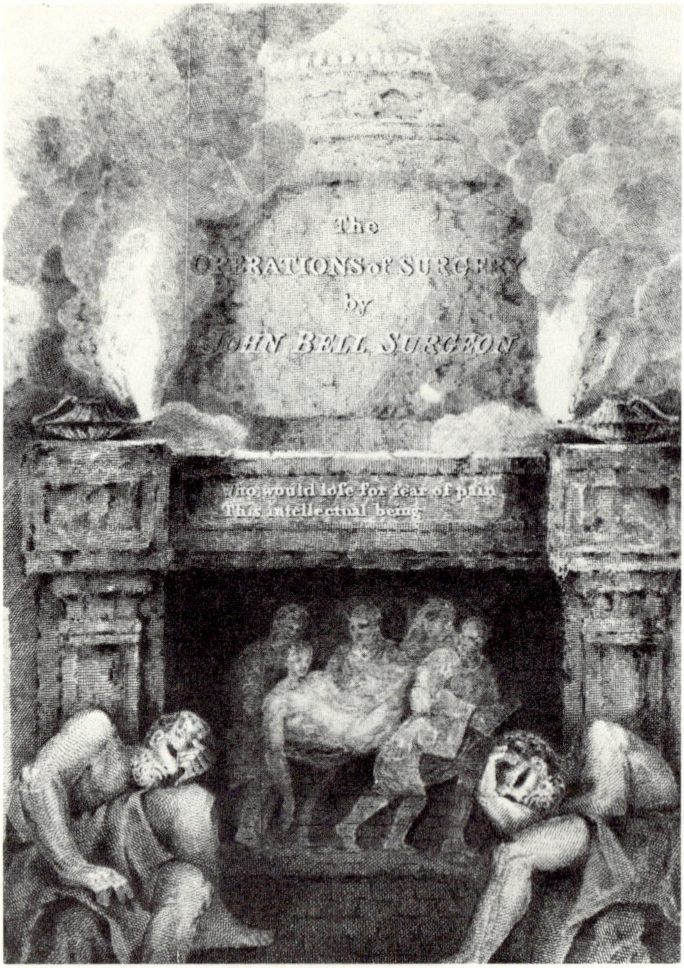

16.1 John Bell's defense of surgery before the days of anesthesia: "Who would lose for fear of pain / This intellectual being." Frontispiece, Bell, *Principles of surgery* (London, 1806), vol. 2.

the test. On October 16, 1846, Warren excised a tumor from a patient's neck, the anesthetic being administered by Morton, who had not divulged the nature of the agent. The patient, Gilbert Abbot, was anesthetized in the sitting position; he suffered no pain except, as he afterward recalled, a scratching sensation. Warren remarked, "This is no humbug."

The Boston papers carried news of the operation the next day. The first professional release on the subject was that of Bigelow in the *Boston Medical & Surgical Journal*, November 18,

1846, a paper he had already presented at two scientific gatherings in Boston. Whereas the word "ether" does not appear in the title, Bigelow remarked that the odor of the fluid used by Morton was "readily recognized" as sulfuric ether. Bigelow listed a surprising number of patients who had undergone extraction of teeth and excision of tumors, as well as amputations, in the month's interval since ether was first used.[3] Within a few weeks many letters addressed to the editor were printed in the *Journal*, expressing criticism over the secrecy, patenting, and other matters surrounding the introduction and employment of ether anesthesia.

Ether was not a recent discovery, having been synthesized from sulfuric acid and alcohol in about 1540 by Valerius Cordus, who called it sweet oil of vitriol.[4] It was long known to have medicinal properties and to produce somnolence on inhalation. "Ether frolics," in which the gas was inhaled for its exhilarating and hilarious effects, had been popular among medical students in America. At one of these parties Crawford W. Long, a surgeon of Jefferson, Georgia, noted that several participants bruised in the celebrations were insensitive to pain, and he decided to try ether as an anesthetic for surgery. His first patient, James Venable, experienced no pain in removal of a small tumor from his neck on March 30, 1842. Long performed a somewhat similar operation successfully in June 1842 and an amputation of a toe in July 1842. Other procedures under ether were successfully carried out by Long in 1843 and 1845.

Long, a graduate of the University of Pennsylvania (1839), was only twenty-seven at the time of his first operation with ether and was not identified with professional associates, who would have appreciated the importance of publishing his experience. Yet he must have been aware of its significance for surgery. He did not print an account until 1849, however, stating that his resolution to publish had been interrupted by a busy practice and that he had only succeeded in composing a few lines.[5] His fees of two dollars for each operation were so modest that it is difficult to believe he suppressed the information for financial gain. It was, indeed, a serious omission.

Long was not alone in neglecting an opportunity of great promise. Among the medical students who participated in ether frolics at the Massachusetts General Hospital in 1836 was Wyman, who shortly thereafter was to reveal unusual innovative talent in his adoption of trocar aspiration for pleural exudates. Many years too late (1877) he recalled a significant experiment performed in the youthful celebrations in which ether was given

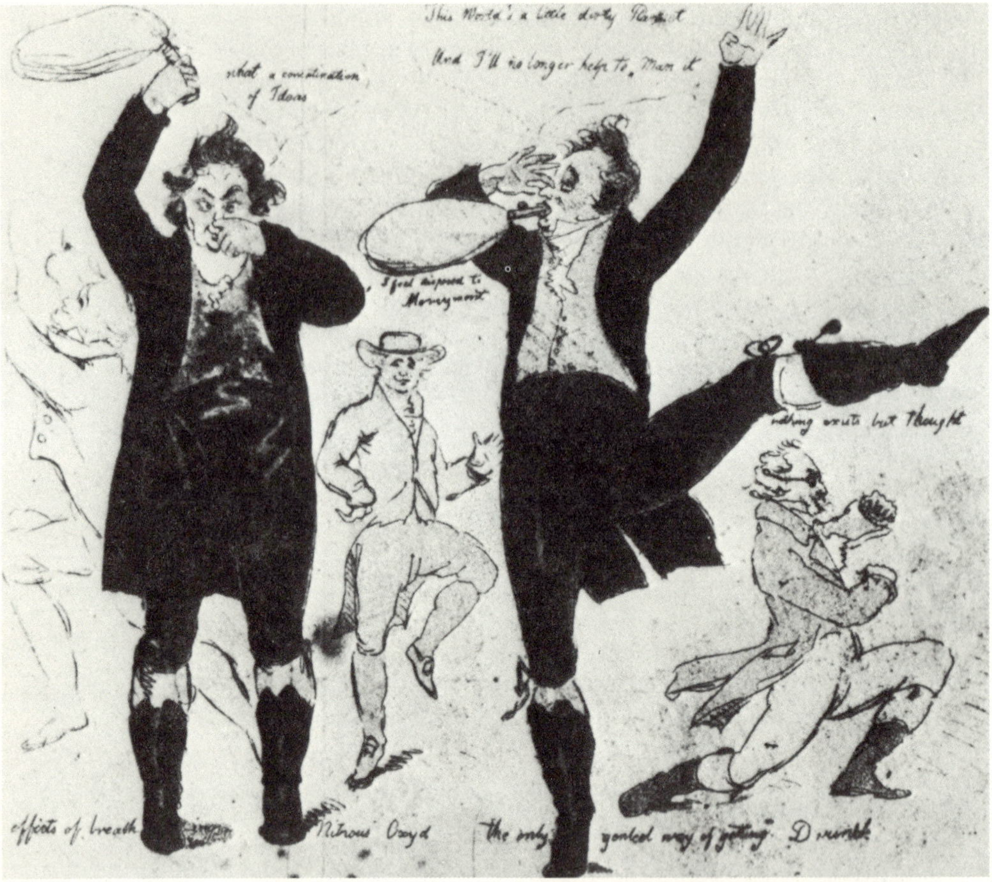

16.2 Nitrous oxide frolic. Caricature (1808). Courtesy Edgar Fahs Smith Memorial Collection, University of Pennsylvania.

to rats in a glass globe until they became entirely motionless. Concluded Wyman: "But with all our experiments we never thought of trying the sensibility under ether, even by pricking with a pin! It was a great oversight."[6]

The twenty-two-year-old chemist Humphry Davy published (1800) a large monograph on nitrous oxide, a gas discovered by Joseph Priestley in 1772. Davy tested the effects of inhalation of the gas on animals and human beings; over a period of several months he breathed the gas three to four times a day and described its anesthetic effects. He noted its exhilarating and hysterical laughter-producing qualities, an observation responsible for the term "laughing gas." Moreover, Davy did suggest that the gas could be employed to ablate pain in surgery.[7]

In 1844, two years before Morton's administration of ether, Horace Wells, a dentist of Hartford, Connecticut, began to use nitrous oxide to allay pain in dental operations. In watching a public demonstration of the effects of laughing gas, he had noted that a volunteer was unaware of a severe knee cut sustained during the showing. As a trial Wells had one of his own teeth extracted under nitrous oxide the next day, and without pain. Warren provided Wells an opportunity to demonstrate "painless" tooth extraction before a Harvard medical class in January 1845; the patient, a young boy, screamed out, students hissed, and the demonstration was a failure. The dentist would have been better advised to have chosen a cooperative, mature adult for the demonstration. Wells's suicide came three years

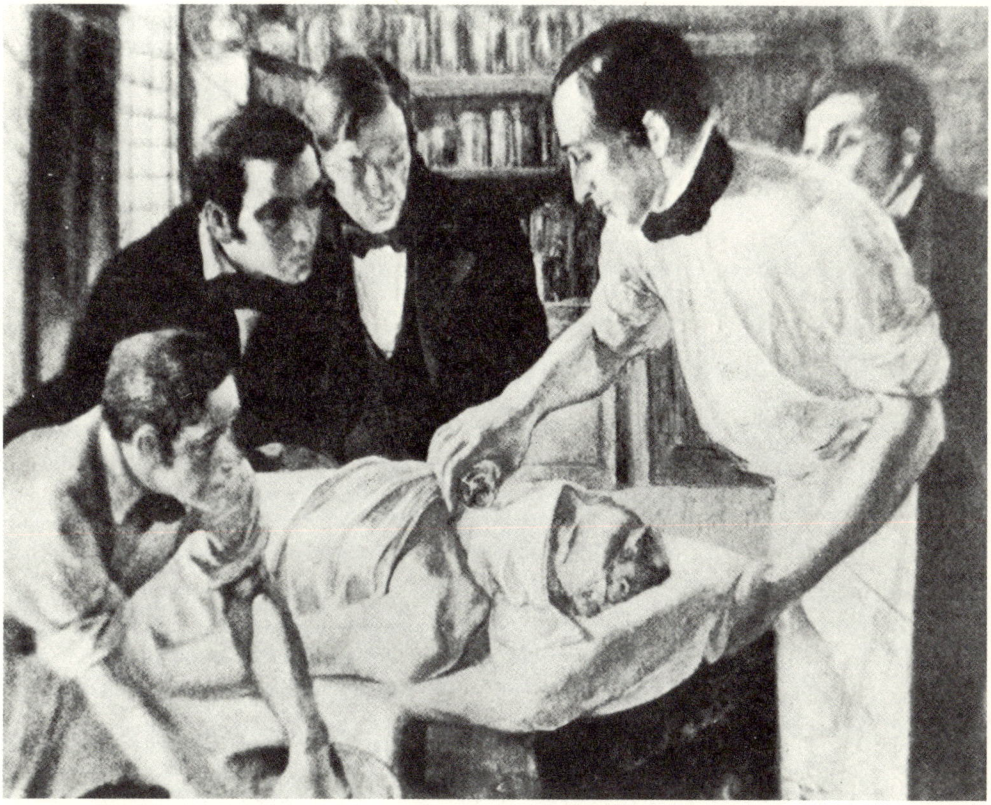

16.3 Crawford W. Long operating and administering ether anesthesia (March 1842), at Jefferson, Georgia, as portrayed by Maurice Siegler. From Frank K. Boland, "Centennial of Crawford Long's first use of ether in surgery," *Surgery* (1943), 13:280.

later following fruitless attempts to gain recognition of his claims to priority and mental derangement aggravated by constant self-experimentation with chloroform.[8]

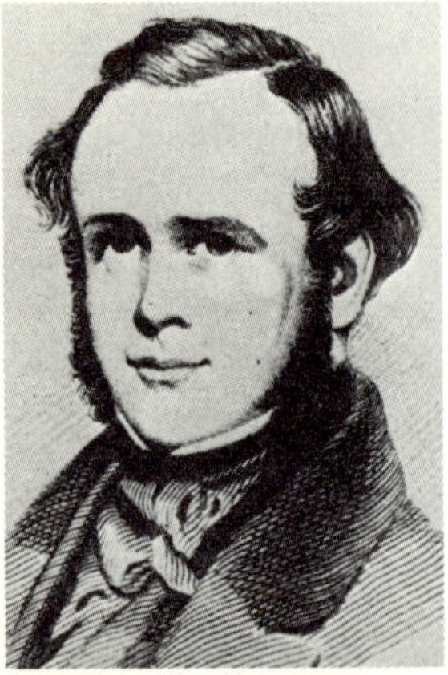

16.4 Horace Wells gave nitrous oxide anesthesia for extraction of teeth (1844).

Few discoveries have been so readily accepted as anesthesia. The world had waited long for an effective lenitive to the painful ordeal of operations. A few weeks after the first public demonstration in Boston, ether was in use in many hospitals throughout the world. However much it contributed to the relief of pain in surgery and easement of the surgeon's anguish too, the discovery did not greatly further the borders of elective surgery; that extension waited upon recognition and acceptance of chemical and thermal antisepsis.

The Priority Question

The American people, grateful and appreciative, wished to express their thanks through Congress to the discoverer of anesthesia. Unfortunately, the participants were unwilling to share the honor, and the proposed magnanimity of their fellow citizens was never realized. The Congress was in a mood to award $100,000 to Morton, but there were other claimants with loyal supporters. Sharing is one of the most beautiful and winsome words in the English language. Honors, rewards, and opportunity are readily and ungrudgingly shared by generous and high-minded persons.

Morton's secrecy concerning the exact chemical nature of his Letheon, correctly recognized by many to be ether, is disappointing in a claimant to an important discovery, as was also the circumstance that he and the chemist Jackson took out a patent on their joint discovery. Jackson's subsequent treachery in omitting mention of Morton in a surreptitious letter to the French Academy of Science in November 1846 describing the discovery as his alone serves to eliminate Jackson as a bona fide contender for recognition and honors in the ether controversy.[9]

Wells (1847) addressed a letter to the French Royal Academy of Medicine dated February 23, 1847, presenting his claim to priority for anesthesia; Morton made two representations of his claim to the French Academy of Science.[10]

The priority controversy over the discovery of anesthesia continued into this century.[11] There can be little question of the greater influence of Morton's successful demonstration of the efficacy of ether on October 16, 1846, in allaying the pain of operation and speeding acceptance of anesthesia. Wells had only one scientific publication on nitrous oxide (1847). However, survival of the practice continues to be an important determinant in the adjudication of priority. Now, more than 130 years later, it probably would be in the spirit of fairness to cite Wells with Morton for division of the honor of discovery. In fact, as will be shown later, the use of ether has disappeared in many clinics, and nitrous oxide, used in 65 percent of anesthetic procedures, is the more durable legacy.

Acceptance of Anesthesia

Within a short time of the announcement in Boston ether was in use in operating rooms throughout the United States, as appreciative and enthusiastic letters attested. In New York Mott removed a cluster of tumefied glands from the axilla of a woman's neck after she had inhaled ether (December 8, 1846). Her insensibility to pain lasted throughout much of the protracted procedure.[12]

The first use of ether in an operation at the University of Pennsylvania was apparently on October 20, 1847, for the treatment of fistula-in-ano; the surgeon was Horner, professor of anatomy. This was a full year after the demonstration at the

16.5 Morton administers ether anesthesia at Massachusetts General Hospital (October 16, 1846). Courtesy National Library of Medicine.

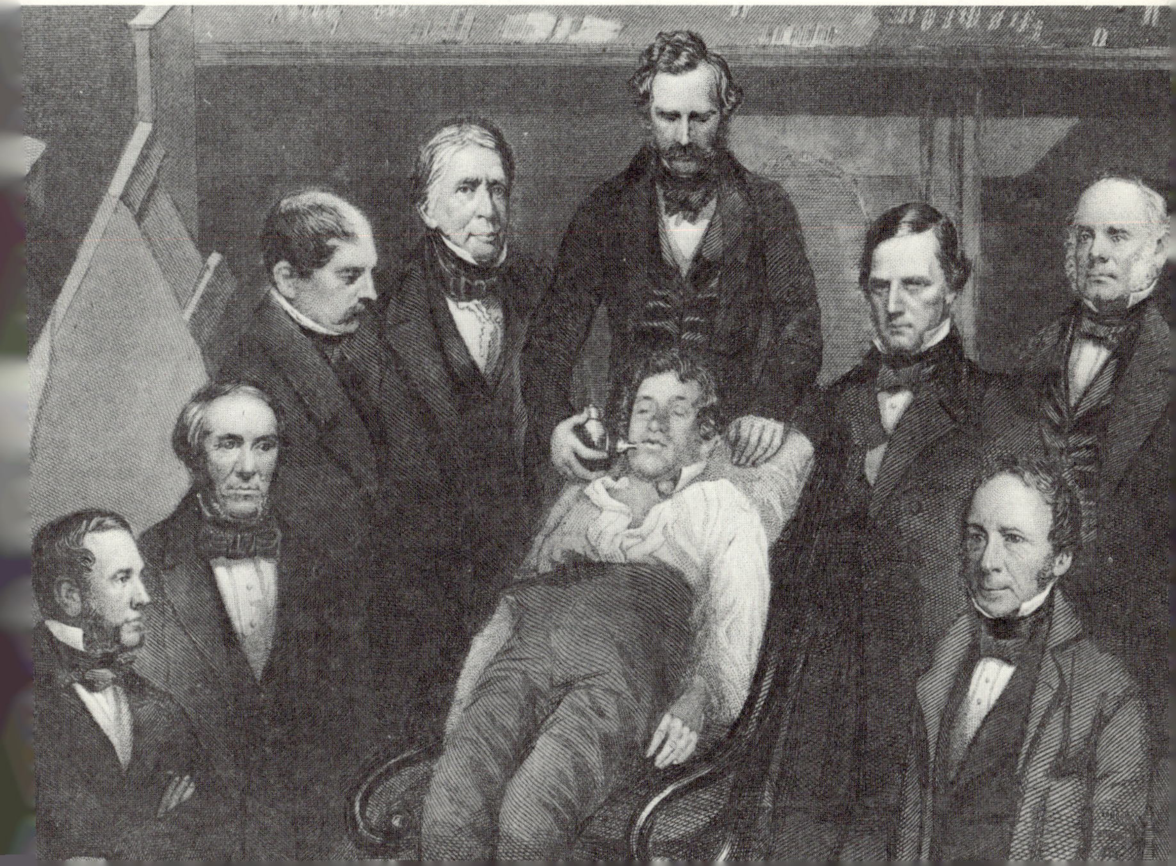

Massachusetts General Hospital. Anesthesia obviously did not catch on in Philadelphia as quickly as it did in Boston, New York, London, and Paris. Meigs, professor of midwifery at Jefferson Medical College, manifested keen disapproval of ether for childbirth, emphasizing increased risks. To illustrate the point during his lecture before some 300 students, he had a large male goat anesthetized with ether. The goat apparently died during the administration and its corpse was placed in a small room outside the lecture hall. On conclusion of the lecture the door to the room was opened: "Out came Billy, very drunk, charged between Wallace's [the assistant's] long legs into a mass of delighted students."[13]

Jacob Bigelow, a botanist, sent a letter to an old friend, Francis Boott, in London on November 28, 1846, describing ether inhalation for the relief of pain in operations, enclosing his son's description of the method. Boott sent the news at once to *Lancet* and to Liston, and on December 19 Boott himself employed ether in the extraction of a molar tooth from Miss Lansale at his house, the extraction being performed by James Robinson, a dentist. This was two days before Liston's famous amputation of a thigh under ether anesthesia at University College Hospital.[14]

F. W. Cock has provided a vivid account of the event of December 21, 1846. As preparations were under way for Liston's operation, William Squire, an assistant who was to administer the anesthesia, inquired whether someone in the audience of students would volunteer to be etherized.[15] None replied. Squire then chose a large powerful hospital porter and asked him to lie down and suck at the mouthpiece connected with the ether bottle, which he did. A few moments later the porter jumped up and dashed wildly beyond the railings into the crowd of students, who scattered like a flock of sheep chased by a dog.

At 1:00 P.M. the amphitheatre was crowded — "crammed to the uttermost." Liston entered at 2:15, saying to the assembled students and colleagues, "We are going to try a Yankee dodge today, gentlemen, for making men insensible." Liston took from his operating case a long straight operating knife of his own design with notches on the handle indicating the number of times it had been used. The house surgeon put the saw, two or three tenacula, and the artery forceps named after the operator on a chair close by and covered them with a towel. The assistant then threaded a wisp of well-waxed hemp ligatures through the buttonhole of his operating frock. The patient, a thirty-six-year-old butler, was brought in on a stretcher; the anesthesia tube was inserted in his mouth while Squire held the patient's nostrils.

Squire announced that the patient was ready. "Time me," said Liston. When the operation was over, the time for severance of the extremity varied among the five reporters from twenty-eight seconds to twenty-five seconds. The quickest time was clocked by one of Liston's dressers, an observation which found favor with Liston. Within five minutes after the patient entered the operating room he had already been wheeled out, asking when they were going to begin the operation. Said Liston, "This Yankee dodge, gentlemen, beats mesmerism hollow."

Cold water dressings were applied to the amputation stump at short intervals until 7:00 in the evening, when the flaps were brought together with a few stitches and two small arteries in the wound were religated. The patient's wound suppurated; he was dismissed from the hospital on February 11, 1847.[16] Complete lack of antiseptic precautions and a crowded amphitheatre, despite the use of open wound management, undoubtedly accounted for the hospital stay of fifty-three days.

Chloroform

Simpson began to employ ether in his wide obstetrical practice in Edinburgh in January 1847. He was not, however, completely happy with its use and started experimenting upon the anesthetic qualities of a number of substances. The suggestion to try chloroform came from David Waldie, a chemist in Liverpool.[17] An experiment was carried out in Simpson's dining room on the evening of November 4, 1847. Simpson and his two assistants inhaled the vapor simultaneously; all three were quickly somnolent or unconscious. Simpson concluded that chloroform induced anesthesia rapidly and had some advantages over ether.[18]

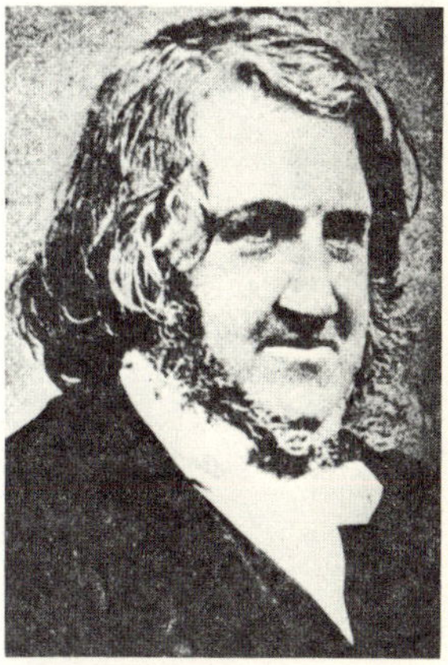

16.6 James Y. Simpson, Edinburgh obstetrician and surgeon, administered chloroform anesthesia (1847).

Despite opposition from Scottish churchmen to alleviating the pains of childbirth, and from some medical men who believed anesthesia unsafe, Simpson popularized the practice among his colleagues. Queen Victoria's acceptance of chloroform in the delivery of her eighth child established it as a fashionable and proper procedure. The need for caution with prolonged chloroform anesthesia became quickly evident. In his sojourn in France during the American Civil War, Sims experienced considerable difficulty with chloroform in operations for repair of vesicovaginal fistula.[19]

Intratracheal Anesthesia

In his *Fabrica* (1543) Vesalius described studying the movement of a sow's heart with open thorax. He made an opening in the animal's trachea and inserted a tubular reed through which he blew to inflate the lungs. When the pig took a breath of air, the heart action became strong. This technique permitted Vesalius to examine the motion of the heart with the anterior chest wall partially removed. When the lungs collapsed, the heart weakened; when the lungs were inflated, the heart beat was strong again. Robert Hooke (1667) demonstrated that a dog with the anterior thoracic wall removed may be kept alive for more than an hour by repeatedly inflating its lungs with air through a bellows. Hooke apparently divided the trachea at a high level and inserted a tube into the distal end.[20]

The American surgeon George Fell of Buffalo (1891) used forced respiration to treat victims of accidental morphine poisoning or drowning, following cessation of respiration; occasionally he added tracheostomy. Matas (1900) employed intralaryngeal insufflation for open operations upon the thorax. It remained, however, for Samuel Meltzer and John Auer (1909) of the Rockefeller Institute to simplify intratracheal insufflation. This was accomplished through a tube attached to the trachea, thus producing continuous respiration, keeping the lungs expanded even though the thorax was open. Meltzer in his early New York days (1893) was a physician-surgeon who treated pneumonia and operated for empyema.[21]

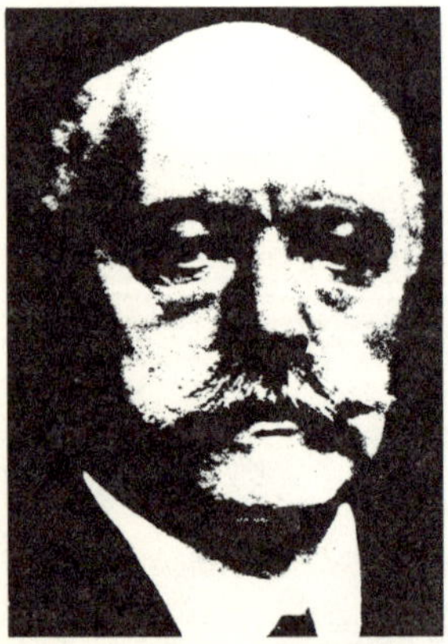

16.7 Samuel J. Meltzer developed positive-pressure inhalation anesthesia (1909).

It seems strange to us now that such persistent efforts were made by Sauerbruch over several decades (1904–48) to perfect a negative-pressure cabinet for operation.[22] Had the surgeons of that day been more enthusiastic over the Meltzer-Auer technique, open operations upon the thorax would undoubtedly have come much earlier. Only when the importance of tracheal insufflation was recognized did operations upon the thoracic viscera become commonplace — first for mediastinal tumors,[23] then for bronchiectasis and lung cancer, followed by operations for constrictive pericarditis and malformations of the paracardiac great vessels. Finally came open heart surgery.

Ethyl Chloride

Johann Heyfelder of Erlangen used ethyl chloride for inhalation anesthesia in 1848. The anesthetic does not provoke the period of excitement that attends induction of ether. A crowing inspiration indicates approximation of the vocal cords, signaling need to discontinue the anesthetic and remove the gauze overlying the nose and mouth onto which the agent is sprayed. When ethyl chloride is sprayed on the skin, it produces a freezing and numbing effect permitting painless incisions. The Swiss surgeon Camille Redard recommended ethyl chloride for local anesthesia in 1891.[24]

Hazards of Inhalation Anesthesia

Simpson (1847) believed that anesthesia had great advantages for the patient and that its administration did not increase operative mortality. Not all surgeons of the period shared this view. Dieffenbach wrote a 228-page monograph *Ether against Pain* in 1847, but he cautioned against the use of ether unless absolutely necessary because of the hazards of suspension of respiration and death.[25]

The pioneer French experimental physiologist François Magendie (1847) was an ardent opponent of anesthesia, contending that the pain of operation was a useful safeguard to the surgeon and that over-etherization was a real hazard to the patient. Bransby Cooper too believed pain was a protection in operations. An English military surgeon J. J. Cole, back from service in India, wrote in 1852 that chloroform was a "highly pernicious agent" in a field hospital.[26] Undoubtedly many of the sequelae attributed to anesthesia following its innovation were owing to sepsis, the nature and origin of which were not fully resolved for several decades.

There was a trying interlude when young residents came into anesthesia without any skill or experience in its administration. Later the nurse-anesthetist supplanted the untrained intern. The administration of a number of anesthetic gases simultaneously became common practice. In addition to ether and nitrous oxide, ethylene and cyclopropane were available. The concentration of any anesthetic gas in the patient's respiratory tract under such circumstances was often unknown, a situation that occasionally led to confusion and disorientation.

Monitoring during Anesthesia

Cushing and George Crile were invited by W. T. Councilman of Harvard to air their views on the importance of blood pressure measurements during operation before the Boston Medical Society (1903). The discussion generated enough interest to warrant appointment of an investigative committee. After a year's interval the distinguished group reported, "The adoption of blood-pressure observations in surgical patients does not at present appear to be necessary as a routine measure."[27]

When a physiologic-surgical conference at the University of

Minnesota failed to explain or resolve an "anesthetic death" under concomitant use of several anesthetic vapors, the problem was taken to Alfred Nier, professor of physics, who was experienced in the capabilities of the mass spectrograph. He, in fact, provided us with a model. Our surgical colleagues Fletcher A. Miller and Varco, working cooperatively with the anesthesiologists, found the device extremely helpful in ascertaining the concentration of inhaled vapors during all phases of anesthesia.[28]

Today many new techniques for monitoring the concentration of oxygen, carbon dioxide, and anesthetic vapors in the patient's lungs and blood during surgical procedures have simplified the task and added greatly to safety in prolonged operations. The sophisticated monitoring systems currently used by anesthesiologists in operating suites and in intensive care units under supervision of both anesthesiologists and surgeons reveal the great interest of surgical specialists in utilizing all available scientific data during major operations and well into the recovery period.

Just before World War II professional anesthesiologists came to replace the nurse-anesthetists. Nurses trained in anesthesia, and directly responsible to surgeons, occupied an important role in many teaching hospitals throughout the United States and were not readily displaced. Today trained nurses are again on the scene but directly responsible to the department of anesthesiology. The opposition of surgeons to professional anesthetists involved prestigious professors of surgery at The Hopkins and other institutions, but the battle for the professional anesthetist was gradually won. The practice begun in London in 1847 by John Snow, the first professional anesthetist, is now accepted the world over.[29] The professional anesthetist is now essentially a clinical pharmacologist knowing considerably more about drugs than the nurse-anesthetist did at an earlier period, however skilled and experienced she might have been in the administration of an inhalation anesthetic.

Intravenous Anesthesia

The "learned and ingenious" Christopher Wren suggested to Robert Boyle in about 1659 that fluids could be administered intravenously through "slender Syringes or Quills, fastened to Bladders." Boyle promptly supplied a large dog for the experiment and Wren injected a "warm solution of opium in sack" into the animal's hind leg. The dog soon became "stupified." It was revived by being kept awake and in constant motion — "whipped up and down" a garden.[30]

The first successful intravenous use of drugs in man for anesthetic purposes was by Johann Major (1667) of Kiel. Two centuries elapsed before Pierre Oré (1874) of Bordeaux produced insensibility in dogs using chloral intravenously and followed with its use in operations upon man and to allay convulsive seizures of tetanus.[31]

After Ludwig Bogendörfer (1924) employed a Ciba preparation of soluble barbital (dial), intravenous anesthesia caught on. George Clowes and associates (1929) at the Eli Lilly Research Laboratories brought out sodium pentothal, still in use. Kirschner (1929) did much to popularize avertin, finding it facilitated induction of inhalation anesthesia.[32] Intravenous anesthesia proved very acceptable to patients, anesthesiologists, and surgeons, reducing the sensitivity of the tracheobronchial tube to anesthetic vapors and doing away with the frightening cyanosis of induction.

Rectal Anesthesia

Marc Dupuy, a Paris intern, wrote on April 5, 1847, of producing unconsciousness in a dog and a rabbit by injection of small amounts of ether mixed with a similar amount of water into the rectum and being able to operate upon the rabbit without pain. Pirogoff performed similar experiments on animals on May 5, 1847. He was so encouraged by the results that he employed rectal administration of ether in surgical operations on patients and with considerable success. Ether instilled via rectum did not provoke irritation of the larynx, as when inhaled, and so was useful in surgery on the face.[33]

Phlebotomy, Precursor of Anesthesia

Copious bleeding, long known to reduce muscle tonus, was proposed by Monro II of Edinburgh as a means to facilitate reduction of luxations. The redoubtable Physick of Philadelphia, who was graduated M.D. in Edinburgh in 1792, "was the first who had the boldness to carry the practice to the extent necessary for complete success," wrote his nephew Dorsey. It was Physick's custom to bleed a patient with a chronic joint dislocation from the veins of both forearms in the erect posture until he collapsed on the floor. At this juncture the patient was insensitive to pain and completely relaxed. The surgeon, using only his hands, could then replace the dislocation without difficulty, even though great force had previously proved ineffective. Colin M'Kenzie of Baltimore wrote Physick that in treating a sailor (1805) with a chronic dislocation of the shoulder sustained in a fall five or six months before, he removed nearly five pounds of blood before the patient fainted; reduction was easily achieved.[34]

In his lectures as early as 1774 Monro II had advised bloodletting "in a large stream, the patient standing . . . to bring on Languor & faintness, when the surgeon [would] begin to attempt ye reduction."[35] He probably repeated the suggestion in lectures during Physick's stay in Edinburgh in the early 1790s. Monro was clearly the father of the idea; there is, however, no evidence that he actually carried through with it. In July 1777 Monro II had been granted the title professor of medicine and

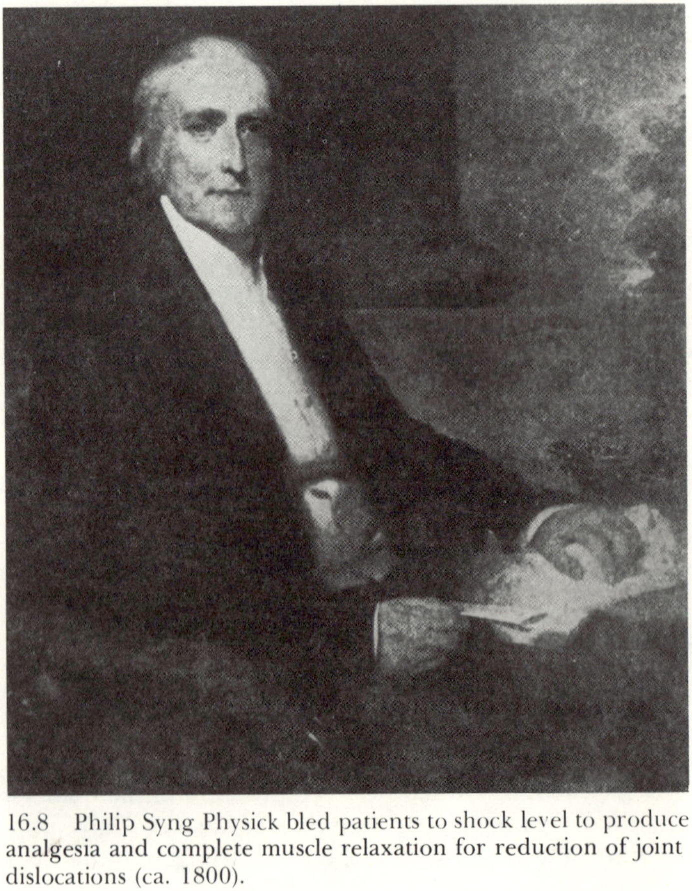

16.8 Philip Syng Physick bled patients to shock level to produce analgesia and complete muscle relaxation for reduction of joint dislocations (ca. 1800).

of anatomy and surgery; whereas he lectured on surgery, he was apparently not an operating surgeon. That extensive phlebotomy succeeded in the reduction of chronic dislocations evidently was established by Physick. In 1822 Astley Cooper was likewise endorsing bleeding as the "most powerful" remedy for reducing dislocations. Monro III said Cooper had confirmed the observation of his father, Monro II, in this practice.[36]

In 1806 Dewees, a colleague of Physick, endorsed phlebotomy to lessen pain and facilitate delivery in cases of difficult and protracted labor. He found that the shocklike state occasioned by the bleeding was followed by relaxation of the perineal muscles and of the cervix uteri. There apparently was also some lessening of uterine contractions, which did not last long.

Dewees wrote that in the summer of 1789 he saw a patient who had had several very difficult and painful deliveries. In the most recent a severe hemorrhage from her lungs quickly reduced her to a state of extreme debility, whereupon she promptly had a painless labor. This observation persuaded Dewees to practice bloodletting on patients in difficult labor. His first planned case (1790) concerned a young girl of fourteen and a half, who had been in labor for thirty-six hours when seen by Dewees. He let 15 ounces of blood and an hour later another 15 ounces; an uneventful delivery followed. Dewees reported a total of twenty-three patients whose relatively painless deliveries attended phlebotomy. One patient (1805) was bled 20 ounces and quickly delivered her tenth child.[37]

Today's surgeons and obstetricians probably could use Physick's method to advantage, collecting and citrating the blood and returning it after the objective of the phlebotomy has been accomplished. Actually the character of the muscle relaxation under the influence of extended phlebotomy undoubtedly exceeded the degree of reduction of muscle tonus later achieved attending ether inhalation, probably equaling that of the anoci-association of Crile and W. E. Lower (1915).

Anoci-Association

Crile (1915) was aware that unless a patient is deeply anesthetized with ether, impulses can still pass beyond neural synapses and reach the brain. To obviate this occurrence, he combined ether administration with prior physiologic doses of morphine and scopolamine, or with local infiltration anesthesia, a situation he described as anoci-association.[38]

Alexander Forbes and Harvard associates (1916) observed

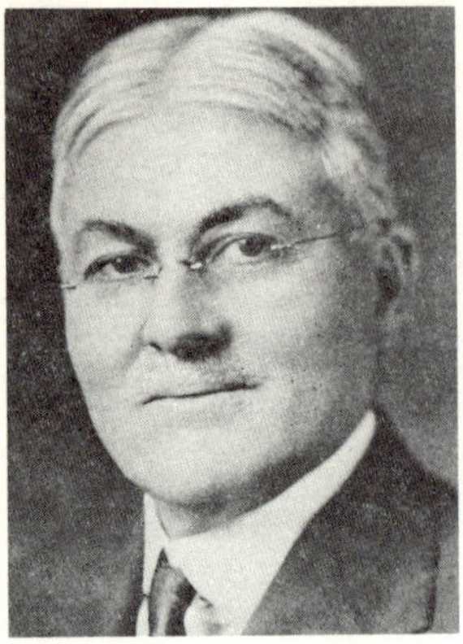

16.9 George Crile created anoci-association (1915); inhalation anesthesia is complemented with regional procaine to enhance muscle relaxation.

that when nerve trunks were electrically stimulated under deep ether anesthesia to the point of abolishing respiration, action currents were still detectable and transmitted centripetally.[39] These observations, indicating that nerve impulses may reach the brain despite deep ether anesthesia, appear to lend validity to Crile's hypothesis.

In abdominal operations before the availability of muscle relaxants, patients were anesthetized with ether to provide satisfactory relaxation for abdominal wall closure. By the simple expedient of injecting the posterior rectus sheath on both sides of the incision with a 0.5 solution of procaine containing epinephrine, the operator could then readily close the wound without tears in the peritoneum and without deepening the ether anesthesia.

Curare and other relaxant analogues have proved a great boon for procedures in which effective muscle relaxation is imperative, notably in abdominal surgery and in some operations upon the extremities. Curare has no effect upon sensory nerves. It affects only motor nerves, causing temporary ensuant paralysis; artificial respiration, therefore, may be mandatory accompanying its use.

Preanesthesia Relief of Pain in Operations

In the first century A.D., Dioscorides wrote his great Greek *Herbal.* Among the herbs and roots he described was mandragora (mandrake), used by physicians on patients when they were about "to be cut, or cauterized." Wine prepared from the bark of the root promoted deep sleep for several hours and insensitivity to pain. Dioscorides observed that mandragora was safe in moderate doses, "but being too much drank, it drives out ye life."[40] Pliny too described the juice of mandragora as a surgical anesthetic, remarking that just the smell of the leaves was sometimes enough to put the patient to sleep.[41]

Dioscorides wrote of juice from the seeds of hyoscyamus which would lessen pain and of the opium poppy, a "pain-easer" that caused sleep but, if too much were consumed, made "men lethargicall & it kills." The two juices were often given together, and were, as G. K. Tallmadge has pointed out, less toxic than either drug used alone. Poppy, hyoscyamus, and mandragora are all mentioned by Celsus in prescriptions for causing sleep and relieving pain.[42]

Drugs with soporific and narcotic properties were a part of ancient folktale, song, and poetry. Poppies, sleep, oblivion, and death are often associated with various forms of the term

"Lethe" in classical literature. Vergil told of "slumbrous poppies" and "Lethe's poppies." From this tradition Morton derived his name for ether — Letheon. A beautiful passage is that in a Latin lyric of the fourth century by the Spanish poet Prudentius. He wrote of drinking of the "cup of all forgetting" when

> The still Lethean waters
> Now steal through every vein,
> And men no more remember
> The meaning of their pain.

Homeric legends as well as Elizabethan drama included episodes in which such liquors played important roles.[43] Often we are not told the ingredients, but Shakespeare's Cleopatra said:

> Give me to drink mandragora . . .
> That I might sleep out this great gap of time
> My Antony is away.
> *Act 1, scene 5*

The lines from *Othello* are equally well known:

> Not poppy, nor mandragora
> Nor all the drowsy syrups of the world
> Shall ever medicine thee to that sweet sleep
> Which thou ow'dst yesterday.
> *Act 3, scene 3*

The formula of Hugh of Lucca's twelfth-century soporific sponge for operations was described by his disciple Theodoric. The method consisted in causing the patient to breathe the vapor given off from a sponge which had been boiled in a decoction of opium, unripe mulberry, hyoscyamus, spurge flax, mandragora, hemlock, lapathum, ivy, and lettuce seed. Such sponges were then dried in the sun and stored for use as occasion would require, being moistened with warm water just before application. At the end of the operation the patient was resuscitated by a sponge dipped in fresh vinegar passed under his nostrils. Guy de Chauliac (1363) repeated Hugh's formula, but did not say that he used it himself.[44] The matter of poorly controlled dosage obviously constituted a great hazard with primitive analgesic and soporific drugs.

Seeds of opium poppies have been found in the prehistoric Lake Dwellings of Switzerland, dating possible knowledge of the narcotic to as early as 3000 to 2000 B.C.[45] It apparently was in use in Egypt by about 1590 B.C. "The most powerful of stupefacients is opium," declared Avicenna in the eleventh century.[46] "Opium still reigns supreme in its power to relieve pain," wrote

Dickson Wright in 1926. Throughout this long history of use by mankind, opium has brought much comfort and inspired great poetry and prose; it has also caused addiction, engendered wars, and degraded nations.[47]

Throughout most of the nineteenth century opium continued to be a favored treatment for patients with strangulated bowel obstruction, as it had been in Sydenham's day. Paget remarked (1835) that colostomy patients "could enjoy the full influence of the drug [morphia] for they were no longer subject to its constipating effects." Kern in 1826 advised *Mohnsaft* (poppy juice) in amputations.[48]

Warren wrote that he had allowed "mesmerites and magnetizers to make their trials"[49] but found opium the only effective agent for relief of pain in operations before the use of ether. For painful procedures such as lithotomy, he gave adult men as much as 8 to 10 grains of opium, obviously a large dose.[50] The senior author has seen a man of seventy-five remain in coma for four days after administration of ¼ grain (16 mg.) of morphine.

Franklin Wright, one of this surgeon's urological teachers after World War I, was very partial to H.M.C., a combination of hyoscine, morphine, and cacodylate, to induce somnolence in suprapubic prostatectomy. Actually, it is an old remedy, known as twilight sleep. A full dose was given three hours before operation and a smaller dose one hour before; if the patient stirred on testing his sensitivity to painful stimuli, he was again given half a dose. Wright performed many such operations without inhalation anesthesia. His prostatectomy was an extraperitoneal suprapubic operation, and the occasional struggles of the patient did not interfere seriously with the operation's progress. The patients rarely had recollections of their operation.

Liberal quaffs of wine or brandy were frequently administered to a patient undergoing amputation in early days. The function of one of Ravaton's four surgeon-aides in an amputation was to administer cordials to the patient. Larrey appreciated the worth of alcohol as a soporific and analgesic for operations during his service in Napoleon's campaigns. Many of his patients too were in a state of shock and hence less sensitive to pain. The American sanitarian reformer and surgeon Stephen Smith (1919) relates that for feeble patients he preferred alcohol to ether in elective operations. For an operation scheduled for 3:00 P.M. he would order, beginning at 8:00 A.M., an ounce or more of whisky in hot milk every two hours until the time of operation. By then, little if any ether was necessary for the performance of the operation.[51]

Morphine and Cocaine Addiction

It is probably not out of place to record here that surgeons have become drug addicts. The German surgeon Nussbaum (1829–90) was a morphinist; he announced (1872) his addiction in a very unusual manner, sending to Langenbeck, president of the German Surgical Congress for fourteen consecutive terms, a paper detailing experiments upon himself with oral ingestion and subcutaneous and intravenous injections of morphine.[52] The intravenous route, he observed, was four times as powerful as other channels. Nussbaum was greatly loved by the people of Munich, and thousands attended his funeral (1890). Halsted's cocaine addiction traced back to Carl Koller's (1884) publication on cocaine for eye surgery and was a well-kept secret until after his death. Apparently the effectiveness of neither of these great surgeons was adversely affected by the indulgence.

Elizabeth Barrett Browning, a morphinist from her late youth, wrote beautiful poetry and had a happy and successful marriage. Coleridge's (1772–1834) addiction to morphine began at age twenty-four and continued throughout his life; it estranged him from his family. His was a significant influence in the English romantic period of the early nineteenth century. De Quincey (1785–1859) too announced his own addiction, begun as a student at Oxford (ca. 1808), in his well-known *Confessions of an English Opium-Eater* (1822); nevertheless, he had a productive literary career.

Halsted had a complete change of personality accompanying his addiction, but his scientific achievement in surgery appeared to have been heightened thereby. Perhaps it is the isolation and self-communing that rivets the attention of victims of the drug habit upon thought processes. Undoubtedly many unfortunates are completely immobilized by the addiction. Every surgeon, sensitively alert to the need to provide his patients relief from pain in the postoperative period, must beware of the habit-forming propensities of such medications when long continued.

Regional Anesthesia

Cocaine was isolated from the Peruvian cocoa leaf in 1859 by Albert Niemann, but it was some years before its potential as a local anesthetic was recognized. Koller, discoverer of the local anesthetic properties of cocaine, published his first paper on the subject in 1884. He related that a 2 percent aqueous solution of cocaine instilled into the eyes of rabbits or dogs caused the cornea to become insensitive to painful stimuli in thirty to sixty seconds; he had tried the drug on his own eyes and a friend's, with similar effects. Koller suggested that the method should provide anesthesia for operations upon the human eye, a procedure he had not yet attempted because his experiments were only two weeks old.

Some of Sigmund Freud's admirers credited Freud with origin of the idea that cocaine possessed local anesthetic properties. In a letter to Dr. M. G. Seelig (1941) Koller wrote of his work on the drug with Freud, stating that the latter was not, and had never claimed to be, responsible for its trial as a local anesthetic.[53]

In 1885 Halsted announced that he had used cocaine with great success in more than a thousand minor surgical operations. His paper was to be concluded in a subsequent issue, which never appeared.[54]

Karl L. Schleich, while an assistant at the Ziegelstrasse clinic in Berlin under Bergmann, appeared before the 1892 German Surgical Congress and read a paper on infiltration anesthesia using dilute solutions of cocaine. The presiding officer was Adolf Bardeleben of the Charité, the competing university surgical clinic; Bardeleben was known to be at times irascible and easily provoked. On the conclusion of his presentation Schleich made a strong emotional appeal to replace "dangerous" chloroform anesthesia with local cocaine infiltration, concluding, unhappily, that those continuing to use inhalation anesthesia in situations where infiltration was applicable actually were guilty of malpractice. When Schleich had finished, Bardeleben asked for a show of hands of those agreeing with Schleich. Not a hand went up. Schleich approached the podium to comment; Bardeleben said the session was over. Schleich obviously had made a significant but overenthusiastic announcement, the merits of which he should have been willing to let the future determine. One might reasonably have anticipated that Bergmann, Schleich's sponsor, familiar with his work, would come forward to endorse his protégé's important announcement. Bardeleben was not a sympathetic leader of young men and apparently was more influenced by Schleich's emotional appeal than by the substance of the presentation. Schleich's report concerned 521 patients operated upon solely under infiltration anesthesia of 1 to 2 percent cocaine; the surgery included hernia repair, breast amputation, and some abdominal procedures; in an additional 16 patients, complemental chloroform also was necessary. Schleich's eccentric behavior precluded his ever obtaining an important academic post, despite his great ability.

At the 1894 German Surgical Congress Bergmann invited the members to witness an operation by Schleich at the university's Poliklinik the next day, an announcement made at the request of Esmarch, the president of the congress. Bergmann reported to the congress the following day that Schleich had performed two operations under local infiltration anesthesia in the sensitive area of the perineum; one operation was for fistula-in-ano, the other for hemorrhoids. A large Bozeman speculum was inserted painlessly into the rectum and the procedures were performed without distress to the patients. Bergmann concluded by saying Schleich's infiltration anesthesia could be recommended for operations in areas that are not too extensive, and it should be acknowledged that in the development of his method Schleich had made a "contribution not to be underestimated." Bergmann's statement came two years after Schleich's presentation at the twenty-first congress in 1892. It was obvious that many German surgeons were apologetic over the unsympathetic reception tendered Schleich on that occasion.[55]

When Heinrich Braun of Zwickau, a former member of Volkmann's department, substituted novocaine for cocaine in 1905, infiltration anesthesia gained in popularity among surgeons. Braun also observed that adding epinephrine to the infiltrate greatly lengthened the duration of the anesthesia.[56]

Spinal (Subarachnoid) Anesthesia

In writing of his clinical experiments and experience with intradural spinal anesthesia, Bier (1899), then of Kiel, began by saying that infiltration and regional local anesthesia had made significant inroads on "dangerous general anesthesia." Heinrich Quincke had introduced spinal puncture for diagnostic purposes in 1891; Bier conceived the idea of achieving regional anesthesia by injecting a cocaine solution into the spinal canal.[57]

In early August 1898 Bier performed the procedure on eight patients, securing evidence of insensitivity to painful stimuli. On August 24, 1898, he asked his assistant, Hildebrandt, to perform spinal anesthesia on him. The cocaine solution was injected, but considerable spinal fluid drained away and Bier observed no loss of sensation. Hildebrandt then submitted to the test, Bier performing the puncture and injection. Within a few minutes Hildebrandt had lost sensitivity to painful stimuli in his lower extremities. After completion of the procedure the two had dinner, drank wine, and smoked several cigars. Bier went to bed, slept well, and took an hour's walk in the morning, following which he noted headache and dizziness, symptoms that ameliorated when he lay supine. Hildebrandt experienced severe headache; he reported for work in the morning, but was partially incapacitated for more than two weeks. Bier concluded that the unpleasant side effects warranted discontinuance of the experiments.

Fourteen years before Bier, Leonard Corning reported (1885) having performed spinal anesthesia on a dog as well as upon a patient. Corning suggested that the method might serve as a substitute for ether for some types of surgery, but he did not follow through with the idea. Matas and associates (1899) in New Orleans used Bier's method "with satisfactory anesthesia" in operations for hemorrhoids.[58]

The French surgeon and anesthesiologist Gaston Labat spent the academic year 1920–21 at the Mayo Clinic introducing techniques of regional anesthesia. By the late 1920s spinal anesthesia was being tried throughout the United States. Labat (1928) emphasized the role of the Trendelenburg (head low) position in combatting cerebral anemia in spinal anesthesia. He felt that probably the most frequent cause of death from spinal anesthesia was the vasodilation attending ablation of vasoconstriction of the lower half of the body, which liberal use of the Trendelenburg position would avert.[59]

George Pitkin (1928), a surgical pupil of the Philadelphia surgeon Wayne Babcock, began experimenting with anesthetic fluids, both heavier and lighter than the fluid in the spinal canal, which has a density in the area of 1.0068. Arthur Barker (1907) of London placed glucose in the anesthetic fluid, thus making it heavier than spinal fluid. By positioning the patient, light anesthetic fluids would ascend in the spinal canal; weighted fluids would descend. Barker reported one hundred instances of its use for operations, including some lower abdominal operations; Barker had three hospital deaths, none apparently related to anesthesia.[60]

Epidural Anesthesia

Caudal or epidural anesthesia was first employed through the sacral canal by J. Athanase Sicard of the Salpetrière Hospital, Paris (1901) in nine nonsurgical cases, achieving anesthesia of the perineal and scrotal areas. No ill side effects were encountered, and Sicard believed that caudal anesthesia could provide adequate analgesia for perineal surgical procedures.[61] A week later, Fernand Cathelin, a Paris urologist, reported that India ink injected extradurally through the sacral canal dissected in a few minutes well up into the cervical area. His trials with caudal anesthesia on patients were not satisfactory; however, he believed the method might prove useful for operations around the anal canal. The method gradually gained favor and was frequently used for surgical procedures about the perineum in the senior author's training period in the early 1920s. Waldo Edwards and Robert Hingson (1942) found continuous caudal anesthesia helpful and practical for delivery of parturients.[62]

Acupuncture

The placement of needles at "pain points" for various body segments, or acupuncture, has long been a favored method of Chinese practitioners to induce analgesia for operative procedures. The method has again enjoyed a wave of popular interest; anesthesiologists, physicians, and surgeons have visited Chinese hospitals to witness its use. The circumstance that complemental intravenous infusion is usually given simultaneously has confused some observers. Its effect, in part, may be similar to hypnosis, the susceptibility of the subject varying tremendously. J. H. Cassedy (1974) has summarized facets of the early use of acupuncture in France and this country. John Z. Bowers (1973) has described the technique and historical aspects of its use.[63]

Today's Anesthetics

In response to a query concerning present trends in anesthesia, F. H. Van Bergen, chief of anesthesiology at the University of Minnesota Hospitals, presented the authors with a computer print-out of the anesthetics used during the last three months of 1974 at the University Hospitals.[64] In that period there were 2,264 surgical procedures. Van Bergen reported that nitrous oxide was used in 65 percent of all anesthesias, regional anesthesia in 25.8 percent; regional anesthesia was supplemented by general anesthesia in 1.94 percent; no anesthesia was necessary in 0.84 percent. Barbiturates, chiefly pentothal, were used in 55 percent of cases.

Endotracheal intubation was used in 61 percent of all inhalation anesthesias; face mask anesthesia or regional block was done in the remaining 39 percent. Muscle relaxants, though used frequently, were not given in 36.4 percent of operations. Curare was rarely used; newer muscle relaxants more commonly employed were gallamine, succinylcholine, and pancuronium. During the period covered by Van Bergen's thoughtful appraisal, ether, chloroform, ethylene, cyclopropane, and rectal anesthesia were not used. Extensive use of monitoring devices in operating suites has mandated exclusion of potentially flammable and explosive agents. That nitrous oxide anesthesia, introduced by Wells in 1844, has come to supplant ether and chloroform may surprise many readers, suggesting in retrospect that Wells did have a valid claim to share honors with Morton in the Massachusetts anesthesia innovation.

This recital suffices to indicate that the modern anesthesiologist is a serious student of pharmacology and that the role of pharmacology is now vastly more appreciated than it was fifty years ago. In his early days as chairman of the university's Department of Surgery in the mid-1930s, this surgeon suggested to his clinical colleagues that the Department of Pharmacology be represented in the hospital activities; the petition was denied, at least two department heads protesting that they were their own clinical pharmacologists.

In the search for better anesthetic agents anesthesia has become one of the most scientific of surgical disciplines. Stress is upon molecular biology accompanied by emphasis upon the physiologic mode of action of anesthetic agents — quite a departure from the empiric selection of anesthetic agents in the mid-nineteenth century.

Summary

Inhalation anesthesia is by general consent America's greatest contribution to the advance of surgery. Remote from academic halls, Long of Jefferson, Georgia, aged twenty-seven, employed ether anesthesia in surgical procedures successfully several times in the 1842–44 period, but failed to publish until 1849. Wells, aged twenty-nine, a dentist of Hartford, began administering nitrous oxide for the extraction of teeth in 1844. Morton, also a dentist, aged twenty-seven, made the first public demonstration of ether in surgery on October 16, 1846, at the Massachusetts General Hospital, a historic day in American surgery. The current trend in surgery today is away from ether, nitrous oxide being the preferred inhalation anesthetic in a large number of university surgical clinics throughout America. Simpson, Edinburgh's famous obstetrician, introduced chloroform anesthesia in November 1847, long since out of vogue. The world had waited so long for an effective antidote to the pain of operations, that anesthesia was accepted readily almost worldwide with little opposition. The dramatic demonstration of ether at London's

University College Hospital by Liston in a thigh amputation, December 21, 1846, has become a surgical legend.

Intratracheal anesthesia became firmly established in 1909 by Meltzer and Auer for intrathoracic surgery. Despite persistent trials, Sauerbruch's (1904) negative-pressure cabinet for such operations never became practical.

Cushing and Crile (1903) made a plea for registration of blood pressure during inhalation anesthesia before the Boston Medical Society; an investigating committee subsequently reported it was unnecessary as a routine measure. The mass spectrograph devised by Nier was found very helpful in monitoring the concentration of inhaled anesthetic gases when several were administered simultaneously, and was first applied successfully by Miller and Varco (1950). The device has been greatly improved in the intervening years, constituting a useful monitoring instrument regularly employed by anesthesiologists everywhere.

Snow of London became the world's first professional anesthetist in 1847. The resistance of American surgeons to acceptance of professional anesthetists was responsible for anesthesia's lag in our country. Universally today, anesthesiologists are essentially practical clinical pharmacologists, playing a significant role in making surgery safer for the patient and the surgeon too. Intravenous anesthesia has simplified induction of anesthesia, eliminating the patient's resistance to inhalation of irritating anesthetic vapors.

The role of extended phlebotomy in producing profound muscle relaxation as well as adequate analgesia was invoked by Physick, Philadelphia Nestor of American surgery in about 1800. Its use permitted easy reduction of chronic dislocations resistant to all other methods. It combined, in fact, the advantages of Crile's (1915) anoci-association, in which employment of local procaine anesthesia with ether inhalation prevented centripetal relay of painful stimuli across more centrally located neural synapses.

Mandragora for the promotion of sleep and relief from pain was known in the time of Dioscorides (first century). Homeric legends and Elizabethan drama include episodes in which drugs with soporific and narcotic properties were administered. Opium was one of Sydenham's (1676) favorite remedies for medical disorders, as it was for Thomas, a Liverpool surgeon of the late nineteenth century.

The local anesthetic properties of cocaine were long known; we owe its introduction for eye surgery (1884) to the Vienna ophthalmologist Koller, subsequently prominent in the profession in New York. Schleich (1892) introduced cocaine infiltration for general surgical procedures, for which Braun substituted novocaine in 1905. Bier invoked regional anesthesia for surgery upon the lower torso and extremities in 1899, injecting cocaine into the spinal canal. Corning had suggested spinal anesthesia as a substitute for inhalation anesthesia in 1885. Caudal epidural anesthesia for operations about the perineum came in the hands of Sicard in 1901. The role of acupuncture as an acceptable anesthetic, uncomplemented by concomitant intravenous anesthesia, still awaits definitive evaluation.

(For notes, see pp. 657–63.)

CHAPTER 17

Antiseptics

BEFORE ADOPTION OF GUNPOWDER, the chief weapons in battle were the spear, sword, arrow, and hurled rock. Those who have searched Homer's *Iliad* find that extraction of the lodged missile, washing the wound with water, and bandaging constituted the essentials of wound care in the tenth century B.C. There are 114 deaths recorded among 147 wounded in Homer's recital, a mortality rate of 77.5 percent, an accomplishment not bettered considerably under conditions of warfare until the last quarter of the nineteenth century.[1]

When gunshot injuries appeared in European warfare, recourse to complicated polypharmacy in dressings became more frequent, usually featuring what is now recognized as an antiseptic agent. The origin of the term "antiseptic" is somewhat obscure. The word appears several times in a curious little pamphlet by Place, published in London in 1721, *An Hypothetical Notion of the Plague, and some out-of-the way thoughts about it*. Place found "the Motion of the Pestilential Poison to be putrefactive, it makes the Use of Antisepticks a reasonable Way to oppose it, and whatever resists and is preservative against Putrefaction, and admits not of the Generation of Insects."[2] Some thirty years later (1750), the British Physician-General John Pringle also used the word "antiseptic," and in 1752 related forty-eight experiments performed over a three-year period in which he established the antiseptic value of mineral acids by noting their ability to thwart decomposition in freshly killed animals. Strangely, despite his field service experience, Pringle did not propose antiseptic agents for wound therapy, a suggestion one might have expected as a natural sequel to these observations.[3] D. M. Macbride (1764), William Alexander (1768), and Thomas Henry (1773) extended Pringle's antiputrescent studies with mineral acids, but also failed to suggest or employ them in clinical trials of wound management.[4]

In 1767 the Academy of Sciences and Arts and Fine Letters of Dijon offered a prize for the best written discourse on antiseptics. The first prize was won by Barthelemy C. de Boissieu, who considered the subject historically and departed least from tradition in appraising therapy. He recommended the cautery for gangrenous ulcer and for *pourriture*. The second prize was awarded to Toussaint Bordenave, who wrote more specifically about antiseptic agents and mentioned turpentine, pitch, aloes, styrax, benzoin, balsam of Peru, and alcohol.[5]

Resins and Balsams

Among the most ancient wound antiseptics were those derived from the resins of plants and trees, especially conifers. Accounts of the production of turpentine, pitch, and tar were given by Pliny (first century), who remarked that terebinth resin dissolved in olive oil lessened suppuration in wounds.[6] Application of pitch cerate to compound fractures is mentioned in Hippocrates, a practice continued by Celsus, Galen, and Avicenna.[7]

Turpentine and Oakum

In the Middle Ages turpentine was a common wound remedy, often combined with other ingredients. It was so recommended in a popular formula of Guy de Chauliac (1363) and by Brunschwig (1497). "But if sinews are cut in a member, there I praise the red Oyl of Turpentine," said the sixteenth-century Swiss surgeon Würtz.[8] Paré's partiality for turpentine has been noted.

The first suggestion of a statistical account of successes with antiseptic agents for wounds is to be found in Woodall's *Surgeons Mate* (1639). He recounted having done 100 amputations at St. Bartholomew's Hospital with not more than 20 deaths — a truly remarkable achievement for that period. Turpentine was Woodall's favorite dressing. Among other early English surgeons who used turpentine for wounds were John of Arderne (1376), Lowe (1597), and Wiseman (1676). Yonge (1679) in *Currus triumphalis, é terebinthô* described 13 cases in which turpentine was applied hot or warm, often on pledgets of tow (probably hemp or flax), to gunshot or other wounds and ulcers to stop hemorrhage. He added that turpentine had many admirable "vertues for Wounds." The German military surgeon Matthäus G. Purmann in the late seventeenth century employed turpentine in his dressings for compound fracture.[9]

A time-honored application among sailors was oakum, produced by picking apart the old tarred flax or hemp rope of ships' riggings. Pepys records in his diary meeting a wounded seaman just ashore, "muffled with dirty clouts and his right eye stopped with oakum" (June 4, 1666). Oakum was extensively used for dressings in the American Civil War. Lister (1871) found that it had antiseptic qualities and, except for the smell, made an advantageous covering for granulating sores after a washing with carbolic acid.[10]

A letter written in a bold and fine hand extolling the use of spirits of turpentine in the treatment of hospital gangrene was addressed to the Surgeon General, March 20, 1864, by George P. Hachenberg, Assistant Surgeon to the Union Army during the American Civil War. Hachenberg wrote that turpentine, applied every three hours over the entire wound surface, was a successful antiseptic as well as hemostatic dressing. Apparently Hachenberg's letter was never published, but his therapy was reported in British and French journals of the day and F. H. Hamilton alluded to it in his *Treatise on Military Surgery* (1865).[11]

In a laboratory appraisal Waid Rogers (1966) observed that concentrations of 0.002 ml. per liter of Barber's gum spirits of turpentine exerted a bacteriostatic effect upon cultures of *Staph. aureus*, as did concentrations of 0.0005 ml. per liter for *E. coli*.[12] The layman has not forgotten the traditional antiseptic and styptic value of turpentine for fresh wounds: carpenters still dip a cut finger into turpentine.[13]

Myrrh and Frankincense

Among the native gum-resins valued and exported by ancient peoples of the Middle East were myrrh and frankincense. Besides their familiar use as perfumes and incense and for embalming, myrrh and frankincense had medicinal applications. According to Celsus, they agglutinated wounds. Both were common ingredients of wound applications throughout the Middle Ages. The French chemist Antoine-F. de Fourcroy (1786) wrote that myrrh, powdered or dissolved in alcohol, cleansed foul ulcers and stopped the progress of caries.[14]

Styrax and Benzoin

Two of the oldest and most popular balsams in wound therapy were styrax and benzoin (known as "Benjamin" in many old English accounts), obtained from different trees of the styrax family in Southeast Asia. Pliny remarked that styrax cured scrofulous sores. It was a favorite wound remedy of the French surgeon-accoucheur Guillaume Mauquest de la Motte (1732). Styrax was still in use during the Napoleonic Wars, being favored by Larrey for contaminated war wounds. He wrote that he preferred it to alcohol for dressings in such cases because alcohol stopped wound suppuration! As late as 1868 William Adams of the Royal Orthopaedic Hospital, London, called benzoin "the old Friar's balsam of well-deserved notoriety."[15]

Balsam of Peru

An Indian medication for wounds, brought back from New Spain by the conquistadores, was mentioned at least as early as 1553 by the Portuguese physician Amatus Lusitanus. This so-called "balsam of Peru" was enthusiastically acclaimed in 1565 by Nicolo Monardes, a physician of Seville. His account, "Englished" in 1577 as *Joyfull Newes out of the New Founde Worlde*, declared: "Any maner of woundes beyng freshe it doth heale them in any parte of the body . . . so that there be no more in it but a simple wounde." Initially worth a hundred ducats an ounce in Rome, Monardes said it had become an inexpensive household remedy. By 1620, it was a recognized surgeon's aid in Germany.[16]

In 1876 Eduard Wiss counseled not to forget balsam of Peru in the fervor for new remedies. Frequent references in early twentieth-century literature show its popularity, particularly in Germany, even after the vogue for Dakin's solution. An experienced German surgeon postulated that the shortage of balsam of Peru in World War I was responsible for many infections that balsam could have controlled.[17]

An Appraisal

Long traditional usage of a mode of therapy is not necessarily a proof of its efficacy — witness phlebotomy. Before turning from the subject of resins and balsams to other venerable but less ancient antiseptics with well-known bactericidal properties, it is important to consider what results were actually achieved by these primitive applications in wound management. The wound of compound fracture, dangerous and familiar, was the one selected by Lister for his tests with concentrated carbolic acid dressings; documented comparison is available in at least three trials in earlier periods with resins and balsams.

Management of Open Fracture

In the history of surgery few wounds were as badly managed as those of compound (open) fracture. "Any blockhead" can do an amputation, wrote the Scottish physician-obstetrician Thomas Kirkland in 1780. The skillful man is the "one capable of curing without operations."[18] A great force obviously is necessary to drive a splintered bone through the muscular and cutaneous integuments, resulting almost inevitably in heavy contamination of the wound. The risk attending incised wounds in the preantiseptic era was measured almost solely by the surgeon's standard of cleanliness. The mortality rate of simple fractures was minimal, that of compound fractures was always large.

Early Proposals of Conservatism

The treatment of open fractures advised in the Hippocratic writings has a conservative modern ring; the wound was to be kept moist and a goatskin placed beneath the extremity to carry fluid away from the wound. Pitch cerate and wine dressings were applied, with the admission, however, that "they do neither much good nor much harm." A twentieth-century surgeon and classicist, Frederick B. Lund, has interpreted the Hippocratic attitude as, "whatever method is adopted, these cases are extremely serious and the wise physician will do well to escape them if he can do so gracefully." From the time of Hippocrates to Paré, the usual management of compound fracture was to saw off protruding segments of bone which could not readily be replaced.[19]

During the sixteenth to the late nineteenth centuries primary amputation was generally the approved method of treating compound fractures resulting from gunshot. It was the accepted practice in the American Civil War (1861–65) and the Franco-Prussian War (1870–71). Dissident voices favoring conservative management were distinctly in the minority but included such well-known figures as Würtz (1596), labeled the "Father of Conservative Surgery,"[20] Schmucker, and John Hunter.[21]

Paré expressed his mistrust of conservative management as follows: "But when the affect shall be compound by diversity of Symptomes, as a wound with an ulcer, inflammation, contusion and fracture of a bone, you must hope for no other from Tents or Lints, nor charmes than death." When compound fracture was complicated by fever, Paré advised amputation because of the great threat to life imposed by such an injury. Both Paré and Pott have been cited as advocates of primary amputation for compound fractures. However, Paré did not advise early amputation without trial of conservative practices. It is of interest that when these two eminent surgeons each suffered compound fractures involving tibia and/or fibula, they accepted conservative treatment.

Paré sustained a compound fracture of the leg, a few inches above the ankle, from a kick by a horse in 1561. He knew well the likelihood of disaster and the need for primary amputation, but asked his associate, "that he would handle me, as if he knew mee not." Conservative management was carried out and Paré survived with a good leg. The wound was dressed with *unguentum rosatum,* much commended by "joynt consent of the Ancients." It contained *oil omphacino, aqua rosacea, pauco aceto,* and *cera alba.* The primary dressing was untouched for six days; Paré believed that air had an unfavorable influence upon wounds. He poured oxycrate or rose vinegar over the dressing many times a day, to keep it moist, and "thick and astringent red wine, for the strengthening of the part, and repressing the humors; which two things wee must have a care of in Hippocrates opinion, in fractures especially with a wound." Paré favored use of phlebotomy for serious wounds only and submitted to being bled after his fracture.[22]

Two centuries later, 1756, Pott received a similar injury. He had already acquiesced to the verdict of amputation by his associates, but when his teacher Edward Nourse arrived on the scene advising nonoperative management, Pott was happy to accept the suggestion. Unlike Paré, Pott was not bled for his fracture. The outcome was successful, yet within seven years Pott joined the lists in protest against Bilguer, a surgeon-general of Frederick the Great, who had issued a directive to all Prussian military medical personnel, making a waiting policy mandatory after compound fracture of the extremities from gunshot.[23]

In a series of papers that evoked considerable debate (1761–91), Bilguer extolled conservative management, relating that of 6,618 wounded soldiers under his care in a military hospital, 653 died (9.7 percent), a commendable percentage for that day for patients hospitalized because of wounds. Bilguer stated that many more would have died if amputation had been frequent. In fact, he believed he had spared 1,800 patients with severely damaged extremities from undergoing amputation. Bilguer had no survivors among amputees. Obviously he was not the surgeon that Larrey was. Bilguer also failed to give the survival rate of patients with compound fractures treated conservatively. His dressing was a concoction of lime water, camphorated spirits of wine, and sal ammonia (ammonium chloride). He also used oil of turpentine dissolved in lime water, a suggestion gleaned from the writings of Heister[24] — a wound dressing with bacteriostatic, if not bactericidal power.

Among prominent civilian surgeons defending nonoperative management of compound fractures in the eighteenth century was the Irish surgeon and ophthalmologist Silvester O'Halloran. He estimated recoveries in amputation as being 30 percent and found the indiscriminate use of amputation more of a detriment than a service to mankind.[25]

By the early nineteenth century a number of surgeons, particularly in France and Belgium, were proponents of conservative management. These included Boyer, who, however, was unwilling to go as far as Gerard Van Swieten, founder of the Vienna Medical School. The latter (1776) opposed immediate amputation and advised trial with "antiseptic fomentations." Foucard of Pont-Sainte Maxence, France (1850) reported a remarkable instance of a boy of eight who, caught in the revolving wheel of a mill, sustained four fractures of both thighs and legs, three of which were compound. The patient obviously was in severe shock. His wounds were dressed with diachylon, a cerate of turpentine and lead acetate; he recovered.[26]

Silence on Compound Fracture

Malgaigne, an accomplished surgeon and great historian of surgery, was also a courageous and forthright critic. His exposure in 1842 of the miserable accomplishment of Paris surgeons with amputation startled his colleagues, alerting them to the need of studying the methods of other surgeons, notably the English. Malgaigne wrote a monograph on fractures (1847) and an earlier (1839) statistical account of fractures and dislocations observed at the Hôtel-Dieu since 1790. He failed in these publications to say anything concerning the management of compound fractures.[27]

One looks in vain in textbooks of surgery or monographs on fractures in the late eighteenth to the mid-nineteenth century for factual accounts of the outcome of treatment of open fracture. It is as though the great surgeons of that period were in collusion not to expose their tragic results. The texts of Cooper, Liston, Fergusson, and Gross are silent on the subject. Erichsen's widely read *Science and Art of Surgery* (1860) gives no indication of the mortality of compound fracture. On the contrary, he outlines in some detail the mortality of amputation, indicating that amputation of the thigh was one of the gravest of surgical procedures. The mortality of limb amputation for injury in 53 cases at the University College Hospital, where Erichsen worked, was 35.8 percent; for thigh amputation, 60 percent; and for leg amputation, 17.6 percent. The mortality of limb amputation for disease in 121 cases was only 18 percent. Erichsen alluded to Malgaigne's report on the formidable mortality of amputation in nine Parisian hospitals, but added that "of 24 cases [thigh amputation] recorded by South, Laurie [Lawrie] and Peacock, as occurring at St. Thomas's Hospital, at the Glasgow Infirmary, and the Edinburgh Infirmary, every one proved fatal."[28]

In a critical and extended review in his 1850 monograph *Chirurgie conservatrice*, Alexis Alquié strongly urged conservative management of compound fracture. He was able to show very definitely the huge mortality of amputation for fractures of thigh, leg, and arm. However, he failed to deduce factual evidence that conservative management, as then practiced, resulted in salvage of a large number of patients. Alquié did say, "One should prefer uncertain conservation to the uncertainty of sacrifice amputation."[29]

Three Successful Predecessors of Lister

In the early nineteenth century two obscure country surgeons in England and an internationally famous French military officer achieved outstanding results in the conservative care of compound fracture, using antiseptic management. The materials they employed, resins and balsams, were as ancient as surgery itself, but the factual reports of their consecutive successes, at a time when the mortality generally was forbidding with this injury, should have alerted the profession several decades before Lister's search for an effective antiseptic for the wound of compound fracture. Their experiences, however, were either overlooked or misinterpreted.

Serious accidents were frequent in the West Riding of England, wrote John Crowther in 1802. The area, said he, "abounds with coal mines and stone quarries, and is full of manufacturers, many of whom are employed in the direction of dangerous machines worked by steam-engines." Fractures apparently were taken care of largely in the homes of patients. Yet Crowther stated that he and his brothers, William and Robert, had treated 28 consecutive compound fractures without mortality in a space of slightly more than two years (April 28, 1798, to October 5, 1800).

The Crowthers' mode of treatment was wood tar (which comes from beechwood), made liquid by heating in "an iron or earthen pan." A large "pledget of tow" constituted the primary dressing. The Crowther method was to "take hold of each end, dip the middle part into the hot ointment, then lift it out, and apply it directly to the wounded part." If one pledget did not cover all the laceration, another was applied. The hot-tar dressing was next covered with a roller bandage impregnated with "alegar or vinegar," and a paste board was put over it to lend stability. The board was moistened in warm water to permit shaping of the dressing; splints were placed beneath for immobilization. Crowther indicated that this form of management had been practiced "with the greatest success by our ancestors, in Eland, near Halifax, time immemorial, being handed down from father to son."[30]

Upon the fall of Napoleon in 1815, his great surgeon Larrey, despite his fame and popularity, was stripped of all his positions except Honorary Surgeon in Chief to the Old Guard, whose

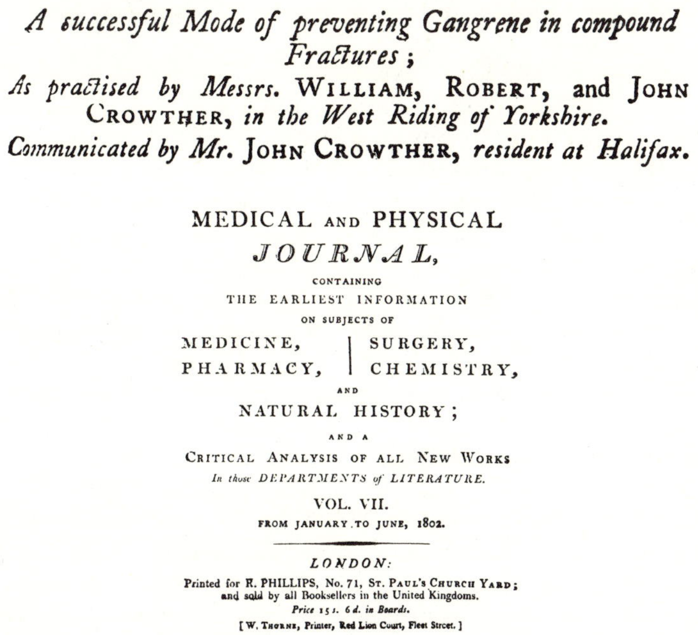

A successful Mode of preventing Gangrene in compound Fractures;

As practised by Messrs. WILLIAM, ROBERT, and JOHN CROWTHER, *in the West Riding of Yorkshire.*

Communicated by Mr. JOHN CROWTHER, *resident at Halifax.*

MEDICAL AND PHYSICAL

JOURNAL,

CONTAINING

THE EARLIEST INFORMATION

ON SUBJECTS OF

MEDICINE, SURGERY,

PHARMACY, CHEMISTRY,

AND

NATURAL HISTORY;

AND A

CRITICAL ANALYSIS OF ALL NEW WORKS

In those DEPARTMENTS of LITERATURE.

VOL. VII.

FROM JANUARY TO JUNE, 1802.

LONDON:

Printed for R. PHILLIPS, No. 71, ST. PAUL'S CHURCH YARD; and sold by all Booksellers in the United Kingdoms.

Price 15s. 6d. in Boards.

[W. THORNE, Printer, Red Lion Court, Fleet Street.]

17.1 The Crowther brothers in the West Riding of Yorkshire treated 28 successive compound fractures with tow dressings dipped in hot tar without mortality (1798–1800).

hospital was the Gros-Caillou.[31] It was in the latter capacity (1821–24) that Larrey introduced conservative therapy and successfully treated twelve successive compound fractures with topical application of styrax. A linen dressing coated with styrax was placed over the wound, then a soft *charpie*, and next compresses soaked in wine or camphorated vinegar. The extremity was immobilized in a splint and all was encompassed with a many-tailed Scultetus bandage. During the long convalescent period the dressing was changed only once or twice. Larrey presented one of his patients at a September 1824 séance of the Academy of Surgery, a soldier of the Guard whose leg had been badly broken when he was thrown and dragged by his horse during maneuvers. The final report of the twelve patients was published later that year.[32]

Larrey's achievement was described in several reviews during 1824–25, including one in Italian, but only the role of immobilization was emphasized.[33] None took note of the special circumstance of local application of benzoin compound to the wound. Centuries of use of various balsams for wound dressings had served only to cause confusion and create a deep-rooted skepticism of the value of antiseptic agents in precluding infection. Larrey's use of styrax apparently went unchampioned, although in a Paris thesis (1873) Ludovic Biencourt stated that Larrey had completely changed the management of compound fracture,[34] and well he might have, had the method been subjected to trial. Strangely enough, French surgeons did not even debate the validity of Larrey's contention.

The Shropshire village of Oswestry on the border of Wales was the home of a remarkable surgeon, Edward Bennion, who died there in 1844 at age eighty-seven. It is a mining region, where, as in the Crowthers' area, serious accidents were common. Bennion apparently never published concerning his extraordinary achievements in the management of open fractures. His reputation, outside his unusual local fame, rests on the testimony of an eyewitness, a Mr. Davies, who came to London to attend Adams's lectures at the Grosvenor Place School. Davies described Bennion's technique to Adams, saying it was a "matter of common observation that Mr. Bennion's cases generally did well whilst the compound fractures treated by the other surgeons in the district were generally fatal." Adams mentioned Davies's account in a lecture before the Medical Society of London in 1857, some thirteen years after Bennion's death, and Sampson Gamgee of Birmingham repeated Adams's description in his monograph *On the Treatment of Wounds and Fractures* (1883).[35]

According to these two accounts, Bennion, after bringing the broken ends into apposition, covered the wound with "a large bit of lint, saturated with compound tincture of benzoin. . . . He never disturbed the first dressing or bandaging unless urgent symptoms indicated the necessity of so doing." In the absence of such symptoms, the dressing remained in place for a month.

Hoping for more information about this obscure but competent country surgeon who employed an antiseptic with unusual success for open fractures at least a quarter of a century before Lister's use of phenol, the authors enlisted the help of a number of English friends. Charles Talbot of the Wellcome Institute of Medical History turned up the obituary of an Oswestry surgeon, who (it read) "was perhaps best known as the son of the cele-

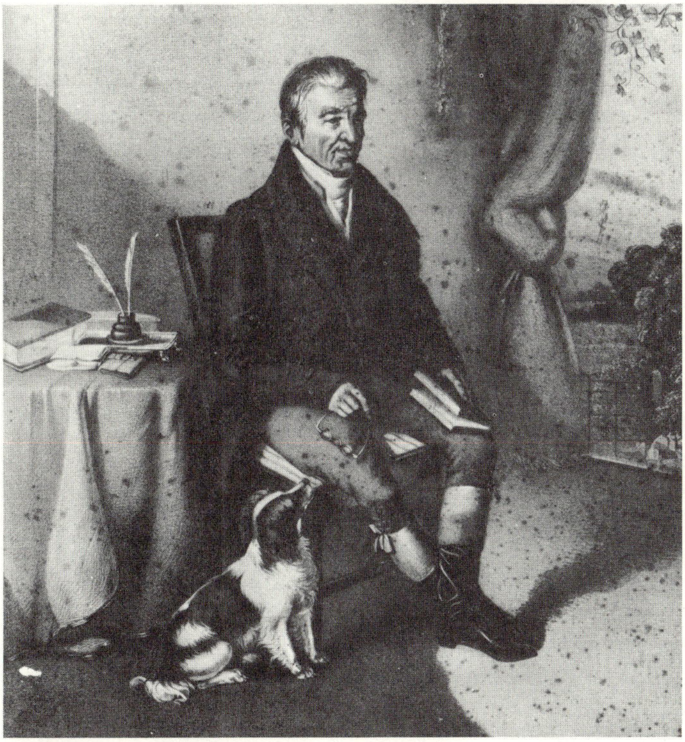

17.2 Edward Bennion's success in treating open fractures with compound tincture of benzoin (ca. 1840) drew wide attention in Oswestry, Shropshire. Family portrait, courtesy Kathleen M. Whitfield.

brated Dr. Edward Bennion, whose fame for surgical skill extended over this and many neighbouring counties."[36] John Shepherd of Liverpool found graves of three Bennion surgeons in Oswestry, one the father of Edward Bennion. Finally Miss Kathleen M. Whitfield, a direct descendant, sent a picture of her distinguished ancestor and other pertinent information.[37] The inscription on the portrait is in both English and Welsh. The family was of Welsh descent. Appropriately, a celebrated orthopedic hospital stands today in Oswestry, the Robert Jones and Agnes Hunt Hospital.

In 1876, Bryant of Guy's Hospital confirmed the virtue of compound tincture of benzoin as an antiseptic agent. In 1861 he had reported upon 302 compound fractures with an overall mortality of 31.7 percent; for femur, the mortality was 64.7 percent. Later, when he used compound tincture of benzoin, Bryant was able to report 14 consecutive compound fractures without a death.[38]

From this brief account, it is obvious that Lister had antecedents in the Crowthers, Larrey, and Bennion, who had acquired successful techniques for treating compound fracture, even though they did not understand why their methods succeeded, and several decades before the pathogenic character of bacteria was recognized. Had their discoveries received adequate trial at the hands of contemporaries, successful management of compound fracture could have come several decades earlier.

Alcohol and Elective Surgery; Glycerine

No other antiseptic agents command so great a literature in wound therapy as do wine and alcohol.[39] Wine obviously was considered a panacea for many ills, including melancholy and sadness, for the relief of which Noah trifled with its use. Galen favored dressings of wine for all wounds because of its desiccating and drying effect, a thesis supported later by a succession of medieval surgeons of the Bologna School of the thirteenth and fourteenth centuries. Among its distinguished representatives were Hugh of Lucca, Theodoric, Saliceto, the latter's pupil Lanfranc, who settled in Paris, and Mondeville of Montpellier. All this illustrious band subscribed to primary wound closure and wine dressings.[40]

With the advent of distillation in Europe (thirteenth century),[41] alcohol, brandy, and aqua vitae became available and were employed in dressings by many military surgeons. Guy de Chauliac (1363) used full-strength "biting wine" (brandy) for the purpose. Following abandonment of scalding hot oil as the primary treatment for gunshot wounds in 1536, Paré remained a lifelong devotee of turpentine, oil of roses, egg yolk, and aqua vitae for wound management.

Giuseppe Lanzoni of Ferrara (1692, 1715) reported upon wounds successfully treated with topical application of brandy, which was apparently Heister's (1750) most frequently mentioned wound remedy, although he also applied myrrh, oil of roses, turpentine, balsam of Peru, and other agents.[42] Johannes Juncker (1724) and Theodor Kappenhagen (1745) referred to brandy as the finest therapy for putrid ulcers in that it dissipates the flow of pus and arrests hemorrhage from wounds. The latter listed seventeen indications for the use of strong spirits, including management of fresh and suppurating wounds. According to a hospital memorandum of Les Invalides in 1763, alcohol (*eau de vie*) was made available to the surgeon major of the hospital each day for the dressing of wounds. The unused portions were returned to the pharmacist and immediately put under lock and key.[43]

Alcohol in Elective Surgery

Nélaton's important work in Paris upon the problem of wound infection has not received the attention it deserves from students of surgical history. By 1863 he had adopted alcohol soaks for wounds of elective surgery.[44]

The French surgeons, chiefly Nélaton's associates, who reexplored the use of alcohol for dressing of wounds in the midnineteenth century, had a deep sense of its antiquity. In reporting their research, essentially experiments upon animals, J. F. Batailhé and A. Guillet (1859) suggested that they were "fellow workmen of Hippocrates, Galen, Dionis, and Ambroise Paré, in fact, of almost all surgeons till the end of the past century." Jules Le Coeur of Caen (1864) said, "We must return to the practice of the ancients."[45]

When S. A. Chedevergne and Jean de Gaulejac, Nélaton's associates, independently reported his success with alcohol dressings, they too made reference to its use in ancient practice. Nélaton used alcohol in strong concentration, pouring as much as one-half to a full liter into deep wounds at each dressing, enough to render many patients intoxicated. He was partial to camphorated alcohol with an alcohol concentration of 56 percent, but also employed stronger concentrations. Nélaton recognized that the antiputrescent effect was owing solely to its alcohol content.[46]

In succession, alcohol dressings were applied by Nélaton to wounds of trauma, in the management of compound fractures with open wounds, and in elective surgery. His emphasis was on use of alcohol to prevent infection in elective surgery. His operations of election of some magnitude, largely for tumors, were attended by amazingly low hospital mortality rates. Chedevergne, in summarizing the experience of Nélaton at hôpital des Cliniques for the first half of 1864, reports upon 48 elective operative procedures with 3 hospital deaths, only 1 death being from wound sepsis.[47]

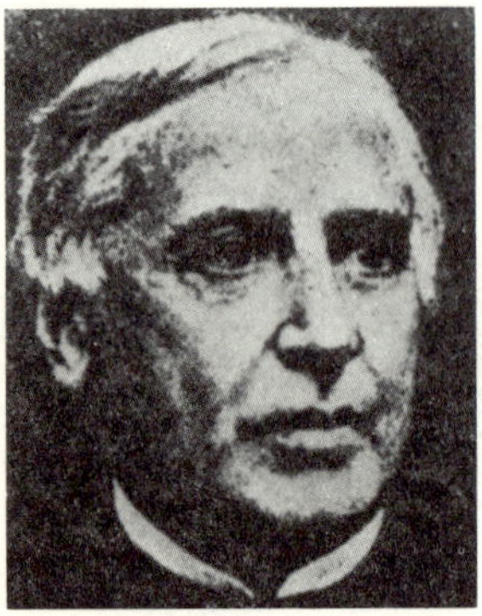

17.3 Auguste Nélaton, celebrated Paris surgeon, performed elective surgery placing large alcohol soaks in wounds, with hospital mortality of less than 5 percent (1863–64).

Among Nélaton's 54 operations for 1863 reported by de Gaulejac, there was 1 hospital death. Eliminating the lesser cases in this series, there remain 28 major elective operations, among which the only death was recorded (amputation of the penis), accounting for a hospital mortality of 3.5 percent.[48] Nélaton's overall hospital mortality for elective operations, many of which were major, rarely exceeded 4 percent, with a mortality from infection of less than 2 percent. Watson Cheyne's (1882) critique that Nélaton's cases "were, however, not very severe" is not well taken when one recalls that any incised wound was fraught with great danger and dreaded by patients and surgeons alike.[49]

In 1865 dressing wounds with alcohol was called the "ordre du jour" by the editor of a distinguished Paris medical journal. Why did not this unusual accomplishment command wider attention and acclaim by the profession? When a commission was appointed by the Paris Surgical Society to adjudicate the promise and performance of alcohol in elective surgery and for contaminated wounds, observations and recommendations for the adoption of Nélaton's practice were enthusiastically presented by Marc Sée (read by Labbé). Their pleas were set aside by the commission on the basis of argument and without a recommendation for prospective trials (1867). One of the arguments lodged against use of Nélaton's procedure was that it did not consistently forestall erysipelas in wounds. The primary problem obviously was that Nélaton's antisepsis was incomplete, the sole focus being upon the wound, with no similar care of hands, instruments, and operating materiel, despite his attempts to avoid contamination.[50] Unfortunately, the complication of erysipelas as well as parotitis occasionally attended operations well into the twentieth century, disappearing only when sulfanilamide became available (1935) to combat and thwart streptococcal infection.

The aging Velpeau and Hippolyte Larrey were members of the commission that passed the unfavorable verdict upon the enthusiastic endorsement of Nélaton's alcohol dressings by Labbé and Sée. Interestingly enough, Velpeau (1866) entertained hopes of better days for wound management, but was not prepared to approve of alcohol. Hippolyte Larrey's disapproval was undoubtedly an extension of his father's (Dominique Larrey's) opposition to putting alcohol in wounds because it stopped suppuration. It was the elder Larrey's thesis, as it had been of surgeons for generations, that suppuration encouraged wound healing.[51]

Had Nélaton been a more assertive surgeon with a penchant to overcome opposition, he would undoubtedly have established the virtue and protective role of alcohol in elective surgery and for contaminated wounds. By 1864 he was a famous man with the largest surgical practice in Paris, perhaps in the world. He was tired and old for his fifty-seven years, and not very well. Three years later he withdrew from active practice because of failing vision and impending heart failure.[52]

Nélaton's accomplishment was not exceeded until the role of bacteria in wound infection was recognized and the need for a complete antiseptic program understood and adopted. Had he and his associates been alert to the teachings of Pasteur on putrefaction (1863) and the earlier significant work of Semmelweis (1847), Nélaton undoubtedly would have had a broader view of the problem of wound infection. It is of interest that Chédevergne, employing a microscope, observed dissolution of pus on contact with alcohol. He failed to recognize the presence of bacteria in such exudates.[53]

Use of Alcohol outside France

Although it was in France that alcohol for wound dressings found widest application in the pre-Listerian era, Augustin Prichard of Bristol published his experience with brandy and alcohol for wounds in 1860, including two cases of compound fracture treated successfully.[54]

At the first International Medical Congress, in Paris, August 1867, the Portuguese surgeon Antonio M. Barbosa spoke of the use of alcohol for wounds. He reported a mortality rate of 24.2 percent in 243 amputations at St. Joseph's Hospital in Lisbon during the 1855 to 1866 period. In the preceding two years there was only 1 death in 14 thigh amputations, a laudable achievement for that day. In two of the eleven wards no deaths resulted from amputation over the twelve-year period of study. Better ventilation and less crowding in those wards were cited as the responsible factors. Barbosa attributed the low mortality rate in elective surgery to use of alcohol dressings. He added that alcohol had been widely used in elective surgery throughout Portugal before its application by Nélaton — the Portuguese surgeon Amaral had used it at the beginning of the eighteenth century and employment of camphorated alcohol for wounds and ulcers had persisted at Hospital de Coïmbre.[55]

According to the records of the Radcliffe Infirmary, Oxford, in 1870, beer was brewed on the premises and strong beer was placed in wound poultices. Strong beer, not fit for drinking, was given to the surgeons to be used in their wound dressings. Use of whisky in wound dressings was an old country practice and a good one, wrote the Scotsman David Blair in 1870.[56]

Glycerine

The Swedish chemist Karl W. Scheele discovered glycerine, a trihydric alcohol and a weak antibacterial agent, in 1779. Michel E. Chevreul (1823) studied it more fully and named it.[57]

A strong endorsement of glycerine for wound therapy came from Jean-Nicolas Demarquay (1859), who found it of value in treating *pourriture d'hôpital* at hôpital St.-Louis in 1855, and for surgical and chronic ulcerating wounds and burns. A.-J. Desormeaux (1862) used a 90 percent glycerine starch ointment for all types of wounds with much satisfaction, finding it effective in suppressing suppuration. In the discussion that followed Desormeaux's presentation before the Paris Society of Surgery, Hippolyte Larrey said the advantages of glycerine had been exaggerated. Others agreed. By 1875 it was no longer vaunted as a panacea for wounds.[58]

In 1929, M. E. Lichtenstein of Chicago mentioned the antiseptic and hydroscopic properties of glycerine, which he had used in "several thousand dressings." He quoted studies (1918) showing that in 100 percent concentration, glycerine was quite effective against *B. coli* attending a three-hour exposure.[59]

Honey

There is much testimony but little evidence that honey is useful in wound management. It is an old remedy for a number of purposes.

Honey was employed in 319 of 966 prescriptions in the Ebers Papyrus (ca. 1550 B.C.). Celsus said that honey encouraged wound agglutination.[60] When added to such substances as turpentine or alcohol, it ameliorated the irritant effects.

Mercuric Chloride

Known also as corrosive sublimate, mercuric chloride is a powerful but slow-acting antiseptic. Its antiseptic action apparently is increased if alcohol (70 percent) is used as the vehicle. Solutions of 1:10,000 to 1:2,000 have been employed for irrigation and cleansing of wounds. Use of mercuric chloride is limited by its toxicity and corrosive action.

Paracelsus in the fifteenth century described preparations of corrosive sublimate and employed it for wounds. According to Brasavola, it was "unknown to the ancients." He prepared it by adding ammonia to Albucasis' formula — chalcanthum, mercury, and vinegar. His contemporary Jerome Cardan (1501–76) also used *argentum sublimatum*, which he made by subliming a mixture of mercury with vitriol in a glass vessel. Venice was the chief distributor of mercuric chloride in the sixteenth century. It was available in London, Amsterdam, and France in the early eighteenth century.[61]

Lister invoked mercuric chloride in wounds in a dilution of 1:500, but concluded that carbolic acid was better. Mercuric chloride was popular as a hand-dip and for preparation of the operative site by many European and American surgeons at the end of the nineteenth century. In 1890 Behring reported that neither it nor carbolic acid had a strong antibacterial effect in blood serum.[62] Halsted believed it interfered with wound healing when used for wound irrigation but continued to employ it for involucral cavities of bone. A. C. Abbott (1891) found that 1:1,000 mercuric chloride was ineffective for destruction of the staphylococcus.[63]

Silver Nitrate

One of Lister's countrymen, John Higginbottom, a surgeon of Nottingham, in 1826 asked the rhetorical question whether silver nitrate implanted into the wound of a compound fracture would not in fact convert it to the state of a simple fracture. After nearly forty years of trial and experiments, Higginbottom answered his own question, saying yes, silver nitrate "reduces the dangerous circumstances of a compound fracture to that of a simple fracture, the wound being healed by the first intention."[64] This was 1865, two years before Lister's famous paper on the use of carbolic acid for compound fracture.

Higginbottom at first applied a lunar caustic stick to minor ulcerated pricks and wounds. He also used silver nitrate in 1 percent solutions and extended the therapy to burns and erysipelas. For treating lacerated wounds and compound fractures, he found a 30 percent solution successful.

Although Higginbottom was the keenest proponent of silver nitrate in the preantiseptic era, its therapeutic properties had been recognized for at least two centuries before his advocacy; its discovery, probably by the alchemists, is still a matter of conjecture. The mysterious Basil Valentine, usually identified as a monk living in Erfurt in the fifteenth century, is sometimes credited with the first fabrication of silver nitrate. Paracelsus may have used his work.[65]

Silver nitrate was called in French medicine *pierre infernale* or *caustique perpetuel*, and by the Germans, *Höllenstein*. By the seventeenth century notes of its use began to appear in medical literature. Thus, the *Lapis infernalis* was advised by Alexander Read of London (1635) for removing foul matter of ulcerated cavities on the surface of the body, and the records of the Hôtel-Dieu, Paris, show that an order was placed in 1661 to purchase the ingredients to make "a remedy called infernal stone," needed by the apothecary.[66]

Silver nitrate early became popular for treating lesions about the eye. Antoine Maître-Jan (1707) and Charles de Saint-Yves (1722) employed it for tumors of the eyelids. In 1884 Carl Credé of Berlin reported that instillation of a weak solution of silver nitrate into the eyes of infants at birth was prophylaxis against the possibility of contracting gonorrhea from passage through the birth canal.[67] The measure became a legal obligatory precaution for the accoucheur.

François Quesnay (1764) recommended *pierre infernale* to prevent purulent suppuration in wounds. Joseph Lieutaud (1776) used silver nitrate for ulcers and spoke of its rapid action. Busmann, in a Göttingen publication (1798–99), said that he disliked calling such a marvelous remedy *Höllenstein* (infernal stone); one of his patients had dubbed it *Wunderstein*. Home (1797) used nitrate of silver dissolved in water as a lotion for various kinds of ulcer, although his choice for indolent ulcers was powdered rhubarb. Astley Cooper (1823) likewise used a wash of silver nitrate for ulcers and cauterized the surface of punctured wounds with lunar caustic.[68]

The Halogens

Hypochlorites

Lime water was a wound therapy of old usage, applied by such surgeons as Albucasis, Brunschwig, and Gersdorff. Mauquest de la Motte (1732) treated gangrene with *eau de chaux*, and Barthélemi Vigarous used it at Montpellier in the latter part of the eighteenth century for ulcers and wounds.[69]

After Scheele isolated chlorine in 1774, the French chemists became eager to find practical applications for hypochlorite. Chlorine gas was recommended by Fourcroy (1791) to disinfect cemeteries and stables and by the physician François Chaussier (1814) to disinfect dissecting rooms. French surgeons of the Napoleonic era including Percy employed *eau de Javelle* (hypochlorite) against *pourriture d'hôpital* in military hospitals.[70].

It was primarily the pharmacist Antoine-G. Labarraque (1810–23) who stimulated acceptance of hypochlorites by Paris surgeons. In 1826, Lisfranc advocated *chlorure de chaux* for indolent ulcers, burns, and operative wounds. In 1827 the English surgeon Thomas Alcock suggested hypochlorite instillation for compound fractures. His publication on the subject, *Chlorurets*, received a scathing review in *Lancet*, the editors accusing him of "making a volume of the ephemeral archives of the French."[71]

Semmelweis established the value of hypochlorite in his preventative antiseptic program (1847–49, 1861). He used it as a hand-wash for accoucheurs and their assistants and for chemical sterilization of all materials likely to come in contact with the parturient canal. The last to promote hypochlorite in an enthusiastic manner were Carrel and Henry D. Dakin in World War I.[72]

Iodine

Bernard Courtois, a chemist engaged by Napoleon to make nitrate, dicovered iodine in 1811. Studies of its elementary nature were carried out by Davy and J. L. Gay-Lussac, French chemist and physicist. J. F. Coindet, who first advocated iodine internally for goiter (1820), also first endorsed its external use for scrofula.[73]

John Davies of Hertford (1839) believed iodine to be the most efficient of all topical applications for burns, ulcers, erysipelas, and "lacerated, contused, and punctured wounds." For fresh wounds he found application of tincture of iodine curative. Davies's suggestions found wide acceptance.[74]

In France A. A. Boinet (1846) reported excellent results attending local injection of iodine for wounds. In his *Iodotherapie* (1855) he related three cases of compound fracture treated successfully with topical iodine. Amédée Bonnet of Lyons (1852) used iodine and tincture of potassium iodide as dressings for wounds and abscesses. C. J. Marchal (1859) said he had applied iodine in dressings for gangrenous and fetid wounds at Val-de-Grâce prior to 1848.[75]

Before adoption of surgical rubber gloves, iodine was used as a finger-dip by many surgeons, including César Roux of Lausanne, Mikulicz, and Senn. Antonio Grossich (1908) recommended tincture of iodine for preparation of the skin of the operative site.[76]

Bromine

Antoine Balard of the School of Pharmacy, Montpellier, first isolated bromine from salts in the Mediterranean in 1826. It was used shortly thereafter by Pourché of the medical faculty of Montpellier in treatment of scrofula, but seems to have received little attention as a wound remedy until the American Civil War. In 1863, Middleton Goldsmith, a Union Army medical officer, in a *Report on Hospital Gangrene*, made a glowing account of the efficacy of bromine in the management of war wounds. Of 308 patients with hospital gangrene treated with bromine solutions, 8 died (2.6 percent); of 30 treated by other methods, 13 died (43.3 percent).[77]

Creosote and Carbolic Acid

Creosote

The German naturalist Karl Reichenbach in 1832 announced his discovery of "creosote," distilled from beechwood tar. The appellation was taken from two Greek words meaning "I preserve flesh." With the help of a country doctor and an *ancien* pharmacist, the material was applied topically in a 2 percent aqueous solution to various lesions, including suppurating wounds, of twenty-three patients. All, said Reichenbach, were cured except one, a patient who died of a compound fracture. When creosote was applied to fresh wounds from sharp instruments or other agents, suppuration did not occur.[78]

Translations and reviews of accounts of creosote rapidly appeared in the medical journals in several countries. The *Bulletin général de thérapeutique* ran five articles on the subject in 1833 and mentioned the impatience of physicians when the material dispatched to Paris by Reichenbach was unaccountably held up at the border. The review of Reichenbach's paper in the *London Medical Gazette* (1834) struck a cynical note: "We must of course be prepared to hear this new remedy cried up in all quarters, until it is displaced by something more new."[79] By the end of 1833 creosote was being widely used by German and French surgeons for suppurating wounds and for caries of bone.

Carbolic Acid (Phenol)

The German chemist Friedlieb Runge (1834) discovered carbolic acid two years after the announcement of creosote by Reichenbach.[80] Creosote and carbolic acid were tried only intermittently for wounds until after mid-century when interest was stimulated by the work of E. Corne and Demeaux and by Crace Calvert.

In October 1859 the *British Medical Journal* announced a "great stir" in "scientific assemblies of Paris regarding the application of a mixture of coaltar and powdered gypsum as a disinfectant and deodoriser" introduced by two French practitioners from Libos, France. Corne had originally suggested the material for application to the night-soil of Paris; Demeaux had tried it for suppurating wounds. A commission of the Academy of Sciences headed by Velpeau, who instigated trials at La Charité, agreed that the agent did aid the healing of suppurating surfaces, as well as being an effective deodorant of fetid wounds. Across the Channel a somewhat similar powder, known as M'Dougall's, was already being employed for a disinfectant, as the Scottish medical press hastened to point out.[81]

Frequent application of phenol to wounds began with Jules Lemaire and Gilbert Déclat in France, who wrote extensive monographs (1860–65) sketching its uses for wounds. The Italian Enrico Bottini (1866) indicated that he had treated 600 patients with suppurating wounds or ulcers with topical 2 percent carbolic acid "with almost uniformly good results."[82]

The English-born chemist Calvert spent much of his early life in France and did research under Chevreul in Paris. On returning to England, he undertook experiments at Manchester as early as 1851 to determine the antiseptic and antiputrefactive powers of carbolic acid. By 1862 scattered reports began to appear in British medical journals on successes with the antiseptic for gangrenous and fetid wounds.[83]

In 1863 Calvert reported that Thomas Turner, a surgeon at Manchester Royal Infirmary, had read a paper at a branch meeting of the British Medical Association on the uses of carbolic acid as a remedial agent. Turner had applied the preparation locally for hemorrhoids, gangrenous wounds, and fistulas and observed it promoted separation of dead tissue. Calvert also alluded to experiences of Hughes of London with phenol and to Lemaire and Gratiolet's work on the arrest of putrefaction with the acid. Calvert's report provoked further discussion on carbolic acid, particularly in its distinction from creosote, as letters to the *Lancet* attest.[84]

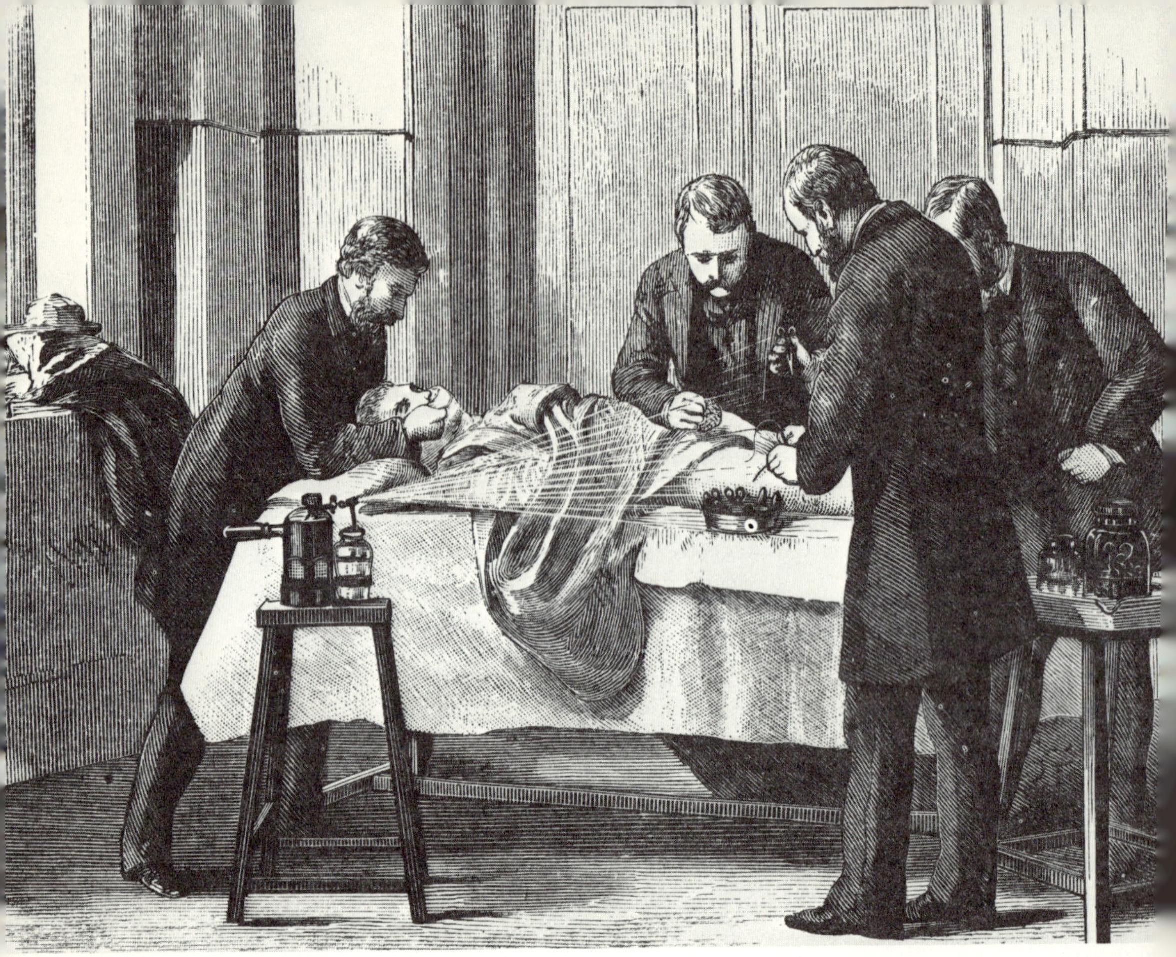

17.4 Use of the Lister carbolic acid spray. From W. W. Cheyne, *Antiseptic surgery* (London, 1882). Courtesy National Library of Medicine.

In a dissertation, August 1863, James Watson reported that carbolic acid had been helpful in two cases of sloughing ulcer at the Edinburgh Royal Infirmary. J. R. Wolfe of Aberdeen (1865) deduced from experiments with cotton-wool dressings saturated with the acid that it lessened the risk of purulent and of erysipelatous infection in his surgical wards.[85] Lister's 1867 publication on carbolic acid for compound fracture tended to overshadow other antiseptic usages.

Miscellaneous Antiseptics

Ferric Chloride

Late in 1854 two boxes of ferric chloride were dispatched to the French Army in Constantinople by a pharmacist, A. Burin du Buisson, who had shared investigations of the material with Pravaz, Pétrequin, and others in Lyons. It was his belief that ferric chloride would have merit as a hemostatic agent and in treating suppurating wounds in the war theatre.[86] His thesis was substantiated by the experiences of Salleron and other French army surgeons in the crowded hospitals during the Crimean War, where *pourriture d'hôpital* prevailed in endemic form for two years with an intensity never seen in peacetime. A great number of other local antiseptic agents were tried, including camphorated and aromatic vinegar, lead acetate, saturated solutions of zinc and aluminum sulphate, and tincture of iodine, but ferric chloride was reported the most effective in combatting infection.[87]

Beneficial effects of ferric chloride in suppurating wounds were described shortly afterward by a number of French surgeons. Its use as a prophylactic measure in elective operations was dramatically proclaimed by Bourgade at the 1867 International Medical Congress. He reported 95 operations of election in the Hôtel-Dieu at Clermont-Ferrand with no hospital deaths. On completion of the surgery the wound was washed out and covered with a dressing soaked in 30 percent ferric chloride. Included in a miscellany of operations were 8 leg amputations, 5 near the ankle, 4 of the arm, 5 of the forearm, and 3 partial foot amputations. There were no thigh amputations. In 11 of the 95 cases, redness developed at the wound edges. Only once did erysipelas supervene, but it was controlled.[88]

The popularity of ferric chloride as a topical application did not last. Some said it provoked continued suppuration. Reyher is quoted as remarking that the surest way to necessitate amputation of a limb fractured by a bullet was to apply a *charpie* soaked in ferric chloride to the wound orifices.[89]

Nitric Acid

Among other antiseptics used in the American Civil War was nitric acid, successfully employed in wound therapy by Alfred North of the Union Army. William Detmold, a consulting surgeon for the Union Army, alluded to its importance in the management of hospital gangrene in 1863. He referred to nitric acid as the "actual or potential cautery." J. Julian Chisolm in the Confederate Army also advocated nitric acid for hospital gangrene.[90]

Zinc Chloride

Burnett's disinfection fluid, a solution of zinc chloride, was applied to injured fingers by employees at Portsmouth Dockyard years before Campbell de Morgan of the Middlesex Hospitals

(1866) reported upon an extensive experience with zinc chloride in management of the wound after breast removal for cancer. The practice had originated at the hospital in 1864 when Charles H. Moore employed a 6.6 to 8.8 percent solution to minimize the likelihood of local recurrence. De Morgan and colleagues extended local application of zinc chloride to other wounds. Lister (1868) employed it for compound fracture, but concluded it was inferior to carbolic acid.[91]

Current Attitude toward Antiseptics in Wounds

Allusion has already been made to successful use of a variety of antiseptic agents in the wounds of compound fracture by a number of individuals in the early decades of the nineteenth century. It was the basis of Lister's antiseptic program. At the end of World War I, Fleming (1919) announced that all antiseptics instilled into wounds did more harm to the tissues than to the bacteria.[92] The profession failed to accept this advice until the sulfonamides and antibiotics, which respectively became available in the 1930s and during World War II, proved their superiority and the inutility of placement of antiseptics in wounds. Nevertheless, there is good clinical evidence that antiseptics in wounds of compound fracture were beneficial. The incompleteness of the pre-Listerian antiseptic system limited its usefulness.

Summary

The New Testament parable of the Samaritan pouring oil and wine into the wounds of a man who fell among thieves on the road to Jericho has served to focus sharp notice upon use of antiseptics in contaminated wounds (Luke 10:33–34). Perusal of the practices of well-known surgeons serves to indicate that turpentine was favored by Guy de Chauliac (1363), Brunschwig (1497), Paré (1545), Würtz (1563), and Woodall (1617). Antiseptics were consistently placed in wounds by a few military surgeons in the American Civil War (1861–65); in the Union Army Goldsmith employed bromine (1863), North favored nitric acid (1864), and Hachenberg preferred turpentine (1864). In the Confederate Army Chisolm (1864) too employed nitric acid. Disappearance of hospital gangrene and a greatly improved mortality record with wounds so treated were noted by all these observers. Nélaton of Paris (1863–64) poured alcohol into wounds of elective surgery up to the point of intoxication, with an overall hospital mortality of about 4 percent. It was Lister

(1867), however, who drew the attention of the profession to consistent and inclusive antiseptic wound practices. He had several antecedents who placed antiseptics into the wounds of compound fractures, notably the brothers Crowther (1802) of Halifax, England, Larrey of Paris (1824), and Bennion (ca. 1840) of Oswestry, England. Placement of antiseptic agents into wounds throughout the first three quarters of the nineteenth century finally gave way in the mid-1880s to the prophylactic surgical wound practices of Semmelweis (1847). In World War I there was a rebirth of interest in placing Dakin's solution into contaminated wounds, actually the hypochlorite of Semmelweis. With availability of sulfonamides and penicillin, dependence upon this practice also ceased. At the end of World War I, Fleming announced that all antiseptic agents did more harm to wound tissues than to the bacteria in them. Despite denials of any useful or effective role of antiseptics in wounds, one cannot peruse the surgical literature of wound management without being persuaded that, though superseded by prophylactic surgical antisepsis, which provides a more complete type of protection from wound infection, chemical antisepsis did play an important role in lessening the hazards of wound infection. The writings of Paré (1579), Woodall (1655), and of Chédevergne (1864) and Gaulejac (1864), both pupils of Nélaton, provide both testimony and convincing evidence on this score.

(For notes, see pp. 663–71.)

CHAPTER 18

Early Hospital Practices

THE FIRST HOSPITALS in Western Europe were essentially almshouses, providing refuge for the sick and the poor. As Christianity spread westward, hospices for the ill and the helpless and for travelers were often provided in small infirmaries within monasteries or near a city church, tended by members of the religious community. Some of the world's greatest hospitals originated as such monastic charitable institutions — Hôtel-Dieu of Paris and St. Bartholomew's of London being among those that have survived over the centuries. Many of the first hospitals were built in juxtaposition to cathedrals, because of the church's commitment to relieve poverty, illness, and distress.

Hospitals for Roman soldiers were built in the military camp towns of the Roman Empire and usually located near an outer wall. Designs of these symmetrical establishments are depicted by a number of medical historians, including Charles Singer (1928), who maintained that the early hospitals of Europe were essentially a contribution of Rome and its military organization.[1] J. D. Thompson and Grace Goldin (1975) have collected and sketched hospital and ward designs of the Roman military hospital at Vindonissa, Switzerland, in a comprehensive historical study of hospital design. Their handsome monograph fills a hiatus long in want of elaboration.[2]

The need for refuges grew as pilgrimages and the crusades brought many weary travelers to foreign lands. About 380 A.D. the Roman matron Fabiola turned her home into a haven for the sick and developed a cluster of buildings outside Rome for pilgrims. The projected plan for an infirmary at St. Gallen, Switzerland (816–17) provided special accommodations for the very ill, a place for attending medical men to live, and even a bloodletting house.[3] At Cesarea (370–79), Constantinople, and other cities of Eastern Europe far more elaborate hospitals were constructed than the first Western institutions with which our study is primarily concerned.

Leprosy and other diseases were carried by travelers and traders from the East to Europe and Britain. Toward the end of the thirteenth century almost every town in France had its pest or leper house and soon thereafter such establishments became common in England. Nursing, but no therapy, was supplied in these segregated areas. They represented a "great social and hygienic movement, a wave of genuine prophylaxis as well as of human charity." With the appearance of syphilis in Europe and complications thereof, it became necessary that hospitals, staffed with medical men, be prepared to treat patients with chronic illness. Such arrangements became operative in Strasbourg in 1500, in Leipzig in 1517, and at the Hôtel-Dieu of Paris in 1536.[4]

According to Garrison the first hospital in America was built by Cortez in Mexico City. Quebec's Hôtel-Dieu dated from 1639. Montreal's two-room log hospital opened in 1644; it was protected by a palisade with mounted guns for fear of Indian raids. Manhattan Island had a hospital in 1663. Toward the end of the fifteenth century ornate and beautiful hospitals were functioning in many large Italian cities.[5]

An assessment of the nature of hospital care in a few great hospitals that have long been in the forefront of medicine's advance will serve to reveal how surgeons dealt with the problems of their patients over succeeding periods in time. Two of the oldest and most famous hospitals in the world are the Hôtel-Dieu in Paris and St. Bartholomew's in London. More undoubtedly has been written of these two celebrated hospitals than of any others. If one applies the criterion of physicians in attendance, a desideratum that has come to distinguish hospitals from almshouses, neither the Hôtel-Dieu nor St. Bartholomew's is quite as old as often suggested.

French Practices

Tradition places the date of the origin of the Hôtel-Dieu around 650.[6] It was once called the Hospice Saint-Christophe, later the Hospice Notre-Dame. By 1157 it was known as the Maison-Dieu de Paris. In 1184 the Hôtel-Dieu was partially demolished to make room for the Cathedral of Notre Dame then under construction (ca. 1160–1250).

Hospital care with physicians in regular attendance, the true definition of a hospital, would place the origins of the Hôtel-Dieu as a hospital near the beginning of the thirteenth century. Until then medical attention was given only by canons and nuns. In October 1221 a surgeon named Hubert devoted his activities to the Hôtel-Dieu "for charity and the good of his soul." Vincent des Bois, a physician, followed his example in 1231. Regular organized medical care started during the next century. After the fourteenth century patients at the Hôtel-Dieu were cared for by two surgeons appointed by the king and paid from the public treasury; a physician and a midwife were also in attendance. After the fifteenth century the hospital administration regulated and paid for professional services.

The Hôtel-Dieu was the only hospital in Paris before the Renaissance. In 1519 La Charité was built; in 1607, the Hôpital St. Louis. During the Middle Ages the Hôtel-Dieu acquired seven large rooms, having benefited from donations of kings and noblemen and wealthy citizens and through legacies and decrees. By an edict of 1168, for instance, every canon of Notre Dame across the square from the Hôtel-Dieu, on dying, donated his bed to the hospital, literally a mattress of straw with pillows and sheets, or an equivalent value in silver.[7]

The Hôtel-Dieu of the sixteenth century was architecturally a thing of beauty, with two facades. A number of disastrous fires in the eighteenth century, culminating in the holocaust of 1772 which burned for eleven days and took a number of lives,[8] finally necessitated the rebuilding of the hospital, a project which had been discussed repeatedly over the years. The old Hôtel-Dieu was replaced with a less attractive structure. It was called the Grand Hospice d'Humanité during the French Revolution. The Hôtel-Dieu was completely rebuilt in 1877.

In the early days at the Hôtel-Dieu, the brothers and sisters rose at 5:00 A.M. and, after matins, washed the hands and faces of the patients and made their beds. Meals were served twice a day, at 11:00 A.M. and 6:00 P.M. The patients were given meat four times a week. The common dish was mutton soup or stew; eggs, cheese, herring, and dried fish were usually available. Three quarts of milk sufficed for an entire ward for a whole week. Wine was served regularly. Each patient had his own wooden bowl and spoon, a goblet, and a wine pot. Nursing sisters retired at 7:00 P.M., and old women took over for the night to watch the

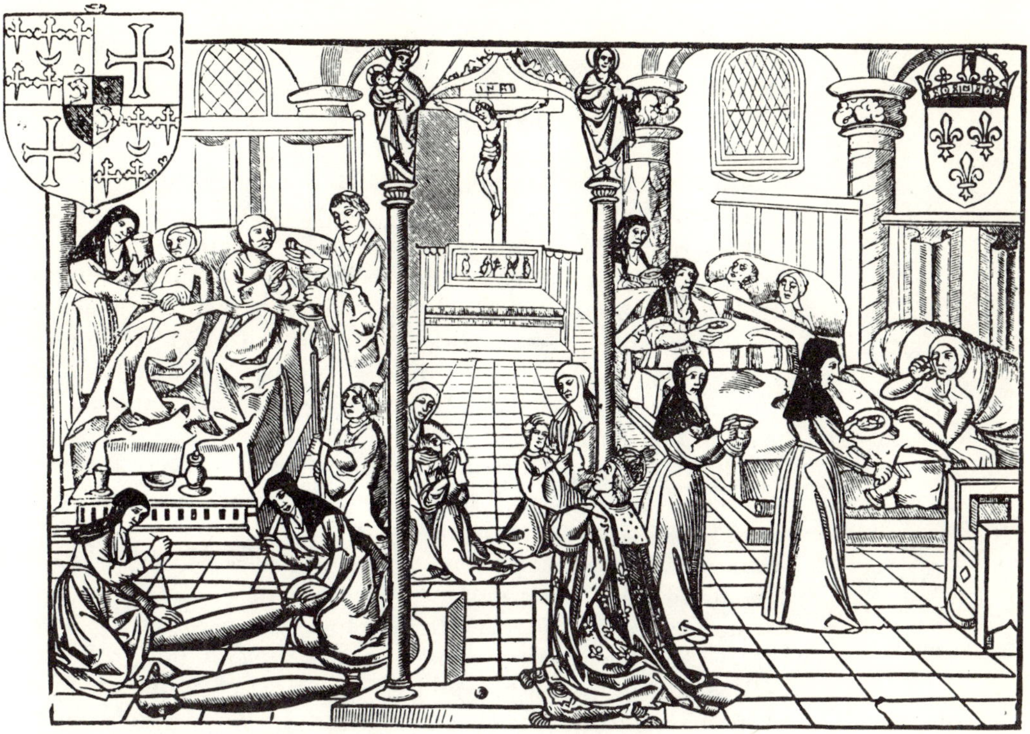

18.1 Early scene, Hôtel-Dieu, Paris. Care of the living and the dead. From a sixteenth-century woodcut reproduced in Casimir Tollet, *Les édifices hospitaliers* (1892). Courtesy National Library of Medicine.

dying and accompany patients to toilets, an onerous duty for there was no system of lighting in the hospital until 1487. The night attendants were given three pints of wine to fortify them for their vigil.[9]

There was no heat in the wards; stoves were provided only for surgical patients and in the maternity wards. In the main, ventilation was good because of the high ceilings. The linen was washed in the Seine River, and the sisters stood in the water to do the washing, even in winter. The river supplied drinking water for the hospital and carried off its waste.

There were 800 to 900 patients daily at the Hôtel-Dieu during the thirteenth century. Ordinarily at least two patients occupied a bed, as was usual in inns for travelers of that period. Also, following the custom of the period, they were naked. Men and women and children were often intermingled in the beds.[10]

During the years 1366–68, according to E. L. Coyecque, 22,500 patients died at the Hôtel-Dieu, or 7,500 each year. By the fifteenth century the number of patients had doubled. The mortality from famine, war, and pestilence averaged 10,000 to 15,000 per year at the hospital; occasionally as many as 30,000 patients died there, never less than 3,000 a year. From 4 to 6 or more patients were crowded together in great beds — the dying, the convalescents, and patients with contagious diseases, together with those only mildly ill. Vermin were frequent. The beds were enclosed by curtains, which were eventually recognized as a sanitation hazard. It was felt by the hospital administrators that the overcrowding was considerably better than allowing prospective patients to die on the street. In 1592 it was estimated that 63,000 patients died of the black death (bubonic plague) in the Hôtel-Dieu. There was considerable venereal disease in the wards by late 1495.[11]

The room for parturient women at the beginning of the seventeenth century was as it had been at the time of François I (1494–1547), cellarlike, eighteen or twenty steps down, on the edge of the Seine, which sometimes overflowed into the delivery room. In 1649 this room was relocated in a segment of the hospital over the bridge; there were four or five women to a bed. In 1663 another move was made to a building on the Left Bank, beneath the ward in which injured patients were hospitalized. In 1664 the delivery quarters were placed in Salle St. Joseph, with windows opening on an arm of the Seine where the hospital latrines converged.[12]

Jacques Tenon in his famous report of 1788 described the miserable state of the Hôtel-Dieu's delivery rooms, where in the years 1776 to 1786 between 1,400 and 1,600 women were delivered annually. Their names were kept in a special register under lock and key to protect the secret of their identity, for many came to hide a birth out of wedlock. No visitors were allowed. Since there were no cribs, the infants were placed in their mothers' beds and were sometimes smothered by the multiple occupants. Most of the deliveries were performed by midwives.[13] Despite the sad situation, the Hôtel-Dieu had the only school for midwives. It was here that Saviard, Mauquest de la Motte, and Levret learned obstetrics.

At the time of the Frondé insurrection during the long reign of Louis XIV there were nearly 4,000 wounded and sick patients at the Hôtel-Dieu, which had optimal accommodations for no more than a quarter that number; 14 patients were reported to have occupied one bed. In the eighteenth century there were 1,219 beds in the hospital, of which 733 were great beds, able to accommodate several patients; the 486 beds for single occupancy were not infrequently filled by two persons. When the

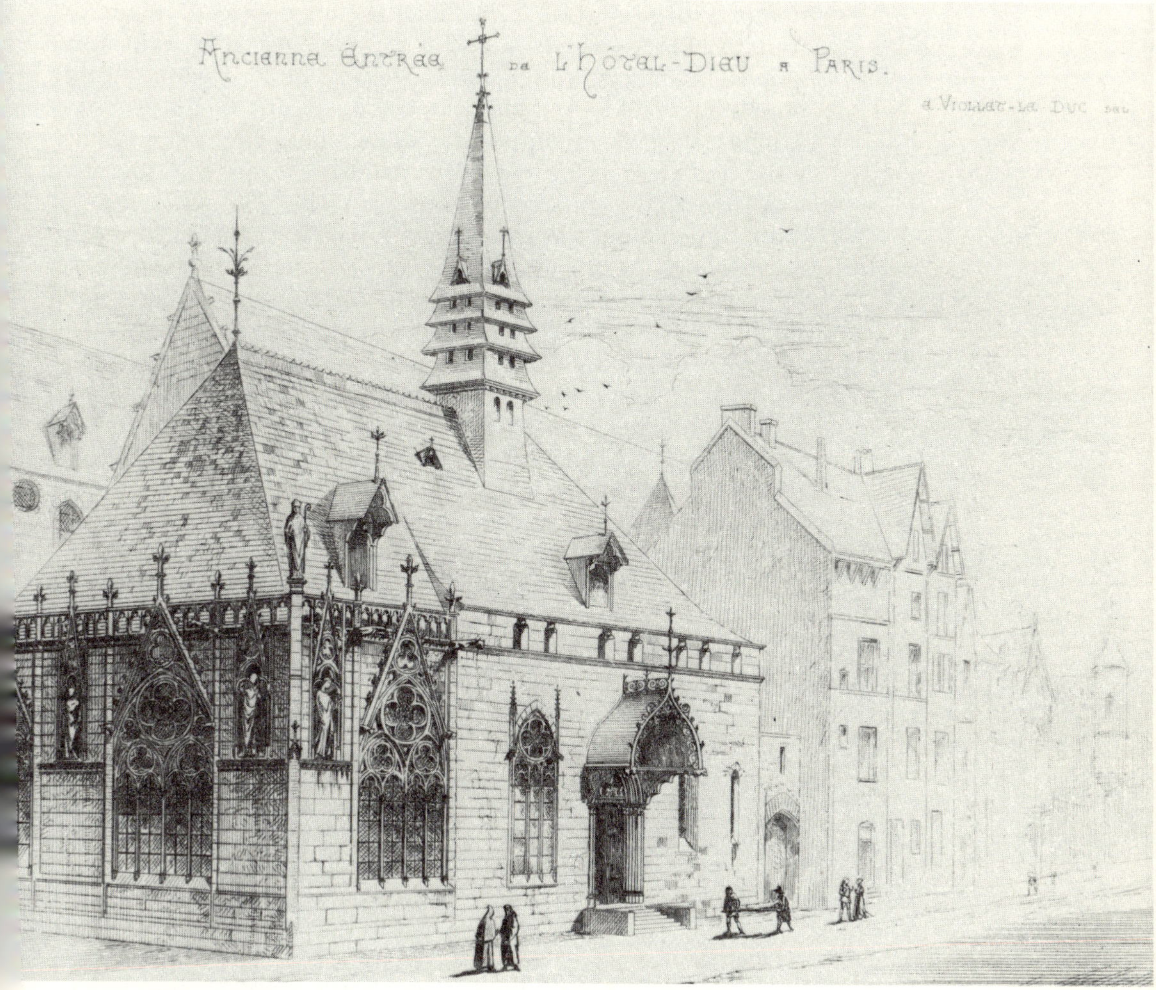

18.2 Entrance to Hôtel-Dieu, fifteenth century, as produced in Armand Husson, *Étude sur les hôpitaux* (1862). Courtesy National Library of Medicine.

straw in the beds was changed, it was heaped in the middle of the room and was carried away in armloads; the odor was terrible. A certain number of beds in each ward were usually set aside for the dying. D'Alembert, writing of the Hôtel-Dieu in the *Encyclopédie* in 1765, said, "It is the largest, has the greatest number of patients, and is the richest and the most frightful of French hospitals." In the late eighteenth century, of every nine patients admitted, two died (22.2 percent mortality).[14]

The younger J. Collins Warren of Boston published a description of a surgical ward at the Hôtel-Dieu from a 1776 unnamed source. There were 106 beds for 273 patients. "The walls were soiled with expectorations and the floors with evacuations of the bowels and bladders, as also with blood and discharges from the wounds. The wood supply and the washing were kept in this ward, and every afternoon there was also an outpatient clinic."[15]

A Paris architect, Bernard Poyet, wrote in 1785 of the need to move and rebuild the Hôtel-Dieu, a recurring theme throughout the eighteenth into the nineteenth century. He said that there were 20 rooms in the present edifice, some large, others small; the large wards accommodated most of the patients. He had counted 1,067 beds, but said he was unable to enter some rooms. The least number of patients in the hospital was 2,000 to 3,000 a day; often there were as many as 4,000 to 5,000 and, in periods of epidemics, the number went up to 7,000. Poyet presented plans for a new circular-form hospital, suggestive of some of today's latest structures, each unit to have only two floors, the second floor to be occupied solely by servants of the hospital. Tenon recommended that each ward have only 24 beds,

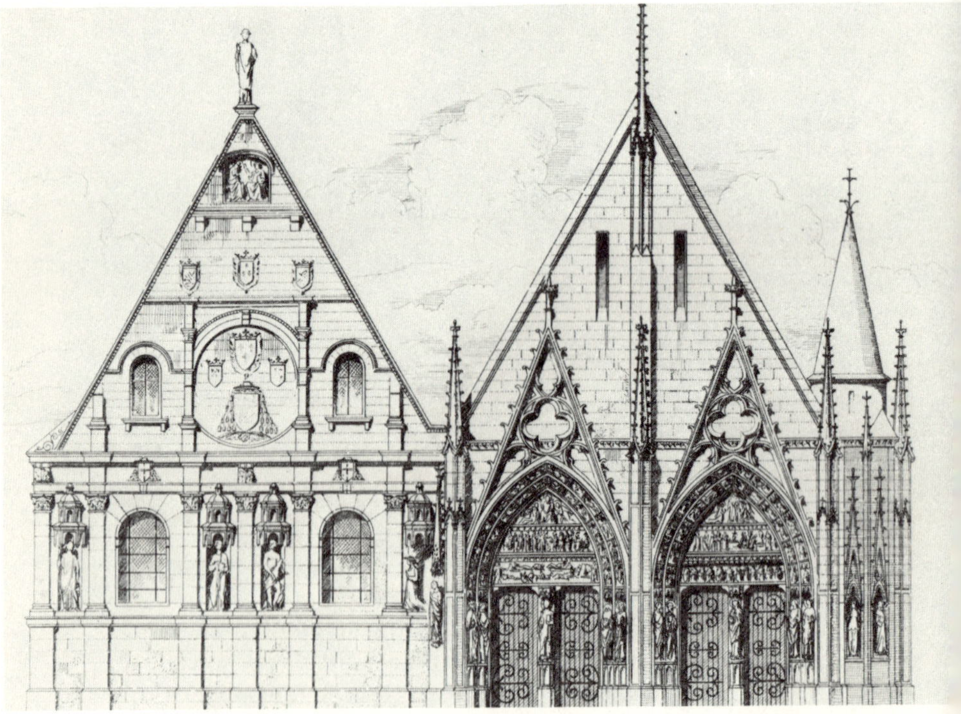

18.3 Facade of Hôtel-Dieu before the fire of 1772. From Husson, *Les hôpitaux*. Courtesy National Library of Medicine.

with separate rooms for patients undergoing operations.[16] He urged the need for pavilion hospitals.

The title page of a pamphlet by Regnier (1789) stated that nearly 100,000 patients had died at the Hôtel-Dieu over the past fifty years, many of whom could have been saved by better hospital administration. Regnier said that after the great fire of 1772 there was much agitation over the location and condition of the hospital; up to 8 patients in a single bed, the sick and the dying mixed with the dead. The beds were provided with feathers instead of mattresses. Some rooms were so dark that bleeding could not be done in them, and the air was offensive to breathe. Almost all the patients, sick or convalescing, walked on bare feet and were bare-legged in the midst of winter. Regnier said he had written the king in 1776 suggesting a plan for reform of the hospitals, urging better administration.[17]

Emperor Joseph II of Austria visited the Hôtel-Dieu in 1777 on his first trip to Paris and manifested his disapproval. On returning to Vienna, the emperor ordered a reform of the Viennese hospitals and sent Hunczovsky to France and England to observe their hospitals. The young surgeon spent two years in France and three months in London studying problems of wound care. He summarized his observations in an extensive treatise (1783), an important source of information on hospital methods of the period. He noted that the Hôtel-Dieu had 1,233 beds and usually 3,000 to 4,000 patients. Repeated bleedings were done for fever, as often as five to seven times in thirty hours. The diet was meager: soup three times a day; 4,000 pounds of bread were baked daily on the premises.[18]

Hunczovsky was extended the privilege of operating during his prolonged visit to French hospitals. He remarked that he had seen patients with compound fractures treated with encouragement of suppuration "almost to the grave." He noted that at La Charité fistula-in-ano was treated by setons rather than with the knife, a procedure apparently preferred by the patients.[19]

The training period for surgeons beyond an internship, he wrote, was a minimum of six years, occasionally as long as fifteen. The senior surgical resident, the *gagnant matrise*, performed considerable surgery and supervised the wound care of 20 to 100 wound surgeons who did the dressings.

In the early days at the Hôtel-Dieu physicians were dominated by the clergy, according to Coyecque. After the thirteenth century the Hôtel-Dieu was essentially a place of practical instruction relating to licensure and achievement of the *robe de maître*.[20]

The names of the Hôtel-Dieu's physicians and surgeons from

the early thirteenth century on have been listed by Coury (1969). As one examines his tabulations, it is obvious that the Hôtel-Dieu surgeons of the early centuries did not match the lustre of those at St. Bartholomew's in London. The first surgeon named is Hubert, already alluded to, who volunteered his services. Jacques Petit (1611–1708) never left the premises of the Hôtel-Dieu during his fifty years of service.[21] Paré was a surgical apprentice at the Hôtel-Dieu for three years (1534–36) but failed to identify a single surgeon of the staff by name in his writings. As a barber-surgeon, he could not qualify as a member of the faculty.[22] It was at least another century before the Hôtel-Dieu had surgeons on its staff known to us because of contributions to their discipline. Yet France had many distinguished surgeons during the period — Lanfranc, Henri de Mondeville of Montpellier and Paris, and Guy de Chauliac in Avignon, the most erudite surgeon of his time, to mention only a few.

It was not until late in the eighteenth century that the Hôtel-Dieu school brought distinction to French surgery. Many notable names appear thereafter.[23] Obviously, other great hospitals of the period were vying for the services of renowned Paris surgeons. In 1780 Louis Desbois de Rochefort (1750–96) organized the first real clinical teaching in Paris at La Charité. Students deserted the Hôtel-Dieu to flock to his clinic. After the Revolution bedside teaching in surgical clinics was organized also at the Hôtel-Dieu. The first years of the nineteenth century Coury characterized as the golden era of French surgery. This was the period when the surgical teaching under Dupuytren eclipsed that of all other departments at the Hôtel-Dieu. His fame was international. The hospital was crowded not only with patients but with visiting students and surgeons from all over the world.

An unidentified German author (1824) wrote that nosocomial cutaneous infections were common at the Hôtel-Dieu. He had seen many patients upon whom Dupuytren had applied six to eight leeches, often as many as thirty, without effect. Suppuration was frequent. In some cases, besides employing leeches, Dupuytren made several incisions in attempts to prevent tissue destruction from phlegmon. The author mentioned an intern whose injured hand was treated with many leeches followed by incisions, but all failed to stop tissue destruction from cellulitis. The author stated that cleanliness at the Hôtel-Dieu was reasonably good, but that the close proximity of beds of patients with chronic ulcer to others was a likely source of contagion.[24]

Ulysse Trélat wrote a critical and historical memoir on hospitals in 1828, relating that at the Hôtel-Dieu overcrowding was a recurring problem before the construction of other community hospitals. The need to accommodate 4,000 to 5,000 patients in far fewer beds had made it mandatory to place 4 to 6 in a bed. The sick and the dying were regularly huddled together. However, by 1843 when the American surgeon Stewart wrote of Paris hospitals, he was able to report of the Hôtel-Dieu: "The double beds have all been suppressed, and single ones of iron substituted. The sexes are likewise accommodated with separate wards, and the diseases classed according to their medical or surgical character."[25]

Georg Cless, a visiting physician from Stuttgart of the same period, wrote in admiration of the Hôtel-Dieu's long wards with waxed floors, rows of iron beds covered with white linen, and the nursing sisters in white and black robes silently performing their ministrations. There were then 1,000 beds; more than 12,000 patients entered the hospital yearly. Cless said that two pots of *tisane* daily (medicinal tea, probably largely barley) was the only nourishment given the acutely ill, and soup was considered the proper diet for convalescents. The patients sometimes complained they were dying of hunger. Quite a contrast to the beef, mutton, and veal allotted patients in the seventeenth century! Another German visitor, the surgeon Hueter, was more critical. He recalled that in 1860–62 in Paris hospitals he had observed "wounds of Navy patients washed regularly from the same wash basin with sponge and water, the basin containing ultimately a mixture of pus from the wounds of the patients, thus spreading wound diphtheria."[26] This untidy and unsanitary practice apparently was almost universal among French, English, German, and American surgeons into the late 1870s.

When the subject of hospital salubrity arose at a session of the French Imperial Academy of Medicine in 1861, it precipitated six months of heated discussion. The debate was triggered by young Léon Le Fort's question on why disarticulation of the hip, although performed in other countries, was rejected in Paris. He backed his report with international statistics and revealed that this formidable operation had been done only once in Paris (by Roux, 1847, unsuccessfully). Noted physicians and surgeons joined the discussions. Some felt that the better hygienic conditions in British hospitals accounted for their lower mortality, justifying the performance of operations too dangerous for Paris. The ailing Malgaigne entered the fray, reiterating that the hospitals of Paris were probably the most detestable in Europe and recalling his shocking revelations of 1842 on the death rate of amputations in Paris. In the end Velpeau said he did not believe the operative mortality was acutally greater in Paris hospitals than elsewhere.[27]

Although much of the emphasis was on ventilation, location, and construction of hospitals, some significant facts were brought out in the Academy sessions. Pierre Chalvet's findings of organic molecules on the rarely washed walls of operating rooms were mentioned, as was the research of Pringle, Ollivier, Bernard Gaspard, and Magendie. The physician Pierre Piorry spoke of the experiments of Chaussier, who found animal materials in expired air and in perspiration and excrement. Piorry stated that the name "septic virus" should be given to these infectious materials which, said he, had formerly been called putridity. The disasters and high mortality in the French army of 1841, Piorry believed, were owing essentially to a septic virus.[28]

Following a presentation by Trélat (1864), the Academy of Surgery also took up the subject of hospital hygiene and, after much debate, reached the conclusion that operative mortality was in direct proportion to omission or disregard of hygienic precepts. It was recommended that the principal guides of Tenon (1788) be followed with regard to hospital practices and construction. The most important facet of the long discussions emerged when the anatomist and surgeon Joachim Giraldes stressed the work of Pringle and Pouteau, saying that the chief danger in hospitals was not the lack of oxygen or the prevalence of carbonic acid in the atmosphere, but such matters as animal exhalations, vegetable spores, and purulent globules on walls and in the atmosphere.[29]

In 1864 Émile Vidal, a Paris physician, concluded that isolation of parturients with infectious diseases was mandatory, as demonstrated by the success of strict isolation in military and marine hospitals. He believed that pavilion hospitals were best for management of infectious fevers. This report came exactly ten years after Spencer Wells in Smyrna strongly advocated isolation, while prominent physicians on the scene in the Crimean War felt there was no need for it. The Lyons surgeon Louis X. Ollier, best known for his arthroplastic work, also (1868) wrote of nosocomial infections. He said that 20 percent of surgical deaths, at times, were owing to erysipelas, and that approximately 7 percent of all hospital deaths were owing to this cause.[30]

In his monograph (1843) on hospitals and surgeons of Paris, Stewart wrote that since the revolution of 1830 the medical profession had become discountenanced in European society, that it was difficult for its members to gain posts of honor or positions in the French government. Very few persons in the upper class of French society entered the practice of medicine, peopled largely by young men from the lower and middle classes for whom the government provided free instruction. Many of the eminent surgeons and physicians of France of this period, said Stewart, came "from the lowest castes of life, and many from the uttermost depths of poverty."[31]

As late as 1637 a Protestant could not be admitted as a student to lectures of the faculties in the University of Paris, a regulation involving both teachers and students. Raynaud (1862), famous French physician, writing of medicine in the time of Molière, said that the first requirement of the University of Paris was the matter of religion: students and faculty must be Catholic. Raynaud related that the Duke of Orleans, brother of King Louis XIII, urged that a certain Brunier, son of a prominent physician and a Protestant, be admitted to the University. The Duke wrote a warm letter of recommendation to the Dean, Hardouin de Saint-Jacques, signing the letter "your good friend, Gaston." The king also joined his brother in the recommendation, but to no avail. By 1648, said Raynaud, some relaxation of this requirement had come about.[32]

Emile Bégin (1880) lamented that hygiene and legal medicine had little or no representation in the faculties of medical schools in France, although, in the persons of Antoine Louis in legal medicine and Vicq d'Azyr in hygiene, France had once enjoyed special strength in these disciplines. Bégin said Vicq d'Azyr proposed a special chair of hygiene for each medical school in France and presented plans for construction of hospitals, advising hospital sizes of fifty to sixty beds. His plans were stopped by the French Revolution, but he set a plan of organization in motion helpful to his successors.[33]

When Jean Rameaux (1839) wrote of the status of hygiene at the beginning of the nineteenth century, he emphasized the role of Johann P. Frank of Vienna in 1778 and alluded to climate, mores, customs, religion, behavior, and temperance as factors of civilization that affected the longevity of a nation's people. William Falconer discussed these suggestions philosophically in a large monograph (1781), arriving at similar conclusions. Frank's *Conseils de salubrité*, the author felt, had great influence on public health in Europe.[34]

Writing of the importance of hygiene in France, Aimé Martin (1803) characterized large cities as "the tombs of the human species." Maintenance of community rules of salubrity, said Martin, demanded police authority for reinforcement.[35]

British Practices

Among the first charitable institutions in England was a leper house founded at Canterbury in the eleventh century by Archbishop Lanfranc, who came with William the Conqueror. Another such haven was established a few years before at Rochester. There are earlier records of hospitals for wayfarers and of refuges for the aged and infirm during the Saxon period; these hostels were often identified with monasteries. There were no inns, and hospitality was a duteous obligation. The earliest London hospital that has survived to the present day is St. Bartholomew's, founded in 1123 in intimate association with an ecclesiastic bishopric and priory. It has been called the "Mother Hospital of the Empire." St. Thomas's, founded in the early thirteenth century, was London's second great hospital; it was moved in 1862 and again in 1871.[36] It too has a famous history. It suffered several bomb attacks with extensive damage to its structure in World War II. Over many years staff members of St. Thomas's and Guy's, founded in 1721, shared hospital privileges, a spirit of permissiveness extended also to students of both institutions; the final separation took place in 1825. Westminster was founded in 1719, St. George's in 1733, and the London in 1740 — a few of London's world-famous hospitals.

The story of St. Bartholomew's begins with Rahere, a courtier and cleric, who went to Rome to do penance for his follies. There he saw a "vision full of dread and sweetness," in which St. Bartholomew directed him to construct a spiritual house in London. On returning, with the aid of the Bishop of London, he sought King Henry I's permission to acquire land in Smithfield for a monastic house and a hospital for the sick poor. This was an area just outside the city walls, where debtors and malefactors once paid for their defections and misdeeds on the gallows, and also the sporting arena for joustings and horseracing. London then was a walled city whose gates were closed at night.[37] Rahere's tomb is in St. Bartholomew's Priory Church, adjacent to the hospital.

St. Bartholomew's survived deprivation of its name and property by Henry VIII (ca. 1535) in the dissolution of religious houses, when monasteries, infirmaries, and hospitals in England came under the possession of "the King and his heirs forever." Over 600 foundations were destroyed. The period was a sequel to Henry VIII's break with the Vatican and the establishment of the Church of England as the country's official religion. Corrupt influences in the hospitals and infirmaries, as well as the king's avarice, contributed to the closures. All the personnel dependent on support from the institutions vanished, including monks, friars, nuns, brotherhoods, sisterhoods, and an army of bakers, brewers, embroiderers, rope-makers, sextons, and others; begging was the sole alternative open to them. The sick were carried to their homes, not alone from St. Bartholomew's Hospital but from many infirmaries too. The problems of state and the decay of trade overshadowed all; the dying and the ill were forgotten. The king proposed a name change of St. Bartholomew's Hospital to "The House of the Poor in West Smithfield in the Suburbs of the City of London of King Henry VIII's foundation." In Acts of Parliament this proposal has been followed, but in the daily life of the hospital St. Bartholomew's retains its original designation.[38]

A few years later the City of London restored the hospital and a period of benefactions by bequest followed, the history of which is to be found in parish records. For centuries the hospital buildings of St. Bartholomew were scattered one-story structures of timber, lath, and plaster. All that now remains of the medieval complex is the tower of St. Bartholomew the Less, a beautiful chapel; the Henry VIII gateway was added in 1702. The hospital was completely rebuilt in the eighteenth century. The new St. Bartholomew's, as planned by the architect James Gibbs, consisted of four buildings of brick with stone facing, four stories each, surrounding an open courtyard or square, called "one of the great, if not the greatest outdoor rooms in England."[39] The cost of rebuilding (1730–59) was defrayed solely by voluntary contributions.

Three surgeons with salaries were appointed in 1549, but no physician is mentioned until 1568. The surgeon Thomas Gale, writing in 1562, said, "I did see in the two hospitals of London called St. Thomas's Hospital and St. Bartholomew's Hospital to the number of three hundred and odd poor people that were diseased of sore legs, sore arms and feet and hands with other parts of the body so sore infected that a hundred and twenty of them could never be recovered without loss of a leg or an arm, a foot or a hand, fingers or toes, or else their limbs crooked so that they were either maimed or else undone for ever." In the years 1645 to 1656 the number of patients occupying beds in the hospital annually averaged 684, with an annual mortality of about 10 percent.

In what had once been free care for all, a number of abuses arose. Some hospital employees demanded fees of entering patients to cover possible future expenses. If a patient died, the beadle would receive a shilling for notifying the patient's friends, the porter a shilling for the certificate to the parish where the patient was to be buried, and the bearers each had to be paid 2 shillings for carrying the body as far as the hospital gate. A shilling was also due the matron for a black cloth which served as a pall, and the steward required a shilling for certifying to the patient's death. These monies, labeled "caution money," apparently were returned if the patient was fortunate enough to survive. Flagrant abuses of this practice led to its revocation. William Marsden, a surgeon, in 1828 organized a crusade setting aside the system of governor's letters which helped patients gain admission to hospital.

In 1678, only 8 outpatients a week could be seen at the hospital; in 1696, the outpatients numbered 50 a week; in 1744, there were 250. By 1878 the number of outpatients seen during the year had risen to 250,000, a figure that was maintained.[40]

In the early days patients were brought water by sisters to wash their faces, hands, and feet. The food was poor but probably no worse than what they had at home.[41] "The brethren themselves slept on a rug upon the floor with a pillow as a concession to human weakness and one or more rugs to cover them; the sisters fared no better," nor did the patients. Later the beds were raised from the ground and curtains were added. A man was hired "to keep them free from bugs." In 1815 iron bedsteads were installed.

Four sisters, professed nuns, were an integral part of the original foundation of St. Bartholomew's; later there were twelve. The number dropped to six after the Great Fire of 1666 had depopulated the city and few patients came to the hospital. By 1686 there were sixteen sisters, thirty-one in 1802. The hospital had thirty-three night nurses, "watchers," who lived outside the hospital, on call. In 1789 John Howard gave a good report of St. Bartholomew's Hospital, stating that each ward had a sister and a nurse. By 1818 the hospital had a regular nursing staff; in 1868 the nurses were no longer required to scrub the wards and passages. A training school for nurses was opened in 1877.[42]

In 1766 an anonymous booklet summarized the contemporary dietary and drug treatment at St. Bartholomew's, St. Thomas's, Guy's, and St. George's. The similarity was striking; twenty-four to fifty pages were devoted by each hospital for the listing of medications, most of which had no specific merit. An antiscorbutic remedy at St. Thomas's Hospital did include oranges; an "excellent dentrifice" at St. Bartholomew's contained myrrh, alum, dragon's blood (a red-colored resin), and cream of tartar whipped into a fine powder. Turpentine was a common ingredient in dressings for wounds or ulcers, and tar was applied to children's "scald heads" (an early term for ringworm).[43]

The number of leeches prescribed by the apothecary shop of St. Bartholomew's had increased from 24,700 in 1821 to 96,300 in 1837. Paget, a member of the hospital staff in 1834, related that leeches were used for nearly all active inflammations and congestions and for injuries of hand, chest, and abdomen and after operations such as hernia or lithotomy. A full hard pulse, hot skin, quickened respiration, and flushed face were enough to justify application of leeches and phlebotomy.[44]

Unlike the Hôtel-Dieu, with its relatively lean professional years in its beginnings, St. Bartholomew's from early days was represented by a succession of men whose careers have withstood the neuter and rust of time. John of Mirfield (d. 1407), a cleric or secular priest residing at St. Bartholomew's, wrote the first known treatise from the hospital, *Brevarium Bartholomei* (1380–95), a compilation from many early authors. This enormous production offers nothing original but gives a good idea of accepted theories and practices in medicine and surgery during the fourteenth century. Mirfield included many popular pre-

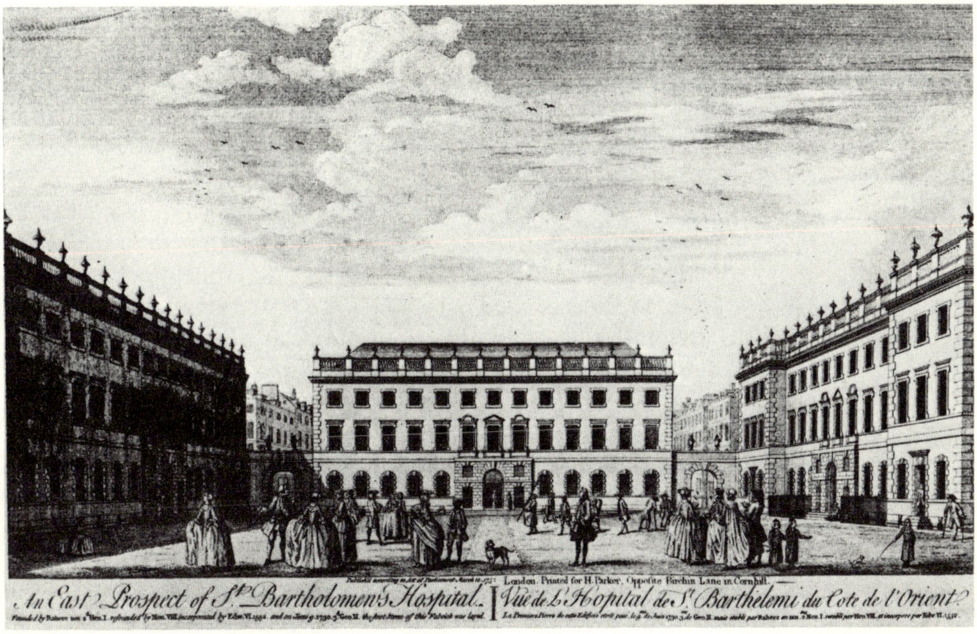

18.4 St. Bartholomew's Hospital (1752).

scriptions, as well as some folk charms and incantations which he did not endorse.[45]

Thomas Vicary, surgeon to Henry VIII, was elected governor of St. Bartholomew's in 1548. He has been immortalized in the portrait by Holbein commemorating the union of barbers and surgeons under Henry VIII in 1540. Clowes, appointed to the staff in 1575, was the hospital's first famous operating surgeon. He published several books on surgical subjects, including one on gunshot wounds (1588) and a monograph on syphilis (1579), in which he related that of every twenty patients admitted to St. Bartholomew's fifteen had syphilis. The naval surgeon Woodall operated at St. Bartholomew's from 1616 until his death. In 1617 he had recognized the value of oranges, lemons, and limes in the treatment of scurvy, more than a century before James Lind's (1753) epoch-making controlled study. Woodall had the enviable record for that day of an amputation mortality not exceeding 20 percent.[46] Harvey (1578–1657) lectured at St. Bartholomew's for more than thirty years and also assumed responsibility for the care of patients in the wards.

Pott, surgeon to St. Bartholomew's for almost forty years, identified coal smoke as the cause of chimney-sweep cancer (1775), an affliction hitherto regarded as hereditary, the first suggestion of a carcinogen. While recovering from an open fracture above the ankle, Pott began to write that remarkable group of durable essays treasured by several generations of readers. Abernethy was a fabulous lecturer, who had the rare quality of making medical students feel their lecturer was the first man in the world and each student second by only a degree. His refusal to interrupt a lecture to respond to an urgent request to see George IV is said to have cost him a royal appointment. In 1796, in operating upon a high-lying femoral aneurysm, Abernethy divided the artery between two ligatures, a truly important innovation. He was elected assistant surgeon to the staff in 1787 and is generally regarded as the real founder of the medical school. Lawrence, who did outstanding work in ophthalmic surgery, was long a member of St. Bartholomew's surgical staff (1824–65), as was Paget (1861–71). Paget was a superb observer, and his descriptions of Paget's eczema of the nipple with subsequent mammary cancer (1874) and of osteitis deformans (1876, 1881) are well known to students of medicine today.[47]

Despite this rich heritage of great names and accomplishments, the surgeons' position at St. Bartholomew's in 1754 has been described as one of "complete thraldom to the physicians." Surgeons examined patients, but apothecaries were not permitted to honor prescriptions of the surgeons save for mercurial purges. Even Pott found he could only prescribe lotions, ointments, and plasters. A lecturer on midwifery was appointed in 1787, but no accoucheur was in charge of beds until 1869. A dentist was appointed in 1836. Ophthalmic surgeons were appointed in 1870, an anesthetist in 1875, an oral surgeon in 1882, a laryngologist in 1906, and a dermatologist in 1908. The orthopedic department started in 1911; there had been bonesetters, however, as early as 1585. Specialization, obviously, was consistently discouraged until late in the nineteenth century.[48]

George Callender, reporting on two years of hospital practice at St. Bartholomew's Hospital in 1873, stated that among 179 operations there were 5 deaths (2.8 percent mortality); among 17 amputations there were no fatalities, nor among 22 compound fractures. He commented, that "in a limited way," antiseptic treatment was used very generally.Washing and cleansing traumatic wounds with carbolic acid lotion or with chloride of zinc was common practice, as was use of balsam of Peru for open sores. In 1878 Callender observed that, whereas pyemia had been completely eliminated, an occasional case of erysipelas still appeared. He said mortality after operation was only a tenth of what it had been in comparatively recent years. Among 100 compound fractures, there were only 2 deaths. According to Holmes Coote (1870), erysipelas remained one of the scourges of hospitals, indicating its occurrence was largely influenced by the presence of many suppurating wounds. He said the surgical staff at St. Bartholomew's Hospital was then divided with reference to use of antiseptics and disinfectants. Some advised restraint in their use.[49]

Hospital Critics

Tobias Smollett (1721–71), a well-known Scottish novelist, graduated in medicine and at one time practiced in London. He helped William Smellie write the third edition of his treatise on midwifery. In his *Adventures of Roderick Random* (1748) and *Peregrine Pickle* (1753) Smollett exposed the deplorable conditions of hospital ships and censured apothecaries, physicians, and surgeons for taking no heed of public welfare. He scoffed at the situation at Bath, where children with large cutaneous ulcers were allowed to bathe with others. Continued Smollett, "I am as much afraid of drinking the water as bathing in it." He believed that regurgitation of water from the bath into the cistern drinking water was a real possibility. This was the period when the water supply was so unhealthy that children at school were encouraged to drink beer and wine; moreover, the water was believed to invite vesical calculi.

William Hogarth, Thomas Rowlandson, George Cruikshank, and other famous English artists of the eighteenth and nineteenth centuries used their talents to satirize cultural and medical evils of the day.

Charles Dickens (1812–70) also lampooned the medical profession. His characterization of the midwife, Sarah Gamp, in *Martin Chuzzlewit* (1844) attached a critical label to hospital nursing of that period, which Moynihan believed still lingered in memory as late as 1921, attaching an unjust obloquy to the word "nurse."[50]

Treves related (1919) that he entered the London Hospital in 1871, became a house surgeon in 1876 and an assistant surgeon in 1879. Nursing at the hospital, no worse than at other London hospitals, said Treves, was "deplorable and, from any standpoint, very bad nursing was a calling for the derelict. . . . There was only one sponge in the ward, and with this deadly instrument, the nurse — who was not always sober — washed every wound in the evening, using not only the same sponge, but the same basin and water." The discontinuance of these absurd wound practices obviously was the primary responsibility of the surgical staff. Treves wrote in glowing terms of the nursing supervisor, Miss Luckes, aged twenty-four, who made nursing at the London Hospital after 1880 a respectable and effective enterprise through the simple device of complete dedication to her task.[51]

The *Lancet* (1865) established its own Sanitary Commission to investigate the state of infirmaries and workhouses in London, noting that important changes for the better had come about in recent years, in which "the medical profession has borne an active part." In its report the commission alluded to the vast differences in the support of national hospitals, infirmaries, and workhouses, the latter being the subject of neglect. Reported the commission, "in truth, the whole business is a sham, . . . Our voluntary hospitals can but lightly touch the surface of the wide field of London misery." The commission singled out the scandalous conduct of night nurses for special criticism — "*nothing* will make them quite safe and reliable."

The commission (1874) expressed satisfaction with the status of the surgical wards of St. Bartholomew's Hospital. Their report stated that one sister and three nurses were assigned to every twenty-eight surgical cases during the day and one nurse at night. The house surgeon was solely responsible for all opera-

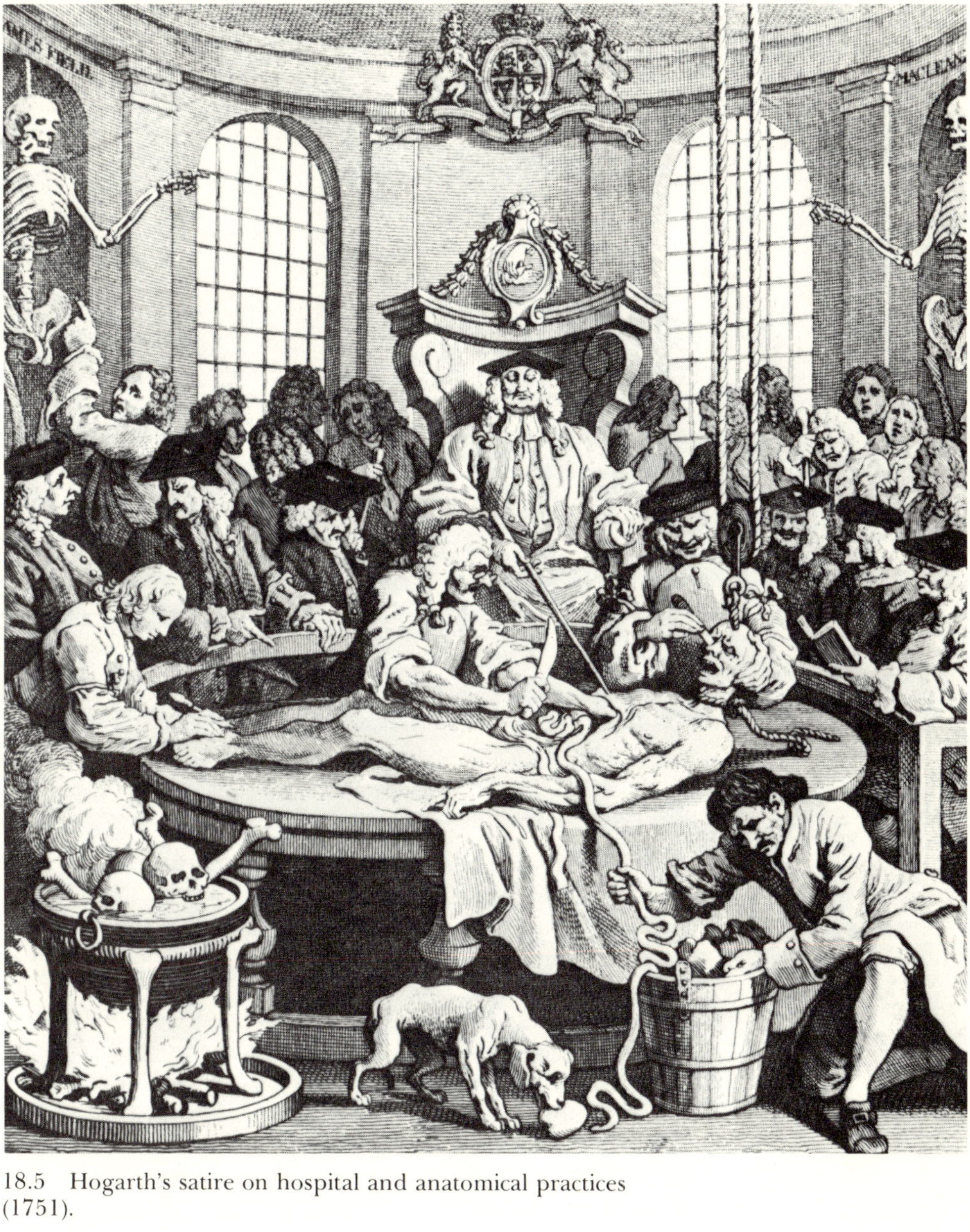

18.5 Hogarth's satire on hospital and anatomical practices (1751).

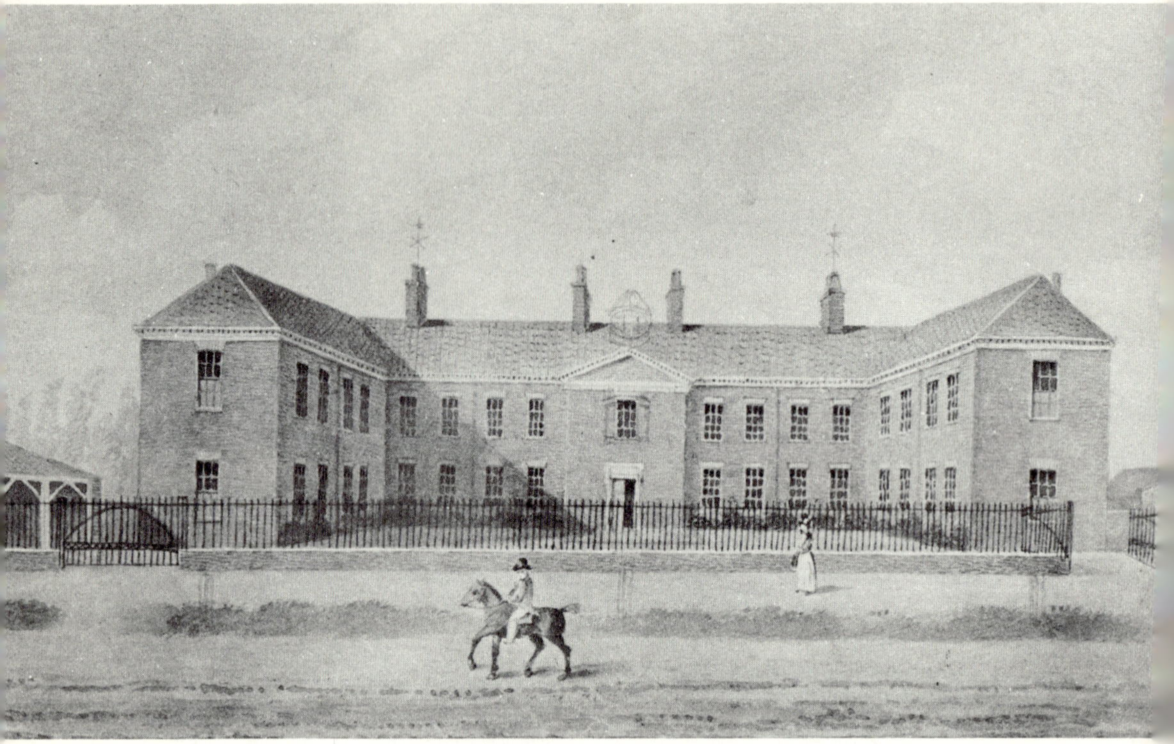

18.6 Norfolk and Norwich Hospital (1772). Lithograph by James Sillet in Norwich Castle Museum. Courtesy A. Batty Shaw and Norfolk Museums Service.

tive cases for a week after their performance, the dressers assisting. However, Callender saw his patients every day and dressed the wounds himself for the first few days, or personally superintended dressing changes. The commission said the five dressers at St. Bartholomew's were greatly overworked, their number being inadequate to attend to large numbers of inpatient surgical cases; moreover, they had no decent accommodations within the hospital, despite the circumstance that they were on twenty-four-hour duty. The commission concluded by saying that ventilation and observance of hygiene and well-known rules of surgery "are the chief factors in successful treatment of surgical cases in St. Bartholomew's Hospital."[52]

Specialty Hospitals

St. Peter's Hospital for Stone was founded in 1860. In the June 16th issue of the *British Medical Journal* an editorial appeared labeled "Hospital Distress," charging that special hospitals were founded primarily to benefit aggressive self-serving individuals and not primarily for humanitarian purposes. The chief objection from the profession stemmed apparently from the circumstance that general hospitals were deprived of segments of good teaching material that drifted into the special hospitals and their outpatient departments.[53] Specialty hospitals usually develop strong staffs of clinicians that advance the stature of their specialty. Similar complaints had been previously leveled against Moorfield's Ophthalmic Hospital, St. Mark's Hospital for Rectal Diseases, and Woman's Hospital under the direction of Sims in New York City. A surprisingly large number of great surgeons in their specialties were trained at St. Peter's Hospital for Stone and at St. Mark's for Rectal Diseases.

Hospitalism

Simpson (1869) coined the word "hospitalism" to characterize prevailing unsanitary conditions in which patients newly entered contracted erysipelas and other contagious diseases. He was one of many surgeons of that period who believed that hospitals should be periodically destroyed. Syme repudiated the designation "hospitalism," believing it damaged public confidence in hospitals.

Erichsen (1859) of the University College Hospital wrote that erysipelas in hospitals could be transmitted by instruments, ward nurses, and surgeons. In a later paper (1874) he defined hospitalism as a "septic influence capable of infecting a wound or of affecting the constitution injuriously." Erichsen alluded to Le Fort of Paris who commented on the maternal mortality of parturients. Said Le Fort, of 900,000 women delivered in hospitals, the mortality rate was 3.4 percent; of 1 million delivered in their homes, the mortality was 1 in 112 or 0.9 percent, 38 times greater among women delivered in hospitals. Erichsen related that the mortality of ovariotomy in British general hospitals was 60 to 80 percent, in the hands of surgeons like Keith and Spencer Wells only 18 to 24 percent. Erichsen was unwilling to concede that differing hospital mortalities were explicable solely on matters of hospital size. He emphasized overcrowding and suppurating wounds as primary causes of hospitalism. Erichsen (1874) knew of the work of Semmelweis (1847) and the striking reduction in maternal mortality he achieved among parturients at the Vienna General Hospital. Erichsen stressed avoidance of participation in postmortem examinations and the necessity of washing the hands with a solution of chloride of lime before participating in delivery of parturients.[54] It is strange, indeed, that he did not apply the Semmelweis techniques to operative surgery.

William Farr (1864), the statistician who aided Miss Nightingale in her drive for hospital accountability of mortality, crossed swords in a running debate with Timothy Holmes, a well-known St. Thomas's surgeon, on the matter of hospital and surgical mortality. Farr said there were those who claimed "the mortality of patients in hospitals may be, and in fact is, increased by the fame of the surgeons, by the selection of cases, and by a variety of causes; but that hygienic conditions is a matter of subordinate importance, if it is of any importance whatever, in these populous houses full of the sick."[55]

German Practices

When German physicians of the thirteenth and fourteenth centuries went abroad to improve their orientation in medicine, they frequently went to Padua and Bologna, the principal seats of medical scholarship in that period. They also went to Montpellier in France, rarely to Paris.[56]

In his monograph on hospitals and lazarettos Virchow (1869) provided an interesting history of old hospitals. Concerning

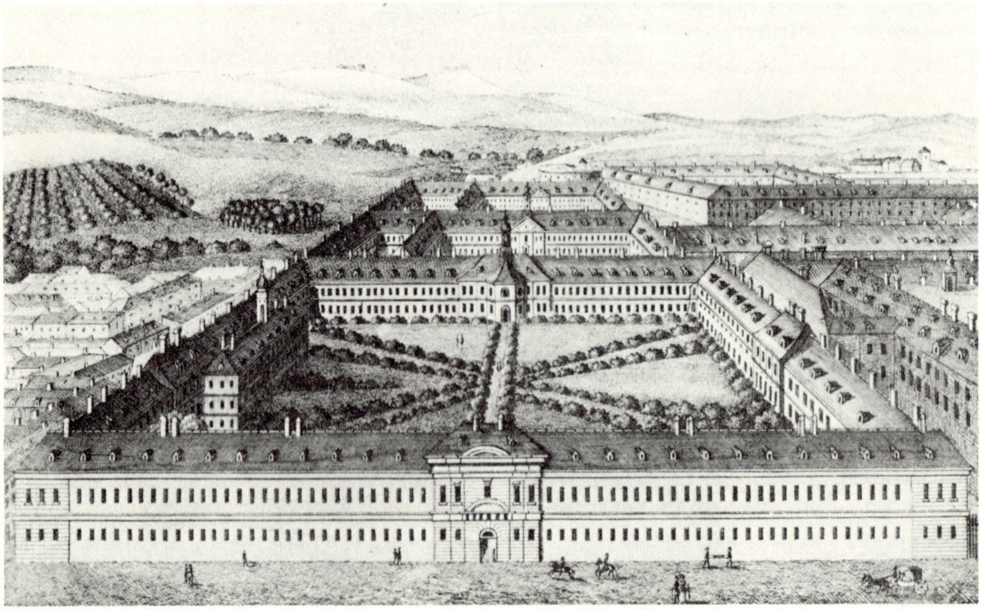

18.7 Vienna's Allgemeines Krankenhaus (ca. 1800).

hospital care of patients and sanitation, he recommended "before all, a good and abundant air and an abundant, ample supply of good water, and good food"; he added, "These help more in many cases than all medical endeavors or, more correctly said, air, water, and food are of more importance than the physicians and the nurses who are the soldiers in the care of the sick."[57] Virchow obviously missed the hard evidence brought forward by Semmelweis of the efficacy of prophylactic antisepsis in the prevention of puerperal fever. In fact, Virchow labeled Semmelweis as "the chap who speculates"; nor was Virchow then ready to accept Listerian precepts.

Ignaz Neudörfer (1869) believed one reason mortality was higher in large city hospitals was because autopsies were performed there, whereas country surgeons did not go directly from necropsies to patients. Lister's practices, said he, had not controlled hospitalism; Neudörfer's suggested remedy was that hospitals admit fewer patients and have a surgeon on hand to receive them.[58]

A. M. Adam, a Scotsman (1860), wrote of his experience on visiting the General Hospital in Munich. He was impressed that the floors received a new hard varnish once a year; the clinical wards had a similar finish twice a year because of the large number of students who daily trod the floors. Adam observed that at the Vienna Hospital only the floors of Josef Skoda's wards were varnished. He remarked that Florence Nightingale too was partial to this practice for hospital wards. Authorities at the Munich Hospital had resisted the introduction of iron bedsteads, patients complaining they were cold, although conceding they were less likely to harbor vermin than wooden bedsteads. Meanwhile the patients slept in those "immemorial wooden boxes which the Germans dignify by the name of beds." Hospital mortality at the Munich General Hospital was 5 percent, perhaps the lowest in Europe at the period.

Munich was the first city in Europe to establish an obstetrical hospital, in 1589, as did Paris in the seventeenth century, Dublin and London in 1745, and Vienna in 1752. The Munich Lying-in Hospital had been rebuilt in 1856, with good ventilation, and wards of six beds each, yet the mortality of puerperal fever was high in the hospital, traceable in some instances to obstetrical assistants performing postmortems. Adam knew and approved of Semmelweis's practices and alluded to F. H. Arneth's paper on the subject in the Edinburgh *Monthly Journal of Medical Science* of June 1851 and to the discussion on puerperal fever at the

Edinburgh Medico-Chirurgical Society in June and July 1851, including remarks by Simpson.[59]

Friedrich Oppert (1859) of the Polyclinic in Berlin warned against overcrowding and advocated high ceilings for improved ventilation. He noted that central heating was rarely available in English and German hospitals, fireplaces being the conventional source of heat in English wards, and *kachelofens*, large wood- or coal-burning stoves, in Germany. Oppert advised that food in hospitals be cooked in large copper kettles at 1 or 2 atmospheres of pressure, not in iron kettles that lose their heat when the food is allowed to stand. In a subsequent paper (1868) he cited progress in sanitary improvements in many hospitals.[60]

In a small monograph C. L. Hoffmann (1788) wrote of the justification of one patient to a bed. The author lived in Mainz and stated he wrote his papers against the teachings of Dr. Karl Strack, a teacher at the University of Mainz. Hoffmann also made a plea for postmortem examinations in hospitals, indicating that the permission of the doctor for the postmortem should be sought. He implied that some doctors did not desire postmortem examinations on their patients, feeling that errors might be uncovered.[61]

A physician (1877), identifying himself only as W. H. W., reported in Cincinnati's *Clinics* observations on Berlin hospitals of a period in which pavilion structured hospitals were popular in Germany, built in pleasant surroundings with shrubs and trees. The reporter anticipated finding a high level of acceptance of such institutions, but, said he, "the unfortunate of Berlin have no more love for the public house of the sick than in our country!"[62]

In writing of wound care in the military hospitals of Mannheim and Weissenburg in the Franco-Prussian War of 1870, Billroth related how the nurses went from patient to patient and bed to bed with a wash basin and a sponge to wash and swab the wounds of patients. The water quickly assumed the appearance of a mixture of blood and pus. Billroth (1872) wrote that he preferred wound irrigation but had difficulty enforcing the practice. He spoke with great warmth of the devotion of the nurses despite their dangerous practices in wound care. Billroth favored a plan in which the nurses were directly responsible to surgeons rather than to nursing authority. A table of organization obviously was lacking; acceptable principles of wound care had not been elucidated and the majority of surgeons probably still approved washing wounds in the manner carried out by the nurses. Billroth had not yet accepted antiseptic practices, favoring open wound treatment. At the Rudolf Virchow Hospital in Berlin, which had thirty to forty hospital pavilions, the house staff made rounds on bicycles as the distance between the pavilions was great.[63]

Many university clinics provided 300 beds for the professor of surgery. Separate and independent hospitals for each clinical discipline was the accepted administrative procedure. During this surgeon's tour (1927–28) of Central Europe Payr had 500 surgical beds at Leipzig. In addition, professors of surgery usually had a private clinic nearby of 50 or more beds at which too often was spent a disproportionate part of the professor's time, certainly not an exemplary pattern of commitment for young surgical house officers to emulate; this was also a practice and involvement that impaired the professor's opportunity to contribute to the patrimony of his discipline.

Listerian practices found general acceptance earlier in Germany than elsewhere, owing to their advocacy by two esteemed professors of surgery, Volkmann (1874) of Halle and Nussbaum (1875) of Munich. Hegar of Freiburg (1876–77) was the first to adapt Semmelweis's prophylactic surgical antisepsis to abdominal surgery, performing fifteen successive ovariotomies without mortality, a great achievement for that period.

Following the observations and experiments of Pasteur and Chamberland (1878–79) and of Koch (1881), substituting thermal for chemical aspects of antisepsis, Neuber of Kiel (1883) adapted these methods for the preparation of operating gowns and operative materiel in practical surgery, techniques accepted and extended by Bergmann (1889) and Schimmelbusch (1892) in Berlin. These practices gave German surgeons a definite lead in extending the borders of surgery, achieving results that convinced laggard surgeons of other nations, slow to accept prophylactic surgical antisepsis, of their folly.[64]

American Practices

The Pennsylvania Hospital in Philadelphia, the oldest American hospital still functioning, came into being in the mid-1750s, two decades before the American Revolution and a decade before Philadelphia's first medical school (1765). New York's Bellevue Hospital began as a prison and almshouse in 1811 and qualified as a hospital in 1850. Boston's Massachusetts General, one of America's most venerable hospitals, originated in 1811 and became functional in 1821.

Anesthesia was on trial when Stephen Smith (1823–1922) was

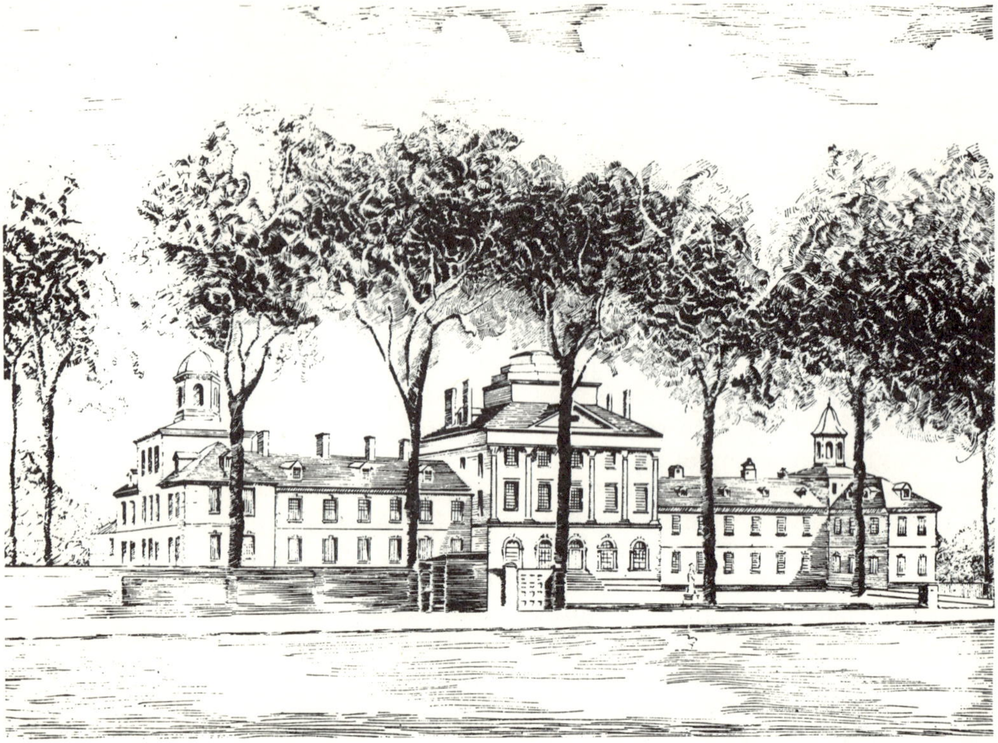

18.8 Philadelphia's Pennsylvania Hospital (1766). Gift of Robert Rosenthal, St. Paul pediatrician.

a medical apprentice in Buffalo in 1847 and his preceptor, Hamilton, was conservative over its employment because some deaths had attended its use. The shocking cruelty of operations without anesthetics almost drove Smith from the profession. Seventy years later he described one of his first experiences, illustrating the conventional practice of the time: A workman with a strangulated hernia was placed on the operating table without any preparation other than removal of his exterior clothing and sponging the surface over the hernia. The surgeon came in haste, without a hospital apron; several attendants held the patient down; there was a conspicuous display of the knife as the first incision was made with frightening rapidity, followed by violent screams and struggles. Later amid shrieks a second incision was made. Finally the patient, worn out by the struggles and shock, yielded; all parties were completely exhausted.[65]

By the early 1850s, when Smith entered Bellevue Hospital as a junior member of the resident staff, it had become an important surgical hospital. His duty was to carry the "pus-pail." Wound dressings, saturated with pus, were changed as often as three times daily. Smith said, "Good pus was thick like cream and was called 'laudable pus,'" believed to indicate healthy healing. Celerity being the order of the day in operating, all preparations were made with that object in mind. Instruments were placed for ready availability without any special cleansing; if dropped during operation they were used again. The patient was often put on the table unbathed and grimy with dirt; superfluous hair was sometimes shaved off. The only preparation of the surgeon's clothes were measures to keep them from getting soiled. Hands and fingernails were not prepared and assistants came from other ward duties with hands dirtied from multiple sources. Casual onlookers at operation were permitted to introduce unclean fingers into wounds. Sponges were merely washed. Sutures were carried in convenient pockets or buttonholes. Ligatures were left long, one end emerging from the wound.[66]

Robert Weir (1838–1927) has written a chatty account of how wounds were managed at the New York Hospital in 1856 when he started there at age eighteen as assistant to the "junior walker." It is essentially a repetition of Smith's experiences at Bellevue, and much like Treves's description of wound therapy at the London Hospital at a somewhat later period (ca. 1870), and Billroth's experience in the Franco-Prussian War. The senior walker was expected to lay out the required instruments, which were stored on a velvet-lined shelf. These he placed on a table and covered with a towel. The sponges, washed out from a previous operation, were kept in a wooden pail of fresh water and were handed to the surgeon during the operation by one of the walkers. "Sometimes" the surgeons and house surgeons washed their hands before operations; however, they did put on clean aprons or gowns, and did not wear, as did many British surgeons, "old coats, stained by the bloody daubs of previous operations." The skin of patients to undergo thigh amputation for compound fracture was washed "with the nice-looking sponges that were filled with disease germs from previous operations which had been quietly multiplying while resting in their pailful of water. Fingers, laden with germs in large quantities on them or under the nails, were stuck into the wounds we made and we further introduced . . . infections and often fatal germs by the brilliant and apparently clean instruments we employed." Blood vessels were tied with strings left long, protruding out of the wound. Weir said that before acceptance of Listerian practices, compound fractures of the lower extremities had a mortality of over 38 percent; for major amputations involving the larger extremities, it was 28 percent.

Weir and William T. Bull made a tour of the great hospitals of Europe in the late 1880s to note what improvements had followed adoption of Listerian methods. They "saw and learned a good deal, but returned with a conviction reaffirmed that American surgery occupied as high a level as that of any country."[67]

In Philadelphia Edwin Maxson (1868) regarded the Blockley, later called the Philadelphia General, as an excellent hospital, and the surgical treatment at the Pennsylvania Hospital as superior to any. The new Episcopal with ten acres of ground, modeled after the Lariboisière in Paris, said Maxson, was probably the best hospital in this country, perhaps anywhere.[68] Maxson obviously failed to note the deficiencies in ward and wound care observed by Smith and Weir at New York hospitals of the same period.

From a diary he had kept as resident physician in the years 1883–84, Arthur Bliss (1916) compiled a story of Old Blockley. Antisepsis, said Bliss, was unknown; instruments used in operations were not sterilized nor were dressings. When an instrument was dropped on the floor, it was wiped with a towel and returned for use. Surgeons and assistants wore ordinary street or house clothes. Residents wore uniforms of blue with brass and gold bands; one uniform did for a whole year's service and was "far from surgically clean."

A member of the staff returned from London, where he had observed Lister's work, and tried to initiate Lister's techniques at Old Blockley; colleagues smiled forbearingly but continued their old practices. No wound healed by first intention, but most wounds healed after a long process of suppuration. Puerperal fever was so common that a ward set aside for the purpose had its beds completely occupied. During his term on the obstetrical service, Bliss employed utmost cleanliness in delivery procedures and observed no instance of puerperal fever.[69]

Sea sponges for wound care at the Woman's Hospital in New York in 1891 were bought by the pound. They were put in bags and beaten, then energetically kneaded in water to get rid of shells and spicules until the water came off clean. The sponges were then soaked twenty-four hours in a solution of strong hydrochloric acid, placed under a stream of running water, kneaded again until free of foreign matter, and stored in an aqueous solution of phenol. After use, the sponges were washed in cold water and kept forty-eight hours in a jar of ammonia (1:6 water), then transferred to running warm water until clear, and placed in a solution of carbolic acid (1:20). Sponges were discarded after two or three weeks of use; all sponges contaminated with pus or suspicious matter were burned. Silk, linen, and silver wire sutures were wound around glass reels that had been in a bichloride solution; the loaded reels were boiled in water one hour, then kept in a solution of alcohol.[70]

During his Bellevue days in New York in the mid-1880s Halsted operated in a tent, believing the hospital unsafe for operations, a practice reminiscent of field conditions in the American Civil War.[71]

In 1901 a committee of the Medical Board of Bellevue Hospital reported upon problems involving administration, nurses, food, costs, and living quarters for employees and full-time professional house staff. Many of the latter could not be accommodated in the hospital; on the hospital premises three lived in a room and occasionally five or six, "a state of affairs incompatible with the highest grade of work in the extremely exacting position in which these men are placed . . . who, without pay, are constantly facing grave emergencies." In England, in John Simon's day, apprentices paid their surgical teachers approximately 100 guineas annually for the privilege of assisting; they usually lived with their teacher, being permitted to enter by the backdoor. The committee complained that the per diem cost for ward patients was by far the lowest in New York City, a mere \$1.21.[72]

In considering the air of the operating room as a possible factor in the infection of wounds, Hunter Robb of Cleveland (1909) was anxious to learn whether it was safe to use an electric fan on hot summer days. He came to the conclusion that a fan does not substantially augment the bacterial count. According to his report, before the morning operative session, the floors of the operating room were mopped with a 1:1,000 bichloride solution ($HgCl_2$); basins, tables, and so forth were washed in a 1:20 carbolic solution. Robb's pour-plates of solidified agar were set out, usually twelve to twenty in number, for the tests. These were then incubated for forty-eight hours, and the colonies were counted and the bacteria identified by histological study or by pathogenicity studies in guinea pigs, rabbits, or mice. The pour-plates did reveal a significant diminution in bacterial colony counts when the floor of the operating room was mopped and washed just before start of operations and setting out of the plates. Actually, when the floor was washed with a 1:20 aqueous solution of carbolic acid before starting operations, the bacterial counts were much less than when bichloride was used. When the floors were neither mopped nor washed before surgery, the colony counts were significantly greater. When no antiseptic at all was used on the floor and no fans were running, even so, the bacterial counts on the pour-plates were great.[73]

An inquiry was lodged in 1835 to ascertain why erysipelas was so prevalent in the surgical wards of the New York Hospital. Rearrangement of the wards, improved cleanliness, and additional nurses had an immediate beneficial effect; fourteen years later hospital gangrene made its appearance and matters were again out of hand. Another inquiry followed. With better ventilation, heating, and other items, the situation improved, but a good quality of protection for patients came only when prophylactic surgical antisepsis became the vogue in the last fifteen years of the nineteenth century.[74]

Chicago's Cook County Hospital came into being in 1863 and moved in 1866 to the renovated City Hospital building, later referred to as the Old County Hospital. Its facilities were originally shared by Rush and Chicago medical colleges. Much political maneuvering continued to pursue the hospital well into the twentieth century. There was no microscope in the hospital in 1870 and no clinical laboratory, save that of the pharmacist. The interns, said William Quine, "had friendly relations with laudable pus." Puerperal fever was rampant. Walls and ceilings were freshly whitewashed and scrubbed with antiseptic solutions, "but the old deadly ignorance of personal transmission of infection continued."[75] The Chicago surgeon Andrews (1869) had written in the *Examiner* lauding use of antiseptic dressings in wound management, a practice not to find general acceptance at the hands of American surgeons until a decade and a half later.[76] The old Cook County Hospital was replaced in 1913 by a new structure designed to house 5,000 patients.

After the American Civil War Christian Fenger (1814–84), trained as a pathologist in Denmark, came to have great influence in the Chicago area. Fenger was not remarkable as an operating surgeon, but his teachings and dedication to improving medical education brought into being in that area an extraordinary group of men in all the disciplines of medicine, who played significant roles in upgrading greater medicine in the Midwest, a succession of individuals who lent impetus to medicine's growth at the international level.[77]

Management of the wounds of trauma and gunshot and other obligatory operations were the special role of surgeons before general acceptance of prophylactic surgical antisepsis and high standards of cleanliness in the mid-1880s. When the American Surgical Association, the most prestigious of surgical meetings in the United States, convened in 1882, only James Cabell of Charlottesville spoke out forcefully in defense of Listerian antisepsis, as did B. A. Watson of Jersey City in 1883. Most were opposed. "It deserves notice," said Cabell, "that every person who denounced Listerism in the discussion in Philadelphia 1876, took credit to himself for never having tried it."[78] Skepticism persisted in Britain and in the United States into the mid-1880s, long after acceptance of antiseptic practices throughout Germany in the mid-1870s.

A special feature of American medicine has been the development of large clinics staffed with specialists with expertise in their respective disciplines. The Mayo brothers, William and Charles, in Rochester, Minnesota, set the pattern in the first decades of this century; in its beginnings the clinic was predominantly surgical in nature. Moreover, the Mayos were the first to see to it that all patients had a complete physical examination, long before it became standard practice even in university

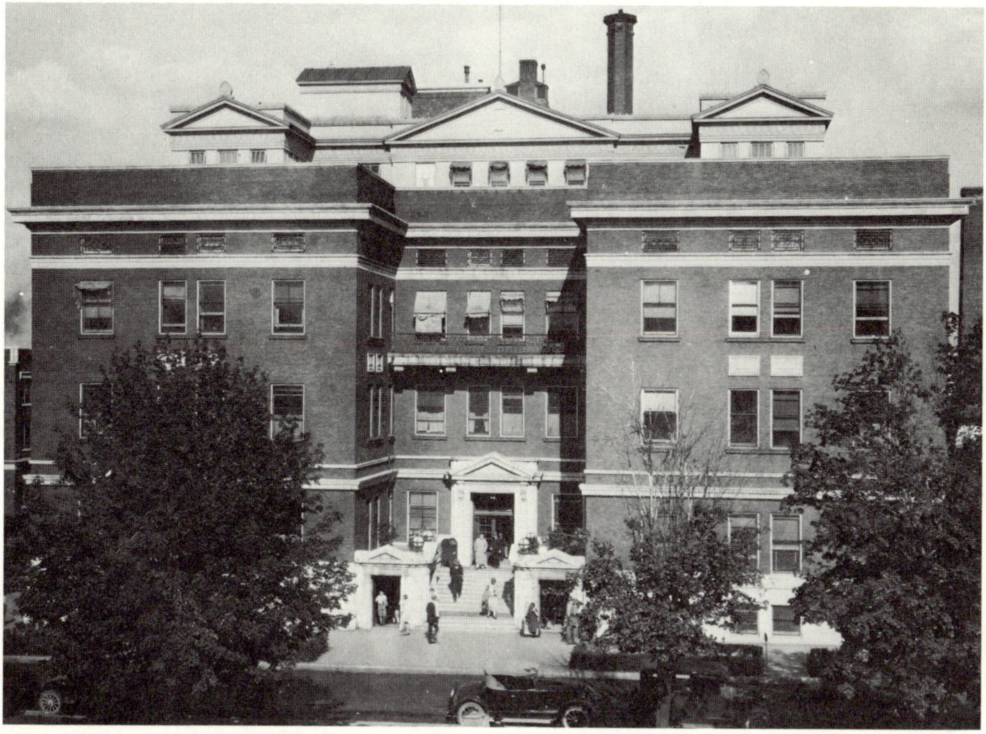

18.9 Mayo Clinic building, Rochester, Minnesota (ca. 1914).

clinics. Group practice has been widely accepted throughout our country, typified by such well-known institutions as the Crile (Cleveland), Lahey (Boston), Henry Ford Hospital (Detroit), and Alton Ochsner (New Orleans) clinics. The scheme, if proliferated throughout the United States, undoubtedly offers the finest type of medical service and probably too at lesser cost in money and manpower than does the promise of a physician in every hamlet in our country. Paramedical care, involving nurses and technicians attached to hospitals and clinics, will certainly provide readier access to primary care of patients in future years.

Only in the last decade of the nineteenth century did hospitals, through improved accomplishment, capture the confidence of the public. Actually, esteem of the public hospitals in America came only with the fruits of intensive research following the largess of Congress after World War II, in which development President Roosevelt, Vannevar Bush, Lister Hill, John Fogarty, James Shannon, and a great number of innovative and creative researchers played significant roles.

Hospital Construction

John Shaw Billings was a keen and ardent student of hospital construction. His views of 1870, 1875, and 1889 reflected a progressive change in attitude, with less emphasis in the final years upon a need for pavilion hospitals. The primary focus on ventilation declined as the germ theory of disease encountered wider acceptance among medical men.

In 1870 Billings had advised construction of temporary hospitals, an attitude probably influenced by J. J. Woodward's Circular No. 6, published on conclusion of the American Civil War (1865), in which Woodward stressed the role of barracks and the low mortality attending hospitalization. In his 1875 report on plans for the future Johns Hopkins Hospital Billings indicated that his 1870 statement had been far too sweeping. He added, the question of the number of stories in the hospital is a different matter than that of permanence. He believed then that 75 percent of patients should be cared for in two-story structures, that patients with infectious diseases should be segregated. The interests of medical schools and their hospitals are inseparable, he said, their first duty being high-quality service to patients, then education of physicians and nurses and the promotion of the science and art of medicine. Ventilation for all seasons Billings regarded as very important. Hospitalism, said Billings, arises from impure air and minute particles from the bodies of patients, harboring disease germs of great vitality. Dilution of the air, he said, will not give security nor will disinfection; he believed isolation was necessary for patient protection and that it should be carried out far more rigidly than was conventional at that time (1875).[79]

On October 23, 1876, Billings wrote Florence Nightingale asking her comment on sketches of the Johns Hopkins Hospital construction plans approved by The Hopkins Trustees. In a subsequent letter, December 4, 1876, Billings expressed his thanks for her letter of December 2, in which she had enclosed twelve sheets of notes and comments on the plans.[80]

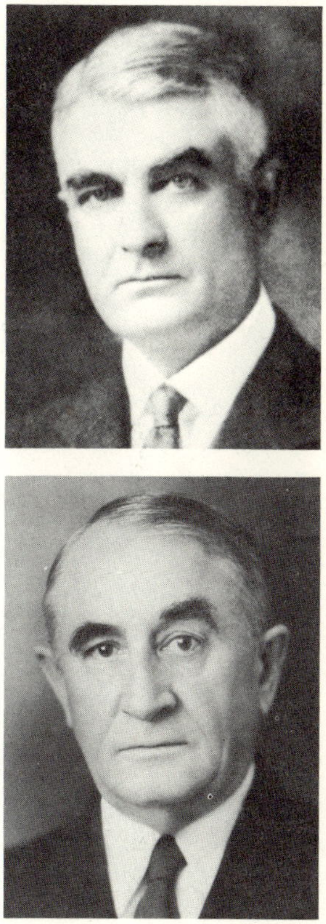

a

b

18.10 **a.** William and **b.** Charles Mayo, founders of famous Mayo Clinic.

The idea of constructing one-story pavilion hospitals is credited to Jean-Baptiste Le Roy of the French Academy of Sciences. His brochure promoting such buildings appeared in 1777. Tenon was an early advocate of the pavilion form of hospital, a conception which rapidly gained approval after experiences in treating casualties in tents and temporary barracks in the Crimean War and the American Civil War. The feeling was that such structures segregated patients, permitted free ventilation, and could be periodically destroyed. Michel Lévy (1862), in the Paris discussions of the salubrity of hospitals, related that in the Crimea he had observed less mortality from cholera in the tent hospitals than in the permanent stone structures. Gustave Chantreuil (1868), a Paris obstetrician, made a plea for dispersion of hospital patients into tents and wooden barracks, especially in the summer, a proposal that he believed would provide superior ventilation and lessen wound infection.[81]

Douglas Galton (1869), a student of hospital construction, speaking at Leeds before the British Medical Association, June 27, 1869, said, "Do not build for a long futurity. Buildings used for the reception of the sick become permeated with organic impurities and it is a real sanitary advantage they should be pulled down and entirely rebuilt on a fresh site periodically." He had little or nothing to say of microbiology. Galton regarded 3,000 cubic feet of air per hour per patient as optimal and recommended smooth enameled walls for hospitals to diminish permeation by organic matter.

In the ensuing discussion Kennedy of Dublin advised removal of windows from corridors to increase airflow and ventilation, thus purifying the hospital atmosphere. He alluded to the advice of the priest in Leviticus (14:39–45) that the plaster and mortar of unhealthy buildings periodically be removed and renewed. Hutchinson spoke the only sensible words of the session: "Hospital efficiency is not increased by increasing ventilation, it is not the quantity of air, but the freedom from the germs of organic disease which should be the chief desideratum." He said, "Nine-tenths of cases might be taken into any kind of hospital and do equally well." Simpson interjected his familiar theme that small country hospitals have a lower mortality in amputation, city hospitals a 25 percent mortality, country hospitals only an 11 percent. He alluded to DeWar at Dunferline, across the Firth from Edinburgh, who had done 53 amputations with one death. Simpson believed that hospitals should conform to barrack structure, to be burned down every two years, a suggestion with which the New York surgeon Lewis Stimson (1875) agreed.[82]

Friedrich Sander (1875), writing of the history, statistics, structure, and arrangement of hospitals, said conditions in hospitals were considerably better than in Tenon's day, a century earlier. The mortality of patients admitted to hospitals before Tenon's report was in the area of 22 percent; between 1804 and 1861, said Sander, the mortality of admissions declined to 14.76 percent. He believed the lesser mortality of amputation in English than in French hospitals was a matter of size of hospitals and numbers of beds. Sander endorsed Florence Nightingale's view that obstetrical wards should never be in general hospitals but in separate structures. He repeated Billroth's statement (1868, 1870) that it has not been proved that "good hospitals" have no pyemia and that poor hospitals have many cases.[83]

In 1871 Félix Rochard proposed the creation of a hospital on an island in the Seine near the Austerlitz Bridge which would combine isolation, ventilation, and uniform temperature. There, said Rochard, major operations would have the best chance of success. A dozen years later Rochard (1883) noted that "hospital atmosphere has changed since antisepsis — there is greater calm and confidence."[84]

Oppert (1859) recommended that hospitals be built at the periphery of industry and activity and not at their center. There should be canals into which the discharges from the hospital could be delivered and an adequate reservoir of water to flood the canals and maintain healthy conditions. He favored small patient wards for all hospitals. In 1868 Oppert remarked upon the noticeable improvement in hospitals since his earlier paper (1859), observing that overcrowding is not so much in evidence. He insisted hospitals should never be overflowing, better to have temporary tents and leave some wards closed periodically. Adds the writer, "Hôtel-Dieu and other insalubrious hospitals should be destroyed."[85]

Y. W. Jastreboff (1885), a St. Petersburg surgeon, recommended application of Lister's scheme to the entire hospital, creating an improved antiseptic atmosphere. Jastreboff would have each section of the hospital separate, with windows never opened and hermetically sealed; the air would be filtered and sterilized — in fact, a prelude to some current-day thoughts on hospital construction. Surgeons and patients would be submitted to disinfection upon entering the hospital; they would disrobe in the first room, take an antiseptic bath in the second, put on purified garments in the third — inconvenient steps that yet remain to be taken up by hospital personnel. F. Rochard commented that "the idea is excellent but its execution would be very difficult," obviously an understatement.[86]

Alphonse Laveran (1890) wrote of frequent communication of pneumonia, typhoid, erysipelas, and infectious fevers to other patients in hospitals. The author stated that the average number of bacteria per cubic meter of air in the sickroom approximated 15,000 to 20,000 colonies. After sweeping and shaking the curtains and eiderdown coverlets, the number increased to 233,000 and in one case to 466,000. He believed that curtains should be abolished in hospitals. He also implicated urinals and defecation containers as sources of infection.[87]

Pavilion hospitals became widespread through Europe in the last decades of the nineteenth century. The idea found expression in several noted European civilian hospitals including the Eppendorfer Krankenhaus in Hamburg and the Bisbebjerg Hospital in Copenhagen; in fact, the pavilion hospital was still very much in evidence, especially in Germany, in the 1920s. However, pavilion hospitals had the serious defect of being costly and they spread the patients out over great distances. They were abandoned almost everywhere when better sanitation and antiseptic hospital practices outmoded their need. For convenience, economy, and efficiency of operation, the multiple-story, high-rise hospital has surpassed the pavilion structure in performance, with constant emphasis on disciplined cleanliness and with conscientious and unremitting heed to preclude and thwart communication of contagion and infection. In fact, Semmelweis (1861) had made such a judgment several decades before the vogue for pavilion hospitals faded away. He had insisted that neither site, age, nor crowded wards were responsible for hospitalism, but rather the methods of hospital treatment.[88] The framework of the hospital edifice has become a consideration secondary to what is done by the attending professional staff. To be certain, there were discerning surgeons in the eighteenth century who recognized and appreciated the importance of cleanliness before microbiology provided convincing proof thereof.

Florence Nightingale focused attention upon the sanitary conditions of hospitals. Unfortunately, she did not believe in the germ theory of disease. And strangely enough, Billings, a great student of medical literature, while concentrating upon ventilation in hospital construction, had failed to appreciate the importance of Semmelweis's observations of 1847. Lister's work and publications (1867–90) centered attention upon employment of antiseptic practices throughout hospitals; yet for the major portion of his professional career his emphasis was upon hospital air as the major source of infection, a view which he ultimately disavowed. The focus shifted from hospital air and overcrowding to a keener appreciation of the need to control infection by delimiting direct contact with infected sources.

Summary

Hospitals staffed by physicians came into being with Paris's famous Hôtel-Dieu toward the end of the thirteenth century; its origins date back to the seventh century — the only Paris hospital before the Renaissance. Originally, like other early hospitals, it provided only nursing care; all were essentially almshouses, places of refuge for the sick, the poor, and for weary travelers. Over many centuries the Hôtel-Dieu was overcrowded, requiring that six to eight patients occupy the great beds while two regularly shared the single ones. Apparently the custom was for patients as well as travelers to sleep naked in such accommodations; in hospitals, the ill and "dying" often huddled together under extremely disagreeable circumstances. Heat in the wards was provided only for obstetrical and surgical patients. The Hôtel-Dieu was described in the mid-eighteenth century as the most frightful of all French hospitals, with 22 percent of the patients dying on its premises.

France could boast of many distinguished surgeons as far back as the fourteenth century; however, the Hôtel-Dieu brought distinction to French surgery only late in the eighteenth. The first three decades of the nineteenth century marked the Hôtel-Dieu's golden era. Until the mid-seventeenth century, religion was the main determinant for both faculty and students at the University of Paris; only thereafter were Protestants eligible to teach or study there.

St. Bartholomew's is England's oldest surviving hospital. Founded in 1123, it had a strong faculty by the mid-sixteenth century. St. Thomas's, Guy's, St. George's, and the London are among London's famous hospitals, as are several specialty hospitals including St. Mark's Hospital for Rectal Diseases and St. Peter's Hospital for Stone. Despite a rich heritage of great surgeons with a distinguished record of accomplishments, St. Bartholomew's surgeons were under "complete thraldom" to the physicians well into the mid-eighteenth century, a posture that the Paris surgeon J. L. Petit had rejected in 1700.

Nursing, especially night care, came under strong criticism from the *Lancet*'s Sanitary Commission in 1865, as it had earlier at the hands of the Scottish novelist Smollett and London's Dickens.

Simpson (1869) coined the word "hospitalism" to characterize the prevalence of unsanitary conditions frequently responsible for propagation of infectious diseases to hospital entrants. Listerian wound practices (1867) found acceptance in Germany in the mid-1870s, a full decade before American and British surgeons capitulated to their use. Elective surgery of the extremities employing Lister's techniques was born in Germany in the 1874–75 period. Elective surgery of the abdomen adopting Semmelweis's (1847) prophylactic surgical antiseptic practices to the minutest detail was initiated in 1876–77 by the Freiburg gynecologist Hegar; he reported a succession of 15 ovariotomies without mortality. In 1886, when Tait of Birmingham, England, reported a series of 139 successful ovariotomies, surgical antisepsis began to find acceptance in Britain and America. Strangely, Tait rejected Listerian practices and affected not to believe in the germ theory of disease.

It is a serious indictment of the profession that despite the work of Semmelweis (1847, 1861), Pasteur (1860–78), Lister (1867–71), and Koch (1876–78) the "pus-pail" survived in the finest surgical clinics of France, Britain, Germany, and America into the late 1870s. The wounds of large numbers of patients in quick succession were swabbed with a single sea sponge dipped into the same container. Surgeons, obviously, were slow to accept factual scientific evidence as meaningful for their own work. Actually it was not a matter of ignorance, but the sad travesty of not believing what they heard or saw and an unwillingness to test the new proposals for wound management.

With proof of the pathogenicity of bacteria established by Koch (1878), there began a deemphasis upon hospital ventilation and a definite swing from the pavilion type of hospital of the Crimean War and American Civil War to the more economical multiple-story structure, a return to Fracastoro's (1546) thesis of controlling infections by eliminating direct contact with infected sources.

(For notes, see pp. 671–77.)

CHAPTER 19

Hospital Reformers, Sanitarians, and Surgical Accountability

IN THE MID-EIGHTEENTH century several persons emerged whose work and writings came to be synonymous with reforms in penal institutions and hospitals. Public exposure of the cruel and unsanitary practices in prisons and houses of correction ultimately revolutionized methods of dealing with incarcerated offenders and derelicts. Similarly, hospital critics demanded regulations to improve hygiene and nursing and to alleviate the miserable and dangerous plight of hospital patients. Finally, recognition of causes responsible for patient morbidity and mortality lent great initiative to the improvement of hospital care, demanding of doctors public admission of accountability and responsibility for their failures and achievements.

John Howard (1727?–90)

In John Howard England had its first great prison and hospital reformer. Self-delegated, unpaid, without training or precedent, Howard swung public attention to the "cause of the prisoner, the sick, and the destitute," championed the importance of sanitation, and set a pattern for future investigators.

An early experience determined Howard's career. When he was vacation-bound to Lisbon in 1756, his ship was seized by a French privateer, and crew and passengers were incarcerated in

Brest as prisoners of war. He was ultimately released to negotiate an exchange of prisoners, but the miseries of his imprisonment left an enduring impression. Elected high sheriff of Bedfordshire in 1773, Howard was shocked to discover the conditions of his small county jail and, seeking comparison with nearby institutions, began an investigation and a mission that was to consume the rest of his life and entail some 50,000 miles of travel.[1] Howard first inspected jails throughout England, Wales, Scotland, and Ireland, bringing before appropriate legislative bodies the inhumanity of prison practices, and with good effect. He then turned his attention to similar institutions abroad, visiting most of the countries of Europe. Howard summarized his observations in a monograph (1777) on the state of prisons.[2] He subsequently conducted a study of lazarettos and hospitals, which appeared in print in 1789.[3]

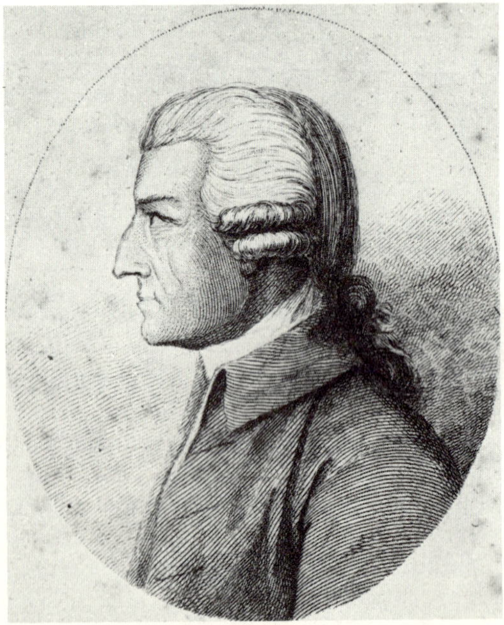

19.1 John Howard (1727?–90), great English prison and hospital reformer.

Said Howard, "At each visit I entered every room, cell, and dungeon with a memorandum book in my hand, in which I noted particulars upon the spot. My description will to some readers appear too minute; but I chose rather to relate circumstances, than to characterize in general terms." He found prisoners in dark caverns with an inch or two of water on the floor in which lay their straw bedding, if they had any. Some jails had no water except what was brought by the keeper — as little as three pints a day per prisoner for drink and washing. In 1777, however, at the city jail of Rochester, England, the keeper told Howard, "The liberality of the public is so great, we cannot keep the prisoners sober." The wardens even sold alcohol to prisoners, a practice that in more recent times has continued with drug traffic in penal institutions. In a Liverpool jail in the winter of 1788, Howard noted men in heavy irons, women prisoners chained to the floor, and no fire. In Liege he said the dungeons were so shocking that confinement in them sometimes took away the victims' senses. "I heard the cries of the distracted as I went down to them." Manacling and chaining prisoners in dungeons, often for minor offenses, was a cruelty that Howard was determined to terminate. He noted that because of a window tax jailers sometimes stopped up the windows and "stifled their prisoners." For his methodical record-keeping Howard carried his own scales to weigh such items as prisoners' bread allotments. Occasionally he approved of.the diet; in Holland meat was given only once a week, but the thick soup of "pease, beans, barley, etc." served daily was hot and "very palatable."[4]

As Howard traveled, his interests broadened beyond the mistreatment of prisoners to the study of disease, "gaol-fever" (typhus) and smallpox, which brought "destruction of multitudes, not only of *felons* in their dungeons, but of *debtors* also." He became concerned over the mode of spread of plague, expressing doubt that air was the principal source of contagion. If this were so, he remarked, why does not every individual in a town become infected? He related an instance in 1665 in which plague was communicated from London to a remote village in Derbyshire through the sending of a parcel of clothes. When asked what precautions he himself used against infection on his trips, Howard said temperance and cleanliness were his chief preservatives, and "in an offensive room I avoid drawing my breath deeply; and on my return, sometimes wash my mouth and hands."[5]

The lazaretto was a place of quarantine where crews and passengers were detained while their ship was under surveillance and attempts were made to fumigate the cargo as well as isolate the personnel. They were in use in such European ports as Marseilles, Venice, and Malta. Howard believed that England could profit from such establishments, properly controlled. Whereas England at the time permitted easy access for Dutch ships to English harbors, goods were not allowed to come directly by ship from Turkey, where plague was at times rampant. Howard explained that as ships docked here and there on their way to England, cargoes were often intermingled, so that Dutch ships might bring Turkish cotton, "a most faithful preserver of contagion." He criticized many of the quarantine measures in the lazarettos and found that many were miserable refuges for human detention.

For first hand acquaintance with a lazaretto, Howard went to Smyrna and purposely took passage "in a ship with a *foul* bill" of health, i.e., a ship sailing from a port where there was known infection or that had infectious disease aboard. On arrival in Venice sixty days later the ship and passengers were put under quarantine, detaining Howard for forty-two days. His lazaretto quarters were so dirty that repeated washings with boiling water failed to remove the smell, as offensive as the "sick wards of the worst hospital." Finally Howard got the room whitewashed with slaked lime and it was "immediately rendered so sweet and fresh, that I was able to drink tea in it in the afternoon, and to lie in it the following night."[6]

Howard's comments on the hospitals of Paris have frequently been repeated. He called Hôpital St. Louis and Hôtel-Dieu "the two worst hospitals" he had ever visited. He often saw five or six patients in a bed at the Hôtel-Dieu, some of them dying. The Hôtel-Dieu in Lyons he called the best hospital in France. He spoke highly of the Leeds Infirmary, which gave, he said, great attention to cleanliness and had "no bugs in the beds." Many were cured of compound fractures there "who would lose their limbs in the unventilated and offensive wards of some other hospitals." He suggested that the fanlights over the doors of the Radcliffe Infirmary wards be open "to purify the air; or, at least, the noxious effluvia would become so sensible through the rest of the house, as might induce the matron, and the gentlemen who only attend in the committee-room, to *insist* upon . . . proper ventilation of the wards." Concerning patients with venereal disease at the Lock Hospital, Howard praised the hospital's enlightened articles of incorporation which concluded, "Suppose the Redeemer . . . had said of us, — 'Leave those sinners to the consequences of their sin and folly.'" Commented Nathaniel Faxon, "It took 140 years and a World War to make us as a people accept this sensible doctrine. The labors and wisdom of John Howard, Sir William Blackstone and Dr. John Fothergill did much to mitigate the terrible laws of England, which executed people for burglary, which imprisoned them for debt."[7]

The physical stamina and self-sacrifice mandated by the rigors of health hazards that Howard endured are almost beyond belief. His last journey took him to St. Petersburg, Moscow, and Cherson (Sevastopol), where he died of an infectious fever characterized by convulsions — a hero and a martyr to a great cause. An impressive monument near the Black Sea honors his contribution to the health of the Russian people. Howard's great work and its telling results, initiating many needed reforms in prisons and hospitals, have an enduring claim upon immortality. Said Howard, "I am the plodder, who goes about to collect materials for men of genius to make use of." Edmund Burke declared that Howard's life was a "voyage of discovery."[8]

Jacques Tenon (1724–1816)

Jacques Tenon was not the first in France to declaim upon the frightful conditions of Paris hospitals or to present plans to rebuild the Hôtel-Dieu, but he was easily the greatest of the early French hospital reformers. His research often paralleled that of England's Howard, whom he much admired. Just as Howard took along his notebook and scales, so Tenon carried his yardstick, and in many ways Tenon's report followed the pattern of his English precursor in what he noted, measured, and condemned.[9] But, unlike Howard, the surgeon Tenon was a scientist with years of experience and observation when he undertook his famous survey of hospitals.[10]

Tenon was the oldest of eleven children of an impecunious surgeon in a small town south of Paris. At the age of seventeen, a frail, timid young man, Tenon took off for Paris to learn his father's profession. His first sight of surgery at the Hôtel-Dieu filled him with horror. Operations were performed in the same room in which other patients awaited their turn, hearing the screams and witnessing the anguish of those on the table. Bleeding was done indiscriminately, one bowl receiving the blood of several patients so that no measurement of a patient's blood loss was possible. Tenon despaired of ever conquering his fright of such scenes and was equally repulsed by anatomy as taught in the sordid atmosphere of the morgue.

Fortunately he found comparative anatomy intriguing and began to make careful animal dissections and to attend Jacques Winslow's demonstrations at Jardin-du-Roi. When this great Danish anatomist saw a heart preparation of Tenon's, he gave him a place in his laboratory, and the young investigator rapidly made his way as an anatomist. Finding that his limited education made advancement in position impossible — he could scarcely write French correctly — Tenon learned Latin and Greek in fifteen months and received a degree in philosophy. After a tour as wound surgeon with the army in Flanders in 1748 Tenon returned to Paris to distinguish himself in a *concours* examination, winning the chair of surgery at the Salpetrière. In 1757 he succeeded to the chair of pathology at the Royal Academy, a position he occupied for twenty-five years. He was chosen to give the dedicatory speech at the inauguration of the newly constructed amphitheatre designed by Jacques Gondoin.

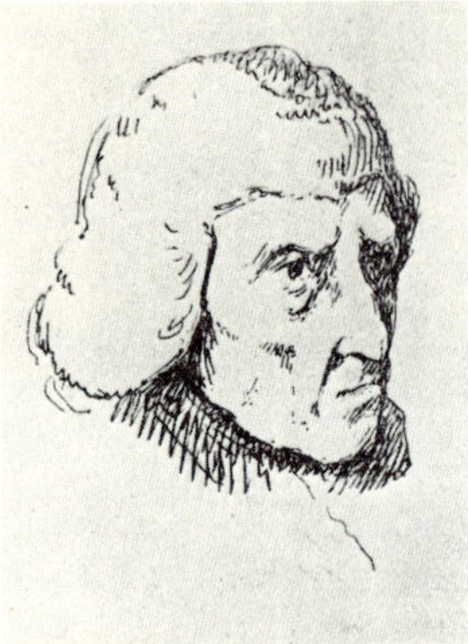

19.2 Jacques Tenon (1724–1816), French anatomist and architect of hospital reform.

For many years Tenon had been quietly studying the problems and shortcomings of Paris hospitals. His research formed the basis of a report (1786) to the Royal Academy of Sciences by a committee of eight on the subject of a new Hôtel-Dieu. Antoine L. Lavoisier and Pierre-Simon Laplace, the great mathematician and astronomer, were among other members of the committee. Public concern was so aroused by accounts of conditions at the Hôtel-Dieu and other Paris hospitals that the Academy of Sciences, with the approval of Louis XVI, sent Tenon and C.-A. Coulomb, a physician, to England to study hospitals, prisons, and workhouses and to find ways to improve Paris hospitals.

Their journey covered fifty-two institutions in eleven weeks. Besides a number of London hospitals, infirmaries, and prisons, Tenon visited hospitals at Oxford, Birmingham, Bristol, Plymouth, Exeter, Salisbury, Winchester, and Portsmouth, and returned to London for further visits. He made a detailed inventory of the care of the sick, including beds, diet, etiquette, attitude toward the patient, hours of meals, and treatment. He investigated the condition of the water in the hospitals and the water supplies, latrines, pumps, stairways, vestibules, anatomical amphitheatres, operating rooms, and ventilation.

A year later appeared Tenon's great *Mémoires sur les hôpitaux de Paris*, an epochal report (1788), outlining specifics for needed reforms. He made many important suggestions and initiated a movement that forcefully brought the lamentable situation in Paris hospitals to the attention of both the profession and the public. The *Mémoires* revealed that in the Hôtel-Dieu there were often four and even frequently six patients in one large bed,[11] just as had been reported in 1651 and 1767; surgical cases were four to each large bed. Parturient women were two to four in such beds. Tenon spoke of this as a dangerous practice that needed correction; patients with puerperal fever, scabies, or venereal disease were huddled indiscriminately together. He said that the women were more neglected in hospitals than men.[12]

Tenon studied the mortality of many of the great hospitals of Europe and Britain and found, as did Malgaigne (1842) over fifty years later, that the Hôtel-Dieu in Paris had probably the highest mortality among hospitals. Tenon recommended that surgical wards should not be near the postmortem rooms, that separate rooms be set aside for operations, for preparing patients for operations, and for postoperative cases, and that obstetrical beds should not be mingled with surgical beds.[13] He recommended the establishment of wards for the reception and care of patients with contagious fevers. Many of Tenon's suggestions are universally in force in hospitals throughout the world today.

Tenon and Howard had great influence in alerting hospital authorities and the public to the urgent need for reform within hospitals. Tenon's broad-based address to the problems served to focus attention upon a number of hospital matters that had gone unregarded, including the need for hospital tables of morbidity and mortality, vital statistics, hospital planning, ventilation, sewage disposal, and general hygienic safeguards. Yet, the emphasis upon direct contact as revealed in the studies of Fracastoro (1546), Redi (1668), Spallanzani (1767–76), and others received little if any consideration. It is clear that whereas the studies of Howard and Tenon did much to improve conditions of hospitals and infirmaries they did not actually get at the heart of the problem. As Semmelweis was to indicate, direct contact between physician and patient and wound was *the* source of wound infection; ventilation and general hospital conditions were secondary matters.

During the period of the French Revolution Tenon disassociated himself from all political involvement and retreated to his country house at Massy, where he occupied himself with research in pathology and anatomy. When his house was raided by foreign troops in 1815, and his papers and specimens were destroyed, Tenon returned to Paris, where he died within a year (1816).

Antoine L. Lavoisier (1743–94)

The chemist Antoine L. Lavoisier took an important role in the struggle to improve public health in cities and among the poor in France. His emphasis was upon ample supplies of good water, air, and food, the abolition of poverty, and improvement of agriculture. He worked with sustained and passionate ardor for the fulfillment of these objectives both as eminent scientist and as active political economist; in the latter role he became embroiled with political revolutionaries that led to his undoing and to the scaffold.[14]

Edwin Chadwick (1800–90)

Edwin Chadwick first awakened British statesmen "to the duty of caring for the Public Health."[15] To defray expenses while training for the law, Chadwick undertook reporting for several civic journals. This task, as well as the calls of his legal investigation, introduced him to the frightful slums of London and the necessity for social reform. In a study of life insurance in 1828, exploring actuarial figures, Chadwick recognized the need for registration of vital statistics including causes of death, and propounded a theory he was never to abandon — a conviction that environment, the circumstances under which people live, affects health and longevity.[16]

His writings drew the approval of young Radicals supporting Jeremy Bentham (1748–1832), the founder of Utilitarianism, the greatest good to the greatest number, the self-evident principle of morality. Chadwick became a member of their circle and an ardent champion of the cause of sanitation and public health. In the year of Bentham's death (1832) Chadwick abandoned his career at the bar to accept an appointment to the Poor Law Enquiry. He applied Bentham's thesis to the reform of the Poor Law (1834) and was largely responsible for passage of the act which established a Board of Public Health in England (1848). Determined, frequently tactless, and impatient to accelerate the movement for improved sanitation, it was not surprising that in the midst of his great career (1854) he was relieved of the opportunity provided by his position on the Public Health Board.

Chadwick's memorable report of more than 450 pages on the *Sanitary Condition of the Labouring Population of Great Britain* was presented to the House of Lords in July 1842; it contained pertinent and devastatingly frank information, culled from statements of government officials, medical men, and a small army of investigators. Included among other information were maps, tables of vital statistics, descriptions of streets, dwellings, schools, ventilation, refuse, privies, water supplies, sewers, drainage, safety regulations, and prevalence of disease and poverty.

From his studies of the average age of death among (1) the gentry and professional persons, (2) tradesmen, and (3) laborers and artisans and among the families of each class, Chadwick declared that the squalor and unsanitary living conditions of the poor accounted largely for their shorter duration of life. In

Bethnal Green, for example, the average age of death among laborers was sixteen and in Liverpool, fifteen; among the gentry and professional classes it was forty-five and thirty-five, respectively. Many of the deaths, especially from endemic fevers, Chadwick believed, could be prevented by improvement of living conditions. He included the report of the famous dunghill of Market Street in Greenock, where in summer the nearby houses swarmed with flies that left the taste of the dunghill on all uncovered food and drink. Chadwick declared that "More filth, worse physical suffering and moral disorder than Howard describes as affecting the prisoners, are to be found amongst the cellar population of the working people of Liverpool" and other cities. Chadwick stated that children began to enter employment in the cotton and other factories at seven to nine years of age, yet the mortality was no greater among them than among those who remained "in such homes as these towns afford to the labouring class" — the factories apparently were drier and warmer.[17]

Some forty years later (1888) Chadwick stated that the death rate in London, which not long before had been 24 per 1,000, had recently decreased to 14 or 15 per 1,000, a reflection, he believed, of improved sanitation. Had sanitation measures been more properly executed, said Chadwick, the mortality since 1856 would have stood at 12 per 1,000. Chadwick believed that the greatest gain of sanitary science was lowering of the death rate by prevention of some childhood diseases. A wash at school and halfpenny dinners for the children, he insisted, do a good deal for the family life among the poor.

Chadwick had become aware of the "deadly error" in high political circles "that sanitation is opposed to the Malthusian doctrine 'that pestilence is the great check to the growing excess of population.'" He built his thesis upon observations noting that illness weakened the population, thereby augmenting the proportion of dependent paupers. Improved health measures, said Chadwick, will prevent greater loss of life than the slaughter of wars. Chadwick also made a plea for soft water and for getting rid of soot. He concluded by saying, "Let us hope that our old England may be the mother of sanitary blessings as well as colonial possessions."[18]

As London's population in the nineteenth century grew to three million, the city's sewage problem became increasingly critical and was a constant source of public irritation and agitation, frequently the subject of hot parliamentary debate. At one time Chadwick believed that the best resolution of the baffling question would be to employ the vast sewage quagmire for agricultural purposes. Meanwhile, each year during the hot summer months an unbelievable stench pervaded London's atmosphere, occasionally interrupting parliamentary debates and court sessions. London was avoided by tourists.

Lack of acceptable sewage disposal for London was editorialized in the *British Medical Journal*, July 3, 1858, the "Year of the Great Stink." The situation was brought to an "olfactory crisis" when Her Majesty Queen Victoria and her entourage and guests, including the King of Belgium and other dignitaries, took an excursion on an Admiralty barge across the Thames to inspect the new ship *Leviathan*. As the *Journal* reported, the queen "was obliged to neutralise the dreadful smell by keeping her bouquet close to her nose." The outing, on June 28, 1858, has been well described by Carleton Chapman.[19]

"It is truly lamentable in a great country like this to see its principal river turned into a regular poisoned chalice," stated a letter in the London *Sun*, June 30, 1858, blaming the College of Physicians for doing nothing about the unhealthy situation. Meanwhile fears were arising that the "pestilential state of the Thames," might bring a devastating plague to London. Chloride of lime and other disinfectants were used to lessen the smell.[20]

John Martin's proposal that London's sewage be drained into the Thames some distance downstream ultimately prevailed, a scheme that took more than ten years to effectuate. The Thames excursion of Queen Victoria's entourage in the early summer of 1858 undoubtedly sharpened the focus of Parliament and public upon a constantly recurring problem and urgent need for reform.

Although he was often called "humorless," occasionally wry twists of wit punctuated Chadwick's grim reports of his investigations. When examining slums in Edinburgh, he interrogated a porter who said he was earning 20 shillings a week and spent half of it for whisky. Chadwick expressed surprise, but added that in the porter's crowded dwelling he had experienced a "coppery taste" in his mouth and hurriedly thereafter "sought correction in a diffusive stimulant, some warm brandy and water."[21] In 1889 Chadwick wrote that the Egyptians had a code of thirty commandments, one of which read, "Thou shalt not pollute the river; wash and be clean," and that the Order of Commander of the Bath which the queen conferred upon him in 1848 was in fact "an order of the washed."[22]

At a banquet honoring his ninetieth birthday and his seventieth year of public service, Chadwick reported that the death rate in a number of English towns had been reduced by 50 percent and that it was no accident that the mortality in Salisbury had been cut from 40 per 1,000 in 1800 to 16 per 1,000 in 1889. When the comment was made that the "present advanced state of sanitation" largely rested on him, Chadwick replied that this nice citation was undoubtedly owing in part to his long years and to his having spent his entire professional life in the service of improving sanitation.[23] Chadwick did much for England and its poor and will always be remembered as a pioneer and leader in the public health movement.

John Simon (1816–1904)

John Simon was already a distinguished surgeon at St. Thomas's Hospital at thirty-two years of age when he became medical officer of the City of London (1848), the first to hold the appointment.[24] Simon retained his position at St. Thomas's and continued to operate on charity patients there until 1876, but the demands of his official responsibilities in public health made it necessary for him to relinquish pursuit of private surgical practice in 1855. He was the first (1852) to do a successful ureterorectal anastomosis for an incontinent urinary fistula caused by congenital vesical ectopia.[25]

Simon wrote well and often brilliantly.[26] Moreover, he was a man of tremendous courage, accompanied by a real capacity of persuasion, talents which came him in good stead with the politicians and statesmen with whom he dealt on a daily basis over many years. Simon retired involuntarily at sixty, having been relieved of his public health responsibilities by internal political machinations.[27]

Simon regarded the practice of court hearings in which scientific experts from opposite sides vigorously supported their partisan interests as moral prostitution and subornation of science. What remedy did he propose? "There should be some tangible head responsible — not only for the enforcement of existing laws, such as they are or may become, but likewise for their progress from time to time to the level of contemporary science, for their completion where fragmentary, for their harmonisation when discordant." He praised the French establishment of *conseils de salubrité*, which existed in most large cities in France and believed this could become a useful English institution.

Said Simon, "There are many men who get no farther in their psalms of life than the question what is there to correct? . . . Everywhere there is the conviction that something must be done. . . . Knowledge, and method, and comprehensiveness are wanted — the precise, definite, categorical impulses of a Parliamentary leader who can recognise principles and stick to them." Added Simon, "And for such a Minister, what a career!"[28]

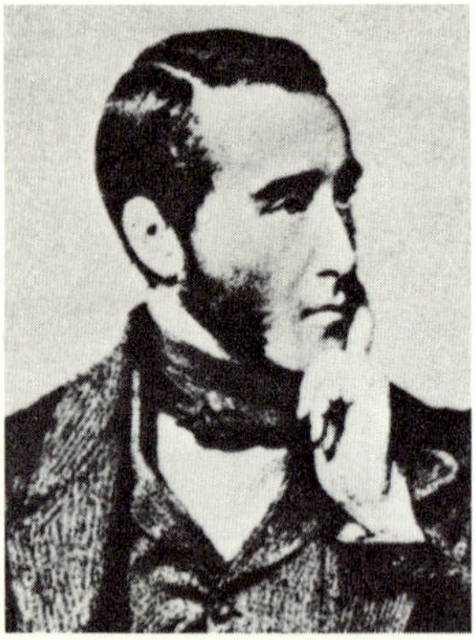

19.3 John Simon (1816–1904), London surgeon and public health reformer.

The public health reports of Her Majesty's Privy Council on the status of health in London reflected Simon's intensive search of the literature for clues to the sources of hospital insalubrity and the nature and causes of wound infection. Nearly half of the eighty pages of his sixth report, that for 1863, dealt with hospital hygiene and statistics. He had sent J. S. Bristowe, a physician of St. Thomas's, and T. Holmes, an assistant surgeon of St. George's, to visit the important civil hospitals in England, Scotland, and Ireland. They subsequently went to Paris and were accorded the opportunity to examine the records of the chief Parisian hospitals. They found, as in England, that very few hospitals kept official records.[29] This neglect in Britain had reached the attention of Florence Nightingale and her advisor Farr, both of whom strongly urged correction of the deficiency. It would appear, however, that Simon was more knowledgeable than they of the real crux of hospital sanitation.

In his report Simon asked, what is a healthy hospital? He concluded, "'A healthy hospital' is a hospital which does not, *by any fault of its own*, aggravate ever so little the sickness, nor oppose ever so little the recovery, of persons who are properly its inmates." He said, "That which makes the healthiest house makes likewise the healthiest hospital . . . the same never-ceasing vigilance against the thousand forms in which dirt may disguise itself, in air and soil and water, in walls and floors and ceilings, in dress and bedding and furniture, in pots and pans and pails, in sinks and drains and dustbins." He wrote of "vibriones" and the "mycelia of fungi," living organisms which had been found floating in the air of the cholera ward in St. Thomas's Hospital. He alluded to the debates of 1861–62 at the Paris Academy of Medicine upon hospital hygiene and the work of M.-G.-A. Devergie and of Chalvet, the young physician who noted there was considerably more floating organic material in the surgical than in the medical wards at Hôpital St. Louis, especially in areas with cases of hospital gangrene. Simon also referred to the work of Heinrich Schröder in Germany and of Pasteur in France.[30]

The report for the year 1863 was sent forward on March 31, 1864; however, Simon added a note (p. 54) dated July 1864: "While this report has been in course of printing, I have had some fresh search made for evidence of infusorial life in the clots and suppurations of pyaemia; but hitherto the search has been in vain."

Simon devoted nearly a page to recounting Semmelweis's experience with puerperal fever and italicized the words, "the real source [of infection] was to be found in the hands of the medical men in attendance contaminated with cadaveric poison." He stressed Semmelweis's advice on thorough hand-washing and disinfecting of hands with a solution of chlorine, which information apparently had escaped Lister completely. Simon's source on Semmelweis was Charles Routh's account in the *Medical-Chirurgical Transactions of 1849*.[31] Although he understood German well, Simon obviously had not read Semmelweis's monograph of 1861, in which emphasis was not solely upon cadaveric contamination of fingers and hands of the accoucheur and his assistants, but upon living organisms in putrescent materials on such materiel as instruments, linens, and basins likely to come into contact with the vaginal canal of the parturient. Had Simon known more of the intimate details of the work of Semmelweis, even without demonstration of the pathogenicity of bacteria, he might well have been the surgeon-sanitarian to interpret and initiate prophylactic surgical antisepsis.

Simon's adjudication of the problem of hospital sanitation is undoubtedly the best assessment available for that period.[32] The emphasis of the day was upon ventilation and so too was that of Simon, yet obviously he was struggling desperately to pinpoint the source of contagion. After discussion of the success of the measures of Semmelweis, Simon commented, "The relation of this fact to the possible 'spontaneous generation' of erysipelas contagium is not, I think, far to seek." Nevertheless, he returned in his report to the importance of ventilation and dangers of overcrowding of patients in hospitals.

Simon also commented on Florence Nightingale's important contribution in her publications *Notes on Hospitals* and *Notes on Nursing*. However, he could not agree, without some reservations, with her discussion concerning the nature of the contagion of disease and interpretation of hospital records. These parts, said Simon, are "not written with the same knowledge of facts as the parts on which Miss Nightingale is herself a high authority — the parts on cleanliness and on nursing."

In 1876 Simon published a small monograph, *Filth-Diseases and Their Prevention*, concerned solely with public sanitation and methods of disposal of human excrement. It justified the comment of William Robinson (1934) that between 1790 and 1832 at the Royal Infirmary at Sunderland, "drainage and sewage were bad and more primitive than at the Palace of Knossos in Crete in 1500 B.C."[33] Simon's book on filth appeared the same year (1876) as Koch's great work in deciphering the manner of transmission of anthrax and two years before Koch's demonstration of the pathogenicity of common pyogenic organisms and of staphylococcal and streptococcal infections.

When John Simon died in 1904 at age eighty-eight, the author of an unsigned obituary notice commented that the "vast good which he did in laying the foundations of enlightened sanitary administration will last as long as civilization."[34]

Florence Nightingale (1820–1910)

Florence Nightingale, the real hero to emerge from the Crimean War (1854–56), was asked by the Royal Commission examining the lessons of the war to testify to her hospital experience. She replied, "I have visited all the hospitals in London, Dublin, and Edinburgh . . . all the hospitals in Paris."[35] The commission's study revealed that Miss Nightingale knew far more of the long neglected art of hospital sanitation than did London's leading surgeons at the sessions, including Brodie, Fergusson, Paget, and Edmund A. Parkes, later to distinguish himself as a sanitarian. Miss Nightingale's contribution to improved sanitation in the British Army rivaled closely her unique and epic benefactions to nursing, now legendary. Her devotion to the care of the sick, both military and civilian, and her initiation of a searching inquiry by the British medical profession and public health officers for improved sanitary conditions in hospitals probably justified the epithet, "the greatest Victorian of them all."

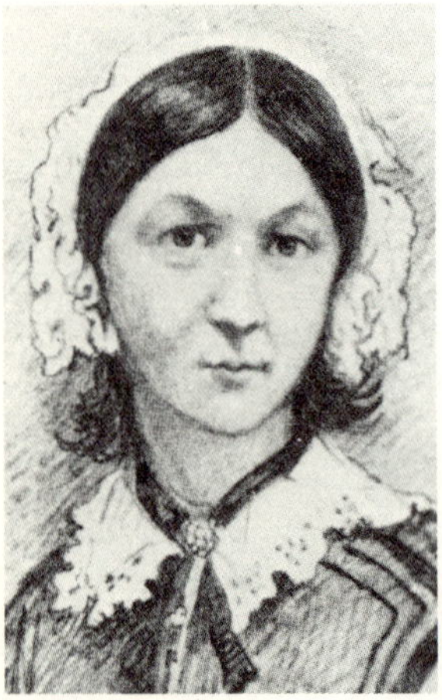

19.4 Florence Nightingale (1820–1910), greatest figure to emerge from the Crimean War. Founder of modern nursing.

Born into a family of wealth and position, Florence Nightingale at an early age engaged in social work in London despite the disapproval of her parents and elder sister. In 1851 she spent three months with the Fliedners at their Institution of Protestant Deaconesses at Kaiserswerth on the Rhine,[36] then made extensive visits to Paris hospitals. In the fall of 1853 she became superintendent of the Harley Street Hospital for "gentlewomen during illness," with a brief interim of nursing cholera patients at Middlesex Hospital. She was considering acceptance of the appointment of superintendent of nurses at the newly rebuilt King's College Hospital in the fall of 1854, when the Crimean War intervened.

In October 1854 the London *Times* published letters from

William Howard Russell, its special correspondent on the war, stating, "There is no preparation for the commonest surgical operations. . . . The French are greatly our superiors. Their medical arrangements are extremely good, their surgeons more numerous, and they have also the help of the Sisters of Charity, who have accompanied the expedition in incredible numbers." The exact number of such nurses, according to Edward Cook, was fifty.[37] It was Russell's report and the consequent public furor that occasioned Sidney Herbert, Secretary-at-War, to urge Miss Nightingale to select a group of women to accompany her and take charge of the care of the wounded at the military hospitals at Scutari, on the Asiatic side of Constantinople.[38] Miss Nightingale was thirty-four years of age. She organized a unit of English nurses[39] and went by way of Paris and Marseilles, arriving by ship at Constantinople on November 4, 1854, ten days after the Battle of Balaklava and the day before the Battle of Inkerman.

She wrote on November 14 to a friend: "We had 1715 sick and wounded in this Hospital (among whom 120 Cholera Patients), and 650 severely wounded in the other Building called the General Hospital . . . when a message came to me to prepare for 510 wounded. . . . I always expected to end my Days as Hospital Matron, but I never expected to be Barrack Mistress."[40]

Miss Nightingale attacked every angle of hospital care in the filthy, disease-ridden barrack hospital at Scutari, which had no kitchen, plumbing, or central heating. Food, clothing, water supplies, and general nursing care all came within her surveillance. Within a few months she had effected sanitary reforms with rigid insistence on cleanliness and established a kitchen and laundry as well as recreation rooms and other measures to cheer and comfort her patients. The drop in hospital mortality was phenomenal, from 42 percent in February 1855 to 2 percent a few months later.[41] Miss Nightingale also went to Balaklava near the battlefields, some 300 miles away across the Black Sea, and carried her reforms there.

She applied an expert's touch and a woman's insight to hospital management and boldly assumed responsibility where things needed to be done. It was said that she never raised her voice in argument; her quiet determination and sheer force of character usually won out. She did not readily take "no" for an answer. After completing her always heavy correspondence late at night, Miss Nightingale would make her final, solitary round of the wards through miles of beds.[42]

She became a legend with the British soldiers and the British people. Longfellow's poem "Santa Filomena" (1857) symbolized the spirit of the soldier's adoration for her and the importance of sympathetic nursing in hospitals.

A Lady with a Lamp shall stand
In the great history of the Land.

"A great commander was lost to England when Florence Nightingale was born a woman," said her biographer Cook. Great as was Miss Nightingale's work in the Crimea, it was acceptance of a life of isolation and solitude from the 1860s on that enabled her, with complete commitment and dedication, to make a significant impact upon practical hospital sanitation and nursing. Her immediate associates, convinced of the worth of her causes, virtually became her slaves in their total commitment to her objectives. Increasingly, Miss Nightingale isolated herself from family and friends and was accessible only to those who shared her interests. That she carried her isolation to extremes is well documented. In May 1875 Miss Nightingale's eighty-seven-year-old mother was ill. The daughter, who was fifty-five, lived a few doors away. She wrote Dr. Andrew Clark to visit her mother and to "call upon me, who am a prisoner to my room." Miss Nightingale's commitment to her daily routine obviously was not easily set aside.[43]

Statistics became her passion, which Farr ardently encouraged. One of her important accomplishments was to persuade reluctant surgeons and hospitals to accept accountability for factual reporting and the keeping of accurate hospital records and annual reports.

Her *Notes on Hospitals* with its plans for hospital construction established her as a leading authority on the subject. She favored the pavilion type of hospital with detached blocks of buildings. They should share "common administration, but nothing else in common." She said the Lariboisière in Paris was an anomaly, "one of the best hospitals in existence, so far as the block plan is concerned, yielding one of the highest rates of mortality." Miss Nightingale advised no more than two floors to a pavilion; no more than thirty-two patients to a ward. The preferable site was in the country, never within the precincts of a town. Her chief concern in construction was for ventilation, light, no overcrowding, and sanitation. Her trust was in soap and water, in the use of boiling water for hospital laundries, and in adequate ventilation and sunlight. She obviously knew of Lister and his work, but up to the end of a long life, she disaffected belief in the germ theory of disease,[44] as did Chadwick. Before 1885, in this respect, they were not alone. Her stubborn resistance to acceptance of prophylactic surgical antisepsis in her attack upon operative and hospital infection is a complete enigma to her loyal admirers.

Stephen Smith (1823–1922)

Stephen Smith, who remained active well beyond his ninetieth year,[45] devoted a goodly segment of his long professional life to questions of public health on a voluntary basis. His crusading zeal began during his internship at Bellevue Hospital, New York, in the 1850s, when he was in charge of the tents on Blackwell's Island, where many patients with typhus were sent for treatment. He noted that patients were continually being admitted with typhus from a single disreputable tenement on East 22nd Street. Smith tried to get the building closed, but the agent refused to identify the owner. The police could do nothing inasmuch as New York City had no health department to which they could appeal. The tax lists were examined and the landlord identified, a wealthy man living in an aristocratic neighborhood and a member of one of the most popular churches of the city. He was informed that his building was a menace to public health, but he refused to make any alterations, saying he obtained no rent from the vagrants who lived in it.

The indefatigable Smith then visited the office of the *Evening Post*, where William Cullen Bryant, the editor, manifested immediate interest and threatened to expose the owner's name and the story of his "fever nest" in his newspaper. Only then did the owner capitulate and agree to make the necessary improvements. Later he thanked Smith, because the renovated tenement brought him high rents.[46]

Following this episode, Smith and others organized the Citizen's Association and struggled to get a public health law through the legislature in Albany. Politicians including the City Inspector, whose office would be abolished by such a law,[47] contrived to obtain indefinite delays and defeated every proposal until 1865. That year the startling report from a corps of young physicians recruited by the association to make a house-to-house inspection of the city revealed the "horrible sanitary condition of New York." Smith, who had organized and supervised the inspection, presented the shocking facts to the Legislative Committee. The Metropolitan Health Bill was the result.[48]

The report, one of the important epidemiological studies of the century, revealed that fully one-half of New York City's one million inhabitants lived in tenements occupying an area of not

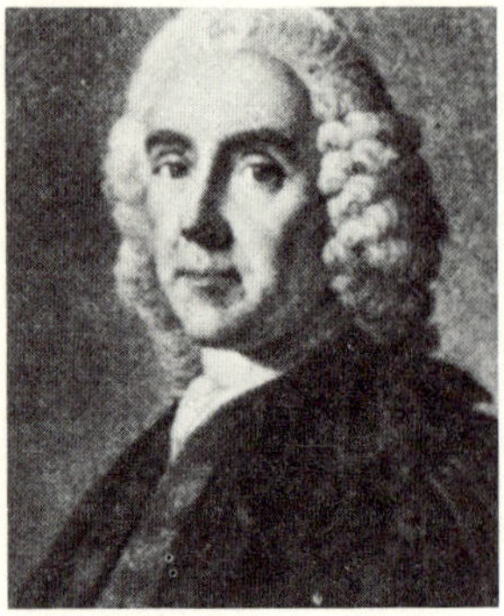

19.5 Alexander Monro I of Edinburgh Royal Infirmary, first to report factually (1737, 1752) on the hospital's operative mortality with amputation.

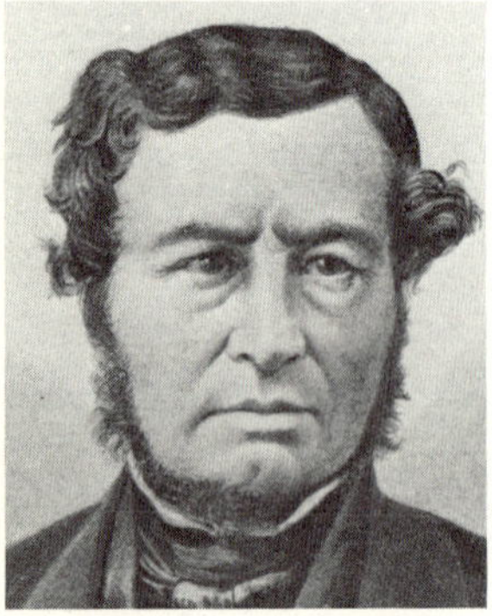

19.6 Joseph Malgaigne (1806–65), noted Paris surgical historian and eloquent spokesman for surgical accountability.

more than two square miles. Many lived in basements, surrounded by indescribable filth. In the Eleventh Ward the streets were covered with "house-slops, refuse vegetables, decayed fruit, store and shop sweepings, ashes, dead animals, and even human excrements." Outdoor privies and cesspools were commonplace in the tenement areas. These receptacles rarely drained into sewers and overflowed into courtyards, streets, and cellars. Cholera, dysentery, typhoid, typhus, smallpox, tuberculosis, and other diseases were prevalent.[49]

The effective legislation to prohibit such abuses invoked in New York in 1865 was subsequently emulated in other cities throughout the country. Smith listed his recommendations for improvement of public sanitation in 1875 as follows: educate the people and the medical profession in sanitary science, encouraging its daily application; educate the professions of architecture, engineering, and allied businesses in sanitary science; promote joint cooperation between the states and the federal government, which bodies should establish guide rules and regulations, assuming a responsible role in the application of sanitary knowledge.[50] It is strange, indeed, that among these very appropriate recommendations there was no mention of microbiology, a circumstance which indicates how retarded acceptance of that discipline was even in the highest circles of sanitation.

Cleanliness and germicides are man's best weapons against infection, said Smith (1911) in his *City That Was*, a small monograph that told the story of his struggles to bring reforms. Filth, whether in rubbish heaps, toilets, garbage, dust, or in secretions of skin and glands, is a culture bed for germs, said Smith, adding that filth is harmless if its bacteria are killed; even so, preventing its accumulation and frequent removal from sight is more appealing. Smith closed his book with a philosophical outlook, alluding to expressions of Wesley and Bacon on the importance of cleanliness, and to the Hebrew Fathers who formulated the Mosaic Sanitary Code.

Surgical Accountability

In 1559, John Geynes, a doctor of medicine at the University of Oxford, was cited by the College of Physicians for having impugned the infallibility of Galen. By confessing that he, not Galen, was at fault, Geynes was admitted to membership in the college the following year. Challenge of authority runs countercurrent to tradition. Until general acceptance of prophylactic surgical antisepsis surgeons were reluctant to release their mortality figures for operations. Monro I (1737, 1752) was among the first to do so; however, his reports on deaths from amputation at the Edinburgh Royal Infirmary were so much better than the prevailing achievement, he did not share the reticence of his contemporaries. Malgaigne (1842) startled the surgical world in revealing that the mortality of major amputations in nine leading Paris hospitals was 52 percent.[51]

Paget (1862) reported that Astley Cooper had visited a distinguished Paris surgeon approximately twenty years earlier, undoubtedly Larrey, who told Cooper he had never lost a patient from amputation at the shoulder joint. When they visited the "dead-house," a body with a recent unhealed wound from an amputated shoulder was to be seen lying on the postmortem table. Said Larrey, the patient died of pneumonia, not of the amputation. Wrote Paget, "We must beware of this dishonesty," yet on that very page he remarked, "Nearly half of those that I have operated on for hernia have died, and more than half after tracheotomy and nearly all after trephining. But these were deaths after operations; not because of them."[52]

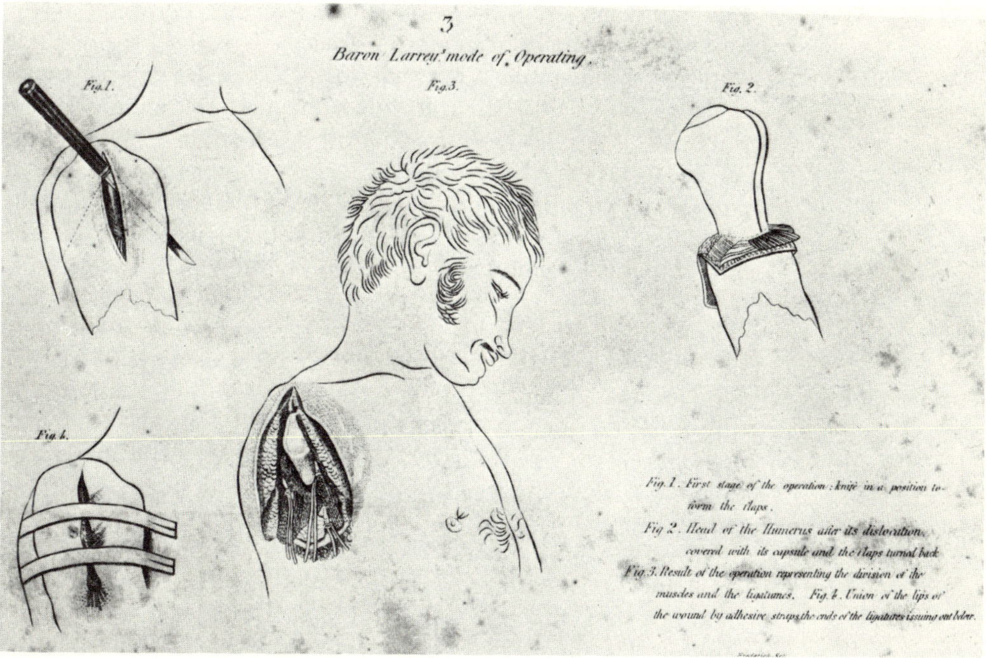

19.7 Larrey's technique of rapid shoulder disarticulation. From Larrey, *Memoires de chirurgie militaire* (Paris, 1817), reproduced in John C. Mercer's translation (Philadelphia, 1832).

Tait, writing on hospital mortality in 1875, asked a large metropolitan hospital for the facts of its amputations for the past sixteen years. The medical board replied it was not expedient to furnish such information. Tait retorted that if they did not supply the figures within a month he would publish their resolution in the *Times*. The board reconsidered. The results, said Tait, "were ghastly." However, sixteen years later the hospital, alerted by this revelation, had reduced its mortality by more than one-half (1890).[53]

Thereafter, statistical appraisals from British, German, and American surgeons appeared more frequently in the literature. Comparison of hospital mortalities was a natural sequel. Today, frank and open reports on hospital mortalities and risks attending operations constitute expected and accepted regular practice.[54]

Summary

Howard, a self-delegated and untrained hospital reformer, began in the mid-eighteenth century a voluntary and unaided program to improve the sanitation of prisons and hospitals in England, a program he extended to Holland, France, Turkey, and Russia. The conditions he described in the prisons were deplorable and pitiable beyond words to portray: starved men and women chained to cold and wet floors without beds. He pursued his studies relentlessly until his death in 1790 from an infectious fever in Sevastopol. Howard summarized his investigations in two publications on the state of prisons (1777) and on lazarettos and hospitals (1789), reports that stirred people and governments to action and initiation of reforms in many countries.

Tenon, France's great hospital reformer, began his professional life as anatomist and pathologist. Over many years he had been quietly observing and investigating hospital conditions throughout France and England; his studies and wise recommendations for reform covering almost every facet of hospitalization and care of patients were published in 1788. It constitutes today, almost two centuries later, a valid guide for earnest students of hospital reform.

Chadwick, trained as a lawyer, was introduced through his legal investigations into the appalling condition of the slums of London. He abandoned his legal career and became a leader in the cause of sanitation and public health, emerging as the person primarily responsible for the important act that established the Board of Public Health for England in 1848. His report in 1842 on the "Sanitary Condition of the Labouring Population of Great Britain" had aroused British statesmen to the pressing need for reform. Chadwick in later years could point with pride to significant changes in death rates owing to improved sanitary conditions among the poor with the abolition of dunghills in cities and villages draining into public streets. He helped put aside the doctrine that filth and pestilence are the main checks to growth of the population. His plea was that improved public health measures constitute the best means of prolonging life.

Simon sacrificed the promise of a distinguished surgical career to become the first medical officer of the city of London in 1848. Simon was unusually well informed, probably the first among surgeons to appreciate the work of Semmelweis and its promise for greater medicine. His reports to the Privy Council of 1854, 1863, and 1864 are models of their kind, informative and well written, reflecting needs for hospital reform, including factual and statistical accounting of hospital and surgical mortality. He was among the first to appreciate the likely role of bacteria in disease, although demonstration of their pathogenicity awaited the findings of Koch (1878). His stress, therefore, on achieving hospital salubrity continued to be on ventilation.

Florence Nightingale is probably the most durable medical hero to emerge from any war. Born to affluence and social position, over the objections of her family she determined upon a career in nursing. At age thirty-four she was summoned by Herbert, Secretary-at-War, to recruit a group of nurses to take charge of care of the wounded at Scutari, where she arrived on November 4, 1854, a day before the battle of Inkerman. Miss Nightingale quickly developed plans of organization in hospital care that won her the affection and admiration of the wounded. Reports of her devoted dedication to care of the sick and wounded, involving long days, concluded by a nightly walk through rows of barrack hospital beds, preceded her return to London, where her productive and tireless labor for ill and wounded British soldiers was already legend.

Miss Nightingale became a recluse shortly after her return, available only to those who sympathized and aided in her struggles to make nursing an honored profession throughout the world. Her trust was in soap and water and cleanliness. She failed to keep abreast of the significant developments in microbiology, disaffecting belief in the germ theory of infection and disease or in prophylactic surgical antisepsis. Urged on by an overwhelming desire to establish nursing as a respectable and worthy profession, she immersed herself in statistics of hospital morbidity and mortality, insisting that surgeons and hospitals accept the responsibility of reporting factually upon hospital and operative mortalities. Memory of her achievements will endure.

Stephen Smith, a distinguished New York surgeon, early in his career became involved on a voluntary basis in problems of public health and sanitation. In a sense, Smith did for public health in the state of New York what Simon, with an official appointment, had done for England.

Suggestions of surgeons accepting accountability for hospital and operative mortalities were slow aborning. Monro I (1737, 1752) had published his striking figures with unusually low operative mortalities attending amputation at the Edinburgh Royal Infirmary, an accomplishment not equaled until general adoption of prophylactic surgical antisepsis. As late as 1862 the celebrated London surgeon Paget was explaining away his operative mortality as owing to unrelated causes. Prophylactic antiseptic surgery extended the surgeon's field and greatly improved his performance. It is readily understandable that surgeons then became willing to supply factual accounts of hospital mortalities attending their operations.

(For notes, see pp. 678–82.)

CHAPTER 20

Germ Theory of Infection and Disease

THE FIRST penetrating insight into the problem of contagion came in the sixteenth century from Fracastoro, a physician of Verona. His famous poem *Syphilis* (1530) was followed in 1546 by a significant treatise on contagion, contagious diseases, and their treatment, which, as Garrison has said, "contains the first scientific statement of the true nature of contagion, of infection, of disease germs and the modes of transmission of infectious diseases."[1]

Fracastoro conceived of infection as owing to invisible organisms (seminaria) that communicate contagion at a distance by air currents or, more importantly, by direct contact. He said that "clothes, wooden objects, and things of that sort, which though not themselves corrupted can, nevertheless, preserve the original germs [seminaria] of the contagion and infect by means of these." He recognized two modes of treatment, prophylactic and curative. Germs, he said, may be destroyed by very hot or very cold agents. Burning may be done by fire or by caustics, "for by these means, the germs are extinguished, and . . . once they have been destroyed, the whole imminent disease is utterly destroyed, since nothing is left over that can generate offspring."[2]

Spontaneous Generation

The first important experiment touching the germ theory and refuting the doctrine of spontaneous generation was that of another Italian physician, Redi of Florence (1668). He found that maggots did not appear in putrefying meat when flies were kept from direct contact with the meat by parchment or fine wire gauze. A few years later came the demonstration of microscopic bodies in raindrops and on human teeth by the Dutch microscopist Leeuwenhoek (1676–83). Their mysterious origin continued to arouse controversy and renew the question of spontaneous generation.[3]

A Welsh Catholic priest living in Europe, John Needham (1748), boiled a meat infusion, corked it up, sealing the cork with mastic, and subjected the vessel to heat. When the fluid cooled, he noted the persistence of animalcules in the infusion, indicating to him that spontaneous generation had occurred. The Italian Abbé Spallanzani felt that Needham had incompletely excluded air from his infusion and subjected the latter's experiments to further trial. Spallanzani boiled a glass vessel for forty-five minutes, then sealed it hermetically by fusing the drawn-out neck of the flask with a flame. He failed to obtain Needham's results and concluded that the theory of spontaneous generation was false. Spallanzani announced his observations in two important papers (1767, 1776).[4] Even so, the myth of spontaneous generation survived.

Franz Schulze (1836), working in Berlin on the effect of air on fermentation, passed strong sulfuric acid through red-hot glass tubes, thus destroying any organic matter entering the flask container from the air. In experiments conducted in the Berlin laboratory of Johannes Müller between 1834 and 1837, Schwann, regarded by many as the founder of the germ theory of disease, showed that putrefaction did not occur in a flask containing muscle tissue and water when heated to the boiling point of water. Even when air, similarly heated, was subsequently permitted to enter the flask, putrefaction did not take place. Schwann's conclusion was that heat destroyed the infusoria from the air, precluding putrefaction.[5]

Charles Cagniard-Latour (1836), Schwann (1837), and Friedrich Kützing (1837), all working independently, announced in print almost simultaneously that yeast cells, living organisms belonging to the vegetable kingdom, accounted for fermentation in fluids; their observations were not taken seriously by most of their contemporaries. Chemistry had become well entrenched scientifically through important research before the biological discoveries of the Pasteur-Koch era, and chemists were wont to believe that every phenomenon was explicable on a chemicophysical basis. The Swedish chemist Johann Berzelius, his German pupil Friedrich Wöhler, and the celebrated German chemist Justus Liebig combined efforts to prevent acceptance of the work of the biologists. Berzelius and Liebig in 1839 wrote contemptuously of the biologists' theory of fermentation. Liebig and Wöhler composed a skit entitled the "Riddle of Vinous Fermentation," which was published anonymously. The chemist Pasteur, with a mind unrestrained by the barriers of a single discipline, and far more expert in use of the microscope than the chemists just mentioned, proved the fallacy of their criticisms.[6] Chemists, physicists, and biologists since that day have come to have greater mutual respect for their fellow scientists in other disciplines and to work cooperatively.

Early in a distinguished career, the German physician, physiologist, and physicist Hermann Helmholtz, extended the matter further (1843) and separated two fluids, a putrefying and a fermenting liquid, from one another by a membrane through which solid material could not pass, yet permeable to fluid. The putrescible material did not appear in the fermenting fluid, nor the converse. Helmholtz concluded that the material responsible for putrescence and/or fermentation must have been a solid substance of colloidal nature.[7]

In 1854–59 Schröder and Theodor Dusch of Heidelberg refined Schwann's experiment by placing cotton wool in the outlet from a glass container in which the infusion was subjected to great heat. The cotton wool filtered the air and arrested the progress of any microscopic particles from access to the infusion, which did not undergo putrefaction. Pasteur amplified their proof. He subjected the cotton wool filter to microscopic examination and was able to demonstrate the presence of bacteria therein. Moreover, he found that bacteria recovered from such cotton wool filters grew out demonstrable microscopic organisms. Additionally, Pasteur observed that the cotton wool filter could be omitted and that merely sealing the end of the tube, much as Spallanzani had done almost two centuries earlier, was equally as effective in preserving sterility of the flasked fluid attending application of heat.[8]

John Tyndall, English physicist, observed that a luminous beam passing through the moteless air of his experimental tube was invisible. It occurred to him that such a beam might be utilized to detect the presence of germs in the atmosphere — air devoid of floating particles would be free of bacteria and incapable of scattering light. Numerous experiments showed optically pure air did not contain bacterial life. Tyndall also noted that ordinary bacteria are killed at temperatures below 100° C, but that the hay bacillus (subtilis) retains its vitality after several hours of boiling. By a process of successive periods of discontinuous heating, he was able to show that such heat killed the hay bacillus suspended in fluids.[9] Microbiologists were quick to seize upon Tyndall's scheme of discontinuous heating to ensure sterility of their cultures.

Microscopy

Of all the aids that have come to medicine from other disciplines, few have influenced its progress as much as the microscope. Yet many famous medical figures had little use for microscopy. Although Leeuwenhoek ground his own lenses and built over 250 microscopes,[10] a century later John Hunter used no greater magnification than a hand lens. Bichat, the creator of descriptive anatomy (1801), neglected the microscope, as did Cruveilhier in his beautifully illustrated multiple-volume atlas of pathologic anatomy (1829–42). When Rokitansky, Vienna's great pathologist, wrote his three-volume handbook of pathological anatomy (1842–46), he virtually ignored the microscope and depended almost entirely on gross descriptions of disease. His emphasis in the body's defense against infection and inflammation was upon humoral mechanisms. Virchow (1846) wrote a scathing review of his older colleague's work and renewed his attack when a new edition of Rokitansky's handbook appeared in 1855, but in a gentler and more appreciative mood.[11]

Many noted microscopists antedated this group of anatomist-pathologists. The German Jesuit Athanasius Kircher used a microscope in his investigations and has been credited with describing bacteria (1658), which Friedrich Löffler later said may have been red blood cells. Leeuwenhoek (1673–83) described clumps and chains of bacteria, identifiable today. Said he, "There are more animals living in the scum on the teeth in a man's mouth than there are men in a whole kingdom." He found the diameter of a grain of sand to be 1,000 times larger than one of these animalcules. Leeuwenhoek's findings that microorganisms are a normal inhabitant of the mouth undoubtedly retarded acceptance of the pathogenicity of bacteria.[12]

An early confirmation of the existence of animalcules was published in 1718 in a thesis on microscopical observations by the

Parisian scientist Louis Joblot. In 1711 he boiled an infusion of hay in water in two flasks for fifteen minutes. One he immediately stoppered tightly; the other was left open to the air. The first solution remained clear; after several days, when unstoppered, small animals developed within it, as in the flask left communicating with air. These came from "eggs dispersed in the air," which the boiling had initially destroyed.[13]

Marcello Malpighi's revealing studies are perpetuated by many eponyms. In 1661 this great Italian microscopist, founder of histology, recognized the capillary anastomoses between arteries and veins in the pulmonary circulation, completing the missing link in Harvey's discovery of circulation of the blood (1628). Hooke, like Leeuwenhoek, built many microscopes, but confined his studies in histology essentially to vegetable matter (1665), as did Nehemiah Grew, the English comparative anatomist (1681).[14]

Had Redi examined microscopically meat with direct access to flies, undoubtedly he would have observed microorganisms in the resultant putrefactive process. Medical history is replete with neglected opportunities that could have led to early significant discoveries. Two centuries were to come and go before Schwann (1837), Matthias J. Schleiden (1838), Christian Ehrenberg (1838), and Henle (1840) laid the foundations for microbiology, which has played so vital a role in medicine's advance. In discussing the value of experiments, experimental medicine, and the requirements of science, Pavlov said that the discipline of microbiology had succeeded in welding medicine into a unified whole.[15]

Ehrenberg traveled widely and collected a large number of plants of various kinds and descriptions, which he drew, named, and catalogued. He became a professor in Berlin and spent the rest of his professional life there. In 1838 he wrote a monumental treatise and an accompanying atlas with colored plates. He classified all the protozoa and bacteria known to him in one group, the infusoria, which he regarded as animal in nature.[16] He too was unaware of the pathogenicity of microorganisms in the provocation of disease.

It is of interest that a large number of microscopic studies of pus and exudates were made by observers who described and pictured microorganisms without recognizing their importance in the generation of the suppurative process. In this group are to be mentioned Julius Vogel (1838), Emanuel Kreipl (1839), and Hubert Luschka (1845).[17]

It does seem strange that Henle (1809–85), who at age thirty-one announced his thesis of the bacterial origin of contagion (1840), should not have pursued his innovative studies. Trained as anatomist and physiologist under Müller in Berlin, Henle, himself a professor of anatomy successively in Zürich, Heidelberg, and Göttingen, became the foremost microscopist among anatomists of his time. His essay upon miasmata and contagion, in which he deduced the role of living microorganisms as the cause of contagion, in some respects reemphasized the thesis that Fracastoro had enunciated in 1546, yet reflected definite gains in scientific sophistication over the interval of three centuries. Metchnikoff, his pupil at Göttingen in 1866, has remarked that Henle remained indifferent to his 1840 proposal of microorganisms as the cause of infectious diseases. Metch-

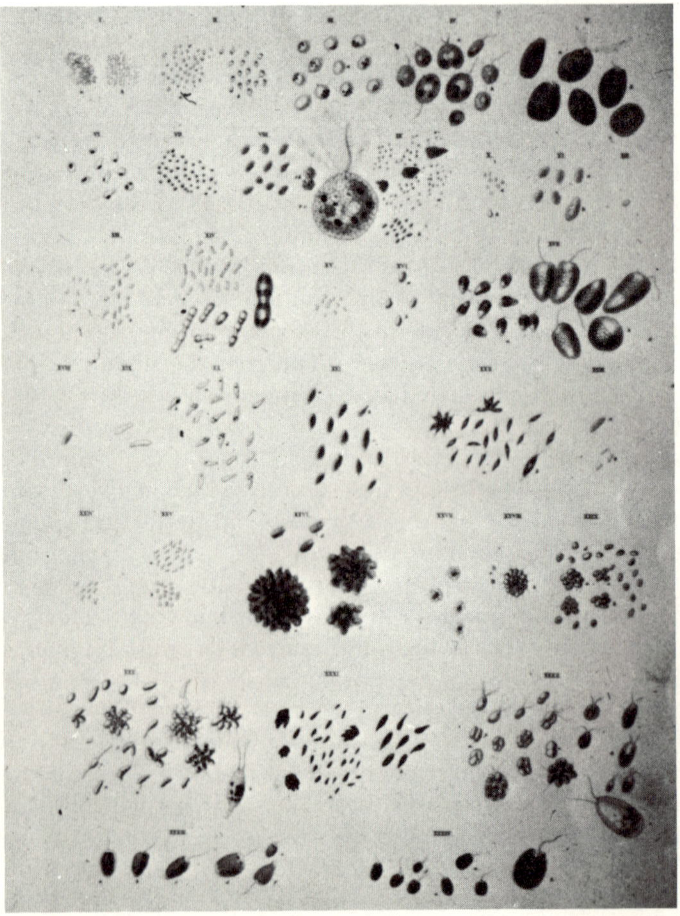

20.1 Ehrenberg's early morphologic studies of bacteria (1838).

nikoff's assignment under Henle was to study the kidney of amphibians and the corpus cavernosum of the penis in man. "At no time did the question of the causes of infectious diseases come up in his laboratory."[18]

Henle was the foremost exponent and interpreter of the microscopic appearance of epithelia, especially the epithelium of the intestine. Broadly trained, a great teacher, and a forward-looking medical scientist-philosopher, he did much to indicate the interdependence of the sciences and to initiate studies which emphasized the factual over the empiric. It remained for his brilliant pupil, Koch, to lend added meaning to what Henle foresaw. Had Henle followed up his earlier 1840 observations upon the contagious nature of miasmata with histologic studies of bacteria, whose relationship to infection he had stressed, the hiatus between the significant work of Pasteur, Lister, and Koch would not have been so long. But such is the nature of progress. Man goes in the direction his interests lead him. Forty years were to elapse following Henle's declaration before chemical antisepsis was replaced by thermal antisepsis for many aspects of surgical operations.

Trained by Virchow in pathology in the early 1860s, Cohnheim foresaw the great significance for medicine's advance on the new front, microbiology, during a period when Virchow still clung to the traditional views of pathologic anatomists. When Welch sought the advice of Carl Ludwig in Leipzig in 1884, he was advised to identify himself with Cohnheim rather than with Virchow — sound advice for that period.[19]

A young Berlin surgeon, Arnold Hiller, in 1875 insisted that "the invisible enemy bacteria" could not be harmful, for did we not live in an atmosphere completely surrounded by them? "We breathe them in 1200 times an hour, over days, weeks, and months — they swarm in our intestinal canals."[20] Koch's work sufficed to convince him. Tait (1886) continued to maintain that bacteria were harmless because he had great success in ovariotomy without observance of the "antiseptic system"; he attributed his good record solely to high standards of surgical cleanliness.[21]

Employment of microscopy was essential for recognition of the role of bacteria in the genesis of wound infection and for understanding the nature of miasmas responsible for hospitalism. Development of cultural methods also was necessary before the pathogenicity of individual microorganisms could be definitely established. Although Ehrenberg had been able to stain bacteria and other microorganisms identifiable today, it took Joseph Gerlach's carmine stains (1858) and Carl Weigert's aniline dyes (1875) to enable microscopists to identify microorganisms accurately and readily. Gerlach's carmine served Virchow through the first twenty-five years of his pathologic studies.[22] Koch elaborated upon Weigert's aniline dye method for the study of bacteria in surgical infections. When Koch in 1881 was able to separate and grow pure cultures of bacteria, the science of bacteriology was well on its way.

Hermann Klencke (1843) had grown out bacteria, on culture, obtained from window panes in hospital wards. The German surgeon H. R. Ranke (1874) was perhaps the first to subject to microscopic examination the exudate from wounds treated by Listerian methods; invariably micrococci in chains were found in the exudate. He called them streptococci, several years before they were described by Pasteur (1879) or Friedrich Fehleisen (1882).[23]

The French physician-microbiologists Casimir Davaine and P.-F.-O. Rayer (1850) demonstrated microscopically the presence of the anthrax bacillus in the blood of sheep that had died of anthrax.[24] Davaine's studies on the rapidity of division of these bacteria antedated Ferdinand Cohn's similar determinations. Davaine stated that the anthrax bacillus divided every two hours; after twenty-four hours 4,096 organisms would divide from a single bacterium; in forty-eight hours, 16,777,216. He estimated there would be 60 billion anthrax bacteria in the bloodstream of a man dying of anthrax. Davaine also dealt with the bacteria of *pourriture*. His characterization identified them as cocci, but whether staphylococci or streptococci is uncertain. Davaine said such bacteria lose movement when heated to 50° C; at 52° C they die. He did not speak of disease germs but of the ferment of putrefaction.[25]

In the Franco-Prussian War, Edwin Klebs, studying wound infection in the Karlsruhe Military Hospital, performed 115 autopsies; in 73 percent of these, septicemia or pyemia was the cause of death, and bacteria were found in almost every instance. However, Klebs labeled all the observed diverse forms of microbic organisms as *Microsporon septicum*. He was not alone in this. Virchow at the same period in time apparently made the same error. It was not until solid culture media, introduced by Koch, were available that bacterial colonies could be differentiated. In a fluid medium such as broth the organisms would have to be identified microscopically; if many were present, this would not be an easy matter.[26] Both morphology and cultural characteristics obviously were essential for the classification of bacteria.

In a series of publications between 1866 and 1869[27] the Strasbourg investigators Léon Coze and Victor Feltz established the transmissibility of infection from man to small animals, primarily guinea pigs and rabbits. They asked, are the responsible toxic agents of infectious diseases simply ferments? They cited the work of Wilhelm Griesinger (1864) and Billroth, both of whom believed that "ferments" (molecular elements) may cause fever.

Coze and Feltz (1866) took blood from a patient dying of putrid infection, mixed it with an equal volume of distilled and filtered water, and injected it into the jugular veins of six rabbits; five of the six rabbits died within fifty-six hours. Arterial blood from one of these sick rabbits was injected without water into the jugular vein of three additional rabbits; all died within six days. In controls, non-putrid blood was well tolerated. From a living patient with typhoid fever Coze and Feltz (1866) obtained venous blood which made rabbits ill when injected intravenously. On successive injections from one rabbit to another, the authors found the virulence of the organisms increased. They (1869) obtained blood from a baby dying of scarlet fever. On reinjection from one generation of rabbits to others, fatal outcomes occurred in much shorter periods of time; sixty-two such injections were made. Leucocytosis was observed in the ill rabbits. Whereas initially the injected rabbits survived four to six days, after the seventh transfer death usually occurred within twenty-six hours. The increase of virulence on repeated intravenous injection is not generally conceded by microbiologists today.

Many trace the beginnings of microbiology to Cohn, professor of botany at Breslau, and his 1872 investigations of bacteria. Cohn (1872) began his book on bacteria, "the smallest of living organisms," by alluding to the work of Leeuwenhoek and said that the Dane Otto Müller (1786) was the first to attempt a classification of bacteria, describing approximately 380 different forms.[28] Bacteria were recognized as animal life up to the time of Agnostino Bassi (1835) and Félix Dujardin (1841). Davaine (1859) was one of the first to identify bacteria with algae, a conclusion with which Cohn agreed.[29]

In writing of bacterial fission Cohn (1872) said that if all the bacteria from the fission of one bacterium survived four and a half days, they would occupy an area the size of all the oceans, or two-thirds that of the entire earth, counting the oceans as averaging a mile in depth. At the end of twenty-four hours the weight of the bacteria from repeated fission would be 1/40 of a milligram; after forty-eight hours, nearly 442 grams (1 pound); after three days, 7,500,000 kilograms. Fortunately the rate of multiplication is not maintained. Cohn stated it was "in the highest degree probable" that "bacteria are in many diseases the conveyors and originators of infection, that they are the ferment of contagion."[30] He studied bacteria morphologically and recognized that this criterion alone was inadequate for accurate differentiation and classification. It remained for Koch and his cultural studies, employing solid media, to provide the missing link.

Sédillot in 1878 coined the word "microbe" which he said meant "small life," a designation that won the approval of the French philologist Littré. Among synonyms for microbes Sédillot mentioned microzoaria, microphytes, aerobes, anaerobes, bacteria, micrococci, and other terms that had been in use for many years and were to survive for many more.[31]

Harmfulness of Pus: Chemical or Bacterial?

The French physician Gaspard was one of the first to assess the role of pus injected into animals by various routes, including subcutaneous, intravenous, and serous cavity injections. He observed (1822) that blood from a dog injected with pus, when injected into another dog, produced symptoms similar to those suffered by the first victim. Gaspard's finding was confirmed by Magendie (1823), who observed that pus, lethal when injected intravenously, was apparently without effect when administered by mouth. In a subsequent publication (1824) Gaspard noted that mineral acids inhibit or retard putrefaction in meat, much as Pringle had shown many decades earlier (1753).[32]

P. L. Panum (1856, 1876, 1878) of Copenhagen studied the toxicity of pus. He was well aware in his later publications of the work of Pasteur and Cohn, yet he was not quite willing to concede that bacteria were solely responsible for the toxicity of infected blood or meat. Edouard Chassaignac, a surgeon of the Lariboisière Hospital, using magnifications as high as 400, examined pus microscopically and described its cellular structure (1859). He identified both protein and fatty substances in the pus. He did not recognize bacteria.[33]

Magendie had shown that filtration reduced the toxicity of infected fluids. To the modern observer it seems a bit strange that the effect of boiling such fluids, as well as filtration, was not critically assessed. The thesis that chemical substances in infected fluid were responsible for the immediate symptoms provoked on intravenous injection of the fluid, long remained the thesis to which many investigators, including several surgeons, were partial. Among these were Adolph S. Stich (1853), Carl Thiersch (1855–56), Bergmann (1872), and Hiller (1875), who subscribed in whole or in part to the old thesis of Gaspard that symptoms attending injections of pus, in part, were a chemical response to toxins contained within the pus.

In 1854 Bergeret had described pus as a liquid containing animalcules which he described as pyozaires. These animalcules, Bergeret believed, usually lived only twenty-four hours; their longevity, he recognized, was influenced by various considerations. Acetic acid, he found, arrested their movement.[34]

An editorial assessment of the existence of micrococci on the walls of hospital wards was presented in the Paris *Union médicale* (1877). Several reports were summarized, including Broca's finding that globules of pus could be squeezed from a sponge on washing the walls of a ward in the Paris hospital of St. Antoine. Chalvet (1860) attributed the blue color often seen around wounds to the presence of microscopic algae. Elisel (1861) of Prague placed pour-plates between beds occupied by children suffering from purulent affections and observed globules of pus on such plates, indicating that the distance separating the beds permitted transfer of bacterial colonies to the plates and that transfer of infection between patients at this distance also was possible. At La Pitié it had been demonstrated that a sponge used to wipe the walls of a surgical ward contained 50 to 60 organisms per microscopic field, suggesting the importance of airborne infection.[35]

Such observations undoubtedly could be repeated for many modern operating suites. Recognizing the difficulty of wrestling with the problem in a realistic and helpful manner, it is not unusual to hear administrative microbiologists attached to operating suites say, "Yes, we know bacteria are present on vertical hospital walls; we are primarily concerned only with those on horizontal surfaces at levels of the operating table, and they do not appear to be a serious threat; it is the shedding of bacteria by the operating personnel that constitutes the greatest hazard of wound infection to patients undergoing operation."

In a séance of the Academy of Medicine Pasteur (1875) spoke of Albert Bergeron's report upon the presence of microscopic organisms in abscesses. The Lyons surgeon had opened eighteen abscesses (hot and cold) with no communication to the exterior and had observed many microorganisms in the exudate.

Pasteur believed the observation was important enough to warrant appointment of a commission to examine the validity of Bergeron's idea that abscesses contained bacteria. The suggestion was declined by the academy because Bergeron had not submitted his report in writing.[36]

Cheyne (1879), who went to King's College Hospital with Lister from Edinburgh, apparently shared Gaspard's earlier view that agents other than bacteria could provoke infection, an outlook Cheyne rejected (1882) after translating Koch's great work on the pathogenicity of bacteria. Alexander Ogston of Aberdeen (1881) concluded as had Koch that bacteria were the causative agents in infection. Ogston stated: "Once micrococci have gained access to a wound, it is not easy to eradicate them." He found that ordinary Lister dressings failed to do so (eight cases). Similarly too after weeks of dressing patients with a 1:16 to 1:8 strength carbolic acid oil (eight cases), boracic lint (four cases), salicylic acid (one case), and chloralum (one case), micrococci were found "in the wounds and ulcers in nearly as great numbers as before; and it was clear these applications, at least as ordinarily employed, although generally sufficient to kill bacteria and bacilli, are powerless to eradicate the micrococci. The only way in which I succeeded in destroying them in wounds, where they had once established themselves, was by cauterisation with strong solution of chloride of zinc, or by strong frictions with five per cent watery solution of carbolic acid — the ordinary 1:20 lotion."[37]

Despite the protests of Fleming (1919) of the inutility of irrigating wounds with Dakin's solution or other antiseptics, the practice continued until specific antibacterial agents, the sulfonamides and antibiotics, became available in the 1935–44 period to thwart infection in contaminated wounds. In fact, many surgeons still continue irrigating wounds in the belief that healing is encouraged thereby.

Transmissibility of Wound Infection

Although microscopy was neglected, a number of significant publications, chiefly by military surgeons toward the end of the eighteenth century and in the early nineteenth century, sounded warnings that went largely unheeded — observations reflecting important gains in knowledge concerning the nature and origin of wound infection. Pringle's experiments published in 1753 showed that putrescence in dead flesh could be prevented and suspended by submersion in mineral acids. Even so, recognition of the nature of the contagion responsible for wound infection and implementation of chemical means to render surgical instruments and materiel for operation reasonably safe were a century away. An "unknown miasma" was the usual label attached to purulent wound accumulations attending operative procedures.

In about 1744 Pouteau, then a young medical student in the Hôtel-Dieu of Lyons, pricked his finger while working on a cadaver. He continued to care for the infected and gangrenous wounds of patients. His finger became inflamed and gangrenous. He fortunately recovered from the severe infection, but through the experience he correctly surmised that wound infection was contagious. He was perhaps the first to write intelligibly on the subject and was also the first to identify the erysipelatous nature of puerperal fever. Many of his observations summarized in a three-volume work published posthumously (1783) have a very modern ring. Pouteau's studies were reviewed more than fifty years later by Delpech when Napoleon's retreating armies filled his hospital at Montpellier with wounded, and hospital gangrene became a major problem in the crowded wards. Using experiments, Delpech enlisted the help of colleagues in a search to understand the problem. He concluded (1815) that suppurating wounds harbored contagious matter which was "animal" in nature.[38]

A courageous surgeon's aide in Napoleon's army in Spain pursued a hazardous investigation in 1810. Ollivier, twenty-one years old, surmising that *pourriture* (hospital gangrene) was transmitted by contact, set out to test his theory. He journeyed alone far through enemy territory to find a military hospital with advanced cases of the disease, then had his right arm inoculated with three pricks of a lancet dipped in pus from a soldier dying of *pourriture*. A few days later an acutely painful spreading cellulitis extended to the axilla. On the sixth day his wound was dressed with camphorated alcohol and cauterized with silver nitrate; in twenty-eight days, after further cauterizations, his arm was healed; he still bore the scar in 1822.

Ollivier sent accounts of his experiments and affidavits of the attending surgeons to his superior officers, but they ignored or discredited his reports. Twelve years later (1822) the embittered surgeon published a remarkable treatise on *pourriture*, documenting his research and supplying a wealth of material from earlier investigators, particularly Pringle, Pouteau, and Delpech. He printed a vituperous exchange of letters with Percy, to whom, "young and confident," he had addressed his first re-

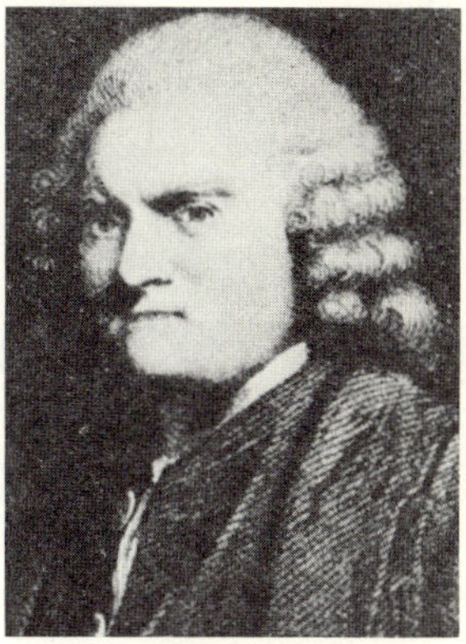

20.2 John Pringle (1707–82), English military surgeon and student of hospital infection, demonstrated that putrefaction in dead bodies of small animals can be prevented by immersion in strong mineral acids (1753).

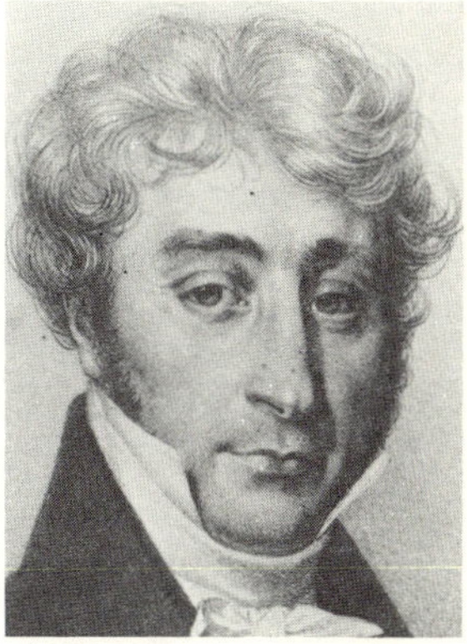

20.3 Jacques Delpech (1777–1832), Montpellier surgeon, concluded that suppurating wounds transmitted a contagion of "animal" origin.

port.[39] He also twitted Percy for authoring articles on such frivolous subjects as "perruque" and "cravate" in Panckoucke's medical dictionary.[40]

Ollivier advised that instruments used in dressing wounds be purified by passing them through a flame, a recommendation repeated many years later by Pasteur. He added that washing instruments with camphorated vinegar was effective, and use of mineral acids averted the contagion. Ollivier urged dressers to wash their hands in soapy water and then immerse them in camphorated vinegar before attending a clean wound; *charpies* should not be reused. He said that contaminated dressings, bedding, and clothing could transmit the disease and patients with *pourriture* should be in a separate ward. He found topical antiseptics ineffective in dealing with *pourriture* and early use of the cautery the only resource.

Thomson, Regius Professor of Military Surgery at Edinburgh, devoted a chapter of his *Lectures on Inflammation* (1813) to hospital gangrene, giving excerpts from several British naval observations. He believed that the contagious nature of the disease was proved by a number of facts: (1) it may be communicated to persons at a distance by sponge, *charpie*, bandage, or clothing; (2) it attacks slight wounds of persons dressing infected persons; (3) it progresses from a single individual through a succession of patients; (4) it attacks recent as well as old wounds shortly after exposure to an infected patient; and (5) it tenaciously persists in only one ward of a ship and will not spread from there if isolation measures are taken.[41]

The enlightened practices of British naval hospitals of the late eighteenth and nineteenth centuries are revealed in a number of contemporary accounts. In 1797 Rollo reported that a sponge could spread sores when "unguardedly used for different sores"; he also related applying silver nitrate to such lesions. He attributed the Woolwich Hospital amputation record of twenty-one cases, one a double amputation, with only three deaths to the "cleanliness, ventilation, and smallness of the wards." A sentinel was posted to prevent "all intercourse . . . except what is indispensible" from wards in which infected sailors were isolated.[42]

Isolation wards maintained in the Royal Naval Hospital at Deal ordinarily prevented the spread of gangrene, wrote Alexander Hutchison (1826). According to navy instructions, instruments from diseased wards were always put in boiling water after use. He also mentioned such precautions as putting fouled bandages into boiling water and dipping sponges and bandages in dilute sulfuric acid after each use; separate sponges were advised for individual patients.[43]

It has been noted (chapter 18) that swabbing the suppurating wounds of many patients with a single sponge was common practice in military and civilian hospitals in the mid-1870s in France, England, Germany, and the United States. The instruction and warnings of Rollo (1797), Thomson (1813), Ollivier (1822), Hutchison (1826), and others had been completely ignored.

A heroic autoinfection, reminiscent of Ollivier's experiment, was that of Karl Garré of Basel, in 1883. Garré rubbed a culture of *Staph. aureus* into the skin of his left forearm, much as one rubs in an ointment. For a control he rubbed sterile jelly into the skin of the right forearm. Six hours later he experienced a burning sensation in the left forearm; swelling followed and within a few hours there were pustules at the site. By the fourth day a large carbuncle appeared, surrounded by a ring of pustules. Garré survived, but it was a bold and almost fatal experiment.[44]

Dissection Wounds

"They took their lives in their lancet-hand," wrote Kipling in his stirring tribute to the surgeons of old going out to fight the plague.[45] The implication was more significant than the poet probably realized. "A pin-prick is a door open to Death," said Velpeau. Before the appearance of the sulfonamides and penicillin, puncture of fingers in dissection of dead bodies was a potentially hazardous occupational accident, as Dorsey observed in 1823. Louis C. Chouvet in a Paris thesis of 1865 described thirty cases from the literature and of recent occurrence in which serious infection followed dissection pricks. Many had proved fatal. Death in such instances was far less frequent after it became common practice in the nineteenth century to embalm cadavers, according to John Shaw, who said there was no longer any fear of dissection at Great Windmill Street. The bodies were injected with a solution of nitre and salt and students could keep them eight to ten weeks with scarcely any smell.[46]

Pouteau's personal experience with a dissection wound, which led to his interpretation of the nature of contagion, has been mentioned. One of the best known of fatal dissection wounds was that sustained by Jakob Kolletschka (1803–47) of Vienna, a close friend and colleague of Semmelweis. He was pricked on a finger by an assistant while performing an autopsy and died March 13, 1847.[47] It was this tragic occurrence that stimulated

Semmelweis's interest in ascertaining the origins of puerperal fever and eventuated in his achievement of prophylactic surgical antisepsis. Another famous death from a dissection wound is a fictional one — that of the physician Bazarov in the last chapter of Turgenev's *Father and Sons* (1861). Bazarov had asked permission to perform the autopsy on a patient who had died of typhus; in doing so he cut his finger. Silver nitrate was applied four hours after the injury, but Bazarov died a few days later.

William Hewson (1739–74), who worked with both the Hunters and won the Copley Medal of the Royal Society, died of a dissection wound, as did Gosset (1792–1854) of silver-gilt suture fame. The Austrian surgeon Hunczovsky (1752–98) died of sepsis from a finger infection sustained during an operation. His trip abroad in 1783 to report on French and English surgery for Joseph II is referred to several times in our account.

Many instances of death following dissection wounds may be found in the obituary reports of physicians. Phlebotomy also took its toll of infected pricks. John Muter of Glasgow (1839) reported the instance of a young soldier who injured his right wrist while placing a body in a coffin. Swelling developed; Muter wished to make an incision but the family objected. A few days later the swelling was incised, but the patient died.[48] In his zealous pursuit of anatomical dissections early in his career, Monro I of Edinburgh sustained a scratch on his hand that threatened to be a fatal dissection wound but from which he recovered despite a cellulitis extending to the shoulder. Paget (1871) described his own personal experience with a dissection wound, an erysipelas-like infection accompanied by abscesses and edema. The usual remedy of such wounds in his student days, said Paget, was to apply leeches, give purgatives, and perform phlebotomy. Six weeks after the original infection Paget developed what seemed to be a crisis, followed by sweating, and his pulse and temperature declined; quinine, sedatives, and morphine brought improvement. After three months of illness, he recovered.[49]

The senior author has been witness to two such occurrences at the University of Minnesota before availability of the sulfonamides. In the mid-1920s, while performing a mastoidectomy, William Murray, professor of ophthalmology, pierced his left thumb. A short time later, Strachauer, our professor of surgery, amputated the ophthalmologist's arm, but the patient died. Shortly thereafter, an assistant in the Department of Anatomy, Lucretia Wilder, while working with rabbits and a streptococcal culture, spilled a drop on her forearm; the rabbit scratched the site while Wilder was preparing to make an intravenous injection. A few days later she died of septicemia. One of President Coolidge's two sons sustained a blister on his heel while playing tennis and succumbed from the infection.

Rags and Dressings

Lister still alluded to use of rags as dressings in 1871, as he had in his first publication on surgical antisepsis in 1867.[50] A century earlier Pouteau remarked that reused linen dressings, inadequately washed, could sow disease in wounds and recommended substitution of disposable paper compresses; he opposed the common hospital practice of employing convalescent patients to prepare dressing materials. Yet at the Radcliffe Infirmary, Oxford, in 1845 and later, old linen sheets were torn up to make wound dressings, and gifts of linen rags for this purpose were solicited by advertisement as late as 1869.[51]

S. J. Brugmans (1816) reported that old wound dressings, bleached in France and imported for hospital use in Holland, often gave rise to erysipelas in surgical patients. Hospital gangrene could be communicated by contaminated soiled linen or lint, noted Boyer (1815). Little notice was taken by physicians or surgeons of William Henry's experiments on the role of direct contact in spreading contagion. Henry was a Manchester chemist with an M.D. degree from Edinburgh. He demonstrated (1832) that when night clothing worn by patients with scarlet fever was sterilized by dry heat of 204° F for one hour it did not communicate the disease to susceptible persons. Whereas Gamgee began applying gauze dressings to wounds in the 1870s, rags washed and partially sterilized by boiling remained a not infrequent source of surgical dressings through the nineteenth century.[52]

Rags collected from diverse sources eventually assumed international trade significance involving great sums of money; such materials were often conveyors of contagious diseases, including smallpox, measles, and scarlet fever. In 1867 a Scottish Public Health Act and, in 1875, a similar law in England imposed a heavy penalty on any person who "gives, lends, sells, transmits, or exposes, without due disinfection, any bedding, clothing, rags or other things which have been exposed to infection from any dangerous infectious disorder." Before 1878 authorities in Austria had forbidden importation of rags.[53]

In the 1880s the subject of rags as an international hazard to health was often discussed by public health officials. At the Fifth International Congress of Hygiene and Demography at The

Hague in 1884 W. P. Ruysch indicated that outbreaks of typhus were traceable to release of supposedly sterilized rags. He alluded to a number of outbreaks of disease resulting from their use in the years 1868–71. He stated that rags imported into Holland had conveyed smallpox, Asiatic cholera, anthrax, and diphtheria. Ruysch emphasized that disinfection of large bales of rags was not easy; increased vapor pressure at 121 to 128°C for two hours was necessary for bales weighing 1.2 tons.[54] For years to come sanitarians continued to repeat facts from Ruysch's startling exposure.

William M. Smith, health officer of the Port of New York, stated (1885) that in that port alone 175,000 bales of old rags worth several million dollars entered annually, despite the circumstance that they were known to be "fruitful sources of the dissemination of some forms of contagious disease." Rags, he said, came from the slums of many cities of the world including Cairo and Alexandria in Egypt, Naples in Italy, and India, communicating infection to a large number of persons. When the public health regulations in the United States required that rags be sterilized by high steam pressure and subjected also to a sulfuric acid steam (1884), the situation improved somewhat. However, one of the difficulties was that the process of disinfection of rags in bales by superheated steam had been patented, making it mandatory either to pay the patent fees or devise new methods.[55]

At the 1886 meeting of the American Public Health Association held in Toronto, a twenty-page report was presented by the Committee on the Disinfection of Rags. Instances were reported in which smallpox and other diseases had been conveyed through exposure to rags. Clothing from victims of smallpox apparently had been put into ragbags. Employees at the paper mills who pulled the bales of rags apart not infrequently became victims of the infection lurking therein.

Especially involved, obviously, were the ragpickers themselves. In 1874 there were 117 rag stores in Marseilles alone, of which 46 were in one district, where the mortality from smallpox was three times greater than in any other area of the city. Of 157 deaths from smallpox, 64 occurred in the houses of ragpickers or houses in close proximity.[56]

As late as 1886 George M. Sternberg, surgeon general and a distinguished microbiologist, wrote a five-page journal letter to Dr. J. H. Raymond at The Johns Hopkins, concluding, "In the absence of any prevailing epidemic I would not treat baled rags differently from other merchandise. If for any reason the health officer at the port of arrival considers such merchandise dangerous, it is evidently his duty to disinfect it. This can be done most effectually by steam." He then suggests that his letter be printed in full.[57] Obviously, Sternberg must have been under pressure from importers to simplify the procedure of rag importation.

C. F. Withington (1887) reported that in 1880 the paper industry had used 189,917 tons of rags, of which Massachusetts consumed one-third. The total value of the rags was over $55 million. The United States imported rags from sixty-five different countries in 1884, which had proved a source of infection for measles and scarlet fever. He said that 225,000 people in France made their livelihood through traffic with rags; 100,000,000 kg. of rags were used in France in 1879, one-third of which arrived at the Port of Marseilles.

Some hospitals disinfected rags with phenol; others used chloride of lime, obviously not a healthy practice. Ragpickers plucked rags out of ashheaps. The rags were often placed in a "duster," a large enclosed box, and heavy iron spikes were used to pull the rags apart to rid them of loose dirt. A health officer in Copenhagen (1890) reported the bacterial count to be fifty times higher in the atmosphere where rags were unpacked than in other parts of the factory building.[58]

As late as 1915 rags and mills that converted rags to paper were recognized as a source of infection in Paris; apparently the suggestion of international regulations adopted at the Fifth International Congress (1884) had proved ineffective. In 1915 Wurtz addressed the French Academy of Medicine on the "Suppression of the chiffonage [rag industry] in Paris." In Paris alone in the year 1903, he stated, the rag industry netted four million francs, and the global industry probably produced eight to nine million. The greater susceptibility of workers in the rag industry to diverse diseases, contrasted with the general population, notably to tuberculosis and typhoid fever, was noted.[59]

It continued unfortunately in several areas to be common hospital practice well into the twentieth century to resterilize and reuse dressings despite tragic lessons of the past. This brief recounting serves to indicate that the rag industry, a distinctly unclean and filthy operation, endured almost up to World War I, serving medical purposes, despite ready availability of sterilizable gauze.

Laundries

In 1877 the *Lancet* Special Commission on the Spread of Disease through Laundries reported that the laundry done by washerwomen, who often served twenty to thirty families, was a frequent source of smallpox. Contamination during ironing was emphasized. Several instances were cited. The editorial expressed alarm; in a few weeks five companies had been founded to provide "sanitary laundries." After the elapse of twenty-one years the editor returned to the subject, concluding, "the most dangerous operation is the sorting and marking of the linen before it is washed." This danger concerned largely small private laundries. The major laundries had facilities for disinfection. The hazard of pinpricks from pins left in contaminated linen was mentioned by E. Beaugrand (1868), who believed that laundresses had a high mortality rate during epidemics.[60]

The keenest impetus to the establishment of laundries in the United States apparently was the Gold Rush in California, in the absence of women to do such work. However, in 1860 commercial laundries were still virtually nonexistent in the United States. Wealthy people had their washing done in their homes or by individuals outside, and approximately 40,000 women declared their occupation to be laundresses in the 1860 census. Washboards, tubs, and boiling water, when available, were part of the usual process. Machines for home use with a revolving barrel turned by a handcrank could be purchased for $10 or more.[61]

M. C. Schroeder and S. G. Southerland (1917) deplored the situation existing in hand laundries in New York City. They found the Chinese laundries on the average better than others. The bacterial count of linen submitted for handwashing was not diminished by the laundry process. Steam laundries were an improvement, but in many respects left much to be desired.[62]

At the London Hospital in 1851 six persons washed 2,400 pieces of linen each week. It lay in cold water for one to two hours, then was placed in a mixture of 9 pints of soap and 1 pint of soda to 10 parts hot water and finally in a hot-water kettle under pressure for one hour; after that it was handwashed in cold water. A hydraulic press eliminated most of the moisture with the help of dry ovens. This technique varied somewhat from hospital to hospital in London.[63]

A correspondent in *Lancet* (1861) praised the laundry facilities at the Salpetrière in Paris. The wet laundry was no longer hung to dry on stretched lines in a heated room — the moisture was removed by hot-air ovens, ranged around the walls. The high temperature apparently did the trick. The author alluded to the washing arrangements at the Lariboisière Hospital in Paris and the Bethanien in Berlin, in both of which 2,000 pounds of wash could be dealt with satisfactorily in six hours. If handwashed, the laundry would take two to four times as long.[64] Oppert (1868) advised adding soda as a bleach to keep the wash white. He expressed approval of the methods at the Salpetrière and the Lariboisière, where the dirty linen was first washed in cold water, omitting handwashing, then thrust into steam where the water was under pressure and at a high temperature, mixed with lye, and percolated for four hours. It was then turned over to women for an additional handwash[65] —an unnecessary source of difficulty.

Susanna Meredith (1877), in the London area, disgusted with the usual means of cleansing hospital laundry, established a laundry of her own where scientific methods were employed to clean the soil of patients' clothing and bedding. Having seen "living things" in garments boiled in tanks for twenty minutes and dried in closets over 200° F, she applied steam at high temperatures and dried the material quickly at nearly 300°.[66]

In recent decades fairly uniform and consistently effective techniques of laundering have been adopted by hospitals for operating room gowns and dry goods.

Soap

At the time of World War I the role of soap in cleansing wounds was intensely investigated. In a Paris thesis of 1937 André Vincent studied the concentrations of soap necessary to influence favorably the treatment of infected wounds. He recalled that Lucas-Championnière (1910) had urged that the utility of soap as an antiseptic agent deserved study. Camescasse (1917) and Ratynski (1917) both explored the role of soap in the cleansing of wounds. They soaped the surface of wounds, leaving a 20 percent aqueous solution of soap in wounds, and also tried the efficiency of alcoholic solutions of soap.

Koch (1881) had observed that a 2 percent solution of soap was effective against anthrax bacillus, but not against other organisms. Koch noted too that meat putrefied in a 10 percent soap solution. One of the virtues of soap in wounds, said Vincent, is that it is capable of dissolving pus and fatty substances, mechanically cleansing and reducing bacterial counts, apparently an effective detergent in wounds.[67]

Richard Reithoffer (1896) stated that whereas Koch (1881)

had found potash soap 1:5,000 would inhibit growth of anthrax bacilli, soap had little effect on other bacteria.[68] Surgeons have learned that vigorous mechanical brushing of the hands with warm water and soap does reduce bacterial counts significantly, but find it necessary routinely to employ antiseptic agents to enhance the effectiveness of the scrub before donning sterile rubber gloves.

P. G. Unna of Hamburg (1885) wrote of medical soaps for various skin conditions. He described phenol and sublimate soaps. He concluded that camphor and naphthol are preferable to phenol as additives to soaps; phenol communicates an unpleasant odor.[69] Tincture of green soap was the usual scrub agent for preparation of the hands during the 1920s. The ideal soap, meeting microbiologic standards of effective bactericidal action, is still being sought.

Summary

Biologists did not take to microscopy as readily as physicists and chemists. Microscopy begot microbiology, probably man's greatest benefactor, and certainly the discipline largely responsible for creating elective surgery and safe conduct of patients through operative procedures. It all began with Fracastoro (1546), who first promulgated the contagion thesis of infection and its transmission by invisible seminaria (germs). Redi (1668) of Florence refuted the doctrine of spontaneous generation by excluding flies from direct contact with meat, protecting it with parchment or fine wire gauze. Maggots did not then appear in the meat. A few years later, the Dutch self-taught microscopist Leeuwenhoek (1676–83) demonstrated the presence of bacteria about his own teeth, but believed them to be nonpathogenic. A century later the Italian Spallanzani repudiated assertions of the Welsh Catholic priest Needham (1748), who believed he had confirmed by experiment that spontaneous generation was a natural phenomenon. Only when the role of bacterial sporulation was understood was the thesis of spontaneous generation set aside for all time. It took not only the convincing evidence provided by a large number of experimenters, including Pasteur and Koch, but also the studies of the English physicist Tyndall (1881) on light diffraction of a luminous beam passed through moteless air, free of dust particles, to prove that optically pure air did not contain bacterial life. Three centuries intervened between Fracastoro and the great triumvirate of Pasteur, Koch, and Tyndall, whose joint labors definitely established the role of bacteria in the transmission of disease and the propagation of infection. Yet along the way, almost a century earlier, a number of surgeons including Pouteau (1760), Delpech (1815), and Ollivier (1822) had presented convincing evidence of the transmission of wound infection from pus, dressings, or hands contaminated with such discharges. The work of scientists, which surgeons had resented and rejected, finally achieved what their debates and arguments had failed to do for the advancement of their discipline.

(For notes, see pp. 682–87.)

CHAPTER 21

Nineteenth-Century Discoverers and Discoveries

FOR CENTURIES puerperal fever and its heavy toll had been an enigma to the profession. Descriptions of the condition may be found as early as the Greek Hippocratic collections. Accounts of epidemics in Europe began to appear by the mid-seventeenth century when an "unknown disease" took the lives of 90 percent of puerperal women in two outbreaks in Leipzig in 1652 and 1665. In one month at the Hôtel-Dieu, Paris, during such an epidemic in 1746, all twenty affected women died.[1] A few astute observers pointed the way to eventual prevention of this dreaded affliction before the cause was fully recognized.

Harvey (1651) described the site of placental attachment of the uterus following delivery as a large internal ulcer.[2] In fact, very few wounds are larger, save those of burns. It is obviously a fertile source for bacterial implantation. The analogy, therefore, between wounds of the parturient canal and surface wounds is acceptable and gives Semmelweis a significant place in the history of wound management.

Among the first to recognize a similarity between surgical wound infections and puerperal fever was the Lyons surgeon Pouteau (1760), who found that "attentive examination" of the bodies of women dead of puerperal fever revealed "ravages of an erysipelatous-like inflammation."[3] Charles White (1773), a

Manchester obstetrician who had studied anatomy under William Hunter, stressed cleanliness in the care of parturients and isolation of any patient with puerperal fever.[4] Alexander Gordon of Aberdeen (1795) was probably the first to establish definitely the accoucheur as a responsible agent in transmitting puerperal fever. Following an outbreak of puerperal fever in Aberdeen and the nearby countryside (1789–92), Gordon published a small monograph on the disease, including the provocative statement that during the epidemic he could "foretell what women would be affected with the disease, upon hearing by what midwife they were to be delivered, or by what nurse they were to be attended, during their lying-in." He maintained that the "cause of this disease was a specific contagion, or infection" that "seized such women only, as were visited, or delivered, by a practitioner, or taken care of by a nurse, who had previously attended patients affected with the disease. . . . Every person, who had been with a patient in the Puerperal Fever, became charged with an atmosphere of infection, which was communicated to every pregnant woman, who happened to come within its sphere. . . . I myself was the means of carrying the infection to a great number of women."[5]

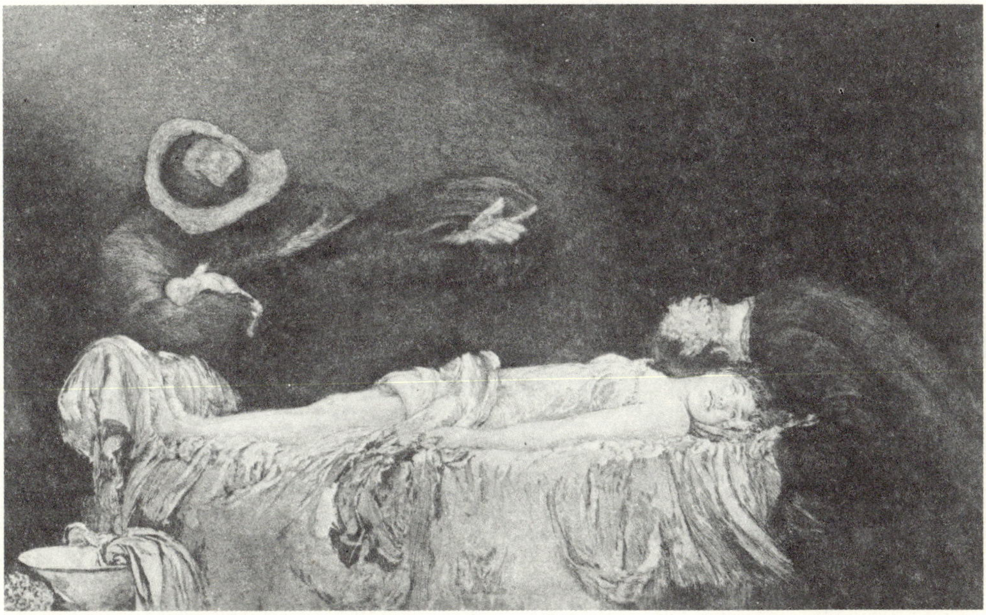

21.1 Max Klinger's 1887 portrayal of "The End" of many pregnancies from puerperal fever before Semmelweis. Courtesy Chicago Museum of Art.

Robert Collins's brilliant work (1826–33) at the Dublin Rotunda Hospital in reducing the incidence of puerperal fever by strict sanitary measures is noteworthy. Many of the precautions he followed were initiated by Joseph Clarke, master of the Rotunda (1786–92), who maintained that puerperal fever originated in "local contagion, and not from any thing noxious in the atmosphere." He also insisted on one patient to a bed. The mortality rate for parturients during the last four years of Collins's seven-year Mastership was a remarkable 0.54 percent. By rotation, one obstetrical ward was empty every ten or twelve days; it was then fumigated with chlorine gas and the woodwork and floors were covered with a paste of chloride of lime for at least forty-eight hours; walls and ceilings were washed with fresh lime. Bedding was usually scoured and heated from 120 to 130° F. Straw in the mattresses was renewed at least after each second occupant and the cover was washed; if a patient died or was thought to have puerperal fever, more stringent methods were observed.[6]

In 1833 the Swedish obstetrician Pehr Cederschjöld announced that use of boiled individual sponges by parturients reduced the incidence of puerperal fever and its mortality. The anatomist and poet Oliver Wendell Holmes (1843) learned from a Boston obstetrical colleague, Humphreys Storer, that a New England physician had been able to halt an epidemic of puerperal fever in his practice in the summer of 1835 by washing his

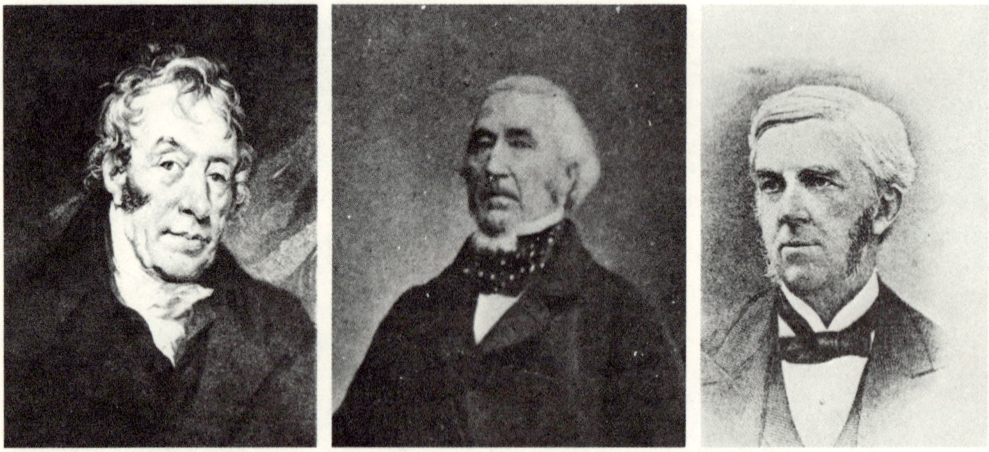

a b c

21.2 **a.** Charles White of Manchester, England, **b.** Robert Collins of the Rotunda Hospital, Dublin, and **c.** Oliver Wendell Holmes of Boston recognized the physician's role in communicating the contagion of puerperal fever.

hands in calcium chloride *after* attendance upon a parturient affected by the disorder. In an articulate and powerful essay Holmes aroused American physicians to the challenge of puerperal fever but did not delineate how the physician communicated the contagion.[7]

Lucas Boër, founder of the Vienna obstetrical school, guided the destiny of obstetrics at the Allgemeines Krankenhaus for thirty-three years (1789–1822) and had the much admired record, long the envy of European professors of obstetrics, of a maternal mortality of only 1.25 percent in 71,395 parturients. Boër was deposed in 1822.[8] Johann Klein, his successor, built a new obstetrical hospital (1832–34) and in 1839 divided the service, assigning half the available beds to supervision by midwives. The medical students attended obstetrical patients only on the division which was supervised by Klein; the parturients were examined by several students, occasionally as many as five, coming directly from performing postmortem examinations. Boër had taught obstetrical maneuvers on a mannequin; the students undoubtedly preferred Klein's method, which permitted active student participation in deliveries. When Semmelweis came as assistant to Klein the mortality of puerperal fever on the service over the preceding six-year period (1841–46) had averaged 10 percent, three times the mortality in the adjacent wards supervised by midwives, where a mannequin was still used for instruction. The disparity remained a puzzle.

Ignacz Philipp Semmelweis (1818–65)

The son of a prosperous merchant in Buda, Semmelweis was sent to Vienna for his education. He had intended to study law, but his friends persuaded him to transfer to medicine. The young Hungarian entered the Vienna School of Medicine, then the most famous in the world, where his teachers included Ferdinand Hebra, Skoda, and Rokitansky. Upon graduation in 1844 Semmelweis applied for a position as a trainee in obstetrics but was obliged to wait two years for an appointment. He spent the interval to good advantage working in medicine with Skoda, from whom he learned the difference between testimony and evidence and the value of factual data and statistics. In February 1846 Semmelweis became Klein's assistant.

Semmelweis's friend and colleague Kolletschka died following a finger-prick sustained while performing an autopsy in early March 1847. Semmelweis was in Venice when this tragedy occurred; on his return he went over every circumstance and facet of the accident, as well as every detail of his friend's postmortem report, while brooding over the personal loss. He reasoned that the postmortem findings were essentially those observed in puerperal fever. By mid-May Semmelweis with Klein's concurrence had instituted a program and prophylactic ritual of hand-washing, including scrubbing with a brush in soap and warm water, followed by a similar wash in chlorine water, until the hands became slippery, for all participants in the delivery. This was accompanied by similar disinfection of all instruments, basins, linens, and dressings likely to come in contact with the parturient's birth canal.[9]

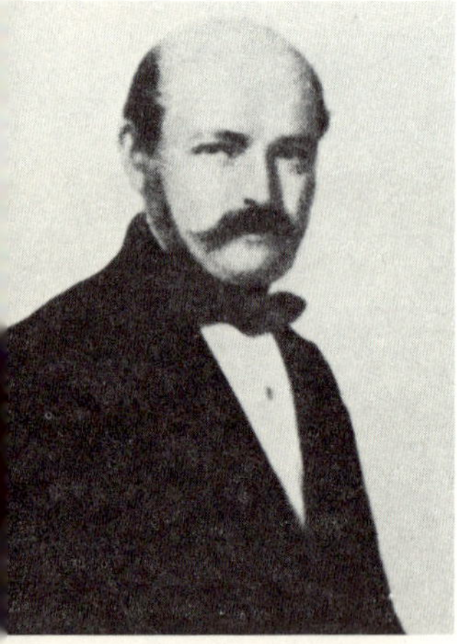

21.3 Ignacz P. Semmelweis (1818–65), conqueror of puerperal fever.

The fruits of Semmelweis's innovation were soon apparent. Within a month (June 1, 1847) Karl Haller, adjunct director of the Vienna Hospital, wrote, "A fresh morning breeze permeates the hospital atmosphere that augurs well for the future." Two years later Haller wrote again, "The significance of this experience for obstetrics and surgical wards is immeasurable and deserves the earnest attention of all men of science and recognition by the highest governmental authority." Hebra, Skoda, and Rokitansky, important Vienna faculty members, also supported Semmelweis and his work. Leopold Auenbrugger's discovery (1761) of percussion had gone unnoticed by Vienna's first medical faculty, an oversight the successors felt keenly must not be repeated in the instance of Semmelweis's contribution.[10] In two years Semmelweis had reduced the clinical mortality of puerperal fever on Klein's wards to 1 percent.

Semmelweis, with the aid of Georg Lautner, an assistant to Rokitansky, was able to demonstrate transmission of fatal puerperal fever to parturient rabbits directly after delivery by introducing pus recovered from the vaginal tract of women dying of puerperal fever. Sepsis did not occur if chlorinated lime also was introduced into the rabbit's vagina. He pointed out that if a patient contracted puerperal fever the patients in beds in immediate juxtaposition thereto did not acquire the infection. He also emphasized that overcrowding in the wards apparently had no relationship to the occurrence of puerperal fever.[11]

All went well until Semmelweis and his work commanded the admiration of the faculty. Then Klein, with the collusion of the ophthalmologist, Anton Rosas, recommended Semmelweis's dismissal to the Minister of Education over the strenuous objection of the Vienna faculty. The year 1848 marked the beginnings of a revolution in Europe that extended from the Baltic to the Mediterranean. The decision of the Ministry of Education may, therefore, have been influenced by a policy of retrench-

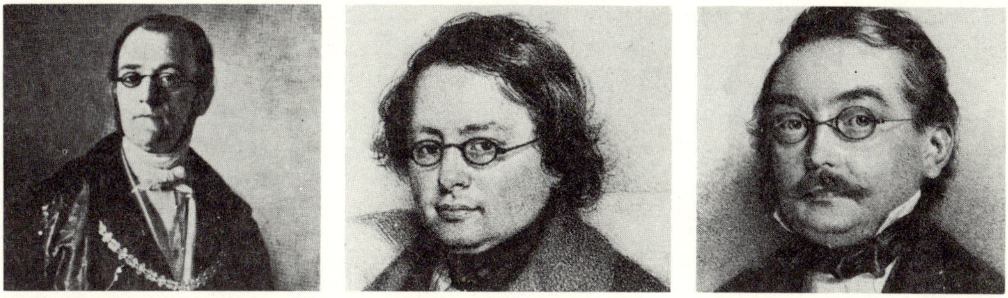

a b c

21.4 **a.** Rokitansky, **b.** Hebra, and **c.** Skoda, important faculty members of Vienna's Medical School, friends and supporters of Semmelweis.

ment against innovation.[12] Semmelweis, greatly discouraged, returned to his native Budapest without acquainting his helpful faculty friends of his intention, an unfortunate circumstance that deprived him of continued support of his friends in the Vienna faculty.

In the beginning Semmelweis (1847) had stressed cadaveric poison on the hands of the accoucheur and his students as the primary source of the contagion. By the time his monograph on the nature and prevention of puerperal fever appeared on the shelves of bookstores in October 1860, Semmelweis had widened the scope of causative agents to include invisible organisms of animal origin. He had observed (1847) that puerperal fever was transmitted from the lochia of a woman dying of cancer of the uterus and subsequently from a patient with purulent infection of the knee. Wrote Semmelweis, "The carrier of the decomposed animal-organic material is the examining finger, the operating hand, instruments, bed linen, atmospheric air, sponges, the hands of midwives and ward attendants that come in contact with the discharges of other ill parturients . . . in a word, the carrier is anything contaminated with decomposed animal organic material that comes in contact with the vaginal tract of the parturient." Semmelweis also described how his chlorine wash provided disinfection and protection for parturients.[13]

Semmelweis was not dealing with a visible surface wound even though its area obviously was very large. Nor did he expand his thesis of preventative antisepsis to other wounds. When Semmelweis returned to Budapest (1850), he did some operative work as a gynecologist. His only report of gynecological procedures concerned enucleation or amputation of uterine polypi achieved without morbidity or mortality.[14]

When Klein died in 1856, Rokitansky together with J. Dumreicher, professor of surgery, J. Dlauhy, professor of public health, and Skoda, professor of medicine, urged the recall of Semmelweis for appointment to the chair of obstetrics at the University of Vienna. The recommendation of this distinguished committee was ignored. It is a tragic story reflecting intrigue and lack of vision. History does have a way of repeating itself.[15]

Had Semmelweis commanded the facile and articulate pen of Holmes or the serenity of Lister in accepting opposition, his cause would have received public recognition considerably earlier. Too many have commented on Semmelweis without having read or studied the presentations of his Vienna colleagues (1847–50) who rose to his defense, let alone perusing his exhaustive and exhausting monumental monograph. It is not an easy task. Semmelweis evolves therefrom as a unique, perceptive, and discerning investigator with an idea very original for its time and, moreover, as one who demonstrated the practicality and validity of his thesis.[16]

Friedrich Wieger of Strasbourg published a favorable exposition of the Semmelweis method. He concluded with the following anecdote: When Semmelweis acquainted an English obstetrician with his technique, the Englishman replied that on his side of the channel the "technique was not new, all his colleagues changed their clothes when leaving the hospital!" In the French Academy of Medicine the Semmelweis thesis of the origins of puerperal fever was roundly debated in sessions from February 23 to July 6, 1858.[17] However, trial, not debate, is the proper manner in which to resolve a question of this kind.

Semmelweis had concluded his monograph by saying that in the not distant future the only instances of puerperal fever would occur through self-infection. Then he added, "If I shall be denied the privilege of seeing with my own eyes the conquest of puerperal fever, the conviction, that sooner or later this thesis will find acceptance, will cheer my hour of death." As Lister's work began (1865–67), the innovations of Semmelweis had found acceptance by leading Austrian and German professors of obstetrics. The *British Medical Journal* (August 26, 1865) considered Semmelweis's death important enough to mention.

It is of more than casual interest that Semmelweis (1844) wrote his Vienna doctorate thesis three years before he announced his prophylactic antiseptic program to combat puerperal fever. Semmelweis listed ten conclusions, the last of which read: "There must be no poison on the physician's hand." His mind therefore was already conditioned to the need for and acceptance of a high standard of surgical cleanliness.[18]

Louis Pasteur (1822–95)

Pasteur published his first paper in 1847 and his last in 1895. His publications, therefore, covered a range of forty-eight years, a stirring half century in scientific discovery.[19] By training Pasteur was a chemist and his early writings related primarily to crystalli-

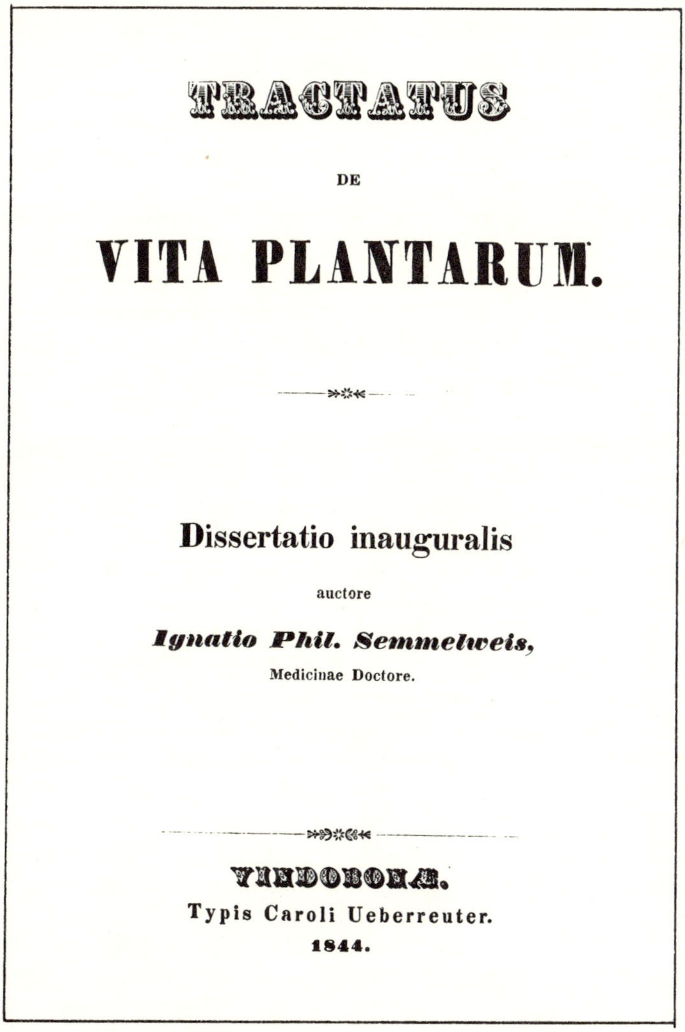
TRACTATUS

DE

VITA PLANTARUM.

Dissertatio inauguralis

auctore

Ignatio Phil. Semmelweis,

Medicinae Doctore.

VINDOBONAE.

Typis Caroli Ueberreuter.

1844.

21.5 Title page of Semmelweis's thesis for medical doctorate. His conclusion: "The physician's hand must be clean."

zation and rotary polarization, subjects which first caught the interest of the shy young scholar from Arbois.

Pasteur's father, a sergeant-major in Napoleon's army with a Cross of the Legion of Honor, returned to the family trade of tanner in the Jura region of eastern France after the emperor's abdication; there he married the daughter of a gardening family. Eventually they settled in a small tannery near Arbois, young Louis's childhood home. Louis inherited from his father a talent for painting and a deep respect for education — some of the portraits he made as a boy are reproduced in his biographies. It has been said that his parents considered the "children's education as essential as their daily bread."

Not a brilliant student in his early years, Louis ranked fifteenth among the twenty-two successful applicants for entry to the Paris École Normale supérieure in 1842. Refusing to enter in this position, he competed again the next year and was readmitted in fourth place. Pasteur's zeal for intensive study probably dates from this period. He had an unusually inquisitive mind directed toward analytic chemistry, despite a grade of *médiocre* in chemistry in his examination for baccalaureate in sciences (1842).

Later that year Pasteur wrote of attending the crowded lectures of the celebrated chemist Jean B. Dumas at the Sorbonne, which, as he recalled forty years afterward, left him "transported, often moved to tears." Dumas became one of Pasteur's first great teachers, a guiding influence in his early career and a trusted colleague throughout life.[20] Pasteur's career was one of patient and complete dedication to uninterrupted work. His technique was to ask of nature sequentially penetrating questions, the answers to which came through devoted attention to original modes of inquiry.

The imaginative chemist Pasteur, resented by many segments of the medical profession because he was not a physician, probably has had as great an influence on medicine's progress as any individual in history. Pasteur ranged far beyond the conventional borders of his profession as chemist. He was essentially a pathfinder, a man of ideas, whose work was not confined within the barrier of compartmentalized knowledge.

Pasteur's advice for success in an endeavor reflects his own extraordinary experience: "Have before you constantly your cherished ideal, and do not swerve or depart therefrom. With constancy of application, you can overcome all difficulties." Pasteur attributed his own achievement to perseverance, but enthusiasm, a keen intuition, and rare talent and ability as an experimenter also played significant roles.

Pasteur began lactic acid fermentation investigations in 1857; his studies of alcoholic fermentation continued to 1860 when he directed his attention more specifically to the thesis of spontaneous generation. These latter studies, employing heat to destroy the vibriones of the air admitted to flasks, also corroborated his earlier pronouncements concerning the nature of fermentation, which he had characterized as a vital action, August 3, 1857.[21]

Pasteur's paper on the presence of organic corpuscles in the air, bearing upon the theory of spontaneous generation, appeared in 1861; additional research in 1863 reemphasized the influence of animal infusoria in the atmosphere upon spontaneous generation.[22]

In a reception at the Tuileries in March 1863, Pasteur was presented by Dumas to Emperor Napoleon III, who manifested interest in Pasteur's studies on animalcules and disease. Pasteur assured the emperor, "All my ambition is to arrive at the knowledge of the causes of putrid and contagious diseases." A few days later Pasteur wrote Colonel Ildefonse Favé of the encounter and affirmed his intention to devote the remainder of his life to resolving the phenomena of putrefaction and fermentation.[23]

Pasteur's first research upon putrefaction appeared in print in June 1863. He showed that some microorganisms were anaerobic and that the oxygen needs of bacteria were not all the same.[24] His studies of 1864 followed up his 1860 research on spontaneous generation, demonstrating that dust from the air contaminated sterile fluids and made them cloudy, probably Pasteur's first allusion to germs in the atmosphere.[25]

It is to be remembered that in his studies on spontaneous generation Pasteur did not introduce antiseptics into his solutions to destroy the atmospheric bacteria responsible for making them unclear; he employed thermal antisepsis (heat) to destroy atmospheric bacteria already present in fluids under study; he filtered the entering air with sterile cotton to exclude particles in the air from the flasks. By acutely bending the long, slender glass tube emerging from the fluid-containing flask, Pasteur was also able to keep fluids therein clear and sterile indefinitely.

The years 1866–68 were devoted in part to consideration of fermentation of wine and vinegar, and the question of why some wines soured. Microscopic studies of the sediment in sour wines revealed the presence of a contaminant, *Mycoderma aceti*. By heating wines during the fermentative process to 55° C, Pasteur found that the souring element in wine was eliminated, a procedure that he subsequently applied to beer.[26] Resolution of the problem constituted an important contribution to the wine industry of France and other countries. What began as a purely scientific inquiry found important practical application in industry. This method was adopted in the early decades of the twentieth century to the pasteurization of milk to destroy bovine tubercle bacilli.

The emperor, accompanied by the empress, visited Pasteur's laboratory in January 1868 to express his appreciation of the fine work of several distinguished French scientists.[27] Later the emperor promised his assistance for a new laboratory, which was started in April 1868. It was at this time that Pasteur was working on silkworm diseases, a study which engrossed him through 1871 and saved the nation's silk industry. Pasteur spent 1872 on agricultural problems and 1872–74 partly on fermentation of wine and beer.

In April 1873 Pasteur was made an associate member of the Paris Academy of Medicine and, as his research led him more directly into the arena of the germ theory of disease, he was frequently in attendance at its meetings. Many of the members had not yet accepted the demise of the thesis of spontaneous generation. In debates at the Academy's sessions, when Pasteur asked for objective factual data, he was met with oratory and argument, responses that elicited his ill-concealed vexation. Some of the discussions became so heated that at one time Pasteur considered resigning his membership. In fact, Jules Guérin, aged eighty, challenged Pasteur to a duel over remarks Pasteur had made concerning preparation of an antirabies vaccine (1880),[28] an occurrence that reflects intolerance of and resistance to innovative ideas. Gradually the members became aware of a new spokesman for science in their midst, whose presentations deserved attention and respect rather than laughter and ridicule.

At the February 19, 1878, session of the Academy of Medicine, the Paris surgeon Le Fort called application of the germ theory to surgical infection completely unacceptable. Pasteur replied that the germ theory ought to be the incessant preoccupation of surgeons and physicians and that microscopically it could be demonstrated that bacteria were responsible for formation of pus.[29]

Pasteur's famous paper on the theory of germs and their application to medicine and surgery, including puerperal septicemia, furuncles, and osteomyelitis was presented to the Academy in 1878; Jules Joubert and Chamberland were collaborators. It was on this occasion that Pasteur said:

"If I had the honor of being a surgeon, impressed as I am with

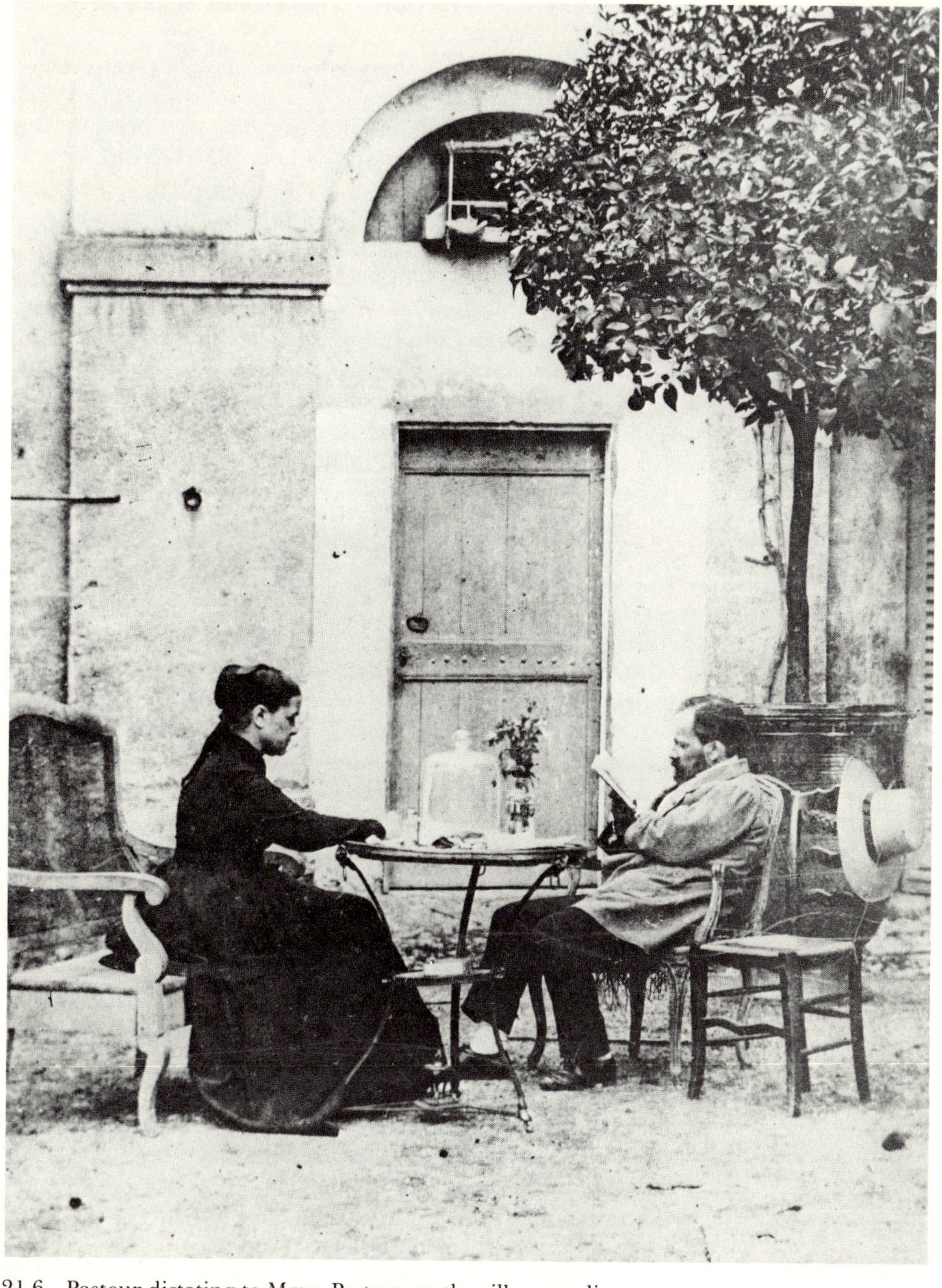

21.6 Pasteur dictating to Mme. Pasteur on the silkworm disease (1868) at an old villa shared with his pupils near Alais. "Shade, water, an orangerie, which made an excellent laboratory" (Émile Duclaux). Courtesy Institut Pasteur, Paris.

the dangers of exposure to the germs and microbes scattered on the surface of all objects, particularly in hospitals, not only would I use only perfectly clean instruments, but after washing my hands with the greatest care and submitting them to a rapid flaming, which would cause no more discomfort than a smoker feels in passing a burning coal from one hand to the other, I would use *charpie*, bandages, sponges previously exposed in air at 130 to 150 [C] degree temperature; I would never use water which had not been submitted to a temperature of 110 to 120 [C] degrees. All this is practical. In this way I would have to fear only the germs in suspension in the air around the patient's bed; but observation shows us each day that the number of such germs is insignificant compared to those scattered in the dust on the surface of objects or in the clearest of ordinary water."[30] Pasteur had written on putrefaction in 1863 but only in the 1875 to 1878 period did he become intimately involved in practical aspects of wound infection, when his work on surgical infection acquired its full intensity and began to have practical meaning for surgery.

It is strange that Pasteur, a great historian of all areas in which he worked, did not know of Semmelweis's accomplishment. Arneth described Semmelweis's work on puerperal fever at a séance of the National Academy of Medicine in Paris in January 1851.[31] At that time Pasteur's interests were in chemistry; however, by 1861, when Semmelweis's monograph appeared, Pasteur's studies in fermentation and putrefaction were well under way. His serious interest in puerperal fever dated only from 1879.

Pasteur's gradual transition of interest from problems in pure chemistry and physics to biologic and microbiologic mysteries has been briefly sketched. Biologic research of that day lacked both the qualitative and quantitative measurements that characterized research in physics and chemistry. Pasteur's primary training in the natural sciences therefore lent his entanglement with biologic problems the new dimension of quantitative evaluation. He reasoned that if studies on wine, beer, and silk manufacture shed significant and useful enlightenment that rejuvenated those industries, could not similar approaches resolve the role of microorganisms in the causation of wound infection and disease, redounding to similar gains for medicine and surgery? It was a question Pasteur had posed to Napoleon III in 1863. Despite his primary interest in basic research, Pasteur was always conscious of the government's attitude that support of research should provide promises of social gain.

When Pasteur announced that the same organism responsible for furuncles also caused osteomyelitis, the communication was received by the Academy of Medicine in silence. Twenty-five years later F. R. Schaudinn and P. E. Hoffmann presented their paper on the *Treponema pallida* before the Berlin Medical Society, May 17 and 24, 1905. On the conclusion of the second session, Bergmann, the presiding officer, said, "The discussion is closed until another syphilis investigator commands our attention." A commentator has since remarked that Bergmann said, "We have just listened to a dissertation on the 20th cause of syphilis. How long must we wait for the 21st?"[32]

What manner of man was this unique scientist, Pasteur? First and foremost, his great love for and dedication to systematic and critical inquiry shone brightly through all his work. Although Pasteur was crippled by the residuals of hemiplegia in 1868 at age forty-six, the intensity of his total commitment to investigation and research did not abate. In his early years the delicate techniques of separation of levo- and dextrorotatory crystals of the salts of tartaric acid had been achieved by his own skillful hands. After his illness of 1868 Pasteur became dependent upon his loyal band of assistants for the technical performance of most experiments. His deductions based upon logical processes of thought, combined with an unusual command of basic knowledge of many disciplines and special skills in resolution of any problem under study, including an accurate head-to-eye-to-hand execution of experiments, ensured consistent reproducibility of results. He touched unknowns in many fields by a penetrating and intuitive insight that served to clarify their nature and to suggest significant therapeutic innovations. Before microbiology matured as a science under the guiding hand of Koch (1876–82), Pasteur had opened the way to therapeutic endeavors with several diseases.

His courage and readiness to participate with vigorous opponents in fierce struggles concerning the validity of their ideas, experimental testing, and establishment of proof were considerations always uppermost in Pasteur's mind. A number of such skirmishes and contentions in which Pasteur usually emerged victorious, established him as a staunch and ready defender of scientific methodology. Pasteur was also an intense and loyal French patriot, a scientist who developed a famous school of productive followers. Blessed with an understanding wife who sublimated her every concern to furthering Pasteur's career, he had in his family life a catalyst for accomplishment as powerful as some of the many ferments with which he had long labored so successfully.

When has any scientist before or since become involved in so many disparate disciplines bringing enlightenment into each? Possessed of great energy and determination, creative imagination, and consecutive and patient industry, such as few men have ever commanded, and a keen sense of social responsibility for the welfare of his fellowman, is it any wonder that Pasteur has come to be known as the greatest benefactor of mankind?

Joseph Lister (1827–1912)

Britain can boast a long unrivaled list of surgeons dating back to the fourteenth-century John of Arderne. In the midst of the nineteenth century came the greatest of them all, the scientist-surgeon Joseph Lister. He grew up in a Quaker family; his father, a wine merchant, was also a well-known microscopist, especially recognized for innovation of the achromatic lens, which enabled a sharper focus to be obtained during microscopic examinations.[33]

Not being a member of the Church of England, young Lister could not attend Oxford or Cambridge colleges. In 1844, at age seventeen, he entered University College in London where he came under the influence of the ophthalmologist-physiologist Thomas Wharton Jones, the great physiologist William Sharpey, and the chemist Thomas Graham. As a student Lister displayed a keener interest in research than in his assigned studies. Upon completion of his medical course he served as house physician under Walter H. Walshe and, later, as house surgeon under Erichsen for nine months in 1851; both were staff members of London's University College Hospital.

By 1852 Lister was already a member of the Royal College of Surgeons of England. At the suggestion of Sharpey he went in 1853 to Edinburgh to spend a few months with the master surgeon, Syme. He stayed long enough to marry Syme's eldest daughter, Agnes, in April 1856[34] and to succeed to the professorship of surgery at the University of Glasgow in January 1860. Although professor of surgery, Lister had to wait almost two years before he was elected surgeon to the Royal Infirmary. When he tried to persuade the chairman of the Infirmary's board of directors that he would be a more effective teacher if granted hospital privileges, Lister met the unique and discouraging reply, "Stop, stop, Mr. Lister, that's a real Edinburgh idea.

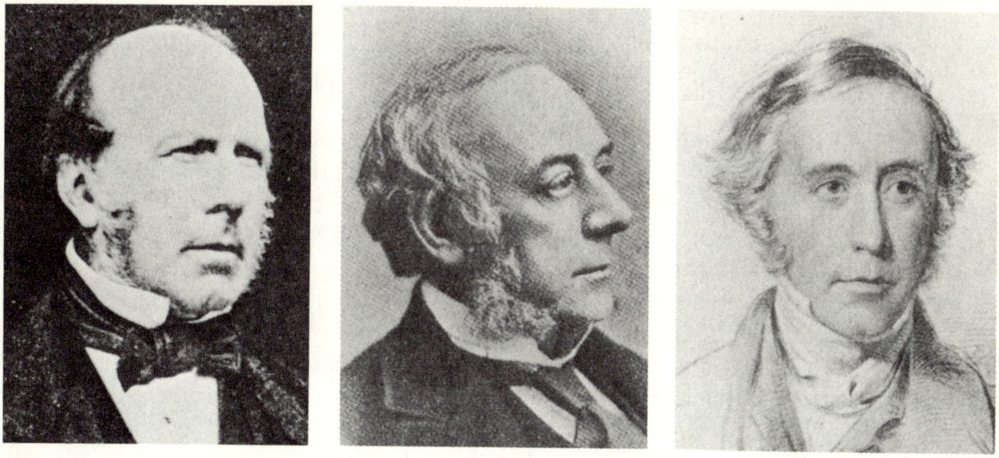

a b c

21.7 Lister's preceptors at University College Hospital: **a.** the physiologist Sharpey and **b.** the surgeon Erichsen; **c.** Syme, his chief at Edinburgh and later his father-in-law.

But our institution is a curative one. It is not an educational one!"[35]

It was at Glasgow that Lister initiated his famous trials with carbolic acid for compound fracture, an accident for which amputation was still an accepted remedy, accompanied by a formidable mortality of 40 to 60 percent. Lister had been alerted in March 1865 by the chemist Thomas Anderson of the Glasgow faculty to Pasteur's work on putrefaction (1863) and to the use of carbolic acid for sanitation at Carlisle. Spencer Wells had given an address on Pasteur's work at the British Medical Association's August 1864 meeting in Cambridge, calling attention to seven important papers by Pasteur of special interest to surgeons.[36] Lister, never an avid reader of medical literature in which he did not already have an active interest, had taken no note thereof, nor did he in subsequent publications on antisepsis allude to Wells's important appraisal.

The work of Semmelweis was initiated before the importance of bacteria in infection was recognized. To be certain, vibrios and bacteria had been described by Ehrenberg (1838) and others; however, there was yet no proof of their pathogenicity. Had Lister followed Pasteur's teachings directly, he would have used methods more like those of Semmelweis, excluding bacteria from wounds by prophylactic measures, rather than attempting to destroy them in the wound.

When in 1866 Lister applied, without success, for the Chair of Systematic Surgery at University College Hospital, he included with testimonials for the appointment a short account of his early experience with carbolic acid dressings, stating that he based his technique "on the beautiful researches of Pasteur." The account, "Notice of a new method of treating compound fractures," was printed verbatim in the New Sydenham Society's *Biennial Retrospect* in 1867, constituting the earliest public notice of Lister's technique.[37]

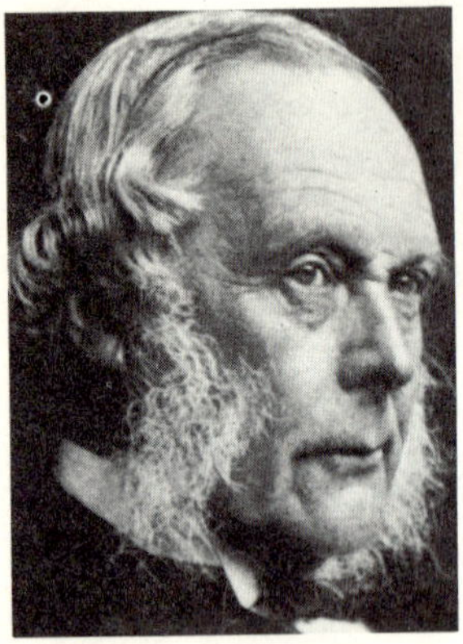

21.8 Joseph Lister (1827–1912).

Lister began (March 1865) by instilling pure carbolic acid into wounds. Later he used lesser concentrations of 10, 5, and 2.5 percent. In 1871 he added the carbolic acid spray on the thesis that the air of the operating room was a significant source of infection. Abraham Wallace, surgical dresser to Lister in Edinburgh, related it had been Lister's practice to irrigate wounds with a syringe containing a dilute solution of carbolic acid at operation and dressing changes. Wallace and John Davidson on ward rounds remarked that a spray would be superior to irrigation, a discussion overheard by John Chiene, assistant surgeon. Chiene reported it to Lister, who implemented the suggestion directly. Lister discontinued use of the spray in 1887.[38] In addresses of 1890 and 1893, he hinted at the possibility of abandoning irrigation of wounds with antiseptic solutions. In his 1896 presidential address before the British Association for the Advancement of Science, four years after his retirement from his third and final professoriate at King's College Hospital (1877–92), Lister capitulated completely to prophylactic antisepsis.[39]

Victor Bruns of Tübingen (1880) had written "Fort mit dem Spray!" Most continental surgeons, however, continued to follow the suggestions of Mikulicz (1889) and Kocher (1894), who favored irrigation of the wound with very dilute solutions of corrosive sublimate. In fact, during World War I there was a return to the Listerian practice with emphasis upon the use of Dakin's solution (hypochlorite) for contaminated wounds, when both Keen and Halsted indicated they had never lost their belief in the validity of the Listerian practice of placement of antiseptics in wounds.[40] One still hears of surgeons employing Dakin's solution in suppurating wounds "to hasten healing." If irrigation is in order, should it not be an appropriate antibiotic suspended in saline solution?

Lister undoubtedly came eventually to employ all facets of carbolic acid antisepsis in his program; however, the two items lent special emphasis in his writings were wound antisepsis and spraying of the atmosphere about the operative field and over the wound in dressing changes. His colleagues and associates have pointed out that Lister deemphasized hand care, merely dipping his fingers briefly into a 5 percent solution of phenol to which had been added a 0.002 percent solution of corrosive sublimate. He deliberately avoided hand-scrubbing with soap and water or with antiseptic agents, reposing his conviction in the belief that scrubbing created crevasses in the palms of the hands in which bacteria would lodge.[41]

Lister did not escape opposition, most strenuous in his own land and in America. His first paper on a new method of treating compound fracture published in *Lancet*, 1867, met with considerable skepticism. Syme, Lister's father-in-law, then professor of surgery at the University of Edinburgh, who had at one time favored amputation for compound fracture, was among the first to fall in line with Lister's suggestion of conservative management of such cases.

One obvious reason for dissident opinions was that wound antisepsis had been in vogue periodically from antiquity and that both Lemaire (1860) and Déclat (1865) had employed phenol (carbolic acid) in wounds, including open fractures, without great benefit.[42] The difference was that Lister's antisepsis was far more complete.

On August 18, 1869, Lister was chosen professor of surgery at Edinburgh to succeed Syme, who had suffered a cerebral hemorrhage.[43] In a paper presented for publication in *Lancet* in December 1869 and published in early 1870, Lister gave an account of his experiences with antisepsis in Glasgow over the prior four years, an account that aroused anger among the Glasgow Infirmary directors. Lister's figures were challenged in subsequent issues of *Lancet* by the Infirmary's secretary.[44]

The practice which Lister advocated gained considerable momentum when two distinguished German professors of surgery, Volkmann of Halle (1874) and Nussbaum of Munich (1875), wrote of their triumphs with compound fracture treated by his methods and the favorable effects both noted on adoption of Listerian practices; hospital gangrene and pyemia disappeared from their hospitals. These welcome reports signaled the beginning of the end of resistance to Listerian practices in Germany. When Lister visited the clinic of Professor Thiersch in Leipzig, in August 1875, the warmth and enthusiasm of his reception was that accorded great military heroes and conquerors.[45] Billroth in Vienna did not capitulate until 1878, favoring open wound management.

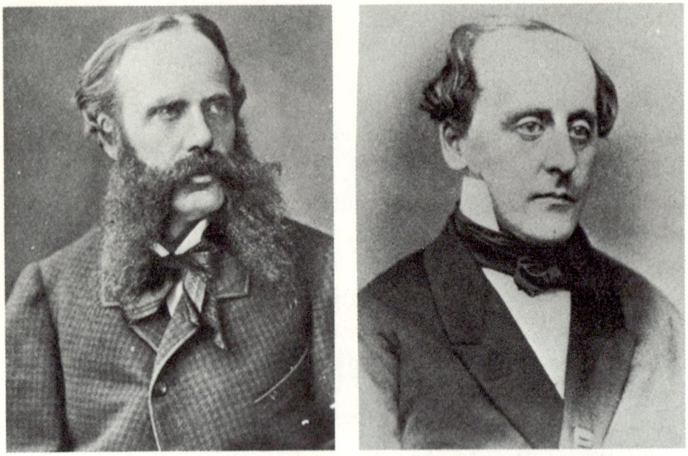

a b

21.9 **a.** Richard Volkmann and **b.** Johann Nussbaum confirmed Lister's observations.

Lister spoke on his antiseptic dressings at the Philadelphia Medical Congress during the American Centennial in 1876. His speech consumed two and a half hours and his answers to questions another hour, but the attention he received excused and perhaps explained his prolixity, commented the *Boston Medical & Surgical Journal*. Despite the interest in his thesis, the discussion at the sessions revealed much skepticism in the American audience. Several surgeons claimed the open treatment of wounds was equally as effective as Lister's measures. Addinell Hewson brought up his technique of adding earth to the wound to produce dryness; Caniff of Toronto found it "impossible to entertain the doctrine of germ putrefaction."[46]

Meanwhile Lister's practices in the hands of European surgeons had met with such success that when he appeared at the podium to speak at the Sixth International Medical Congress in Amsterdam in 1879, he was greeted by tumultuous applause and cheers. The famous Dutch ophthalmologist Frans Donders, president of the Congress, came forward and took Lister's hand, saying, "It is not only our admiration which we offer to you; it is our gratitude, and that of the nations to which we belong." Later under the supervision of the Amsterdam surgeon Jan Tilanus, Lister provided a demonstration of his antiseptic practices. He called on William Macewen, director of the Royal Infirmary in Glasgow, to report his hospital's statistics. The Infirmary had three hundred surgical beds and six surgeons, each of whom treated the same number of patients; not all the surgeons were committed to antiseptic practices. The hospital mortality of surgical patients undergoing operation not treated with antisepsis was 4.6 percent while the mortality of patients treated with antiseptic principles was 2.4 percent — during the last year it was only 1.75 percent.[47]

Even so, when the seventh Congress convened in London in 1881, many of Lister's colleagues remained unconvinced of the merit of his wound practices. In the United States at the first official meeting of the American Surgical Association (1883) more speakers opposed than favored Listerian practices. Two years later (1885) John J. Packard of Philadelphia listed the "great advances in surgery" but did not name Lister; antiseptic surgery, said Packard, was "still *sub judice*." There were, however, no such doubts at the Berlin Tenth International Congress of 1890, where Lister was given a stirring welcome.[48]

Lister's invitation in 1877 to join the faculty of King's College Medical School and Hospital was not warmly encouraged nor endorsed by many of the surgeons of that institution, nor by the medical profession in London. Fergusson, a transplanted Scot and talented surgeon who had occupied the Chair of Clinical Surgery at King's for twenty-two years, died February 10, 1877. A week later the *British Medical Journal* suggested in an editorial that Lister be appointed to fill the vacancy, a nomination that "would once more revive the old glories of King's . . . for Mr. Lister's science and practice is now the most notable circumstance in British, or indeed in European, surgery." An "unauthorized person, probably Sir William Bowman," a distinguished scholar-ophthalmologist at King's, apparently proposed to Lister that he consider coming to King's. On February 18 Lister wrote a letter expressing his willingness to accept the chair provided certain conditions were met. A leak in this exchange developed, followed by a volley of protests and unkind remarks concerning Lister in *Lancet*. Secure in his position at the University of Edinburgh, appreciated by his colleagues, and loved and admired by the large student body, it is surprising that Lister did not withdraw the London application. However, he obviously was a man with a mission. His success in Edinburgh was complete. His teachings had been accepted in most of the important surgical clinics in Europe, but London had remained aloof with little manifestation of interest in his antiseptic practices. Opposition and the prospects of a less pleasant life style did not deter Lister. We can only conclude that he enjoyed opposition, that it sharpened the focus of his attack on problems. Instead of the throng of 300 to 400 attentive and appreciative students in regular attendance at his Edinburgh clinics, when Lister came to London he often lectured to empty seats. John Hunter, for whom Lister had great admiration, is recorded to have said "Gentlemen" in addressing a sole student in the amphitheatre and a suspended skeleton employed for teaching purposes. From 10 to 20 students was the usual number during Lister's early years at King's. On special occasions members of the London faculties of medical schools and hospitals did come to hear him. Modern-day medical students, too, rarely attend extracurricular lectures that will not count when confronted with examinations. Lister's work had yet to find approval in London and students found that to provide Lister's answers to interrogatory boards served their interests very poorly. Before Lister retired in 1892, the numbers of students in attendance at his biweekly lectures had grown considerably. He had found increasing appreciation.[49]

According to Godlee (1914) at the time Lister came to King's College Hospital in 1877, the conditions were much the same as in Lister's student days in London twenty years earlier. A single probe circulated from patient to patient, washed in unboiled water. Most wounds suppurated and none healed by first intention save those of the face. Compound fractures were almost always followed by amputation. The instruments were not boiled; the operating room sister was dressed in unsterile black flannel. The long whipcord ligatures for tying blood vessels were drawn out of a corner of the wound as a drain and pulled away by the dresser when they had cut through the vessel and were loose in the wound. Hernias were rarely operated upon unless they were strangulated. Godlee went on to describe Lister's practices at the end of his active professional career (1892–93). "Lister did not boil his instruments: they were simply placed in a solution of carbolic acid 1:20. He wore no gloves, and his hands, which it should be added were always rough, were sterilized by a mixture of 1:20 carbolic acid in 1:500 sublimate solution," a mixture "much too strong for ordinary hands. Lister used marine sponges which were purified in carbolic acid solution. . . . Lister trusted practically altogether chemical antiseptics."[50]

St. Clair Thomson, a house officer of Lister, said, "Lister never wore a white gown, nor a mask, nor gloves. He frequently never removed his coat, but simply rolled his sleeves back and turned his coat collar up, so that his white starched collar would not be made sodden by the cloud of carbolic spray in which we operated. Sometimes he removed his black frock-coat, and an ordinary towel was pinned across his chest. I myself, for operations, put on an old blue frock-coat which I had worn for years previously in the dissecting room. It was stiff and glazed with dry blood. Yet our cases, as I remember them, healed as rapidly and as smoothly as they do with all the ceremonial and ritual of sterilization and asepsis nowadays."[51]

Demonstrations by Pasteur and Chamberland (1878–79) and by Koch (1881) of the greater efficacy of heat over chemical solutions for the sterilization of materiel and instruments for operations led to its adoption in the hands of a number of German and French surgeons in the mid-1880s, notably Neuber of Kiel (1883), Bergmann (1887) and Schimmelbusch (1892) of Berlin, Tripier of Lyons (1883), and Redard of Paris (1886). Lister, however, clung to chemical antisepsis throughout his career. Stephen Smith said he visited Lord Lister in 1894 at his London residence and found him very pessimistic over the promise of asepsis.[52]

Lister's early writings were on a variety of subjects, suggesting that at different junctures he might have contemplated becoming an ophthalmologist, histologist, hematologist, physiologist, or even a neuroanatomist. His early papers were often presented before scientific bodies and were usually published in scientific rather than clinical journals.

One of Lister's trainees, John Leeson, said that Lister "seemed to us to be surrounded by an atmosphere of indefinable separation that forbade familiar approach which neither time could bridge nor custom abate . . . we were never quite at ease, never quite at our best" with him. Cheyne, who worked in close association with Lister for many years, told Godlee he "never quite got over a feeling of awe of the great man." Lister had few, if any, close friends outside the family circle; his shyness and aloofness did not encourage intimate friendship. His boyhood stammer provided additional evidence of shyness, a defect which he conquered. A devout man, he remained at heart a Quaker. He trained men to become good doctors rather than to do well at examinations; for him, the patient always came first. Lister "never lost his temper . . . but had an infuriating habit of heaving a gentle sigh of christian resignation when faced with slovenly work." He made "little effort to establish ordinary, friendly relations with his professional colleagues." Lister was notoriously unpunctual, yet the most courteous of men.[53]

Lister remained at King's for seventeen years. He was one of the consultants called in when Edward VII developed acute appendicitis two days before his coronation; Edward's abscess was drained by Frederick Treves. In 1897 Lister was the first British surgeon elevated to the peerage. In 1903 he was seriously ill but made a gradual recovery. His eightieth birthday (1907) was celebrated throughout the world. He could then endure only fifteen-minute visits. He made his last public appearance when admitted as a Freeman of the City of London on June 20, 1907.

The Listers had enjoyed an ideal and congenial marriage; they had no children. Both came from well-to-do and successful families. They traveled considerably and while in London maintained a country place. Agnes Lister was her husband's devoted and competent amanuensis,[54] and when she died in 1893 of pneumonia on a vacation trip in Rappalo, Italy, Lister became a lonely figure; he had lost the most important sustaining source of his happiness. It was a blow from which he never fully recovered. In the autumn of 1908 he left his London residence at 12 Park Crescent for a brief visit to the seacoast in Walmer, Kent, to regain his strength. But there he was to remain for the final three and a half years of his life in the tender care of his wife's sister, Miss Lucy Syme. Failing vision, impaired hearing, fatigue, and exhaustion isolated him from his friends, a sad ending to a life devoted to surgery's improvement and man's welfare. "After more than two years spent in a world of darkness and silence, Lister died quietly from pneumonia Saturday 10 February 1912," at age eighty-five. The funeral ceremony was held at Westminster Abbey, but he had chosen to be buried beside his wife in West Hampstead Cemetery.

Lister's will, signed June 26, 1908, is an interesting typed document, not referred to by his biographers, although Lister's generous legacies to various London hospitals and surgical institutions are known. Characteristic was his request that his name should in no way be associated with these sums. Moreover, in willing his diplomas, medals, and caskets to the University of Edinburgh, he declared that the University authorities should be "prefectly [sic] at liberty to dispose" of them, having the medals melted down or the diplomas destroyed, if they so desired.[55]

Having failed to obtain from biographies of Lister, or current historians and surgeons knowledgeable about Lister, any information concerning the house in which Lister spent his final years, the authors made a trip to Walmer in October 1976. The map of the area narrowed the choice considerably and a middle-aged petrol station operator recognized the name Park Place and told us we were almost there. However, 32 Park Place is now known as Coast House. We were fortunate to find the most recent owner at home, who very kindly showed us the entire house. It has two stories. The pleasant outlook faces the sea, and perhaps on arrival there late in 1908 Lister was robust enough to walk occasionally on the sand beach. It obviously was a quiet, delightful retreat with a beautiful garden between the street and the sea. We learned that Lister rented but did not own the house. Sometime after Lister's day Park House was divided into two dwellings, and the rear side is now a separate residence, although this is not obvious from the front. It must have been a very large house for the Lister household of two. The dining and living rooms (or salon) remain undoubtedly as originally designed, charming period rooms with windows looking to sea.[56]

Lister-Semmelweis Priority Controversy

In 1906 Lister replied to an inquiry from Dr. Weckerling of Friedberg in Hessen, Germany, concerning Lister's implied obligation to Semmelweis, a letter exchange quoted in Godlee's biography of 1917. Said Lister, "When in 1865 I first applied the antiseptic principle to wounds, I had not heard the name of Semmelweis and knew nothing of his work. When 20 years later I visited Buda-Pesth, where I was received with extraordinary kindness by the medical profession and the students, Semmelweis's name was never mentioned, having been, as it seems, as entirely forgotten in his native city as in the world at large. It was some time after this that my attention was drawn to Semmelweis and his work by Dr. Duka, a Hungarian physician practising in London."

Concerning Semmelweis, Godlee wrote, "He proved his case conclusively to impartial minds." Continued Godlee, "Semmelweis was thus in two respects the forerunner of Lister. He showed that one particular form of blood-poisoning did not depend upon mysterious and unascertainable causes, but upon the contamination of abrasions and external wounds. He also proved that neither the size of hospitals, nor their age, nor their crowded wards, were responsible for hospitalism, but rather the methods of hospital treatment." Obviously, Godlee had read *Die Aetiologie*. But, added Godlee, meanwhile Semmelweis had been almost forgotten. A few decades later (1938) the British historian of microbiology William Bulloch wrote that Semmelweis's observations "had been discredited and relegated to oblivion."[57] Let us examine the evidence.

Retraction of Opponents

When his *Aetiologie* appeared in print in 1860, Semmelweis had anticipated early capitulation of German-speaking professors of obstetrics to his view; such did not occur. In 1861–62 Semmelweis addressed two open letters to three leading opponents of his precepts, E. C. J. Siebold (Göttingen), Joseph Späth (Vienna), and Friedrich Scanzoni (Würzburg).[58] Two months before his death in October 1861, Siebold wrote, "I gladly forgive my friend Semmelweis for his *Open Letter* of Criticism." Späth (1864) indicated that many professors of obstetrics, while ridiculing Semmelweis and his work publicly, actually were employing his methods in their hospital practices. Scanzoni, Semmelweis's severest critic, published his little-known retraction in 1867. Said Scanzoni, "In the last two decades considerable progress has been registered in this sector [puerperal fever] and it is not incorrect to suggest that Semmelweis' fierce attacks and zealous concern and dedication to the welfare of parturients throughout his lifetime deserves our expression of warm appreciation; that without question he had provided the greatest impetus to improving hygienic aspects of puerperal pathology. . . . Almost all the heads of German obstetrical clinics have lent their attention to Semmelweis' thesis to the end that their united efforts succeeded in effecting a significant diminution in maternal morbidity and mortality from puerperal fever."[59] Unfortunately, when these cheering words of commendation appeared in print, Semmelweis had been dead for two years and the friendly message failed to reach him.

Announcements Abroad

Many reviews and accounts of Semmelweis's work appeared in the British medical press, and he himself presented a summary of his views in *Medical Times & Gazette*, June 7, 1862, sketching his concept and method of control of puerperal fever. Routh, the London obstetrician who had worked with Semmelweis in 1847, lectured and wrote in 1848 that Semmelweis had introduced a new and effective program against puerperal fever. Arneth, a Vienna obstetrician who had worked with Semmelweis, went to Paris and Edinburgh (1851), and later to St. Petersburg, to describe Semmelweis's methods. G. A. Michaelis (1798–1848) of Kiel was one of the early supporters of Semmelweis's practice. He observed that its use stopped an epidemic of puerperal fever, an occurrence he indicated to Semmelweis in a

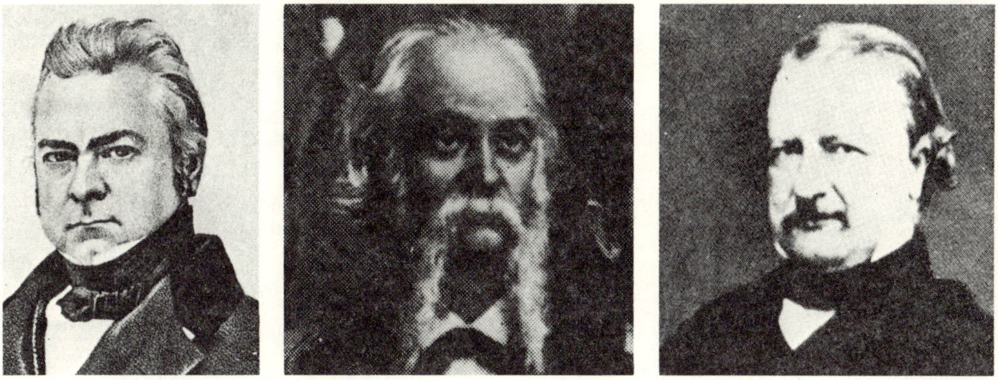

a b c

21.10 Semmelweis's opponents recant: **a.** E. C. J. Siebold, **b.** Joseph Späth, and **c.** Friedrich W. Scanzoni.

letter.[60] As Lesky had remarked, "Scarcely ever had a discovery attained such quick publicity."[61]

Lister's Unfamiliarity with Prior Antiseptic Practices

In his first paper on surgical antisepsis (1867) Lister said, "My attention having for several years been much directed to the subject of suppuration . . ." — but it is nevertheless quite clear that Lister revealed little, if any, acquaintance with the historical background of the abundant literature surrounding use of antiseptic agents for contaminated wounds, even the management of compound fracture.[62] In fact, several of his own countrymen had managed compound fracture successfully with antiseptics, including the Crowthers (1802), Higginbottom (1826–65), and Bennion (ca. 1840).[63]

Lister did not engage in polemical discussions with those opposing his antiseptic practices. Early in his career, however, he had exchanges with Adams (1855), the London orthopedist, in matters relating to his teacher Professor Syme. In this controversy Lister demonstrated himself a very competent and knowledgeable disputant in the correspondence columns of *Lancet* and *Medical Times & Gazette*.[64] This was the same Adams who two years later (1857) brought the name of Bennion and his success in the management of open fracture (ca. 1840) with tincture of benzoin to the attention of the surgical public. It strikes one as strange that Lister, a decade later, apparently had no knowledge of the use of antiseptics in management of compound fracture. It is unlikely that Lister could have completely forgotten Adams, who again in 1868 amplified his report on Bennion's use of benzoin.[65]

In his 1883 visit to Budapest Lister obviously did not appraise the neglect of Semmelweis accurately. The Budapest physicians, superlative hosts, were not about to embarrass their celebrated guest on his visit. Saturday, September 29, 1883, was a festive evening for the Listers, the occasion of a great public banquet given in their honor at Budapest's Hotel of the English Queen, and certainly not the moment to bring up the work of a local hero. Prague's *Medicinische Wochenschrift*, however, was not so reticent; the editors found it "very remarkable that the name of Semmelweis was not mentioned when Professor Lister was in Budapest last week — had they only seized the opportunity for the establishment of a memorial for Semmelweis and placed Lister's name at the apex of the list! Shouldn't their great Hungarian compatriot, Semmelweis, have been remembered on this occasion as the Faculty's proudest ornament?" The bold suggestion of the Prague editor came to fruition nineteen years later (1892), when Spencer Wells, Lister, and other prominent London physicians joined the Budapest movement for an international monument for Semmelweis. Godlee (1917) is strangely silent upon this visit of the Listers to Budapest. Wrench says Lister "met with a tremendous reception. A great banquet was held and a torchlight procession of the students marched past him as he stood surrounded by the most distinguished scientists of the Austrian Empire."[66]

On a visit to the Budapest Library of the Academy of Science in 1973, the present authors, in the company of Ferenc Nemethy of the Semmelweis Historical Library and Museum, found a heretofore unknown letter in Lister's hand, dated October 11, 1883, which reads: "Dear Dr Duka, I am much obliged to you for sending me the illustrated paper. I need hardly assure you how very much gratified I was by the extreme kindness of my professional brethren in Budapest. Believe me, very sincerely yours, Joseph Lister." How unfortunate this letter was not known to Godlee.

At the Wellcome Historical Library in London the authors examined (March 1973) Semmelweis's great book, *Die Aetiologie, der Begriff und die Prophylaxis des Kindbettfiebers*, on loan from the Medical Society of London. It bore the signature of Lajos Markusovszky on the title page. How it got to the shelves of the Medical Society of London is a mystery. At the time of his death in 1912 Lister left the "pick of his books" to the Society, but no catalogue of the Lister bequest has been found. It can only be surmised that the Semmelweis monograph carrying the signature of Lajos Markusovszky may have been a gift to Lister from that great Hungarian patriot, Markusovszky, who presided at the dinner honoring the Listers in September 1883.[67]

Shortly after publication of his monograph Semmelweis sent a copy to Routh. It resides today on the shelves of the Royal Society of Medicine in London and contains the following interesting letter: "Pesth 22-5-1861 Dear Friend: As you have been so friendly in the year 1848 at the meeting of the English Doctors in London to bring forward a discussion of my opinion about the origin and prevention of fever in childbed, I take the liberty, having just finished a complete work upon the same subject, to send it you with the request to mention it again at the same meeting. I have also send my work to Webster, Copeland, Murphy, Simpson, Weber. Thanking you before for your trouble and hoping to hear something of you very soon, Your sincere friend, Ignaz Semmelweis."[68]

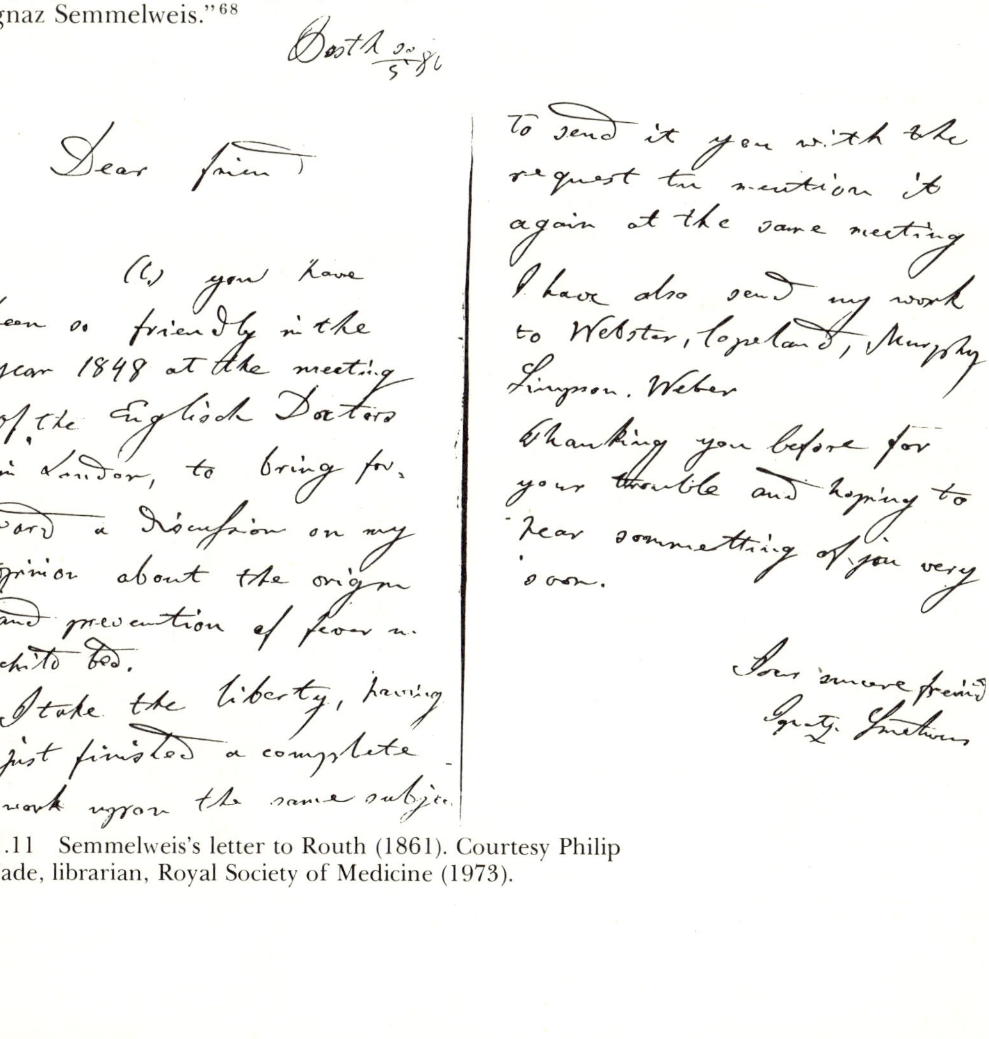
Routh

Dear friend

As you have been so friendly in the year 1848 at the meeting of the English Doctors in London, to bring forward a discussion on my opinion about the origin and prevention of feaver in childbed.
I take the liberty, having just finished a complete work upon the same subject to send it you with the request to mention it again at the same meeting
I have also send my work to Webster, Copeland, Murphy Simpson. Weber
Thanking you before for your trouble and hoping to hear sommething of you very soon.

Your sincere friend
Ignatz Semmelweis

21.11 Semmelweis's letter to Routh (1861). Courtesy Philip Wade, librarian, Royal Society of Medicine (1973).

By 1872 Semmelweis's prophylactic antisepsis had been subjected to trial in the finest obstetrical clinics of central Europe; it was apparent throughout Prussia that a durable impact had been made upon maternal mortality from puerperal fever. The measures of Semmelweis lowered effectively the mortality of puerperal fever, antedating by almost three decades the success of Listerian methods in the hands of a few German surgeons in the management of compound fracture and amputation. The role of Semmelweis's prophylactic practices for surgery had yet to be explored. The earliest confirmation of the validity of Semmelweis's teachings for surgery came from Freiburg, when Hegar announced 15 consecutive successful ovariotomies (1876–77); he observed every detail of prophylactic antisepsis at a time when the mortality of the operation in many competent hands was in the area of 60 percent. Hegar's success occurred a decade before Tait's unique achievement of 139 consecutive ovariotomies without hospital mortality.[69] Moreover, Tait, an opponent of Lister and of the germ theory of disease, did not reveal the underlying feature of his success; we do know he held to high standards of surgical cleanliness. He boiled his instruments and suture material (silk). Since the late 1880s Semmelweis's practices have become the guiding influence and the very marrow of modern surgery, the only change being substitution of thermal for chemical antisepsis of materiel used during operation, for which initiation Pasteur and Chamberland (1878–79), Koch (1881), and surgical students of their techniques were responsible.

Who Is the Discoverer?

In 1969 the senior author outlined three criteria to decide the role of discoverer: (1) who first showed the way; (2) continuance of the practice; (3) influence of the discovery upon contemporary and current practice.[70] On all of these scores, Semmelweis emerges triumphant. In the 1875–85 decade Lister's teachings did lend the first strong forward thrust to acceptance of antiseptic practices. In the terminal fifteen years of the nineteenth century, however, surgeons had swung over completely to Semmelweis's prophylactic antiseptic practices, as did Lister too in the 1893–96 period.

One of Semmelweis's countrymen, Professor István Benedek (1967), historian and psychiatrist, has been critical of Semmelweis for not having been acquainted with Pasteur's work. Wrote Benedek, "Lister could become what he was only with the help of Pasteur. Semmelweis was independent and original. This is undeniably true, but . . . Semmelweis was still living and scientifically active when Pasteur wrote the papers that put Lister on the right track. Had Semmelweis watched carefully, they could have led him too, to see what type of pathological reality was hiding behind his statistical truths. . . . Semmelweis stopped rigidly on his own step without looking around, not to speak of taking another step."[71] Pasteur did write of putrefaction in 1863, but his serious address to pyogenic infection including puerperal fever came only in 1879, when Semmelweis had been dead fourteen years. Semmelweis's health was not good by 1864 and he was in no condition to pursue serious study. There was obviously a spirit of clairvoyance surrounding Semmelweis's innovation not fully understood or appreciated until the appearance of Koch's (1878) work on the pathogenicity of bacteria.

It was Semmelweis's practice to preclude entrance of bacteria into wounds rather than to attempt to destroy them within the wound after entry. Lister's great work gave viable proof to the thesis that bacteria were the cause of wound infection. His role in promoting antiseptic hospital practices was unique; his wound practices lapsed in the terminal decade of the nineteenth century, enjoying a temporary reassertion in World War I with use of Semmelweis's hypochlorite, then known as Dakin's solution. As World War I ended, the value of placing antiseptics in wounds to combat sepsis was questioned, highlighted by the significant observations of Almroth Wright (1915) and the careful studies of his pupil Fleming (1919).[72]

Considering the capitulation of several vigorous obstetrical opponents to Semmelweis's practices by 1867, it is puzzling to note that Viennese surgeons of the era had not heeded Haller's suggestion (1849) that the Semmelweis doctrine had great significance for surgery's advance. Ten years intervened between Lister's first publication on chemical wound antisepsis and the appearance of Hegar's paper adopting all the minutiae of the Semmelweis doctrine for elective abdominal surgery (ovariotomy). Another ten years elapsed until prophylactic surgical antisepsis came to replace the chemical wound antisepsis of Lister. Over this twenty-year interval, Listerian practices led the way in wound care in surgical clinics in Central Europe under the stimulating leadership of Volkmann and Nussbaum.

The importance of discovery transcends national borders. It is only a question of fact and time. Lister's own British colleague Sinclair (1909), one of several of Semmelweis's biographers, said: "Through all the details of prevention and treatment, the temporary fashions and the changes of nomenclature, the principles of Semmelweis have remained our steadfast guide. The discoveries of the bacteriologists from Pasteur onwards, and the work of Lister, only explained and confirmed; they were auxiliary, in no wise conflicting."[73] For several years Lister held to the thesis that air was the chief source of contamination for wound infection. On the contrary, from the very beginning Semmelweis believed that all agents that came in direct contact with the parturient canal, primarily the examining finger, were potential sources of infection.

There was every opportunity for Lister to have known about Semmelweis; however, Lister was not a student of the literature of surgery during the long years of his three professoriates — Glasgow in 1860–69, Edinburgh in 1869–77, and London in 1877–92. Before this period and after his retirement his published writings suggest definitely that he had a ready acquaintance with the literature of the subjects upon which he wrote.

Many have puzzled over the circumstance that the Listers heard nothing about Semmelweis when they were entertained by the Rokitanskys on their first visit to Vienna in 1856, a time when a goodly number of the senior faculty were intent on bringing Semmelweis back to fill the vacancy occasioned by Klein's death. Rokitansky's taciturnity, as recalled by Kussmaul (1822–1902), a well-known German internist, may shed some light on the question. Kussmaul wrote that he spent four months working daily beside Rokitansky, assisting with autopsies. During all that time the only words Rokitansky spoke to him occurred during an interruption of work while the two stood together for a few minutes in the doorway on a fine autumn morning. Said Rokitansky, "Today we have beautiful weather." The astounded Kussmaul pulled himself together and replied, "Yes, it is truly a beautiful day." Perhaps this episode explains why it was unlikely that Lister heard of Semmelweis through Rokitansky in 1856, although the Listers and Rokitanskys had long been family friends.[74]

Markusovszky's Appraisal

Markusovszky, an intimate of Semmelweis, reviewed his book, *Die Aetiologie, der Begriff und die Prophylaxis des Kindbettfiebers*, in the Hungarian journal *Orvosi hetilap* in 1861, an extended and favorable critique.[75] Markusovszky stressed that the work was based on experiments and accurate clinical observations and statistical data accumulated during the resolution of the problem of puerperal fever. The reviewer emphasized Semmelweis's spirit of dedication. He said that publications by earlier authors failed to produce solid facts to resolve the problem. Continued Markusovszky, "the physicians of the sober English nation were closest to the truth in their appreciation of the similarity between surgical and puerperal fever. They considered puerperal fever to be an epidemic, contagious in nature, communicated from one parturient to another through the doctor and linen employed in obstetrical practice. Semmelweis insisted that the disease was transmissible but not contagious." Semmelweis, said Markusovszky, recognized how puerperal fever could be prevented, with great salvage of life for mothers and infants.

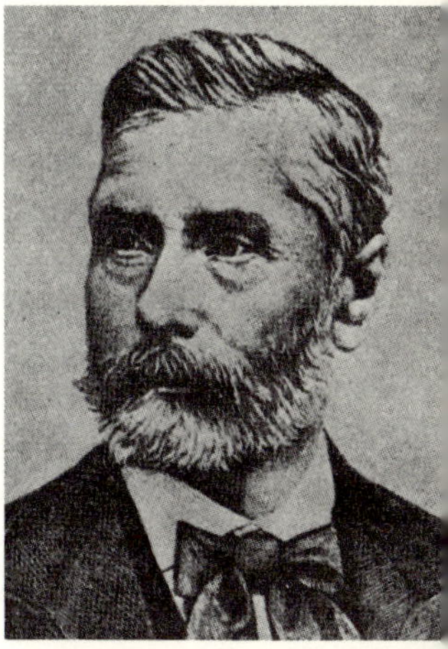

21.12 Lajos Markusovszky, an appreciative critic of Semmelweis's *Die Aetiologie*.

In 1846, wrote Markusovszky, the mortality on the First Obstetrical Service was three to five times that of the midwives of the Second Obstetrical Service, owing solely to the more frequent occurrence of puerperal fever on the service supervised by obstetricians. However, the hospital authorities were not seriously disturbed by the difference, believing that epidemics, a scourge of God, were responsible. Markusovszky supported Semmelweis's contention that overcrowding of the obstetrical service was not a logical explanation of the disparity, for the obstetrical service of the midwives was even more crowded.

Markusovszky related he had shared Semmelweis's apartment in their Vienna days and been an eyewitness to Semmelweis's diligent vigilance. Nothing remained unresearched; he interrogated the women admitted to the service about their general health, diet, and occupation, performing every inquiry and examination with the greatest care. Markusovszky emphasized the importance of the rabbit experiments in which Semmelweis and Lautner demonstrated that puerperal fever could be conveyed to pregnant rabbits following delivery by injecting lochia of women dying of puerperal fever into the vaginal canal of the animals.

The incident pertaining to Kolletschka and his death from an infected finger attending a knife-prick during an autopsy was related by Markusovszky. Semmelweis had rightly concluded that what killed his friend Kolletschka also caused the death of parturients — putrid organic animal material from fresh cadavers conveyed on the hands of students and accoucheurs who examined the parturients. Concluded Semmelweis, "These infected particles which stuck to the fingers of the examiners could be destroyed with some disinfecting agent such as lye (lime), calcium water, or calcium soap. When the fingers of the examiners were clean, the threat could be eliminated, a conclusion substantiated by the results following institution of the program.

"All these pieces of evidence concerning the cause of puerperal fever, its source, the carrier, the uterine site of absorption, and inception of the infection were not developed from theoretical work performed at a desk, but through careful study of patients; by innovations that prevented puerperal fever, observations confirmed by animal experiments." Semmelweis's prophylaxis, concluded Markusovszky, "succeeded in decreasing the mortality of Vienna lying-in parturients from 10 to 0.1 percent, reduplicated later in Budapest. Exclusion of all kinds of decayed animal organic material, disinfection of utensils, and instruments in lime water, and similar washing of the genitals of parturients saved the lives of thousands."

It was Markusovszky who prompted Semmelweis to write his great book. He related that "Semmelweis was reluctant to get at the task, but once started, found himself stimulated, hurrying on from one page to the next, not even rereading the manuscript; off it went to the print shop and the essay planned for 6 folios became a book of 34." Added Markusovszky, "Semmelweis does not put on gloves when dealing with his colleagues; he spoke from the heart; he made no candy-coated apologies." This was the same gentle, versatile, and articulate Markusovszky who presided at the banquet for the Listers at the Hotel of the English Queen, September 29, 1883.

Lister on Semmelweis (1898)

In his biography of Lister Godlee included a letter exchange between Lister and Chiene, then occupying the Chair of Clinical Surgery in Edinburgh (1898). In the first letter Lister extolled Semmelweis and his work but indicated that Semmelweis had very little influence upon wound management in his day, adding: "*Now* people in Germany are glorifying his memory abundantly and most deservedly."[76]

Hebra's Recognition

How did it happen that Hebra (1816–80), a young dermatologist, was the first to recognize the importance of Semmelweis's work? In the authors' view the answer is simple, a circumstance strangely overlooked by historians of surgery. In 1842 Hebra wrote a very knowledgeable treatise on historical aspects of the large operations of surgery, with particular reference to those of his teacher C. Wattmann (1789–1866), leader of the First Surgical Clinic of Vienna (1830–47). Obviously, at age twenty-six, Hebra must have thought very seriously of becoming a surgeon.[77]

The senior author acquired a copy of Godlee's *Lord Lister* in

1922, five years after its publication. It has been rebound twice during the intervening fifty-six years, indicating how frequently its pages have been turned. It is a magnificent biography. Most surgical readers of the English literature of antisepsis are convinced of the primacy of Lister's innovations, as were we for long years. Godlee in his nice factual account does, however, provide inklings that Lister did have predecessors. Pursuit of that quest by the authors over many years does in fact support the thesis that Semmelweis is the originator of current prophylactic surgical antisepsis. It is generally conceded today that one of the most effective techniques in controlling nosocomial infection among hospital personnel is careful handwashing. Inasmuch as Semmelweis stressed handwashing and scrubbing for physicians, nurses, medical students, maids, and parturients, it is probably proper to suggest that he also made an important contribution to the recognition of the source of such infections.

Lister's contribution to acceptance of surgical antisepsis is indeed significant. The facts leave no doubt, however, that Semmelweis was Lister's predecessor and deserves to be acknowledged as the discoverer of prophylactic surgical antisepsis, the sum and substance of modern surgery.

Robert Koch (1843–1910)

The oldest surviving son of thirteen children, Robert Koch enjoyed a carefree boyhood with liberty to roam the Harz countryside, pursuing his interest in natural science.[78] His father, an expert mining engineer, was not affluent, but he was able to send Robert to the University of Göttingen. He entered in 1862, planning to study medicine, apparently with the expectation of becoming a ship's surgeon. Among several distinguished professors on the faculty were Wöhler (1828), who synthesized urea, the pathologist Wilhelm Krause, and the physiologist George Meissner; Koch came to know Henle, the anatomist, well. From these scientists he learned to appreciate the importance of microscopy. In 1865 Koch, aged twenty-two, won first prize for a dissertation upon the structure of the uterine nerves, to which he attached the Latin motto *Numquam otiosus* (never idle).

Upon graduation in July 1865, Koch was appointed as assistant in Krause's pathological museum, a position which afforded him the opportunity of acquiring basic training in pathological and microscopic techniques. He also worked concurrently with Meissner in the Physiological Institute. In January 1866 Koch finished the rigorosum examination with a cum laude citation, delivering a graduation address in Latin on succinic acid in the human body. After a few months graduate study in Berlin, he became an assistant in the general hospital in Hamburg and, in October, physician to an asylum in Langenhagen.

Koch married his childhood sweetheart, Emmy Fraatz, daughter of a Lutheran minister, in 1867. Their only child, Gertrude, was born in 1868. After a brief period as surgeon in the Franco-Prussian War, Koch was appointed a district physician to Wollstein, a small city of 4,000 inhabitants in Polish Prussia, and entered general practice there. He brought his old-fashioned microscope to Wollstein and curtained off a corner of his private office for a laboratory. His wife, knowing how much he needed and wanted a new microscope, scraped and saved enough money from their modest income to provide him with one as a birthday present. Koch purchased a few additional materials including an incubator and, despite demands of a very busy practice, continued his microscopic studies. He addressed himself to the nature of anthrax and the manner of its communication from cattle to men.

On April 22, 1876, Koch wrote his famous letter to the botanist, Cohn of Breslau, who was studying bacterial sporulation. Koch wrote he had worked out the life cycle of the anthrax bacillus and asked permission to demonstrate his experiments. Cohn, greatly interested, invited the young practitioner to come

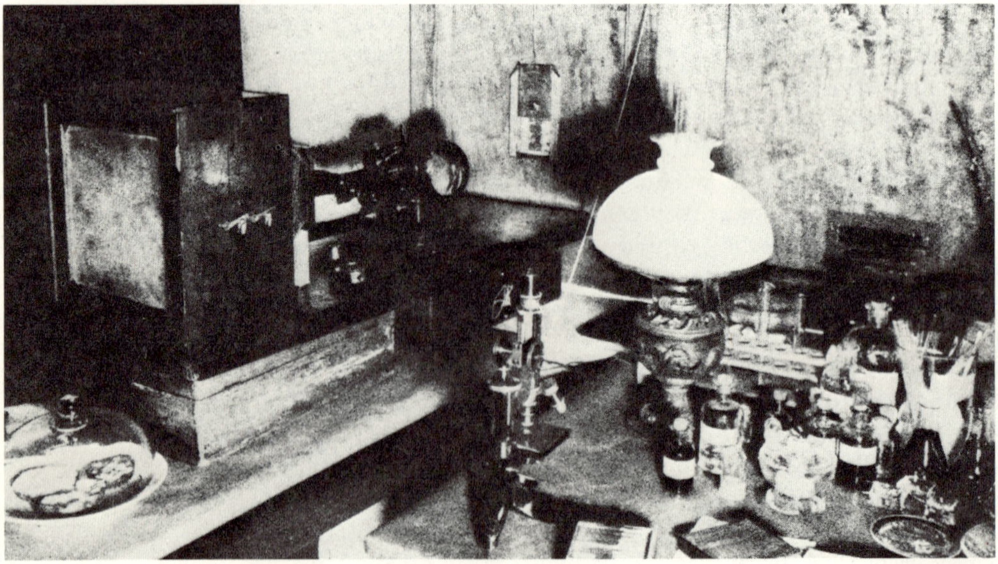

21.13 Koch's original research laboratory in his home in Wollstein.

to Breslau. Koch arrived with all the necessary preparations and animals for the experiments. Three days were occupied with the presentations, viewed by a number of Breslau's celebrated faculty, including Weigert (1845–1904) of bacterial-staining fame; Leopold Auerbach (1828–97), well known for his description of mesenteric nervous plexuses (1863); Ludwig Traube (1818–76) of the Traube-Hering waves; and Cohnheim (1839–84), who demonstrated conclusively (1867) migration of leucocytes through capillary walls in inflammation.

Koch showed how he could cultivate the anthrax bacillus in sterile blood serum or in the aqueous humor of the bovine eye. The short rod, originally present in the blood of animals dead of splenic fever, grew out into long threads or chains of bacilli upon each of which threads a spore appeared. Under proper conditions of temperature and moisture, a short rod characteristic of the anthrax bacillus projected from each spore, as originally observed in the blood of infected animals. Thus Koch was able to demonstrate the complete life cycle of the anthrax organism, the first such description for any bacterium. Early during Koch's demonstrations Cohnheim hurried to his own laboratory, called his assistants together, and told them to "drop everything and hasten to hear Koch." Upon conclusion of the demonstration, Cohnheim declared, "It leaves nothing more to be proved. I regard it as the greatest discovery ever made with bacteria." William Welch, later of The Hopkins, was in Cohnheim's laboratory the following year and recalled Cohnheim's enthusiasm for Koch's work and the latter's frequent visits to Cohnheim's laboratory.[79]

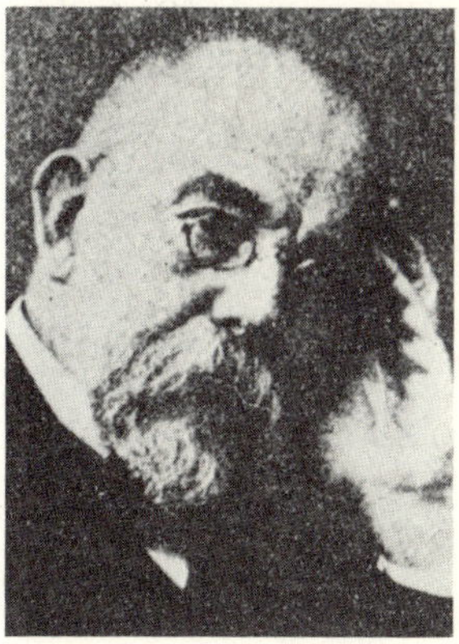
21.14 Robert Koch (1843–1910).

Cohn arranged for immediate publication of Koch's treatise in July 1876.[80] The self-made microbiologist had become famous overnight, at thirty-three years of age. Subsequent studies have not disproved a single facet of this enlightened demonstration.

Virchow in Berlin, to whom Koch next took his observations, received them coolly. In November 1877 Koch's second paper appeared, in which he described his techniques of staining and photographing bacteria, demonstrating the superiority of photography over the use of word descriptions in depicting the morphology of bacteria. Koch indicated how very difficult it is to isolate and identify bacteria by microscopic studies alone. Placing a few drops of the fluid culture on a slide, Koch covered it with a thin glass cover-slip and allowed the preparation to dry. By this means the bacteria became distinctly visible, and Koch preserved the preparation for photographic purposes. He used a magnification of 500–700 in his morphologic studies.[81]

In 1878 Koch published his third paper, on the etiology of wound infection, in which, for the first time, convincing evidence was adduced of the pathogenicity of pyogenic organisms.[82] By then Koch had formulated microbiologic techniques and methods he would use through the rest of his professional experience and which enabled other microbiologists readily to verify his observations because they permitted accurate identification of single microorganisms. Koch listed himself on the title page as district physician for Wollstein.

Koch was persuaded in 1879 to go to Breslau as a city practitioner. He remained only three months and returned to his old position in Wollstein, which paid him 900 marks annually; in addition, he had some private practice. However, he was now, by general consent, recognized as the world's foremost innovative microbiologist and quickly succeeded to an important post as a member of the Imperial Board of Health in Berlin, with a well-equipped laboratory and liberal provision for research support and assistants.

Other important discoveries (1881) followed: the gelatin and beef broth pour-plates which made it possible to detect and separate out various types of bacteria from a fluid culture, and the potato slant bacterial medium.[83] At the London meeting of the Seventh International Medical Congress, Koch demonstrated these procedures to a select group at King's College and also gave a magic-lantern show of his work to a wider audience. Pasteur is said to have rushed forward on seeing the gelatin culture demonstrations, exclaiming, "C'est un grand progrès!"[84]

The potato slant bacterial medium played an important role in Koch's discovery of the tubercle bacillus (1882).[85] In this famous paper Koch characterized the desiderata necessary to establish the specific causative role of a microorganism in disease, a sequence that has come to be known as Koch's postulates: (1) The organism can be demonstrated to be present in every case of the disease. (2) It can be cultivated in pure culture. (3) Animal inoculation from the culture will reproduce the disease. (4) The organism can be recovered from inoculated animals and again can be grown in pure culture. Koch very obviously exacted high standards of performance in his incisive methodology, a responsible component in his extraordinary success.

The most reliable and quick-acting antiseptic agents for purposes of disinfection, according to Koch (1881), were chlorine, bromine (2 percent aqueous), iodine, and 1 percent mercuric chloride, all of which would kill anthrax spores within twenty-four hours. He also observed that aqueous dilutions of 1:1,000 mercuric chloride killed bacteria devoid of spores in a few minutes following a single application.[86] Later Koch's pupil Behring (1890) showed that mercuric chloride did not have a strong antibacterial effect in blood serum; he believed that in the subculture transfer Koch had carried over traces of the antiseptic.[87]

Koch pointed out that most antiseptics fail to destroy bacteria; they only retard bacterial growth. Experiment, said Koch, demonstrates that there is no universal antiseptic agent effective against bacteria and especially against spores. Exposure of hands and instruments to a dilute solution of carbolic acid for a few minutes Koch regarded as useless. His experiments evaluating the efficacy of antiseptic agents were performed largely on mice and rabbits.

Whereas Koch observed that antiseptics have a bacteriostatic and not a bactericidal effect, one cannot peruse the extensive literature on the use of antiseptics in wound management without reaching the inference that they did to some degree assist in controlling localized wound infections, at the same time probably diminishing the hazards of infection introduced by unsterile hands and materiel.

Koch (1881) demonstrated the superiority of heat over chemicals in destroying and inhibiting bacterial action and devised a scheme of sterilization by dry steam. Temperatures of 145° C sustained for three hours, said Koch, are bactericidal.[88] It is to be remembered that the Frenchman Nicolas Appert made canning of foods a safe process by sealing containers directly after heating to destroy enzymes and other agents (bacteria) that led to deterioration of food. Appert's publication on the subject appeared in 1810.[89]

Considerable space was given Koch, then recognized as the world's leading microbiologist, in the *Lancet* report of the Tenth International Medical Congress, held in Berlin in 1890. Koch followed Lister on the program, both receiving prolonged applause. Koch began by saying that as late as 1875 bacteria were generally considered saprophytic; in his small monograph of 1878 he had definitely established the pathogenicity of pyogenic bacteria. He then discussed sporulation of bacteria and the influence of air, warmth, moisture, and chemicals upon bacteria. Said Koch, direct sunlight quickly kills bacteria, including the tubercle bacillus. Even daylight produces the same effect, although more slowly. Moisture is necessary for the growth of bacteria, but hinders their spreading. Bacterial stains have augmented the knowledge of the behavior and structure of bacteria. Therapeutics, predicted Koch, will derive great benefits from bacteriology, but the main item in management will always be prevention. Beginning experiments on human beings rather than on animals, Koch regarded as wrong.[90]

At the 1890 Berlin Congress Koch announced prematurely that he had found a cure for early cases of pulmonary tuberculosis, employing inoculations of tuberculin.[91] The news was hailed the world over as an achievement of the greatest scientific importance. The untimely prophecy still awaits fulfillment. Meanwhile, great strides have been made by preventative and specific curative agents to nullify the threat of the tubercle bacillus.

Even toward the end of his career Koch (1908) continued to be skeptical about the communicability of bovine tuberculosis to man. The subsequent success of the United States Livestock Sanitary Commission and Public Health authorities program (1911–17) with pasteurization of milk and the slaughter of tuberculous cattle established beyond doubt that bovine tuberculosis is transmissible to man.[92]

N. Howard-Jones has written of the Gelsenkirchen typhoid epidemic of 1901, and of the "dead hand of Max von Pettenkofer," who had denied that typhoid fever could be communicated through drinking water. Pettenkofer (1892) had swallowed a culture of cholera vibrio which he stated contained a thousand million microorganisms. His only complication was temporary diarrhea. His faithful disciple, Rudolf Emmerich, joined Pettenkofer in the experiment with far more drastic results than diarrhea, but he too survived. By the time Koch testified for the government in the affirmative against the accused water works officials, Pettenkofer was dead, having blown his brains out with a pistol in 1901 at age eighty-three.[93]

After 1882 Koch was made the head of several commissions. He went to Egypt and to India where he identified and proved the role of the cholera bacillus as the cause of cholera. He also described the cause of conjunctivitis, which had troubled Larrey's troups in North Africa in the Napoleonic Wars.

Over all the years of his married life Koch was completely absorbed in his work. Whereas Mme. Pasteur's sole concern was for the furtherance of her husband's work, there gradually developed some estrangement between Professor and Frau Koch. When their only child, Gertrude, was married, the alienation became complete and divorce followed (June 1893). Frau Koch returned to her native Klausthal. Within two months Koch married Fraulein Hedwig, twenty-nine years his junior, who worked in his laboratory, an occurrence that alienated Koch from many of his former colleagues and friends and deprived him of much of the adulation he had enjoyed at the hands of the German people, a circumstance which may account for the many commitments Koch accepted for foreign travel. In his declining years his strenuous pace of creative work continued and many honors were bestowed upon him, but to a man who had achieved many significant victories over disease for mankind, such acclaims and esteem were lightly borne.

How distinguished scientists in one discipline may know very little of the work of celebrated investigators in a somewhat unrelated area is well exemplified in a statement made by Koch when Pavlov was given the Nobel Prize award in 1904. Said Koch, "It must be on a geographical basis. I know nothing of his scientific contributions." In 1905 Koch too was made a Nobel Laureate, essentially for his contribution to the cause and nature of tuberculosis.

Pasteur is probably best described as an imaginative investigator with a great store of original ideas. Koch was a master of method and was adept at devising original microbiologic techniques both morphologic and cultural. Microbiology was brought to the status of a great scientific discipline by these two giants of the nineteenth century.

After Pasteur and Koch

The science of immunity and immunology links the present with Koch's demonstration of the pathogenicity of bacteria (1876–78). Pasteur had appreciated the prophylactic protective influence of an attenuated virus in the promotion of immunity, an idea tracing back to Edward Jenner's vaccination for smallpox. There emerged in the final decades of the nineteenth century a group of original thinkers and independent investigators, identified at one period in their careers with the schools of Pasteur and Koch, whose work came to have great influence on progress in medical therapy. Émile Roux, Pasteur's keenest pupil, was his successor as director at the Institute. Behring extended Roux's observations, for which he was awarded the first Nobel Prize in medicine (1901). One of the most outstanding and original scientific investigators of this or any period was Ehrlich (1854–1915), whose successive labors and creative genius had great influence on the development of hematology, immunology, and chemotherapy. He shared the Nobel Prize with Metchnikoff in 1908.[94] The latter's work on phagocytosis initiated the phagocytic theory of immunity, work well under way before he joined Pasteur's staff in 1887.

Henle's influence in initiating microbiologic studies provided proof of Fracastoro's (1556) thesis of contagion, alluded to in the preceding chapter. The role of Cohnheim in setting aside Virchow's skepticism of bacteria as etiologic agents of infection and disease did much to advance practical medicine's progress and the science of pathology during a period when the medical profession was contemplating and debating the novel ideas of Pasteur on immunization. Cohnheim's great influence on Welch helped shape the development and outlook of The Hopkins in the future education and training of American physicians and medical specialists. This period also witnessed extensions of interest in microbiology from France and Germany to America and Britain.

Theobald Smith (1859–1934), an original thinker and careful investigator, became one of America's foremost microbiologists, contributing significantly to theoretic and practical aspects of the discipline. In London Wright made his influence felt in the management of wounds and in practical aspects of immunization. He pioneered inoculation for typhoid fever, which at the turn of the century constituted a serious threat to healthy civilians and to armies. His most enduring contribution, many will

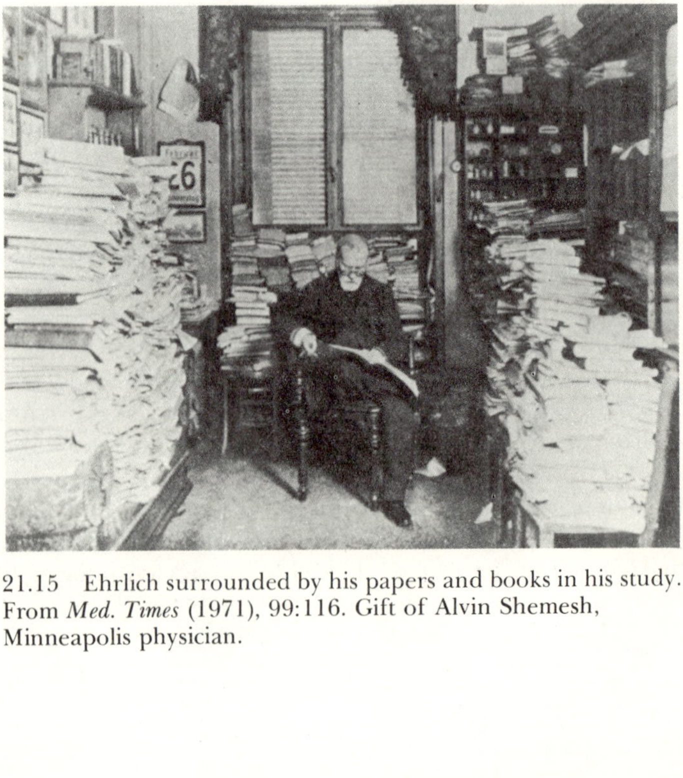

21.15 Ehrlich surrounded by his papers and books in his study. From *Med. Times* (1971), 99:116. Gift of Alvin Shemesh, Minneapolis physician.

agree, was providing an opportunity and training for his most illustrious and innovative pupil, Fleming.

Immunology and anaphylaxis today no longer concern bacterial diseases alone. They lie at the very heart of the success and promise of organ and tissue transplantation. When that challenge is met and conquered through future dreamers of the Pasteur and Ehrlich pattern, greater medicine will have taken another giant step forward.

Summary

In the mid-sixteenth century the great triumvirate of Vesalius, Paré, and Fracastoro emerged, whose writings lent greater medicine a strong forward upsurge. Although wound care prospered from the work of Paré, surgery remained essentially stationary, without important advances or significant extension of its borders. Elective surgery awaited the discoveries of a larger group of inquisitive and scientific men of the mid-nineteenth century (1840–86) for the impetus of much needed clarification.

In operations of urgency, especially in amputation and perineal lithotomy, a few men widely scattered in place and time achieved excellent mortality records while many of their colleagues encountered disasters. The only directives successful surgeons could provide were high standards of surgical cleanliness, adequate hemostasis, and open wound management. Something important was still lacking, and its nature could not be identified, although Fracastoro had provided more than gentle hints (1546) in his suggestion that the sources of infection were invisible "seminaria" (germs) that propagated infection by direct contact with infected sources or through the air. The experiments of Redi (1668) and Spallanzani (1776) shed further light upon the nature of infection, but what constituted the airborne factor and the direct contact source of infection remained a mystery and awaited development of the science of microbiology, the discovery of bacteria and demonstration of their pathogenic character. Bacteria had been described by Müller (1786); Henle wrote a fascinating and informative essay on the origins of miasmata in 1840, a quest he failed to pursue.

In 1847 there appeared on the scene in Vienna a Hungarian student of obstetrics, Semmelweis, whose 1844 botanical thesis contained ten conclusions, the last of which urged that the physician's hands be clean. The nature of puerperal fever was a matter of debate; that it was borne by the physician or midwife was conceded by a few, but exactly how was still an enigma.

Semmelweis noted that the pathological findings in his colleague Kolletschka, who died from a finger-prick sustained in a postmortem examination, were identical with those of women dying of puerperal fever. Without any knowledge of microbiology, which was then not taught in medical schools anywhere in the world, Semmelweis correctly reasoned that an open wound of the skin permitted transmission of the fatal poison. By the time of his important publication of 1861 Semmelweis, without histological aids, had rightly concluded that invisible animal matter was the source of the difficulty. How like the language of Fracastoro of three centuries earlier!

The chemist Pasteur, whose research crossed the boundaries of many disciplines, verified (1860–63) the earlier observations of Spallanzani that spontaneous generation was an unsubstantiated myth. Employing both histologic and cultural methods in later studies, he identified bacteria as the causative agent, a finding amply confirmed by the methodical studies of the self-trained microbiologist Koch (1876–78). Employing the age-old practice of placing antiseptics into wounds, Lister (1867–92) made a significant impact upon surgery's progress, especially in operations of the extremities. When his professorial years were over, Lister capitulated to the prophylactic surgical practices of Semmelweis of 1847. These men with varied backgrounds and talents were the nineteenth-century therapeutic discoverers who resolved the riddle of the nature of infection and who created elective surgery.

After Pasteur and Koch came a succession of brilliant investigators, influenced by their teachings, who sharpened considerably medicine's focus upon immunization and prophylactic therapy. Foremost among these was the many-sided Ehrlich, who made significant contributions to many areas of medicine and to whom we owe chemotherapy. He was a master at formulating theories, which he tested by experiment.

(For notes, see pp. 689–97.)

CHAPTER 22

The Surgical Amphitheatre

TENON (1788) urged that hospitals provide a separate room for operations, but as late as 1815 Dupuytren was performing emergency operations upon patients in their ward beds at the Hôtel-Dieu. The British visitor Crosse watched Dupuytren remove a cancerous breast with the patient seated on a chair in the women's ward.[1] The senior author in 1926 observed the elder Crile surprising patients with "steal" operations in their beds to minimize the shock of operation for severe exophthalmic goiter before effective methods to control thyroid crises had been generally accepted. Elective surgery came only in the mid-1880s when prophylactic antisepsis found favor with surgeons as well as with the public. Before then many hospitals in the nineteenth century provided a room or two for operations, one for septic cases, the other for clean cases; but even this distinction was not consistently recognized.

The Anatomical Amphitheatre

The keen interest of physicians and laymen in witnessing anatomical dissections in the sixteenth century brought anatomical amphitheatres into being. Every student of medicine is familiar with the illustration accompanying Vesalius's great book, the *Fabric of the Human Body* (1543), depicting Vesalius dissecting in public in Padua. One can be very certain, however, that his significant work stemmed entirely from quiet study in a small dissecting room. The first permanent anatomical amphitheatre was that of the surgeon-anatomist Fabricius ab Aquapendente in Padua (1594), where Morgagni performed much of his famous work a century later. Pieter Paaw built a replica of Vesalius's theatre in Leyden in 1597. The idea of a large anatomical amphitheatre was brought to Edinburgh from Leyden by John Monro, father of Alexander Monro I.[2]

In the seventeenth and eighteenth centuries, notably in

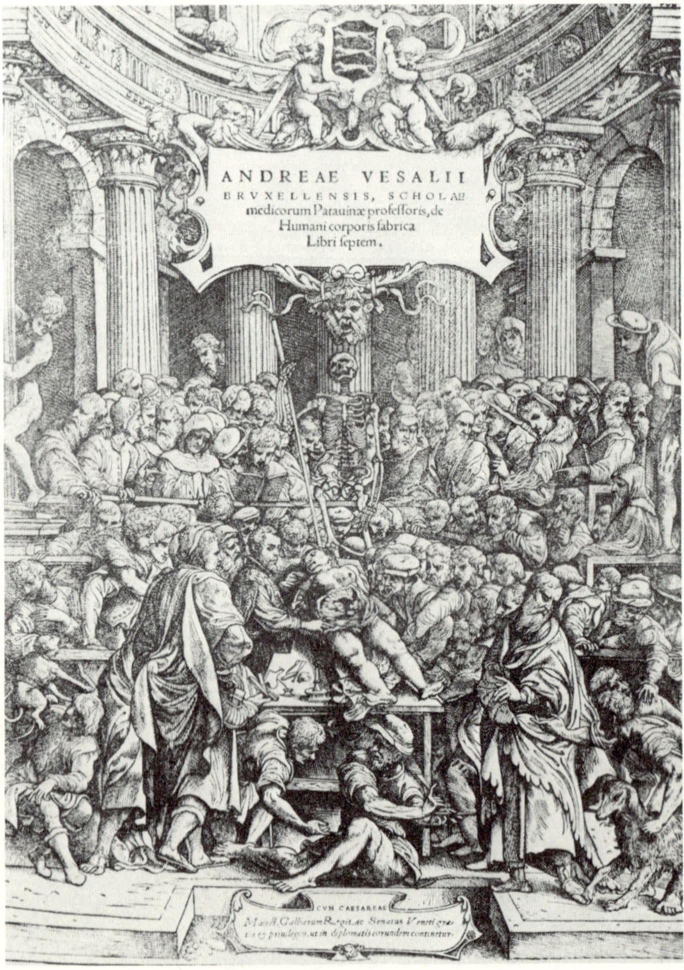

22.1 Anatomical amphitheatre of Vesalius. Title page of Vesalius, *De humani corporis fabrica* (1543).

France, surgeons began to use amphitheatres for demonstrating the anatomy of operative procedures to medical students. As teaching hospitals gradually adopted the amphitheatre it became the main arena of the surgeon's activity, where the professor lectured and performed his operations. This period, before the emergence of surgery as a scientific discipline, was a colorful one, characterized by excitement and tragedy.

Prior to anesthesia (1846), rapid operating was the order of the day. Lisfranc (1790–1847) of Paris practiced his surgical techniques upon a large number of fresh cadavers annually in his anxiety to be able to perform all amputations in a few seconds. Especially famous exponents of celerity in operating were Liston (1794–1847) of London and Fergusson (1808–77) of King's College Hospital, the "surgical flamingo" who could amputate a thigh, close the wound, and complete the dressing in three and a half minutes. It was said of Fergusson that he had "the eye of an eagle, the heart of a lion, and the hand of a lady."[3]

Although anesthesia eliminated the need for hurry, rapid operating remained the vogue in many surgical teaching clinics until surgeons' complete acceptance of the principles of microbiology compelled the separation of operative and tutorial functions. Halsted, emulating the surgical practices of Kocher of Bern, probably did more than any surgeon in our country to eliminate haste in operations. Their teachings demarcate the beginnings of a new era in surgery, characterized by deliberate operating, complete hemostasis, careful and gentle management of tissue — a manner of operating and a technique of wound management that have become the symbol of good surgery everywhere.[4]

Despite the horror and terror of the operating scene before ether became available, heightened by the heart-rending shrieks of the patient, students and physicians flocked to witness such ordeals, impelled by the drive that brought crowds to view the drama of a hanging. Lithotomy cases were often scheduled together on a special morning, when surgeons, physicians, students, relatives, and even townsmen gathered, watches in hand, to observe and time the performance.[5]

Medical history records no finer or more touching example of courage under operation than that of the Scottish peasant woman Ailie, who in 1830 had a breast removed for cancer without anesthesia by Syme in the operating theatre of Minto House, Edinburgh, which was crowded with students. She entered the theatre dressed in her regular clothes, accompanied by her husband, James, and their dog, Rab. John Brown, a participant in the operation as a medical student, told the story twenty-eight years later in "Rab and His Friends" (1858): "Her pale face showed its pain but was still and silent. Rab's soul was working within him . . . blood flowing from his mistress . . . his ragged ear was up . . . he growled . . . but James had him firm. . . . It is over; she is dressed, steps gently and decently down from the table, looks for James: then, turning to the surgeon and the students, she curtsies and in a low, clear voice, begs their pardon if she has behaved ill." Adds Dr. Brown, "the students — all of us — wept like children . . . and, resting on James and me, Ailie went to her room, Rab following." This quiet and exceptionally brave lady succumbed from sepsis a few days later. We are told that when Tait read these lines of John Brown to his class, the eyes of the great but gruff surgeon always filled with tears.[6]

A Few Historic Mastectomies

The seventeenth-century surgeon Scultetus depicted mastectomy for cancer of the breast. After the extirpation, cautery was used. Two other historic mastectomies performed without anesthesia, but not in surgical amphitheatres, are deserving of mention. Fanny Burney d'Arblay (1752–1840), the English novelist, underwent mastectomy of her right breast for cancer by Napoleon's great surgeon, Larrey, September 30, 1811, before he departed on the Russian campaign. The famous patient described her torment and agony in graphic language in a long letter to her sister. The patient was apprised of the time set for the operation only two hours before it was to take place. She was encouraged to eat before the procedure, an indulgence which the arrival of inhalation anesthesia thirty-five years later definitely established as unwise. The progress of the operation, conducted in silence because the patient was fully conscious, was apparently dictated in sign language by Antoine Dubois, Larrey's colleague. A cambric handkerchief placed over the patient's face was so transparent that she could observe and subsequently describe events in detail. Mme. d'Arblay survived twenty-nine more years, dying at age eighty-eight, raising questions concerning the validity of the diagnosis. Alan Steinfeld (1975) reviewed a mastectomy performed on July 28, 1718, by Zabdiel Boylston of Boston, who "in the presence of several Ministers & others" cut his patient's "whole Breast off"! The

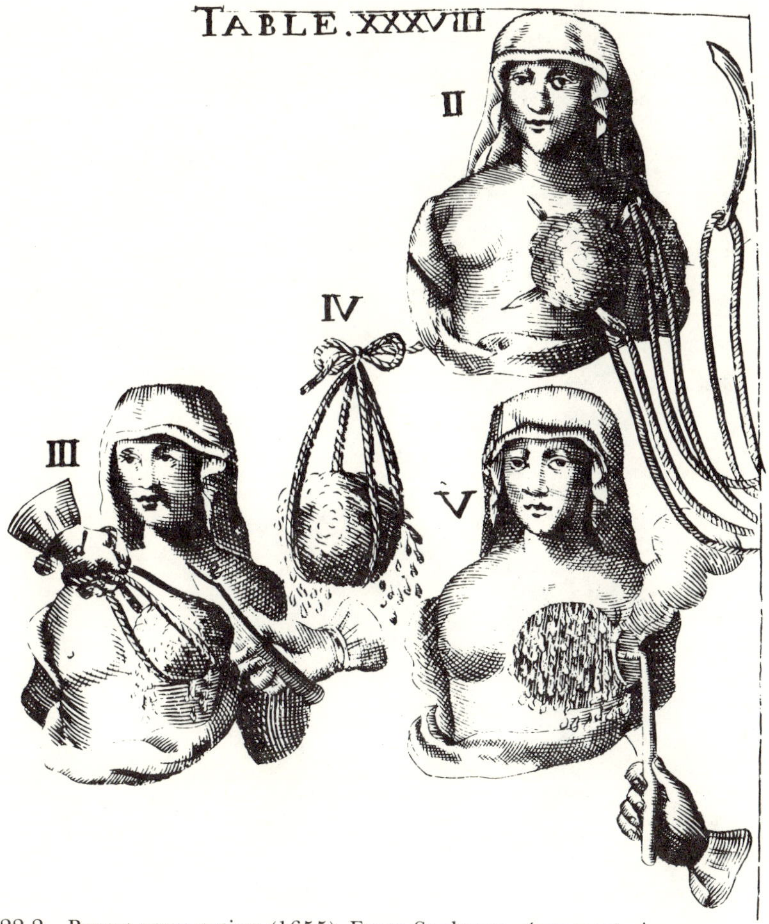

22.2 Breast amputation (1655). From Scultetus, *Armamentarium.*

patient survived the ordeal for thirty-nine years, dying at age eighty-five, again raising legitimate doubts about the authenticity of the diagnosis.[7]

Origins of the Surgical Amphitheatre

Félix's success in operating upon Louis XIV for a rectal fistula (1686) won recognition and public acclaim for surgery, greatly troubling the physicians of Paris.[8] By a series of royal decrees the barber-surgeons were extended the privilege of dissecting dead bodies as well as treating wounds. An amphitheatre for anatomical dissections had been built for the surgeons on a parcel of land purchased from the church wardens of Saint-Côme in the cemetery of the Cordeliers Convent; there Séverin Pineau (November 19, 1616) gave the first public lecture, on lithotomy. Shortly after Félix's fortunate operation upon the Sun King, the amphitheatre of St. Côme was constructed (1694), becoming ultimately the home of the Royal Academy of Surgery (1731), which exerted great influence upon world surgery until its demise in 1792.

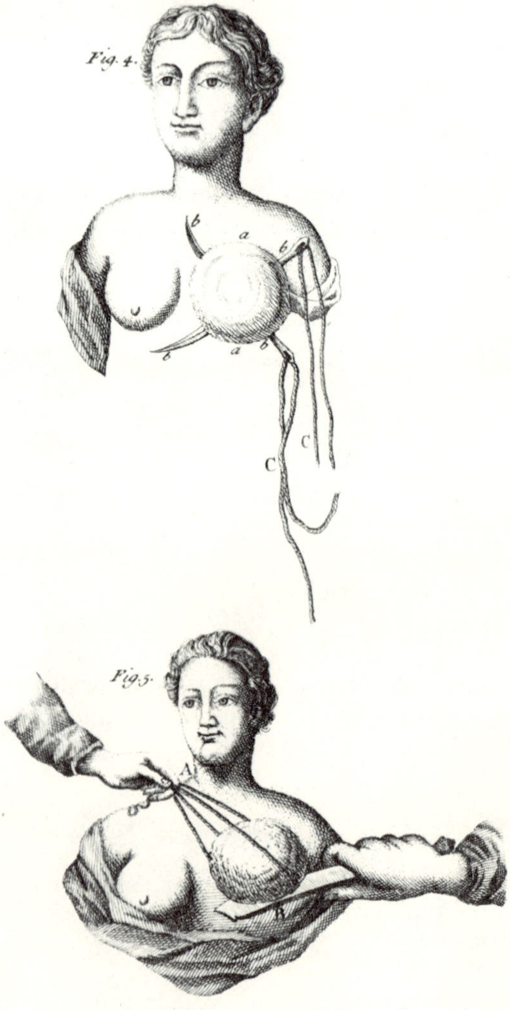

22.3 Breast amputation (1743). From Heister, *General system of surgery*. Courtesy National Library of Medicine.

A century after St. Côme, the beautiful surgical amphitheatre of École de Chirurgie (1780) was designed by the architect Gondoin[9] and built at Louis XVI's expense; it came to house both the College of St. Côme and the Royal Academy of Surgery, and still stands at 5 rue de l'École de Médecine, although no longer a site for surgical instruction. The jealousy of the physicians led to public demonstrations and protests, but the surgeons had won the confidence of the people, at least for the moment. The royal favor helped materially to offset the disapproval of the ranks of the medical faculty, which long had its own anatomical amphitheatre.

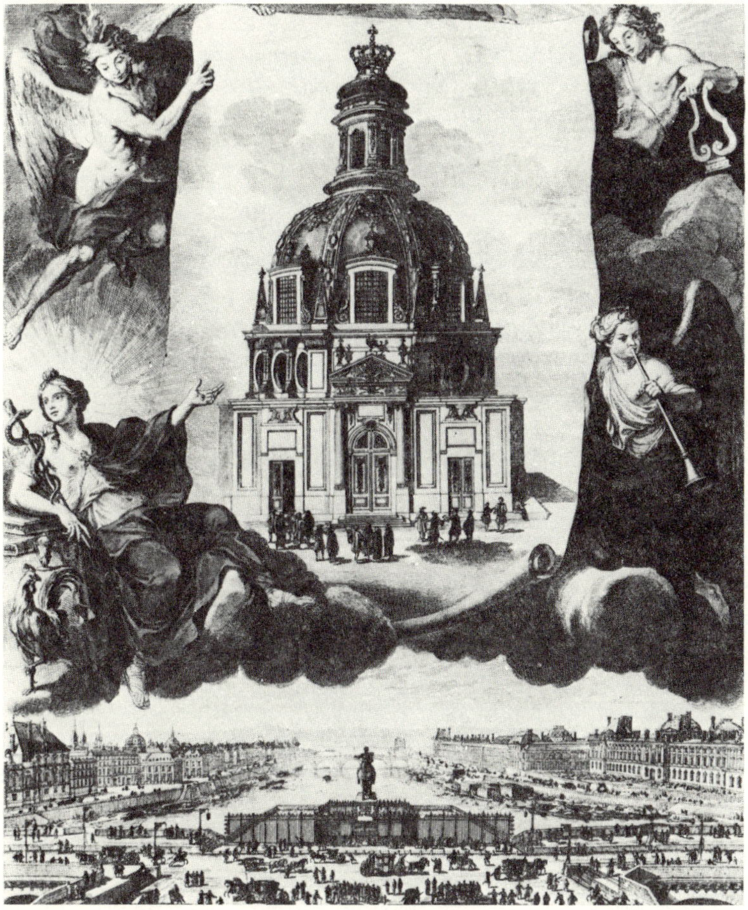

22.4 Surgical amphitheatre of St. Côme (1694), center of activities of the French Royal Academy of Surgery.

During his Paris visit of 1815 Crosse attended Dupuytren's lecture on hernia before a capacity audience of 1,200 students. Six cadavers were laid out on the table in the large amphitheatre to illustrate the anatomy of inguinal hernia, its nature and operative management. Crosse sat far back and felt that good instruction was lost on him, regretting that "what is grand should be so far remote from what is most useful." A Danish physician visitor, Karl Otto, wrote in 1825 that 400 students followed Dupuytren's ward rounds, many taking their stands at the bedsides of interesting cases half an hour before the chief's expected arrival. They reserved places in the amphitheatre with a handkerchief or book as soon as they reached the hospital, but even then it was almost impossible to get an unobstructed view of the lecture demonstrations or the operations that followed.[10] Obviously, large amphitheatre clinics did not provide the best means for demonstration of operative procedures.

Extension of Amphitheatres to Clinical Surgery

The experience of surgeons in teaching the anatomy of operative procedures on cadavers in large amphitheatres was a natural prelude to continuance of the practice in teaching techniques of operations upon patients. As the proficiency of surgeons in operations grew, they urged upon hospital officers the need for theatres in which both operative and tutorial functions could be performed. Delpech became so irate when the hospital authorities refused to improve his inadequate operating room at Saint-Éloi in Montpellier that he returned to operating in the ward. One June day in 1817 in the course of a lithotomy on a fourteen-year-old girl, some students climbed up on the altar in the women's ward to get a better view of the proceedings. In the ensuing scandal, Delpech achieved his demands.[11] Crowding in operating rooms was a common problem; the Norfolk and Norwich Hospital (1821) had a semicircular railing that could be fixed to the floor of the operating room when necessary to "prevent a pressure upon the operator." This seems to have been a particularly adaptable room, for in 1834 an arch and folding doors were added to connect it with the consulting room and to make it "more convenient for the performance of divine service."[12]

Guy's Hospital had a surgical amphitheatre with a skylight as early as 1739. The oldest existing surgical amphitheatre in America is preserved in Philadelphia's Pennsylvania Hospital. It

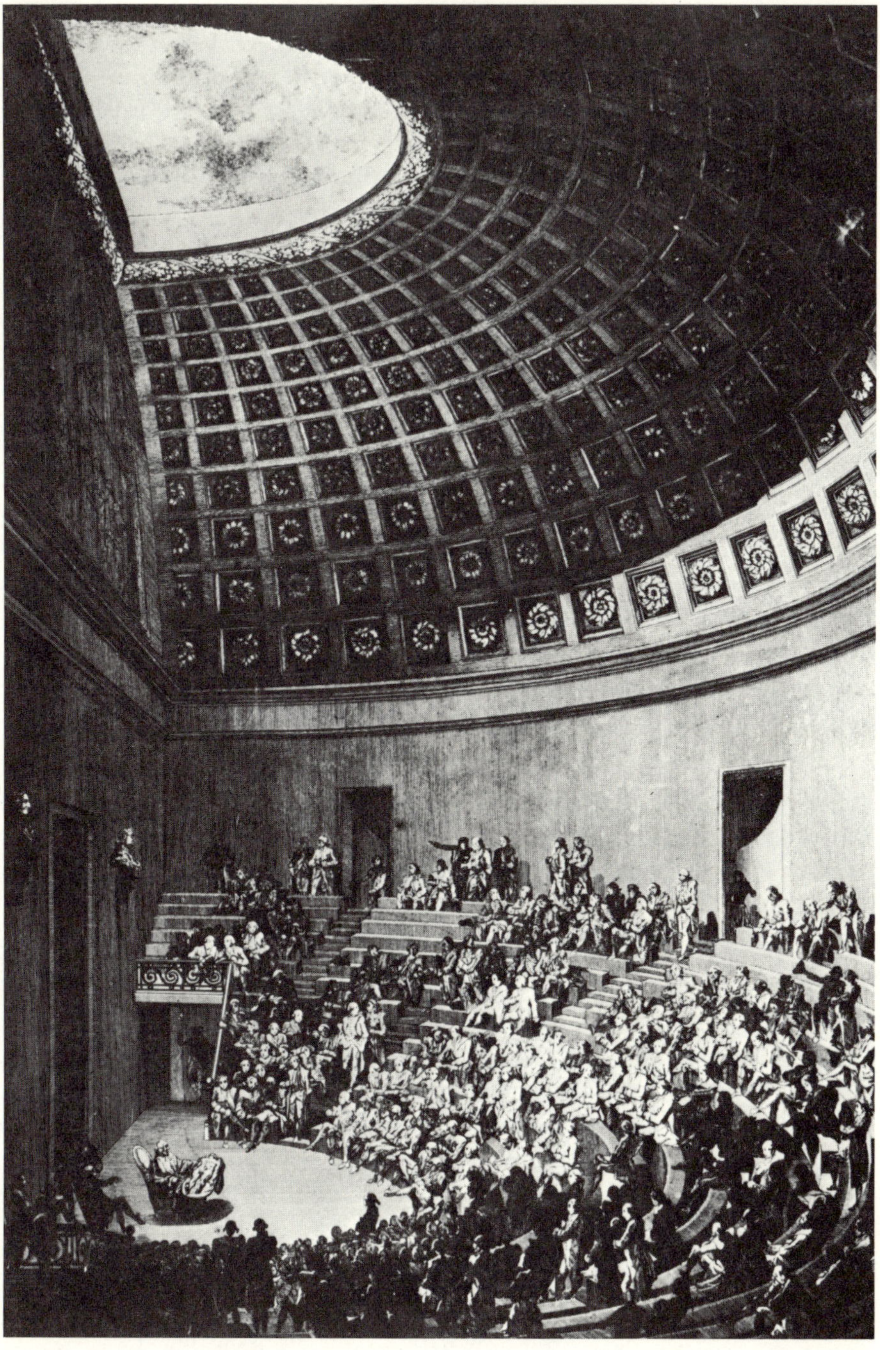

22.5 Grodin's surgical amphitheatre of École de Chirurgie (1780).

was designed to function as lecture and operating room, with a gallery on the operating level as well as on the mezzanine. According to Benjamin H. Coates, the first operation in the "elegant amphitheatre . . . illuminated by a sky light" took place in February 1804. Seymour Schwartz says that Pennsylvania's was not, however, the first operating theatre in America — New York Hospital built one a year earlier.[13]

Throughout the nineteenth century large surgical amphitheatres were commonplace in metropolitan medical centers. The trend gained considerable momentum with the introduction of anesthesia and the acceptance of prophylactic surgical antisepsis, which created elective cavitary surgery. This period marked the summit of the surgeon's dazzling actor-role, in which the spotlight of the public gaze was focused upon him. In 1878, before surgical antisepsis was accepted in America, Stephen Smith, New York surgeon and sanitarian, advised abolition of operating amphitheatres as dangerous to the patient and useless for purposes of instruction. He believed that only the surgeon and his assistants should be present at operations. In his ninety-sixth year Smith described some of his early experiences with pre-Listerian surgeons at New York's Bellevue Hospital: "The Catlin, glittering for a moment above the head of the operator, was plunged through the limb and with one artistic sweep made the flaps or completed a circular amputation. After several aerial gyrations the saw severed the bone as if driven by electricity. The fall of the amputated part was greeted with tumultuous applause by the excited students. The operator acknowledged the compliment with a formal bow."[14] The only thing missing in the scenario was the fall of the curtain on completion of the act.

Tait (1887) reported that when Syme operated for a gluteal aneurysm in the 1860s there were probably seven or eight hundred spectators, filling the old Infirmary theatre to the top of the gallery; Tait philosophized that in the entire audience there were only six or eight men who might someday be called upon to perform such an operation. Syme's entrance, followed by a procession of assistant house surgeons and dressers, "was greeted with a subdued murmur of applause."[15]

Another sensational entrance was that of Wood, who customarily appeared in the operating theatre of Bellevue with a boutonniere of violets pinned over his left breast. He was followed by his house surgeon, the buttonhole of whose operating coat was decorated only with waxed silk ligatures.[16]

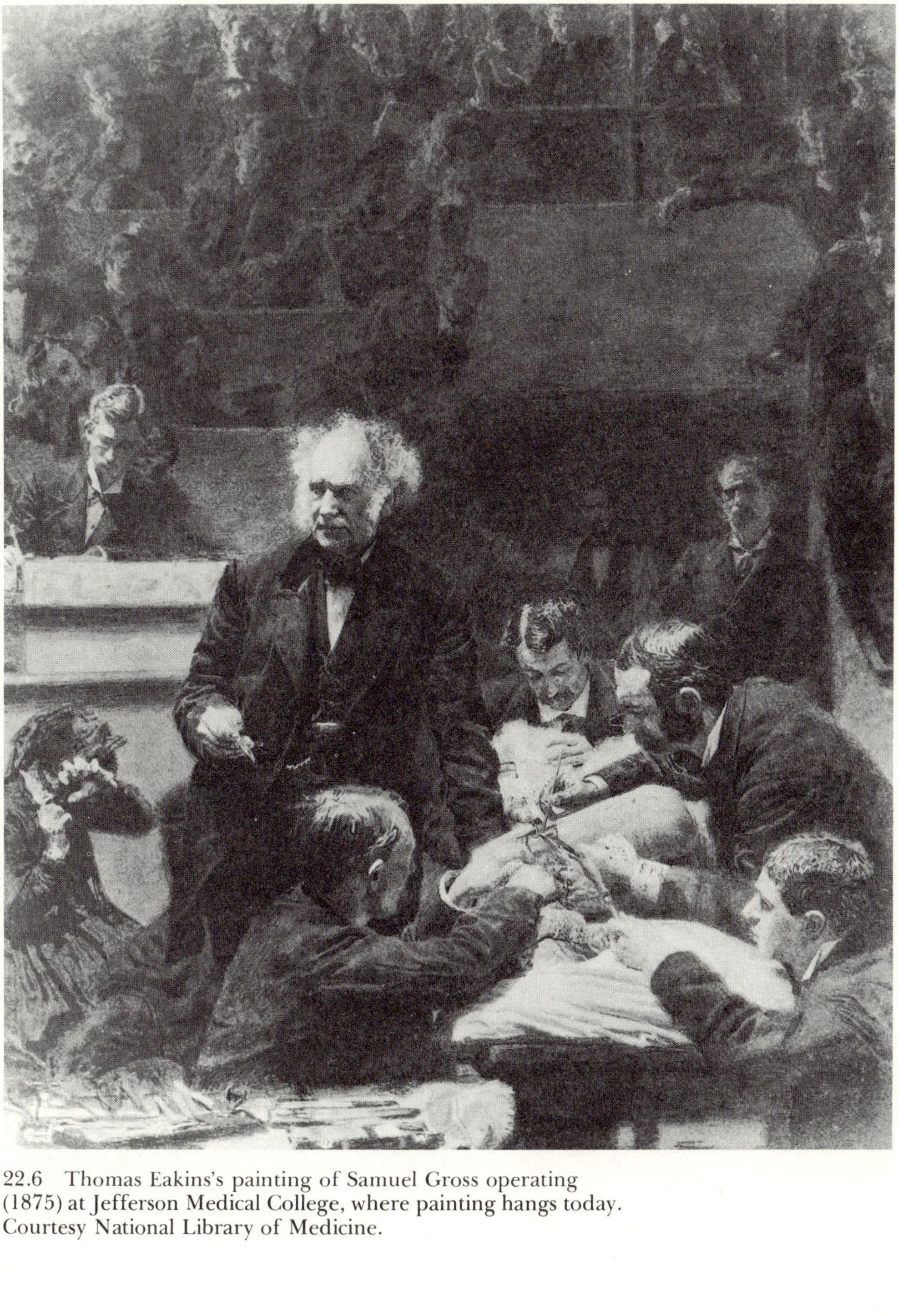

22.6 Thomas Eakins's painting of Samuel Gross operating (1875) at Jefferson Medical College, where painting hangs today. Courtesy National Library of Medicine.

Hospitals Reflect an Improved Surgical Image

As early as 1579 Paré affirmed that surgery had reached its height and that the accomplishments of his day perhaps would never be excelled, a thesis reechoed by Boyer (1818), by Erichsen (1873), and in this century by Lord Moynihan (1926).[17] In the last fifteen years of the nineteenth century there came a dramatic upsurge of interest and confidence in the future of surgery, shared by the profession and the public. Simultaneously, particularly in London, elegant new operating rooms appeared, reflecting a greatly changed attitude of hospital authorities toward surgery, and the readiness of trustees and affluent friends to upgrade the operating arena. Bloodstained operating frock coats had been replaced by clean linens; the new setting obviously was intended to match the sterile dress of the operating personnel and to portray the public's faith in surgery's future.

The Middlesex Hospital (1895) installed teakwood benches in tiers for 130 students, staircases also of teak, and walls of glazed tile; the operating floor was marble terrazzo. Similar develop-

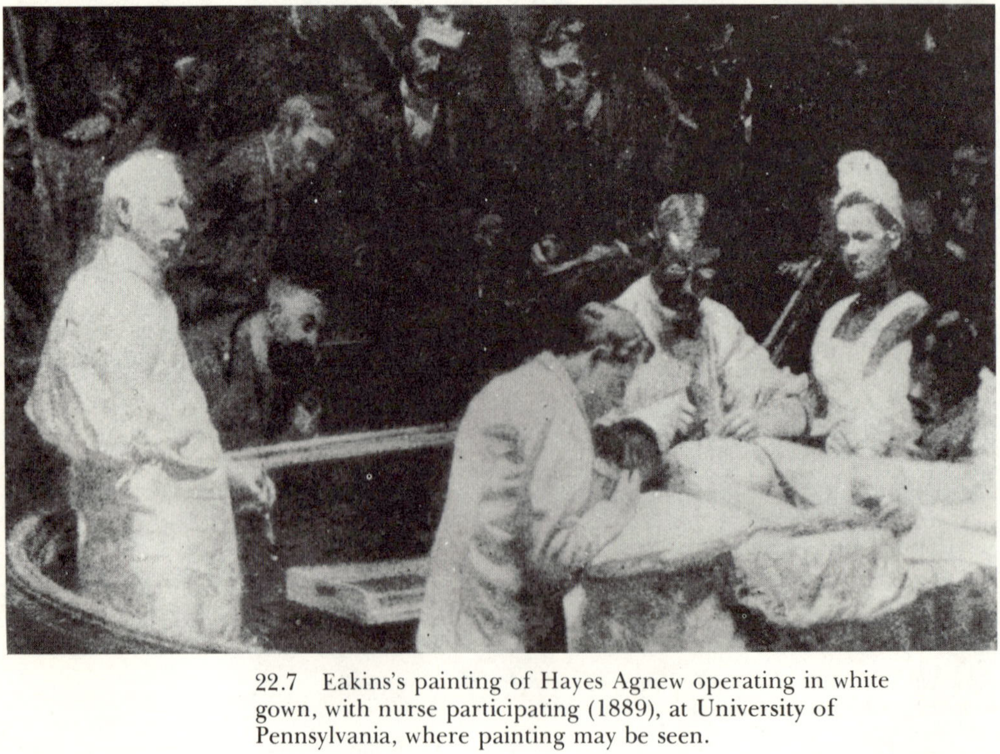

22.7 Eakins's painting of Hayes Agnew operating in white gown, with nurse participating (1889), at University of Pennsylvania, where painting may be seen.

ments were reported at St. George's Hospital two years later. The viewers' benches were white marble, the staircases teakwood, and the floors a marble mosaic. There were large amphitheatres for spectators. In neither the Middlesex nor St. George's was there a separation of audience and operating scene.[18]

Thomas Rhoads (1897) described Keen's Clinic at the Jefferson Hospital in Philadelphia, then one of the largest surgical clinics in America. The operating arena was separate from the wards; the benches, arranged in tiers in the amphitheatre, provided students a good view of operations. Glazed tile 1.5 meters high separated the nearest benches from the operating arena. The coming and going of the large body of students kept a whirl of dust in the atmosphere, "the only danger." The tile floor was scrubbed with hot water before and after each operation and mopped with a 1:1,000 solution of bichloride. Surgeons removed their coats in a private room, rolled their shirt sleeves above the elbows, and put on freshly laundered coats with short sleeves. They scrubbed their hands in view of the students in the amphitheatre.[19]

David W. Cheever in 1899 called the new surgical amphitheatre of the Boston City Hospital "perhaps the best municipal hospital in the world," where marble, glass, and iron had taken the place of wood. The hospital had grown from 230 beds in 1864 to 512 in 1899 and the mortality from amputation had been halved. Cheever said that a patient was now safer in a hospital than at home.[20]

Impending Demise of Surgical Amphitheatres

Even while ornate marble amphitheatres were being constructed, near the turn of the century many great surgeons, including Billroth (1886) and Rudolf Krönlein (1903), both pupils of Langenbeck, foresaw the passing of the surgical amphitheatre. John Duncan of Edinburgh reported that by 1898, surgical amphitheatres had disappeared to become small appanages of surgical wards.[21]

As the risk element lessened, student interest in operations declined correspondingly. The very foundations of the actor-role of the surgeon were badly shaken as advances in microbiology dictated abandonment of his gladiatorlike personification.

During his long professorial tenure at the Ziegelstrasse Klinik in Berlin (1847–82), Langenbeck performed all his duties as surgical teacher in one amphitheatre, interrogating and examining his patients and, on completion of the diagnosis, operating upon those in need of surgery. This procedure continued in many German and Swiss clinics into the twentieth century. Septic and clean cases were operated upon in the same theatre, which served also as lecture hall. During his European visit in 1909, Alexander Primrose of Toronto noted two exceptions: Kocher's clinic in Bern, and the Rudolf Virchow Hospital in Berlin where Moritz Borchardt was chief surgeon; both had special operating rooms set aside for clean cases. Kocher's operations were performed before a student body of two hundred, of whom 70 percent were women. Max Saegesser, erstwhile professor of surgery at Bern, wrote (1974) that throughout Kocher's forty-seven years at Bern, all his professorial functions were performed in the same surgical amphitheatre. When Professor Rudolf Nissen of Basel was a medical student at Breslau, directly after World War I, all instruction by Küttner and his associates took place in the surgical amphitheatre before the operating schedule, as was the situation too at Marburg, Munich, and Kiel. There was no separation of tutorial and operative functions, which occurred consecutively in the same amphitheatre. Nor was surgical bedside instruction available to students.[22]

At the Tenth International Medical Congress in 1890, J. Balandin of St. Petersburg described what was apparently the first use of a glass partition separating students and visitors from the operating arena, "especially applicable when laparotomies were performed." The editor of the *British Medical Journal* (1893) reported a new operating amphitheatre in Madrid designed, built, and funded by the Marquis del Busto and called the Quirofano, which suggests surgical transparency. A long, glass partition intervened between the students and the operating arena. Ordinarily, the surgeon was not heard by those sitting behind the partition; on special occasions his voice was projected through a tube in one end of the glass partition. In 1894 the new Hôtel Necker in Paris had separate amphitheatres for operations and for lectures; onlookers were screened from the site of operative activity by a glass partition. Student viewers were not permitted in the operating arena, a new departure for Paris hospitals. The Royal Free Operating Theatre in London in 1908 had a small viewing gallery installed above the level of the operating room floor.[23]

When the senior author visited Victor Pauchet at Hôpital St. Michel in Paris in 1928, the spectators sat in a gallery immediately above the operating area, screened off by a large glass dome. Between operations, Pauchet came to the gallery and chatted freely with his audience about the operations.

Billroth published his *Lehren und Lernen* in 1876, a book long years in preparation, reprinted, and translated into many languages. He declined to consider a second edition but in 1886 wrote a small text on aphorisms of teaching and learning in the medical sciences in which he complained that in recent semesters his surgical amphitheatre, accommodating 450, was almost empty, with only 50 to 60 persons in regular attendance. When the morning's didactic lecture was over, few if any students stayed to witness operations. The same, said Billroth, was true in the clinics of his surgical colleagues, with only 12 to 15 percent of the anticipated number of students attending. How had this

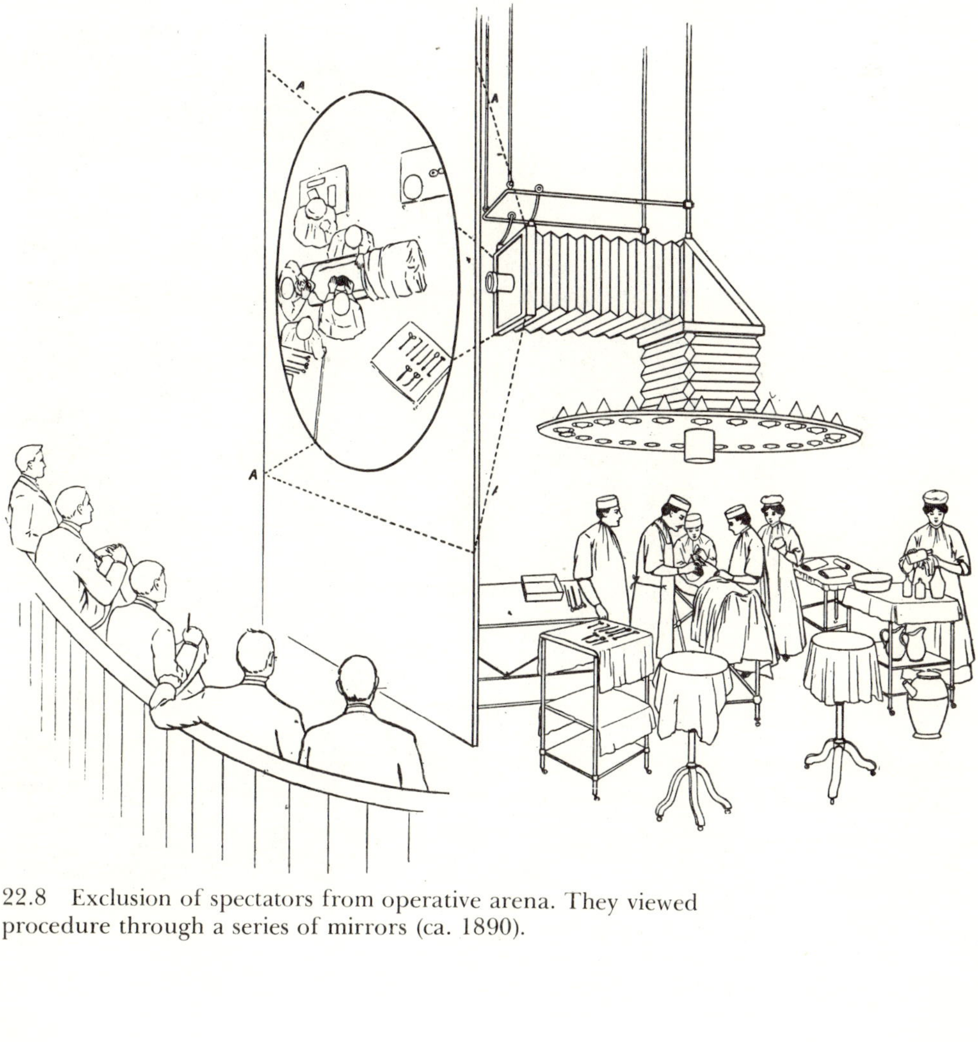

22.8 Exclusion of spectators from operative arena. They viewed procedure through a series of mirrors (ca. 1890).

decline come about? Billroth cited a number of likely causes, including competition from other Austrian and German medical schools, a growing and competent faculty in other disciplines within the school that also attracted students;[24] a more likely explanation, however, was that decreasing risks had removed the sense of excitement and drama from operations in amphitheatres.

Reluctance to Abandon Operating in Amphitheatres

Despite his 1886 admission heralding the demise of the amphitheatre as a place for instruction of medical students, in 1889 Billroth built a new impressive surgical operative amphitheatre

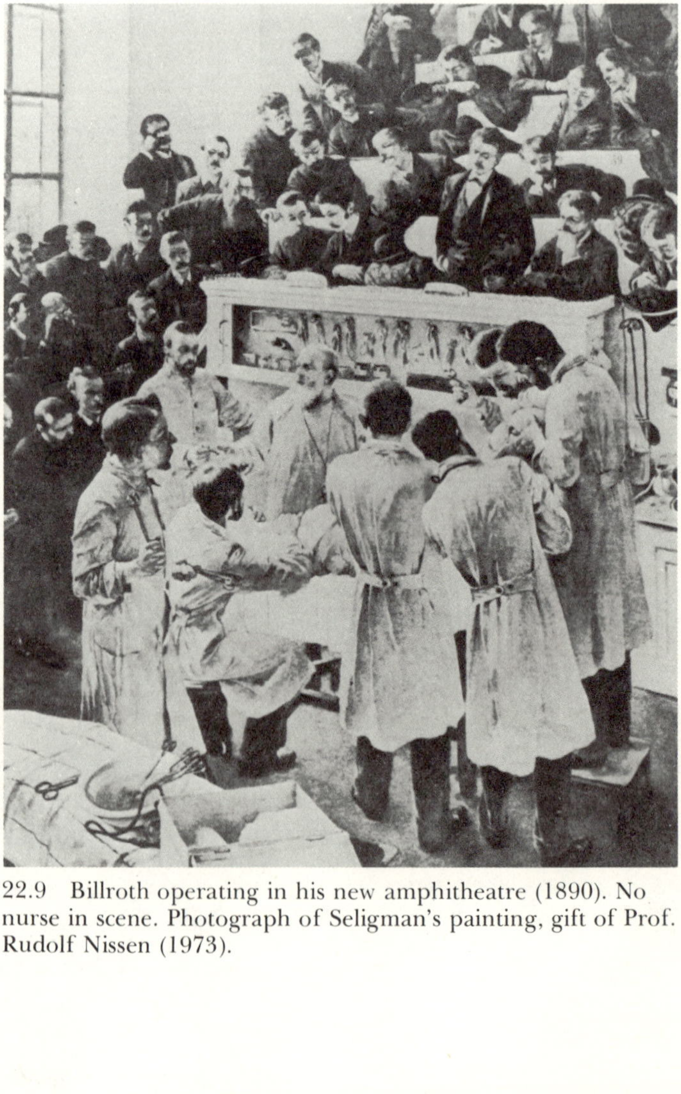

22.9 Billroth operating in his new amphitheatre (1890). No nurse in scene. Photograph of Seligman's painting, gift of Prof. Rudolf Nissen (1973).

with a large seating capacity for students and visitors, portrayed in the beautiful painting by Seligman (1890).

G. T. Beatson (1899) of Glasgow reported in *Lancet* that the most striking activity of the day was rebuilding operating amphitheatres. He believed any system of surgical instruction which deprived students of the opportunity to witness operations was defective. Godlee related that by 1917 not a single old-fashioned combination lecture and operating theatre was to be found in London.[25]

Abandonment of the amphitheatre came more slowly in America and in Germany. J. B. Murphy delighted and instructed a group of spectators in the Mercy Hospital in Chicago at the Clinical Congress of Surgeons in 1913. A photograph of this operative scene shows Murphy, without a face mask, talking directly into his gloved hands before an audience of almost five hundred surgeons.[26] Such large clinics were still in vogue at the 1929 sessions of the same congress in Chicago but were discontinued shortly thereafter because of reported increases in

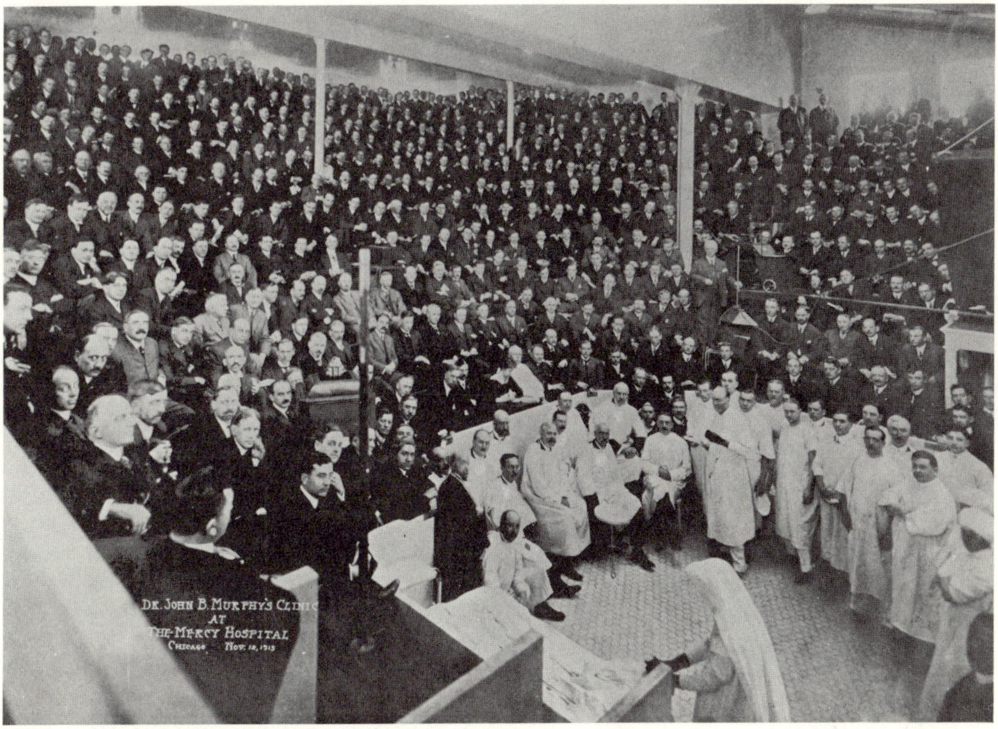

22.10 J. B. Murphy's large operative clinic (1913). Courtesy National Library of Medicine.

wound infection attending operations under these conditions. Screening spectators from the arena by transparent partitions had not yet been adopted in America.

A number of contemporary American surgeons — Jonathan Rhoads, McKittrick, Ochsner, and Loyal Davis — indicated that the surgical amphitheatre in their student days served the dual purpose of instruction and operation. The senior author spent several months at Bern in 1927–28 under Professor Fritz de Quervain, who succeeded to the professoriate in 1917 on Kocher's death. Somewhat more than 10 percent of the students were women, largely Russian. The surgical amphitheatre had been abandoned; the morning surgical lecture took place in a special amphitheatre; and operations were performed in a smaller room on three tables with no viewing stand for spectators. Students rarely attended. B. M. Black wrote that the tendency has been to get away from spectator-viewing galleries in the Mayo Clinic's new operating rooms. William Beck feels that more hard data are needed to validate many current operating room practices.[27]

Alternatives for Operating Amphitheatres

While still a general surgeon at The Hopkins, Cushing emphasized participation by students in the experimental surgical laboratory as the best means of teaching operative technique,[28] a thesis emulated unfortunately by only a few surgical teaching centers. Throughout the senior author's chairmanship of the University of Minnesota's Department of Surgery (January 1930–July 1967), the experimental surgical laboratory served an extremely useful function for our surgical fellows (residents) in acquiring experience and skill in surgical techniques.

Silence during Operation

According to Davis, Cushing insisted upon total silence of all operating personnel to minimize droplet infection of wounds,[29] an injunction noted also by the senior author in several German university clinics in a Wanderjahr abroad (1927–28) and on a visit to Cushing's clinic in September 1928. For this precept the work of Flügge and Mikulicz provided abundant scientific evidence, as will be discussed in the next chapter.

Loss of Stature of the Surgical Curriculum

A portion of the attrition suffered by departments of surgery in curricular assignments among medical faculties throughout our

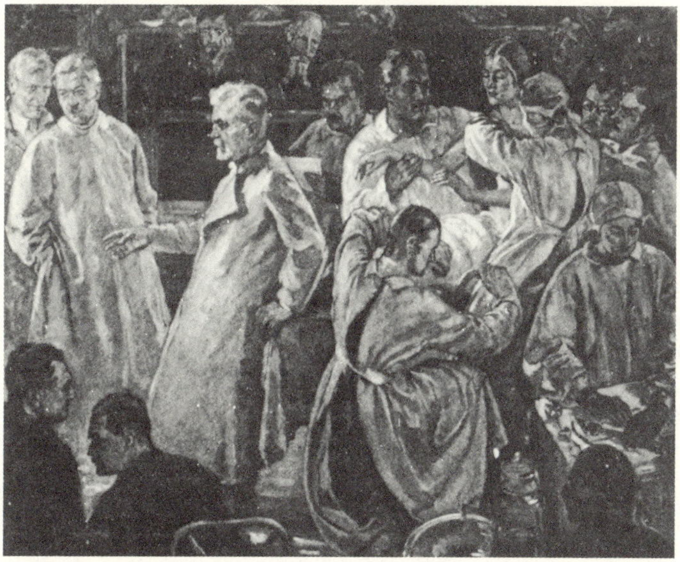

22.11 Operating amphitheatre, Eiselsberg's clinic (ca. 1925).

country in the past decade is owing no doubt to overemphasis upon operative surgery, to which today's medical students also attach a poor rating, whether they are mere onlookers or participants as third or fourth assistants. With no spectators save an occasional viewer through an overhead glass dome, perhaps the professor's fascination and absorption with operative procedures will decline too. Obviously, more effective modes of imparting instruction are at his disposal.

The professor who aspires to be the Paderewski of the scalpel in his clinic, and who with continued practice dazzles associates and onlookers with his operative skill, is unlikely to become the foremost undergraduate teacher of the department. Obviously, his duties are multiple, but he must not regard undergraduate instruction as a distraction and the least important of his many responsibilities. Surgeons need to devise programs that may not be as exciting to students as those of the surgical amphitheatre days but that will prove attractive, informative, and stimulating. Such an atmosphere provides also a healthy climate for graduate training.

Every man is a prisoner of his daily round of duties and responsibilities. No medical academician is more driven than the busy university surgeon. He must determine his priorities, cognizant of his obligations and accountability to students, trainees, patients, and university, as well as his debt to society, school, and profession for the proud privilege and rare opportunity to make a durable contribution to the patrimony of his discipline; and incidentally he has obligations to family, associates, and friends. To survive in this tangled web of life, some of these inevitably are neglected.

Transient Rebirth of the Operating Amphitheatre

When open intracardiac surgery was born (1952–55), the spyglass era of surgery had a transient rejuvenation. Operating arenas provided with an overhead dome screened from the operative action afforded onlookers a good view of the operative field. In an operating suite of more than fifteen separate rooms at the University of Minnesota's Medical Center, four large rooms provided with overhead domes were constructed in 1954 under the direction and supervision of Varco. In the early days of open-heart surgery, the viewing section of the dome room set aside for cardiovascular surgery was always completely occupied when operations were in progress. Medical students, nurses, orderlies, and other hospital personnel often brought their lunch. Visiting ladies who professed a sensitivity to the sight of blood sat in the viewing dome for long hours, often well past the dinner hour, engrossed in the drama of the operating scene. Local businessmen among the onlookers had telephone calls relayed to a nearby office. Surgical celebrities from far-off lands came to view bold, innovative procedures and could readily be recognized among this medley of viewers, truly reminiscent of the heyday of the most exciting period of the surgical amphitheatre in the preantiseptic period of the mid-nineteenth century. Today, save for special occasions, the same viewing domes are empty. Exciting new developments in surgery may rekindle similar flurries of evanescent interest in the operating amphitheatre. Perhaps never again will it command the student, visitor, and surgeon interest it elicited in the latter half of the nineteenth century, an exciting episode in surgery's history.

Summary

The anatomical amphitheatre served the purpose of demonstrating publicly the growth of anatomical knowledge. The surgical amphitheatre was an outgrowth of that activity, used primarily to teach the anatomy of surgical operations. It was a natural sequence that surgeons attached to teaching hospitals adopted the amphitheatre to demonstrate their operations. When prophylactic surgical antisepsis found general acceptance in the mid-1880s, the risk and mortality of operations decreased remarkably; and as the excitement of surgical procedures declined, so did student interest in witnessing operations in progress. Even so, the professors continued to employ amphitheatres for their lectures followed by operative procedures. In London Godlee (1917) observed that the large surgical amphitheatres for demonstration of operative procedures had disappeared. The trend was slower in Germany and America, where professors of surgery used amphitheatres for lectures and for demonstration of operations into the fourth decade of this century; the practice finally died, owing to the general conviction that it enhanced the hazards of wound infection. With the birth of intracardiac surgery in the mid-1950s there was a temporary rebirth of interest in witnessing operative procedures, but in amphitheatres in which the operative areas were screened from spectators by an overhead glass dome. Today the same domes are empty.

(For notes, see pp. 699–701.)

CHAPTER 23

Preparations for Operation

Surgeons' Hands

THE LAST CRITICAL FACTORS looked at by surgeons in considering the nature and causes of infection and failure in operations were their hands. Successively the air was incriminated, then the hospitals within which surgeons worked, and overcrowding. In his unique book of 1579, Paré indicated that "an infinite number of particulars" were important for the success of operations; however, he failed to define these. Nor did Monro I (1737, 1752), who reported the unusual record of accomplishment with amputation at the Edinburgh Royal Infirmary; he stressed hemostasis but did not elaborate on hand preparation. However, Pouteau (d. 1775) emphasized the importance of clean hands for wound dressers, calling the neglect of this observance "deadly for humanity and detrimental to the hospital's interests." He exhorted hospital administrators to enforce the measure.[1]

Surgeons were often advised to wash their hands carefully after dealing with septic cases. Why they failed to appreciate the importance of bringing scrupulously clean hands to open wounds is indeed difficult to understand. The thesis that invisible living organisms, seminaria, were responsible for infection had been projected by Fracastoro (1546), a consideration observed in maintaining a high order of cleanliness by a few surgeons over the centuries, Syme and Mott being outstanding examples.[2] Yet most surgeons continued to look to sources beyond themselves as the primary cause of their failure to deal successfully and consistently with wounds. Strangely, surgeons chose to shun all suggestions of accountability for hospital mortality attending operations into the final two decades of the nineteenth century.

The Nail Brush

The first to lend significant emphasis to strict hand care was Semmelweis, and with great success. He scrubbed with soap and water followed by a similar scrub in chlorine water. Whereas it has been generally believed that he employed gauze for the purpose, a statement by Routh (1849), who had worked with Semmelweis, definitely suggests that Semmelweis did use a fingernail brush. Routh wrote, "when it is remembered that in many dead-houses, from the absence of a *nail-brush*, frequently of *soap* and *warm* water, the hands cannot be properly washed, it is exceedingly probable that a portion of this cadaveric matter is retained under the nails; and it is very easy to understand how, on examination made subsequently *per vaginam*, this poison should be directly and effectively applied." Another colleague, Arneth (1851), and several French clinicians stated that it was obligatory to use a nail brush and a chloride of lime handwash before examining any woman in Semmelweis's clinic in May 1847. The obstetrician Anton Fløystrup (1880) of Copenhagen advocated and used a nail brush in the preparation of his hands for the delivery of parturients.[3]

Gloves in Surgery

The physician Thomas Watson, lecturing in King's College, London, in 1842, on the hazard of the accoucheur's hand carrying puerperal fever, suggested, "In these days of ready invention, a glove, I think, might be devised . . . impervious to fluids, and yet so thin and pliant as not to interfere materially with the delicate sense of touch required in these manipulations. One such glove, if such shall ever be fabricated and adopted, might well be sacrificed to the safety of the mother in every labour."[4] It is now generally conceded that Watson probably was the first in medical literature to suggest wearing gloves for the patient's rather than the surgeon's protection in the performance of surgical procedures. He did not actually use the word "rubber" and apparently did not follow up on his own proposal or appreciate the importance of sterilizing the glove, but certainly the material for the glove he described suggested rubber.

Even before vulcanization of rubber became practical (1839–44), occasional proposals were made that gloves be used by medical men primarily for their own protection from sepsis and syphilitic chancres during dissection or deliveries. "No one should be accused of effeminacy, even if he were to wear thin gloves during the examination of a body of a person who has died of peritonitis," wrote Shaw in 1825, in recounting numerous instances of death from dissection wounds. James R. Liston (1871) had a glove manufactured to be worn by the accoucheurs in the delivery of parturients to protect themselves from syphilis through contact with an occult genital chancre in the parturient canal.[5]

The Rubber Glove

Perhaps the first sterile rubber gloves used in surgery also were worn for the protection of an operative participant. At Halsted's request (1889) the Goodyear Rubber Company made two pairs of rubber gloves with gauntlets for his operating room scrub nurse, Miss Caroline Hampton, whose hands were allergic to the corrosive sublimate hand rinse. She became Mrs. Halsted June 4, 1890. Halsted's first account thereof is to be found in *The Johns Hopkins Hospital Reports* (1890–91) wherein he stated, "the assistant who passes the instruments wears thin rubber gloves which are disinfected in a corrosive sublimate solution. The only hands which come in contact with the wound are those of the operator." Further on he adds, "The hands of the surgeon are, as a rule, the only hands which touch the wound, and these are disinfected in the manner described."[6] One may assume that Halsted at that juncture did not wear rubber gloves for clean operations.

Precisely when rubber gloves came to be worn regularly by all surgeons at The Hopkins is not known. In an exchange with Keen sometime before 1898, Halsted wrote, "I wear gloves if, for example, I am removing a foreign body from the knee-joint or suturing a freshly broken patella, or exploring the abdomen or doing a simple hernia operation, or any other simple operation which does not require a delicate touch or dexterity, and which, if suppuration supervened, might be followed by unpleasant results."[7] Joseph Bloodgood (1899) said that the regular wearing of rubber gloves by operator and assistants during operations was initiated by him in February 1897 for hernia repair and that he was "the first as operator to wear gloves as a routine practice in practically all clean operations."[8]

Robb, an associate of Howard Kelly in gynecology at The Hopkins, had been an ardent student of microorganisms as a source of operative wound infection. He went subsequently to Western Reserve University, Cleveland. Robb reported in the *Cleveland Medical Gazette* (1900) that he had worn rubber gloves in operative procedures "as a routine only for the past five years" and had used them occasionally during operations two years earlier. Robb wrote that he had also routinely worn gowns with sterile armlet sleeves of rubber. He made no mention of Halsted in this account. Robb published a monograph in 1894 entitled *Aseptic Surgical Technique* which went through several editions. Gloves are depicted in Plate II; they extended almost to the elbow. Sterile armlets apparently were drawn on as a last gesture to bridge the gap between the upper end of the gown and the rubber gloves.

Writing from The Hopkins, Robb said in the first edition of his monograph on aseptic technique (1894) that scrubbing of the hands and forearms in green soap followed by immersion in a warm saturated solution of potassium permanganate was, in turn, followed by a wash in oxalic acid until the permanganate stain had disappeared. Then Robb employed a wash in 1:500 bichloride of mercury, and then a saline rinse. Following this, sterile rubber gloves were donned for the preparation of the operative site and the adjustment of the sterile drapes. Then, surprisingly, Robb stated that the gloves were removed and hands and forearms were once more subjected to the tedious wash in bichloride and a rinse. Said Robb, "Now we can proceed with our work." In a later chapter Robb declared, "It is probable that the chances of infection would be very much diminished if the assistants were required to wear them [sterile rubber gloves] at operations." This statement obviously is in conflict with Robb's report in the *Cleveland Gazette* (1900) in which it was related that sterile gloves had been consistently worn by all members of his operating team for the past five years.

In the 1902 revised second edition, Robb wrote, "A somewhat extended experience has convinced me of the great advantages to be derived from their [sterile rubber gloves] use, and I now consider them as essential accessories to an aseptic technique and as eliminating many dangers." He also remarked, "*Rubber gloves* are not employed so widely as they should be. It is probable that the chances of infection would be very much diminished if the assistants were required to wear them at operations, since they can be rendered absolutely sterile, which is not necessarily true of the skin of the hands." Robb obviously recommended

(1902) but did not require or insist that all participants wear rubber gloves in operations. In the fourth edition of the monograph (1906), Robb repeated the statements of the 1902 edition.[9]

The well-known Hopkins gynecologist Richard W. TeLinde (1976) contends that Robb was the first surgeon to urge the routine wearing of sterile rubber gloves for protection of the patient during operation. The published record by a narrow margin would appear to favor Bloodgood in this contested scrimmage; as remarked above, members of his operating team were required to wear sterile rubber gloves from February 1897 on.[10]

In a photograph of 1893 (Fig. 23.1), only Bloodgood of an operating team of five participants wore gloves during a mastectomy. A. McGehee Harvey (1976) reproduced the photograph from James F. Mitchell's 1945 paper on the introduction of rubber gloves for surgery, in which Bloodgood (1893) was depicted operating. Harvey mistakenly identified the operating surgeon as Halsted. Mitchell was a contemporary of Bloodgood and one of the participants in the 1893 operation, all of whom were identified in the caption. The failure to identify the operating surgeon correctly was repeated in a joint monograph by James Bordley and Harvey (1976). The matter is of some historical importance in establishing the originator of consistent use of rubber gloves for protection of the patient from infection in

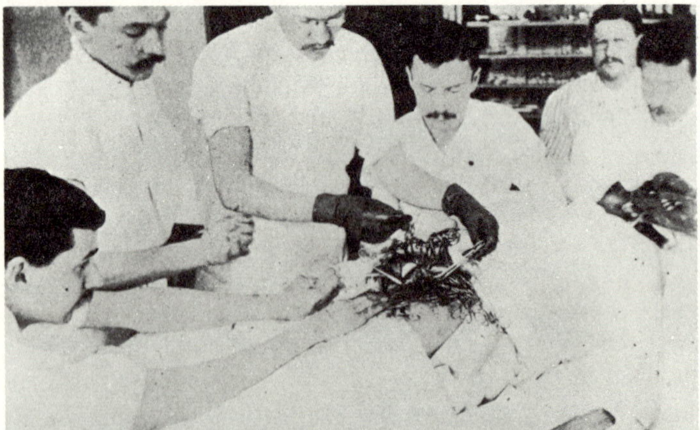

FIG. 1.—A photograph of the first surgical operation in which the operator wore rubber gloves. (Reproduced from a photograph made in 1893 by Dr. James F. Mitchell)
1. James F. Mitchell 2. Chauncey Pelton Smith 3. Joseph C. Bloodgood 4. Harold C. Parsons 5. John (Orderly) 6. Sidney Cone

23.1 An operation at The Hopkins (1893). Only Bloodgood wears rubber gloves. From James F. Mitchell, "The introduction of rubber gloves for use in surgical operations," *Ann. Surg.* (1945), 122(2):902–4.

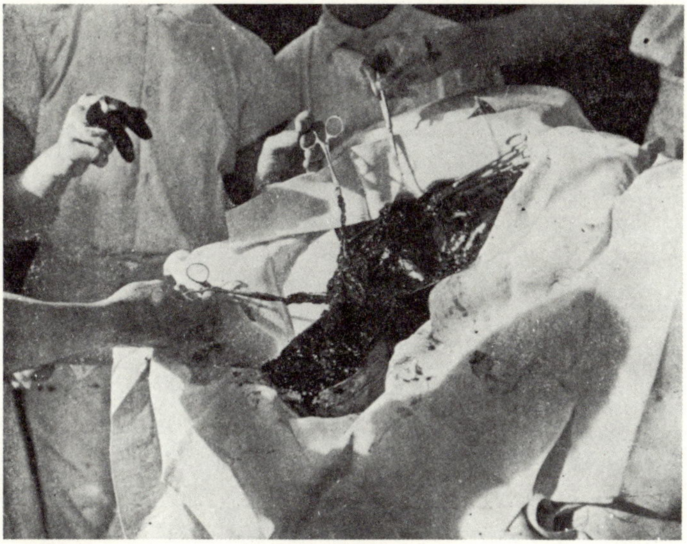

23.2 Mastectomy (1894). Halsted wears a finger cot covering only 3 fingers. Courtesy National Library of Medicine.

operation.[11] The accompanying illustrations in part tell the story. In neither picture does any assistant wear rubber gloves; in one illustration (Fig. 23.2) the operator (Halsted) in a breast removal (1894), not yet convinced that all operating personnel should be gloved, wore a finger cot covering thumb and index and middle fingers of the right hand.[12]

George Blumer (1955), subsequently professor of medicine at Yale and dean of the faculty, was one of Halsted's assistants from May 1, 1893 to May 1, 1894. He related that Halsted had not invoked the use of rubber gloves by the operating team during that period, and that a ritual of hand scrubbing in tincture of green soap, followed by an immersion of hands and forearms up to the elbow in a saturated solution of potassium permanganate and a long (ten-minute) immersion in a 1:1,000 solution of corrosive sublimate was standard procedure. Blumer remarked that the incidence of wound infection attending this preparation was minimal. As Halsted wrote in 1913, "operating in gloves was an evolution rather than an inspiration or happy thought."[13] In any event, it is clear that introduction of sterile rubber gloves for surgery was a Hopkins innovation.

A patent for a rubber glove "for use in surgical or other operations where it is essential to . . . retain delicacy of touch" was taken out in April 1878 by Thomas Forster in England. Even before then various experiments had been made with rubber as

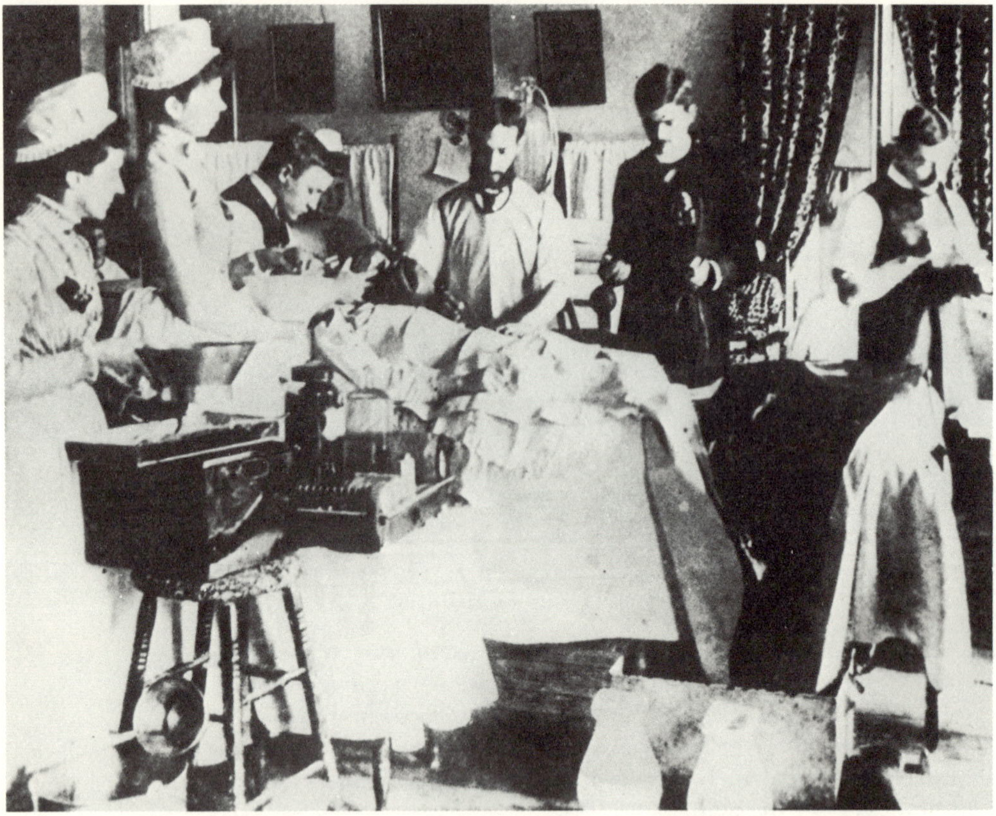

23.3 Operating scene at Bellevue (late 1870s), before rubber gloves were used. Probably the earliest picture showing nurses participating actively in an operation. Courtesy National Library of Medicine.

a protective base for surgeons' hands. In 1834 Richard F. Cooke of Hoboken, New Jersey, sent a letter to Mott, his former teacher, suggesting that "a pair of India rubber gloves would be impenetrable to the most malignant virus." He enclosed a sample of a solution of caoutchouc "dissolved in Guthrie's spiritus of Terpentine," which, he wrote, would produce a thin, rubberlike covering for the hands, suitable for work in the dissection room as well as for vaginal examinations. The rubber film was readily removed by rubbing one's hands together or applying hair powder.[14] William Acton (1848) advised using a similar rubberlike covering to protect the hands in postmortem examinations.[15]

Blatin of Paris demonstrated a rubber glove before the Medical Society of Emulation in 1846. He had devised it to protect the physician when examining patients with contagious fevers or during autopsies. Thomas Cattell, an English surgeon (1847), suggested that gloves made of India rubber would protect surgeons' hands; between use, the gloves should be kept on handblocks.[16]

Acceptance of Rubber Gloves

J. Lynn Thomas of Cardiff was one of the first advocates of sterile rubber gloves for surgeons in Britain. He started wearing them in septic cases in 1898 but preferred a buttonless thread variety for clean operations, because they were cheap and readily sterilized. He saw no need for the surgeon to wear cap or mask — "the experienced mountaineer breathes through his nose when climbing, and the surgeon should learn to copy him when operating." From conversations with London surgeons in June 1898, Thomas gathered that practically no one in the metropolis had taken kindly to gloves, and on that account he ventured to record his short experience confirming their value in safeguarding both patient and surgeon. He observed that suture abscesses had disappeared from the operative wounds since his adoption of rubber gloves and that the gloves did not impair his sense of touch. Thomas preferred scrubbing in running water. Another great advantage of wearing gloves, said Thomas, is that "one does not carry the 'smell of operations' about into drawing-rooms and dinner parties." Moreover, "one can let one's finger-nails grow to a respectable length." In like vein, the French surgeon Tuffier in 1900 brought a lengthy discussion on the use of rubber gloves to a happy ending by reminding his hearers that in their student dissection days, even after vigorous handwashing, the cadaver odor was transferred to their lunch![17]

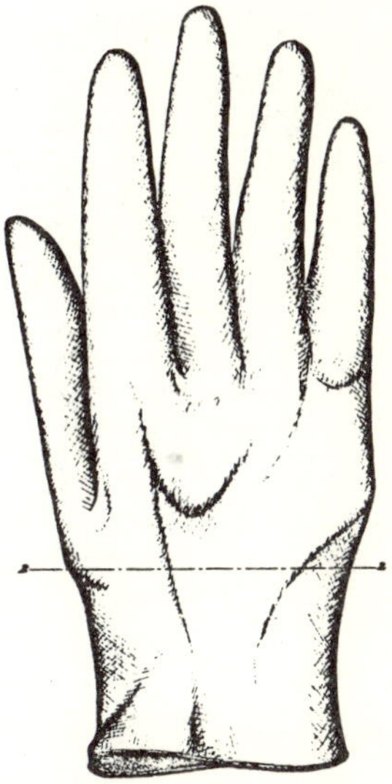

23.4 Thomas Forster's rubber glove as depicted in patent specifications of October 1, 1878. Gift of Charles Talbot.

"A surgeon in order to be *de rigueur* should wear gloves," declared Thomas a few years later (1905). He had by then apparently accepted both mask and cap. The latter, he said, was essential for surgeons with long hair or who are shortsighted or "go in for motoring. . . . When two surgeons, after a motor ride, brush their hairy heads against each other over an operation, one can see with the naked eye a fall of suspicious dust." In the famous 1904 picture of The Hopkins star team of Halsted, J. M. T. Finney, Cushing, Bloodgood, and others, full-length sleeves and rubber gloves were worn, but no face masks (Fig. 23.6). In 1905 Thomas portrayed a surgeon in modern-day operating garb, with sterile gown, rubber gloves, cap, and mask. A surgeon and a nurse similarly outfitted are depicted in Russell Fowler's 1906 monograph.[18]

Cotton and silk gloves had been worn by European surgeons

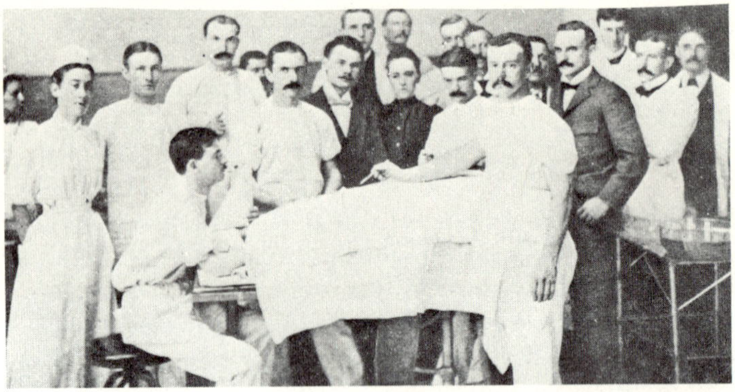

23.5 Kelly operating at The Hopkins (ca. 1897).

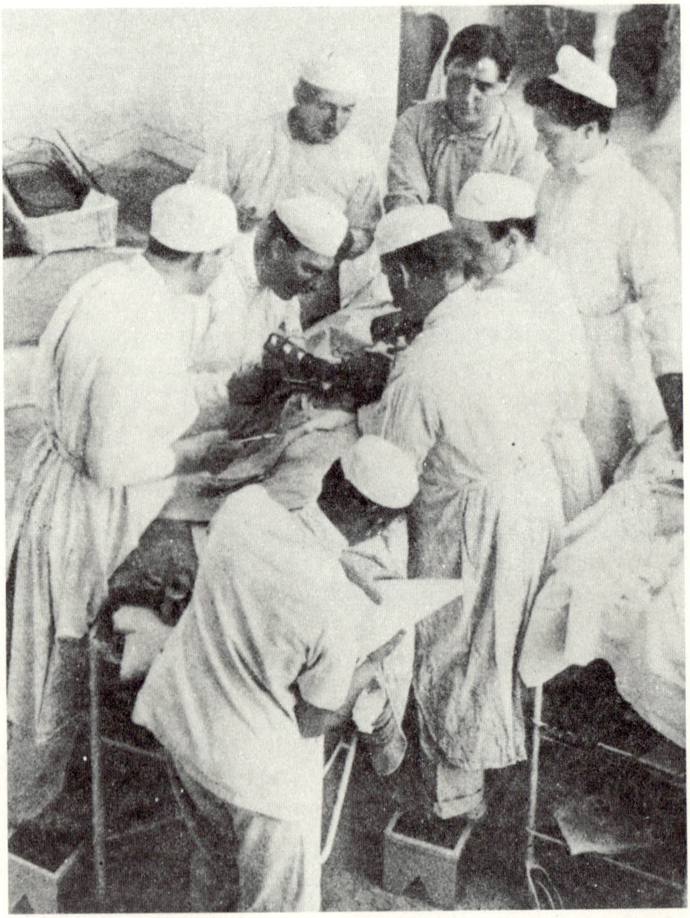

23.6 Halsted's star team operating at The Hopkins (1904).

before the adoption of rubber gloves but obviously, when wet, they readily permitted bacteria on the surface of a surgeon's hands to enter incised wounds. Mikulicz (1897) described cotton gloves ("servant's gloves") which could be washed after use and reworn ten to twelve times; during prolonged procedures, as in the abdominal cavity, he usually changed them three times.[19] A dictum among German-speaking surgeons in the early twentieth century was to use rubber gloves for septic cases and adequate chemical sterilization of the hands immediately before operation in clean cases. Extensive experimentation on the problem was conducted in a number of German clinics, both surgical and gynecological; it was generally agreed it was not possible to achieve absolute sterilization of hands, a result that several decades of experience have since verified. This finding persuaded most surgeons that rubber gloves are an absolute necessity to afford the patient maximal protection.

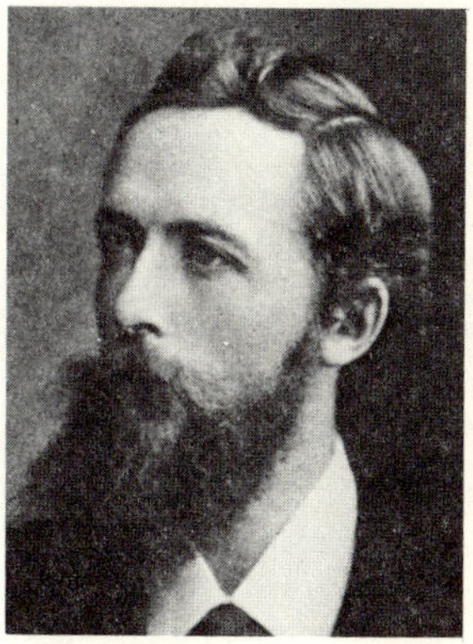

23.7 Johann Mikulicz-Radecki (1850–1905).

Resistance to Rubber Gloves

Herbert Fox and E. A. Schumann (1905) of Philadelphia performed bacteriological experiments demonstrating that the rubber glove was impervious to bacteria and that neither *Bacillus coli* nor *Staph. albus* escaped through the intact glove, even when distended. Yet we know from Primrose's 1909 visit to surgical clinics abroad that the most accomplished European surgeons had not adopted consistent use of rubber gloves in operation. In fact, it would appear that in discarding the old ways, they did not capitulate completely to the new. César Roux and his surgical team at Lausanne, Primrose observed, wore no gloves when operating. At Bern, Kocher and his team all wore rubber gloves, with white linen gloves over the rubber during operations in which the knee joint was opened; when gastrojejunostomy was performed, Kocher alone wore gloves. In Borchardt's clinic in Berlin, all operative participants wore dry, sterile rubber gloves. Bier at the Ziegelstrasse Clinic occasionally wore gloves; his assistants almost invariably did, but not the nurses who passed the instruments. When the senior author visited operative clinics in Europe and Britain in 1927–28, rubber gloves had almost uniformly been adopted everywhere; Professor Sauerbruch at the Charité was an exception, wearing gloves as the spirit moved him; his assistants and the nurses regularly wore rubber gloves. "I know only three surgeons the world over who are in the first rank who do not constantly wear gloves during operations," said Moynihan in 1920.[20]

Many surgeons at first resisted rubber gloves, insisting that they reduced the delicacy of touch. To test this assumption, Carl Black of Jacksonville, Illinois (1916) asked three blind girls to read Braille with and without rubber gloves. A definite decrease of sensitivity to touch apparently attended the wearing of gloves, more marked when they were drawn on dry than wet.[21]

Some surgeons obliged their assistants to wear gloves, while they themselves remained barehanded. One such surgeon was Joseph Price of Pittsburgh, who spent more time preparing his hands than in the operation itself, a ritual perpetuated by his protégé J. W. Kennedy (1921). Robert Morris of New York in 1898 called on the younger generation of surgeons to fight against the use of rubber gloves which would impair their precious sense of touch. By 1920 Morris, although admitting that "the idea of the rubber glove is one of the *finest advances* in surgery," still did not wear rubber gloves in abdominal surgery.[22]

A Manchester surgeon E. S. Bishop (1908) deplored gloves and face masks and insisted that such apparel made the surgeon resemble a high priest of surgery, mindful of the effect of vestments upon his followers. "Let us not convert our theaters into the semblance of Mohammedan harems or Spanish torture chambers, nor terrify our patients out of what little courage they still possess." He said that gloves make the hands sweat, so that if a glove is perforated, the danger to the patient is compounded. "Quiet breathing is not specially harmful [to an open wound]; it is coughing, sneezing, loud talking that is dangerous." If the operator "feels that he is in danger of sneezing, can he not stoop below the table or for a moment leave it?" The author concluded by saying that the only thing in favor of wearing masks is that carrying these factors to perfection will ultimately produce "academic sterility."[23]

To obviate the wearing of rubber gloves, Murphy of Chicago scrubbed his hands with 5 percent tincture of green soap in running hot water, washed three minutes in alcohol, then poured on a rubber solution (gutta-percha), allowing it to dry. He prepared the patient's abdomen for operation in the same manner after first washing it with ether. He admitted that his practice did not provide as much protection for the patient as did intact gloves, but maintained that it was equal or superior to gloves, considering the chances of puncture.[24]

Proponents of Rubber Gloves

McBurney (1898) wrote very enthusiastically of the results from the consistent use of rubber gloves by all participants in surgical procedures over several years at the Roosevelt Hospital.[25] McBurney was the first in New York to adopt their systematic use, said George Brewer, who declared (1898) that introduction of rubber gloves was the most significant item contributing to avoidance of wound infection. Brewer, at the City Hospital and later at the Roosevelt, made a serious study of surgical wound infection for two decades. Before his adoption of rubber gloves in late 1897 he experimented with using no assistants in his operations; the incidence of postoperative wound infection was 30 percent with assistants and 20 percent without. Brewer was very keen about formalin for hand and skin sterilization, using a 1 percent solution. He stimulated concern among his staff by appointing a censor to watch for breaks in surgical technique (1896), rewarding the senior surgical resident with a cash prize of $100 after a six-month residency if he could report no clean wounds had become infected during that period (1915).[26]

The cost per pair of rubber gloves was $1.75 in 1899 and they could be worn for twelve operations according to Horace Packard. He boiled them in distilled water in a sterilizer for two minutes to ensure freedom from ordinary pyogenic bacteria, for five minutes after a "virulently septic case." For scrubbing, Packard placed a tablespoon of lime chloride in the palm of his hand and added a teaspoonful of washing soda and a small quantity of water. The hands were rubbed together until a smooth paste of lather resulted, reminiscent of Semmelweis's hand preparation. Packard rubbed this paste well into the beds of his fingernails and finally rinsed in a bowl of sterile ammonia solution, one tablespoonful per quart of water.

Since using rubber gloves Packard had noted a decreased incidence of stitch abscesses. Moreover, his hands remained in far better condition and had no appreciable blunting of the sense of touch. In 259 elective operations, there were only 8 patients with wound infection, an incidence of 3 percent, a figure that compares favorably with the report of five American university clinics in 1964.[27]

G. W. Theobald (1924) at the Rotunda in Dublin did not consider it important to scrub his hands before operations, insisting that socially clean hands were adequate. He merely immersed his gloved hands in a solution of 1:1,000 biniodide of mercury for a minute. He wore the same gloves all morning, opening doors as he went along to the "labour ward." Before he started another operative procedure, he "re-sterilized" his gloves in the same manner. He reported that he had worn the same gloves for five and one-half hours, first during an hour lecture, thereafter in an abdominal gynecologic procedure, as well as in an intervening obstetrical delivery, immersing them between procedures in the antiseptic solution for a minute.[28] Coauthor J. W. Bigger, a bacteriologist, reported favorably upon the relative freedom of pathogenic bacterial survivors on the gloves used in Theobald's simple antiseptic treatment, a technique which fortunately has not found wide emulation. Theobald cited a letter exchange between Lister and Colonel S. T. B. Williams in which Lister wrote, "he never did more than immerse his hands for one minute in a 1–20 solution of carbolic, and much deprecated a preliminary washing." Primrose (1909) observed that Trendelenburg in Leipzig similarly donned sterile rubber gloves without preliminary preparation of his hands, indeed a startling practice for so eminent a surgeon.[29]

Hand Disinfection

Edgar McGuire (1903) of the Roswell Park Hospital in Buffalo queried whether antiseptics are of any value in hand disinfection. He concluded that mechanical cleansing and scrubbing of the hands before application of antiseptics is most important but that "absolute sterility of the hands is impossible by any method." Rubber gloves add optimal protection, precluding seeding the wound with hand bacteria of the operating team. McGuire said that Bardeleben (1882) introduced corrosive sublimate for hand sterilization, a technique subsequently followed by Halsted and his protégés. Gerhard Leopold, a Dresden obstetrician, demonstrated (1887) the importance of mechanically cleansing the hands prior to use of antiseptics.[30]

Many surgeons employed mercuric chloride for hand sterilization and for wound irrigation, following announcement of its antibacterial activity by Koch (1881). However, as Behring pointed out in 1890, some of the antiseptic quality of mercuric chloride described by Koch was owing to tiny amounts of the chloride transferred unwittingly into the blood serum culture media; mercuric chloride, they inferred, was more bacteriostatic than bacteriocidal in its action. Koch also found oil of turpentine, the favorite wound dressing of Paré and Woodall, to possess bacteriocidal properties. Flügge of Breslau found mercuric chloride in very dilute solution an effective antiseptic in inhibiting growth of bacteria in meat infusions. Schleich is reported to have remarked that in the presence of epithelial cells, fat, sweat, soap, and dirt, chemical disinfection of the hands is nothing but a farcical show and "about as much good as making the sign of the cross over an open wound."[31]

Carl Walter (1969), long a student of the problem of wound infection, found no bacterial growth on 36 percent of gloves following operation. In 3 percent of the instances, more than one hundred organisms per milliliter were present, all from hands with dermatitis.[32]

The history of the arsenal of gallantry clearly reveals a more direct approach to the problem of preventing infection; in the sixteenth century Gabriel Fallopius and others had invoked various devices including the use of lamb's cecum as a contraceptive and as a practical means of preventing the transmission of venereal disease among wayward Casanovas. In fact, Fallopius reported that a medicated piece of linen placed over the glans penis, directly after intercourse and left in place for four or five hours, precluded the development of venereal disease. Said Fallopius, "I call upon the eternal God to be my witness, not one of the 1100 men examined using this method became infected."[33] Fallopius and his patients obviously used up a good deal of luck!

Operating Garb and Ritual of the Surgeon

The dress of the surgeon while operating in the early Listerian period (1870) is familiar to all who practice medicine. The long, black morning coat was worn by all surgical personnel. Between operations, these frock coats usually hung in rows in the theatre, their sleeves encrusted with dried blood and pus. Keen, in comparing military surgery of 1861 with that of 1918, wrote: "we operated in old blood-stained and often pus-stained coats . . . with undisinfected hands . . . we used undisinfected instruments . . . and marine sponges which had been used in prior pus cases and only washed in tap water."[34]

In reviewing his medical student days (1890–95) at the University of Pennsylvania, David Edsall recalled one of his professors "operating day after day in the same unwashable cloth operating jacket," while the other "already an ardent advocate of antisepsis, would regularly scrub his hands thoroughly and after that would reach into his trousers' pocket for his pocket-knife, scrape beneath his finger nails, replace the knife, and proceed to operate."[35]

The substitution of green for white in operating room material was apparently the inspiration of Moynihan. In a letter dated September 9, 1915, he wrote to the *Lancet* that for two and a half years he had used green towels and sheets because they were less "wearisome to the eye" than white and minimized light reflection which should be concentrated on the wound. His theatre had green walls and floor. Moynihan does not mention green operating gowns, but they would be a natural sequence.[36]

Unusual Operative Practices

Before antiseptic practices were accepted, the well-known Paris surgeon Le Dran (1731) related that in performing perineal lithotomy he transferred the knife from his assistant's hand to his own mouth to hurry the procedure. An anonymous admirer of Robert Liston (1899) related a similar expedient used by that great surgeon during amputation. Halsted suggested that some of the poor results of antiseptic practices in New York hospitals in 1884 were occasioned by the practice of the surgeon's taking ligatures from the mouth of an intern.[37]

In writing of the differences in surgical practices of 1861 and 1918. Keen noted that, in the pre-Listerian day, surgeons had no hesitation when threading small needles to moisten the suture with bacteria-laden saliva. He had seen Gross, Philadelphia's celebrated nineteenth-century surgeon, strop his knife on his boot and occasionally on its sole as he prepared to make an incision.[38]

Face Masks

Flügge (1897), Mikulicz's microbiological colleague, was the first to test experimentally the hypothesis that speaking during operations enhanced the likelihood of wound infection by projected droplet infection from the surgeon's mouth and nose. Mikulicz's pupil Wilhelm Hübener placed cultures of *Bacillus prodigiosus* in the mouths of experimental subjects and demonstrated that the wearing of face masks diminished considerably droplet projection of the bacilli upon exposed plates when the subjects spoke during the test. The protection was best when the subject wore a double cotton-muslin mask; in forceful expiration (sneezing), it afforded no protection. Hübener found that masks provided little protection against wound infection when the surgeon was bearded.[39] Long hair and beards obviously are not for surgeons, and probably not mustaches. Hübener observed that contact between beard and mask increased its penetrability.

Flügge's pupil P. Laschtschenko also employed *B. prodigiosus* and observed that when no masks were worn during loud speech, numerous colonies were invariably deposited upon exposed plates 15 to 30 inches away; during coughing, plates were contaminated at distances of 70 inches, and during sneezing, at distances of more than 20 feet. Mendes de Leon (1904) of the University of Amsterdam also underscored the need for surgeons to wear masks and estimated that for each word spoken without a mask, a minute droplet containing, on the average, 4,375 microorganisms could be projected into an open wound. Josef Riese (1936) of Vienna contended that silence during operation offers maximal protection against wound infection and that during his last 1,000 elective operations done in silence, wound infection was not observed.[40]

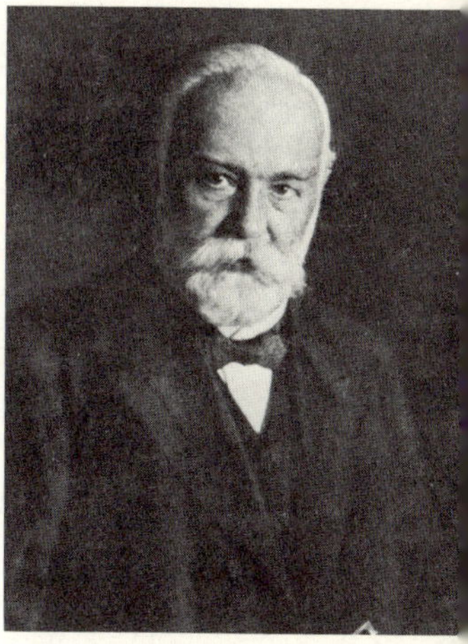

23.8 Carl Flügge (1847–1923) conducted first study of droplet infection.

During the influenza epidemic of World War I, the effectiveness of face masks in protecting against droplet infection was intensively studied. B. C. Doust and A. B. Lyon (1918), using the *B. prodigiosus* technique, concluded that coarse and medium gauze provided no protection but that finely woven "buttercloth" in three layers (probably cheesecloth in a fine weave) was effective at distances of one to six feet. David Haller's and Raymond Colwell's (1918) findings were very similar. Lloyd Arnold (1938) recommended that surgeons use four-ply cellucotton embedded in the masks as an effective filter precluding contamination of exposed plates. He also used *B. prodigiosus* in his tests. M. W. Jennison and H. E. Edgerton (1940), using a high-speed camera with a 1/5,000 of a second exposure, obtained convincing photographic evidence of massive droplet projection during sneezing. J. W. Hirshfeld and P. J. Laube (1941) observed that masks offered no additional protection against droplet infection when the experimental subject remained silent.[41]

Trial in a few university clinics of enforced silence during operations would soon determine the worth of a prescript of silence. Gloves without leaks, silence during operations, and appropriate impenetrable gowns as well as face masks and headdress are probably the most important facets of the surgical ritual, other than sterile equipment, in thwarting wound infection. Professors of surgery did not accept immediately the microbiologists' evidence that large numbers of spectators increased the hazard of wound infection in elective operations. Surgeons have been even more dilatory in accepting the abundant microbiologic proof that the failure of the operating team to maintain silence increases significantly the hazard of wound infection.

The chief source of wound infection during operations is undoubtedly the operating team. Would complete silence of all personnel in the operating arena compete favorably with laminar airflow studies in maintenance of a relatively sterile atmosphere over the operative field? It is an inquiry worth pursuing. Auditory and other aids can no doubt be developed to lessen the burden of enforced silence upon the operating team.[42] Baseball's coach-and-pitcher-catcher system of signals could help resolve dilemmas occasioned by the enjoined silence. The danger from droplets in the surgeon's breath when examining open wounds was recognized in the sixteenth-century by Würtz and honored by Fergusson, who observed total silence during operations, finding it necessary to explain to bystanders after an operation that he and assistants actually were on good speaking terms. Many German university surgical clinics in the late 1920s had *Silentium!* placards posted on the walls of operating rooms. Five decades ago not a word was spoken by Cushing and his team during four- to five-hour operations; the infection rate for Cushing's entire career, says Walter, was only 0.3 percent. Is this not a precept that current-day surgeons would do well to observe?[43]

Preoperative Isolation Units for Major Elective Surgery?

Surgeons need to be constantly alert to the warnings of Pringle (1753) and Simpson (1869) concerning nosocomial infections. If patients admitted for major elective surgery were placed in a hospital room in which strict isolation techniques and a high order of asepsis were scrupulously maintained, minimizing their exposure to potential source of infection, the effort should be rewarding for both surgeon and patient. Assessment of such a thesis would necessitate many preoperative studies being done on an outpatient basis with the elapse of an appropriate interval of time until the patient's newly acquired bacterial flora attending the preoperative studies became less menacing. Moreover, if pertinent exploratory studies indicate that such an approach has merit, hospitals will need to develop preoperative isolation areas for prospective patients undergoing major elective surgery. The suggestion of the Russian surgeon Jastreboff (1885) for hospital construction to implement such a device has been mentioned.[44] If broad-spectrum antibiotics or chemotherapeutic agents, specific for the wide range of bacteria to which patients are exposed during hospital stay, were available, the elaborate scheme we have sketched would already be obsolescent. But while we await more direct agents with suggestions of specificity, clinical trial by a few interested hospital teams could provide the needed appraisal of the likely merit, if any, of preoperative isolation units for major elective surgery.

Sterilization of Instruments and Operative Materiel

By orders of Louis XVI, the tables upon which meat was cut in the kitchens of French military hospitals had to be washed with boiling water twice a day.[45] Regretfully, the operating tools of the surgeons were not included in the directive. The prevailing opinion then and a century later was that the miasmas of the air were the chief source of wound infection. The usual preoperative practice was to remove knives and other instruments from the shelf and place them on a chair or tray convenient to the surgeon. Marine or gauze sponges, without special preparation, were similarly arranged for the operating team, as were towels and drapes. In his early papers, Lister wrote of using "rags" for sponges. All the operative materiel was immersed in varying dilutions of phenol.

In a discussion in 1874 Pasteur made his famous comment, "If I had the honor of being a surgeon, I would never introduce into a human body an instrument that had not been passed through boiling water and better yet through a flame just before operation and rapidly cooled," a statement upon which Pasteur elaborated considerably a few years later, adding washing and flaming of hands and heat sterilization of all operative materiel.[46] The legend of the very successful nineteenth-century veterinarian has often been repeated, who, on his deathbed, admitted to his heirs that the secret of his good fortune with operations was "boilin' my tools."

The early steam sterilizers were built by microbiologists. Koch and his pupils (1881) developed an apparatus for thermal sterilization of culture media; Chamberland built a similar one shortly thereafter, and by 1883 the autoclave, devised to provide moist heat under pressure, was available in many bacteriologic laboratories. Appert (1810) of France had originated sterilization of foods in containers, forerunner of the autoclave. Redard (1886) was among the first surgeons to sterilize linens, drapes, gauze, and surgical sponges by steam heat, rather than with chemicals. Hugo Davidsohn (1888) provided the rationale for the superiority of heat over chemical sterilization as an effective bacteriocidal agent. Gradually heat superseded chemical methods in the preparation of operative materials.[47]

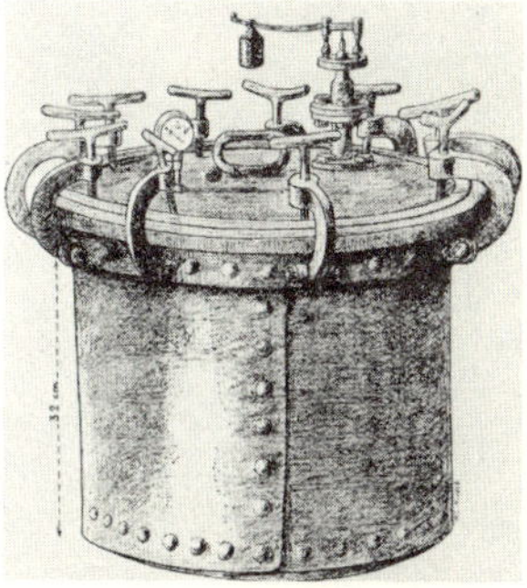

23.9 Charles Chamberland's autoclave (1880).

Writing from memory of his fourth year as a medical student in 1878–79 at St. Thomas's Hospital, Arthur Newsholme (1935) stated that John Simon immersed his instruments in boiling water before operating. Newsholme also related that a notice board in the hospital carried the instruction that students coming from anatomical or postmortem dissections "must wash their hands in chlorinated soda solution" before attending midwifery cases. Leeson had similar memories and remarked that the students took no notice of the handwashing instruction.[48] Semmelweis, although ignored, had not been completely forgotten.

Current Practices

The sterilization in large drums of drapes, gowns, and other materiel for operation has been improved greatly by using prevacuum high temperature steam sterilization at 134° C (274° F) under control of a chamber thermometer and constant monitoring with a chamber vacuum drawing-capacity of up to 70 cms. of mercury. Moreover, the time required to sterilize the "test" packet at the center of the load has been reduced. Pressure steam sterilization, although a longer process, continues to be popular for operating rooms; it is economical and safe. At the University of Minnesota Hospitals instruments too are autoclaved, placed in stainless steel wire mesh trays and encased in two heavy muslin or disposable wrappers; trays of instruments thus processed can be kept sterile on the shelf for more than a week. Disposable knife blades prepackaged and sterile have long been available directly from the manufacturer. Special instruments including motors are sterilized by a mixture of ethylene oxide (12 percent) and freon (88 percent) to reduce the explosive quality of the former.[49]

These current-day refinements represent an evolutionary process ensuring sterility of all materiel used in operative procedures, a vast improvement over the blood-crusted frocks of a century ago and the laundered gowns of a later period. A century and a half ago Henry (1832) demonstrated that the contagion of scarlet fever was not communicated by clothing subjected to dry heat at a temperature of 204° F for one hour, an important experiment of which surgeons should have taken notice.[50]

Inlying tubes long positioned in the airway, veins, arteries, or urethra invite infection. Sterilization of anesthetic equipment constitutes a challenging microbiologic problem, not only of the anesthetic mask and the intratracheal tubes but also of the expansile anesthetic bag. A completely sterile anesthetic set for each case is obviously the desired objective; compromises involving practical considerations apparently cannot always be completely put aside. Cross infection from incompletely sterilized

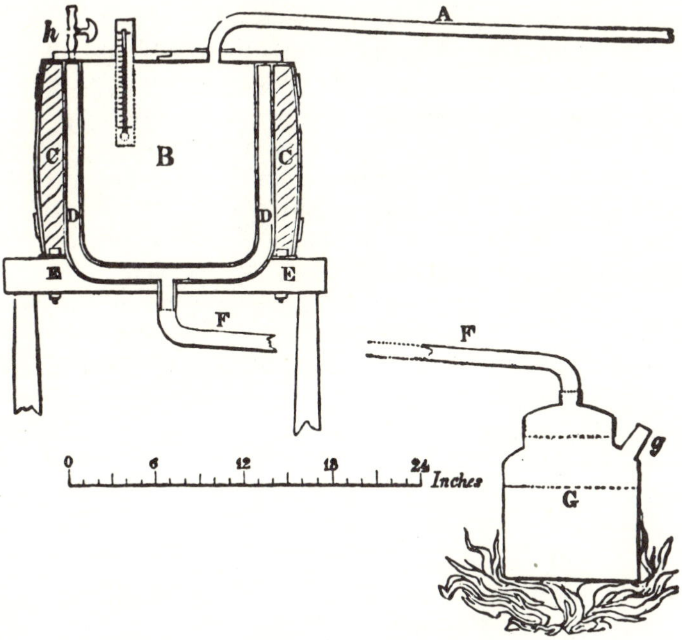

23.10 William Henry's method of sterilizing materials (1832).

anesthetic apparatus constitutes a distinct operative hazard. Operating personnel with psoriasis, chronic eczema, or other dermatitis or any continuing source of infection, such as a rectal fistula, whether anesthetist, nurse, surgeon, or operating room technician, occasionally have to be dismissed from responsibility for health care because they are carriers of infection.[51]

A veritable rash of papers on the air of operating room as a source of wound infection has appeared in the past decade. It was one of the chief topics of discussion at the 1971 Moscow meeting of the International Surgical Society.[52] Lister eventually dismissed the topic as an inconsequential source of wound infection; today the question is again very much alive. Most surgeons are quite willing to concede that it is of secondary importance, that the operating team is the more frequent source. Moreover, airborne infection is not readily dealt with effectively. The most direct attack upon the problem has been made by the English orthopedic surgeon Charnley, who in a succession of papers developed and described a unidirectional (laminar) airflow scheme over the operative field, complemented by provision for suction beneath the face mask to thwart collections of nasal secretions. The present authors raised the question of whether complete silence in the operating theatre might not prove

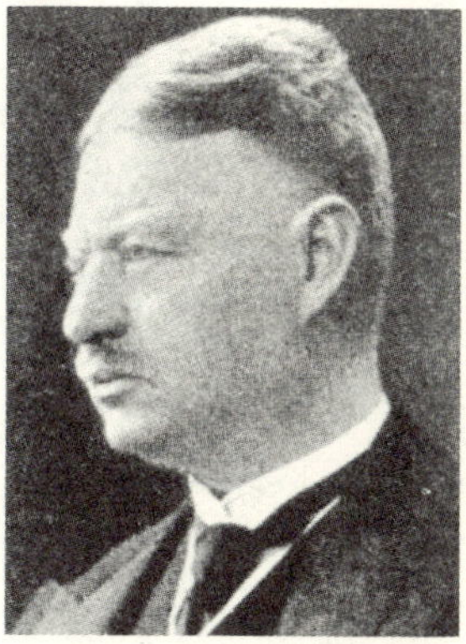

23.11 Gustav A. Neuber (1850–1923).

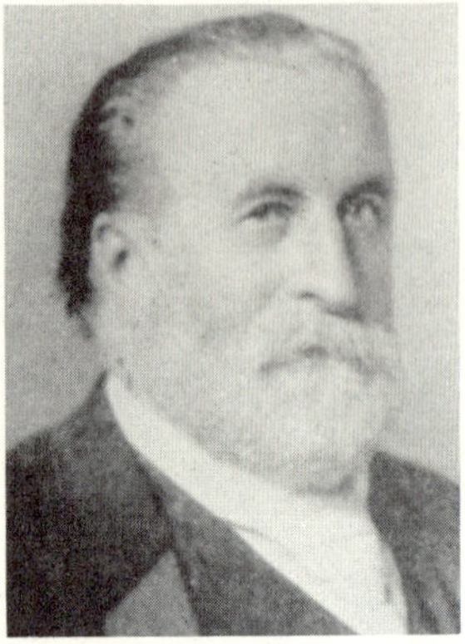

23.12 Ernst Bergmann (1836–1907).

equally effective in minimizing wound infection from the operating team. Charnley and his associate N. Eftekhar[53] also stressed the use of impenetrable plastic operating gowns, an innovation with merit. Joseph A. Moylan and associates (1975) verified the permeability of autoclaved dry gowns, observing that after one hour of operating time the external surface of the gown exhibited bacterial contamination in 23 percent of instances, after four hours, in 76.5 percent, confirming the findings of Charnley and Eftekhar (1969). Moylan and his colleagues did not completely exclude atmospheric air as a source of gown contamination. In fifteen instances they did insert a 4 by 6 inch impenetrable external patch conforming to the abdominal area of the surgeon's gown. These areas exhibited no bacterial contamination, a finding favoring penetrability of the gown as the likely source of contamination.[54]

Summary

Monro I reported unusual success with amputations for the 1737–52 era at Edinburgh's Royal Infirmary, a mortality record not excelled until after the acceptance of prophylactic surgical antisepsis. Monro credited "little circumstances," which he did not define, other than to emphasize complete hemostasis. Without superior cleanliness, the record of an 8 percent mortality could not have been achieved. Pouteau (1783) was a keen advocate of clean hands for wound dressers.

Semmelweis (1847) was apparently the first to emphasize and practice scrubbing the hands with a nail brush in warm soap and water, followed by a similar scrub of the hands with a brush in a hypochlorite solution. Antiseptic treatment of all materiel coming in contact with the vaginal tract of parturients in labor was similarly invoked by Semmelweis. The effect upon the maternal mortality on the obstetrical wards of Vienna's Allgemeines Krankenhaus was impressive, an acknowledgment only reluctantly made by Viennese and German professors of obstetrics following publication of Semmelweis's book in 1861. In 1876–77, the Freiburg gynecologist Hegar was able to demonstrate the worth of the Semmelweis technique for ovariotomy, marking the beginnings of elective abdominal surgery. Before and long after Semmelweis's demonstration (1847), the emphasis of hospital reformers continued to be upon ventilation, espoused by such dignitaries as Nightingale and Paget.

Watson (1842), a physician at London's King's College Hospita, was probably the first to urge obstetricians to wear a glove for the protection of parturients in labor. He did not, however, recognize the need for sterilization of the gloves. Henry (1832) demonstrated that night clothing worn by patients dying of scarlet fever was safe for nonimmune patients after the garments were sterilized with dry heat at temperatures in excess of 200° F. Cotton and silk gloves were in use before rubber gloves were introduced (1889) by Halsted to protect the hands of his operating room nurse, his fiancée Caroline Hampton, whose hands were allergic to the antiseptic corrosive sublimate. Bloodgood of Halsted's surgical staff started the practice of having the entire operating team wear rubber gloves regularly during operative procedures in February 1897. Robb, a Hopkins gynecologist, urged the wearing of sterilized rubber gloves for the patient's protection in operative procedures in 1894, a recommendation not mandated until 1904. It would appear, therefore, that Bloodgood antedated Robb in requiring the entire operating team to wear sterile rubber gloves.

Theobald (1924), obstetrician at Dublin's famous Rotunda, adopted the practice of dipping his unscrubbed gloved hands in a solution of biniodide (1:1,000) for one minute on starting the day's work. His operations were interrupted by lectures, the opening of doors, and other obligations that obviously broke the sterility ritual. Before engaging in another operative procedure, he merely dipped the same gloved hands again in the biniodide solution, a practice no longer in vogue at the Rotunda.

Flügge's (1897) studies on projection of droplets containing bacteria from the mouth during speech, coughing, and sneezing persuaded Mikulicz that face masks covering nose and mouth during operative procedures would minimize droplet projection of bacteria into wounds. Yet the wearing of such masks was not accepted by many European and British surgeons until nearly the beginning of World War II.

Lister introduced the phenol dip for sterilization of instruments and operative materiel some time during the interval between 1867, when phenol was placed into wounds, and 1871, when the operative field was sprayed with phenol. By 1879–80 Pasteur and Chamberland advocated replacing antiseptics with heat for sterilization of instruments and operative materiel, as did Koch in 1881.

Current-day refinements of sterilization of all operative materiel contrasted with the blood-encrusted operating frocks of a century ago delineates the remarkable improvement of the safety factor in operations that came in the final fifteen years of the nineteenth century. There has been a rebirth of interest in trying to achieve a bacteria-free atmosphere over the operative field, a thesis Lister eventually abandoned as unimportant for wound infection. Charnley's unidirectional airflow over the field of operation is being tried out in many areas today. It is probably entirely proper to ask whether mandated silence, required by the American neurosurgeon Cushing of his operating team, may not actually be as effective.

(For notes, see pp. 702–6.)

CHAPTER 24

Surgery of War

GUNPOWDER WAS apparently originally used in China in the manufacture of firecrackers. In his historical study of gunshot wounds, Billroth (1859) said that use of gunpowder was first mentioned in military action in 1338. It is well documented that cannon and small firearms were employed in the Battle of Crécy, August 26, 1346, when Edward III of England and his longbowmen defeated Philip VI of France. When Gersdorff (1517) depicted a surgeon engaged in extracting an arrow from a soldier's anterior chest wall, he portrayed a cannon and three musketeers in the background of the scene. Brunschwig's picture of a "wound man" (1497) features the arrow, sword, dagger, and club as military weapons, but not the cannonball, which was added to later portrayals by Gersdorff (1517) and Tagault (1555) and in several editions of Paré.[1]

Guns

The purpose of military guns and ammunition of all types is to kill or immobilize the enemy. A severely wounded soldier imposes upon the adversary the additional burden of caring for him. In successive wars the initial or muzzle velocity of bullets and fragments has been accelerated tremendously. E, the kinetic energy of a missile, is equal to the Mass of the missile times the square of the velocity, divided by twice the force of gravity (32 feet per second), a formula represented as $E = \frac{M\ V^2}{2g}$ The real

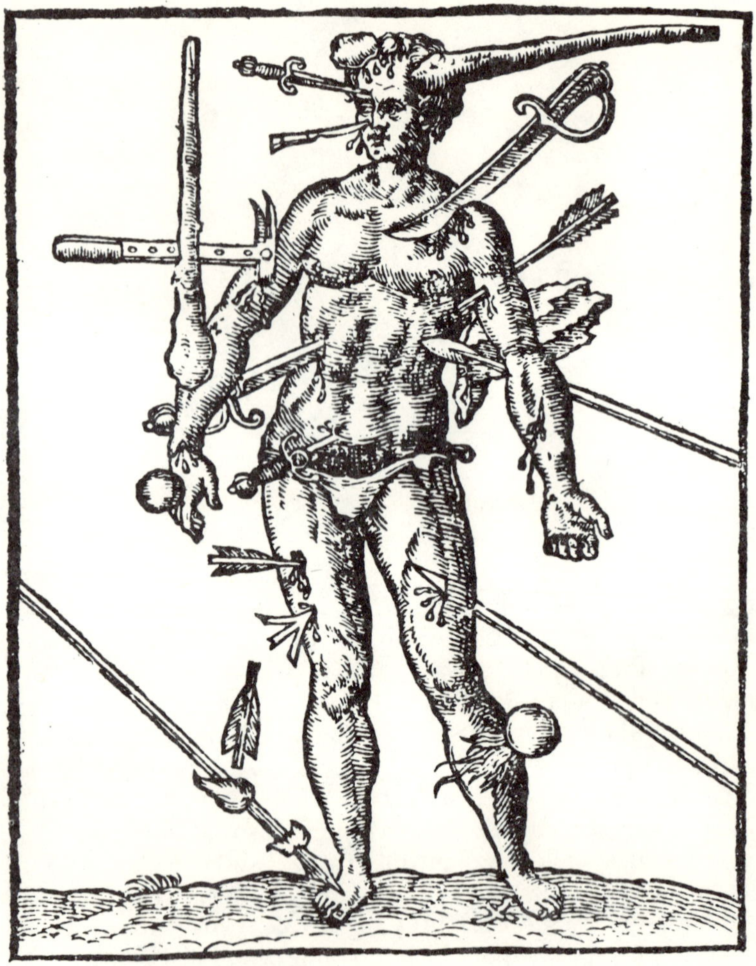

24.1 Paré's "wound man." From Paré, *Workes*.

criterion, however, is the impact force of the missile after its force has been partially spent. The greater the velocity of the missile, the greater the retardation factor in slowing the missile at great distances. It is the explosion of the missile and its fragments on impact that determines its actual kinetic force. The resistance to missiles through air is far less than through denser objects, such as muscle, liver, and bone. In order to study this factor, Kocher of Bern, a consultant to the German armies in World War I, shot through empty tin cans and cans filled with water, sand, or clay, using rifles of medium muzzle velocity in the range of 2,400 feet per second. In the cans whose interior was occupied only by air, the holes of entrance and exit were very much alike; on the contrary, the denser the content of the cans, the larger the site of exit.[2]

The matchlock was first used at the end of the fifteenth century. It was fired by placing a lighted "match" (of rope) near the touchhole that ignited the gunpowder; this weapon was replaced in the seventeenth century by the flintlock, in which the spark was produced by flint striking against steel. The percussion cap, an invention of A. J. Forsyth (1807), superseded the flintlock; it consisted of a small metal capsule filled with fulminate of mercury that exploded the gunpowder on contact.[3] The muskets of this period were muzzle-loaders, used by both Union and Confederate soldiers in the American Civil War (1861–65) until replaced by breechloading guns near the end of the war. Machine guns, firing many bullets rapidly and first used in the Franco-Prussian War (1870–71), were greatly improved through a number of innovations in succeeding conflicts before World War I. The Thompson (tommy-gun) of World War II could fire as many as six hundred bullets per minute. The Browning automatic rifle was first used in World War I, and more extensively in World War II. By incorporating elements of the semiautomatic Garand rifle, self-loading, clip-fed, and gas-operated, the rapidity of its firing action was considerably increased; it in turn was supplanted in 1957 by the M14 rifle with greater firing power.

Shrapnel, dating from the beginnings of the nineteenth century, has become increasingly important in warfare. Land mines, explosive charges placed in the ground and detonated by the weight of a man or vehicle, were frequent weapons in the Vietnam conflict. Grenades and bombs, whether thrown by hand or by guns, are effective assault weapons. Heavy field artillery has supplanted infantry charges. Only when the enemy positions are silenced or immobilized by cannonade or heavy guns do ground troops move in — in the Crimean War (1854–56) a French general said the English charge of the Light Brigade was brilliant, but not military strategy.

The Napoleonic Wars

Napoleon I (1769–1821), a Corsican and an obscure French military officer, came to power after he had dispersed a mob of insurrectionists threatening the authority of the Convention on October 5, 1795, with what he later termed "a whiff of grapeshot." Out of a starving, disorganized army he created within a year an effective fighting force. By speedy, massed sur-

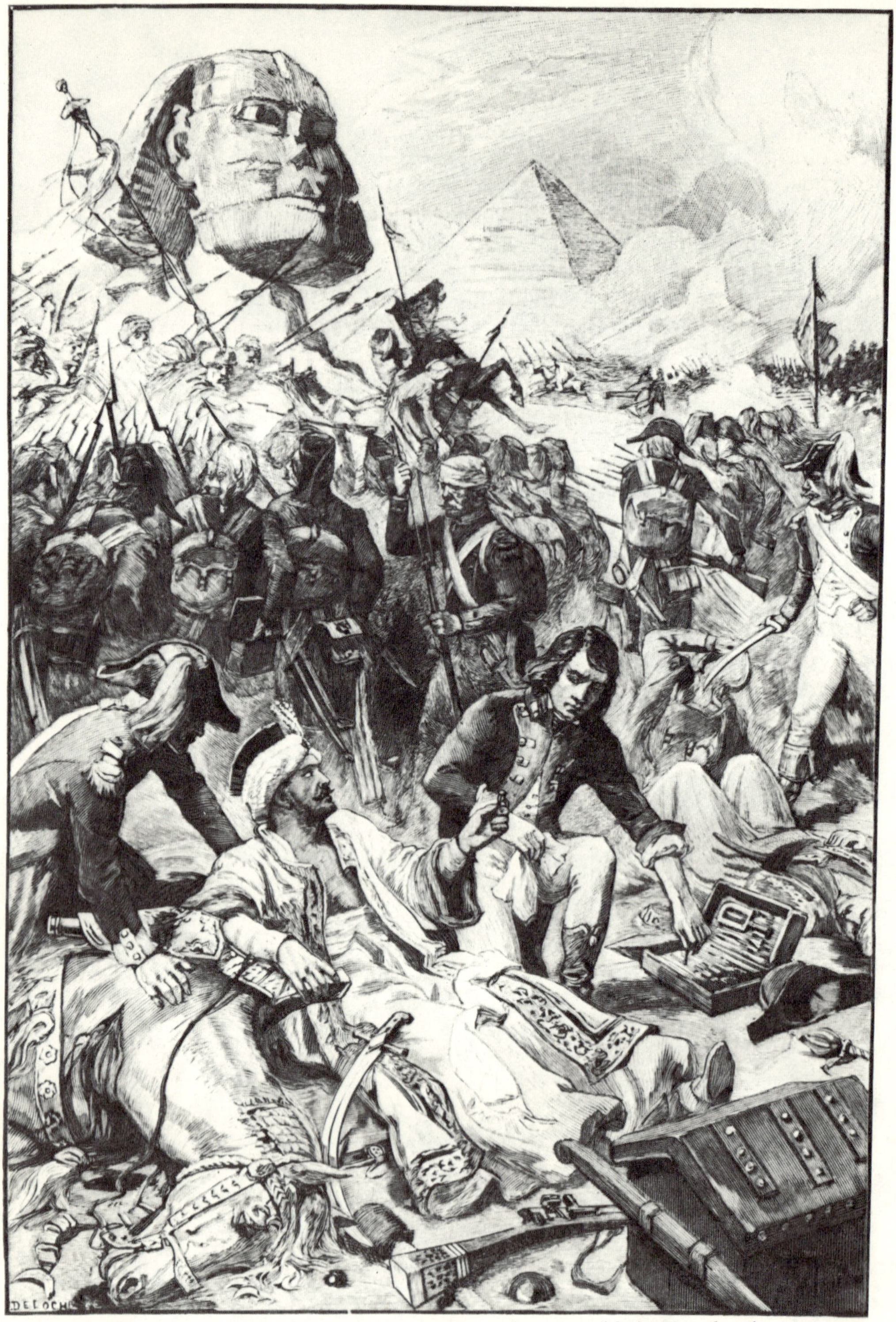

24.2 Larrey operating near the pyramids in Napoleon's Egyptian campaign.

prise attacks he won a succession of startling victories in Italy that drew great admiration throughout Europe for his military strategy.

A portion of Napoleon's success was owing to the important contributions and organizational ability of two competent military surgeons, Percy and Larrey. Percy formed a battalion of ambulance soldiers, with a special company to carry the wounded. He designed wagons to convey surgeons and medical supplies into the field of battle, vehicles later greatly improved by Larrey in speed and efficiency to transport the wounded to rear treatment stations.[4]

When Larrey first employed his "flying ambulances," during the Campaign of the Rhine in 1792, they caused a great sensation among the troops. In the Italian campaign two years later his light ambulance carriages had long open panniers used as stretchers. In Egypt, 1799, panniers were mounted on camels to transport the wounded. Larrey's emphasis on bringing aid to the wounded in the midst of battle won the confidence and affection

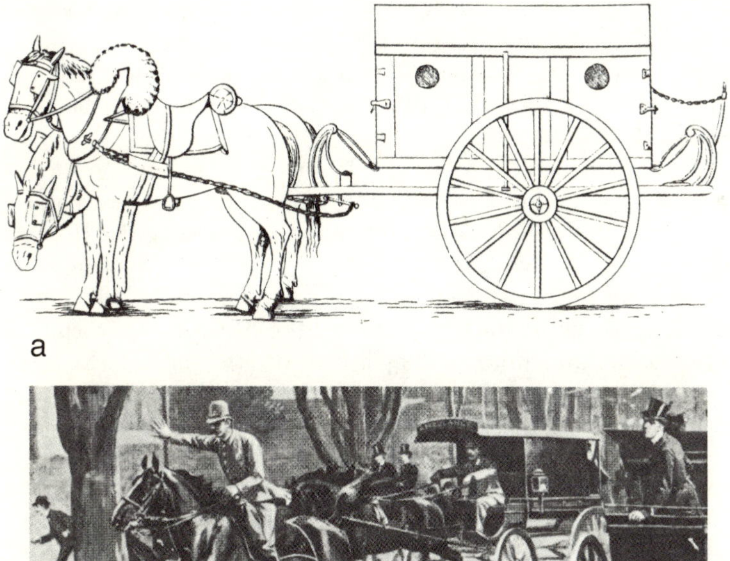

a

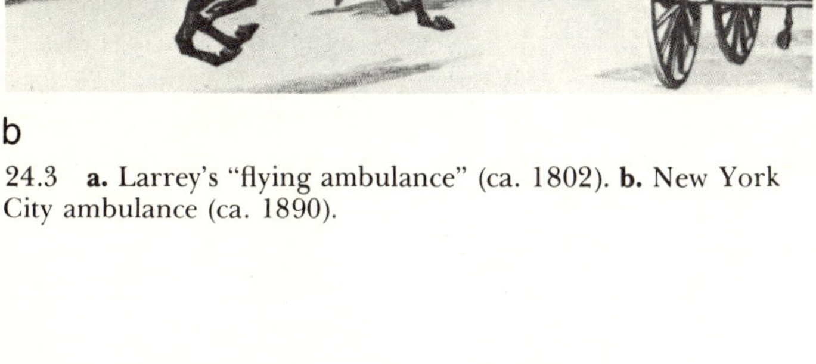

b

24.3 **a.** Larrey's "flying ambulance" (ca. 1802). **b.** New York City ambulance (ca. 1890).

of the soldiers, as did his personal fearless dedication in performing emergency operations and rescue missions under fire. His systematized service of ambulances and movable hospitals, or dressing stations, became an integral part of Napoleon's army organization.[5]

The French people idolized Napoleon after his many early victories and made him "first consul for life." Thereafter, he crowned himself emperor; with victory at Friedland (June 14, 1807),[6] Napoleon was able to negotiate from a position of strength with Emperor Alexander I, arranging a satisfying truce with Russia. After the battle of Wagram (July 6, 1809), Napoleon's ability for rapid and wise decisions appears to have deteriorated. Moreover, his physical well-being had been weakened by a urethral stricture, accompanied by urinary retention and cystitis. There were no more glorious victories for the French emperor.

The invasion of Russia from August to October 1812 was a glaring blunder, with severe battle losses at Smolensk (August 7) and Borodino (September 9). It was here that Larrey performed two hundred amputations in twenty-four hours. Several of Napoleon's military surgeons left accounts of their harrowing experiences in the Russian campaign. Best known are Larrey's *Mémoires*. He wrote: "the horrors of which we were to become victims during this fatal retreat" began on the return to Smolensk, when cold and hunger beset the troops and no shelter could be found in the burned villages; dead horses strewn along the way were the only nourishment. Another surgeon, Joseph Kerckhove, described the high spirits of the healthy young men and veterans as they started the campaign, marching "unhesitatingly toward the formidable enemy," the terrible days of privation, disease, and injuries that followed, and the retreat from Moscow when the sick and wounded were abandoned in the snow without cover, food, or water. By the time Kerckhove reached Germany the inhabitants' fear of typhus prevented almost any care being given to the returning warriors. In the Mainz hospital he found dead and dying lying together in their excrement on the bare earth; some patients had been without food or drink for several days. Finally, "the streets of the town became hospitals."[7]

Napoleon invaded Russia with a military force variously reported to be between 500,000 and 800,000 men, including soldiers of subjugated countries; it has been variously reported that only 20,000 to 40,000 men returned to France. Cold, starva-

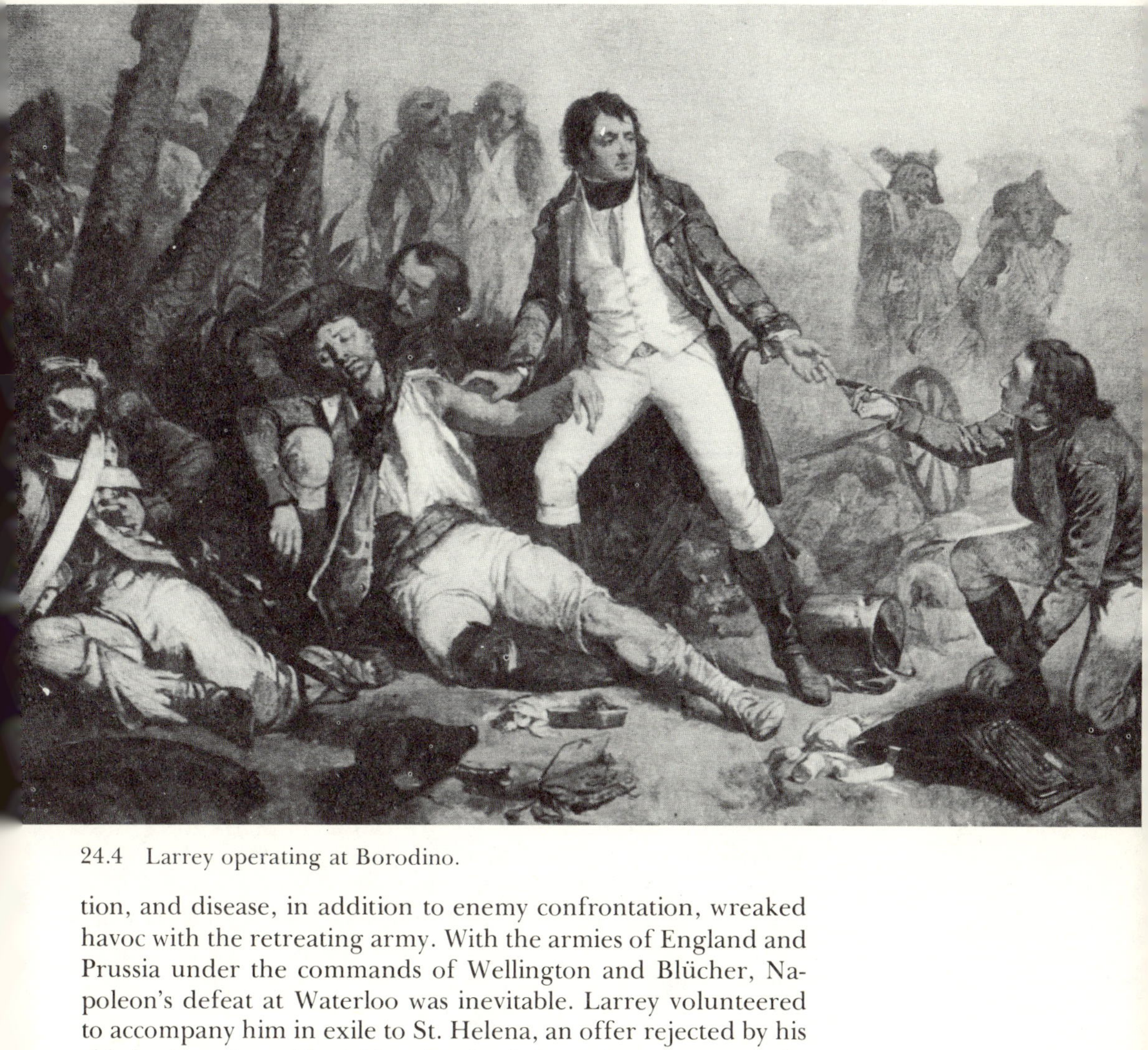

24.4 Larrey operating at Borodino.

tion, and disease, in addition to enemy confrontation, wreaked havoc with the retreating army. With the armies of England and Prussia under the commands of Wellington and Blücher, Napoleon's defeat at Waterloo was inevitable. Larrey volunteered to accompany him in exile to St. Helena, an offer rejected by his chief, who admonished him that he belonged to the army. In his will, Napoleon left Larrey 100,000 francs, a tidy sum but insignificant when compared with the fabulous gifts made to several of Napoleon's military leaders.

In retrospect, despite Napoleon's brilliant military record through 1809, it is clear that the invasion of North Africa was a mistake, as was the Peninsular War in Spain, but his greatest miscalculation was invasion of Russia. Ironically, it was during the period and at the scenes of Napoleon's failures that out-

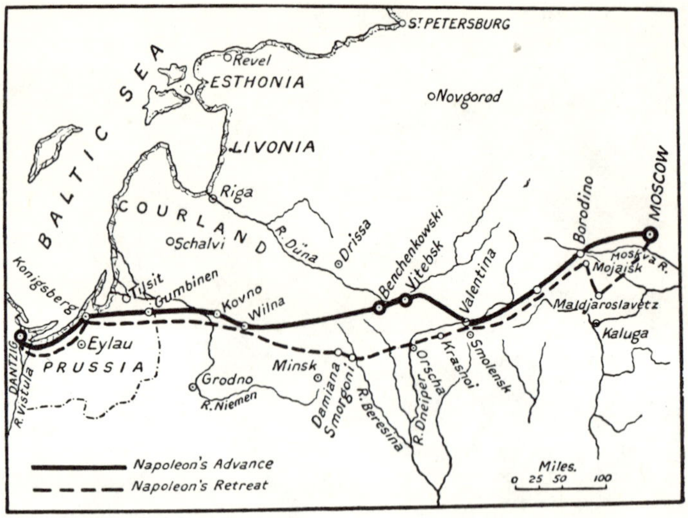

24.5 March of Napoleon's army to and from Moscow.

standing advances were achieved by a number of his military surgeons, isolated and overwhelmed as they often were by the task of salvaging the casualties of his wars.

Ollivier's heroic self-inoculation in a remote Spanish outpost was surely one of the outstanding contributions of military medicine of that era. It won him no distinction at the time but was recalled fifty years later when the nature of infection and prevention of hospital gangrene were coming again under serious consideration. The work of Delpech in treating the wounded of Napoleon's armies from Spain and Russia has been recounted in an earlier chapter. His remarkable account of the transfer of infection in hospital gangrene and the efficacy of cautery in its treatment resulted from careful research in the crowded wards of a Montpellier hospital.[8]

Maurice Treille was the only surgeon left on the field after the battle of Baylen, June 19, 1808, in the Peninsular War. In his care were five hundred severely wounded soldiers lying under the hot sky of Andalusia, without protection of hospital or cover except from olive trees. He had no bandages or medicaments so he irrigated their wounds with water to forestall *pourriture*. Because he could not treat that many patients daily unaided, he divided the men into three groups, alternately irrigating the wounds of one-third of the patients each day while the other two-thirds irrigated their own wounds. Over the three-week interval from June 19 to July 10, 1808, only seven or eight wounds became gangrenous and there were only two cases of tetanus. Treille believed the most effective agent in combatting *pourriture d'hôpital* was the actual cautery. He also suggested two adjunct measures for which he had words of praise, camphor and quinine, but said they were not the equal of cautery. In autopsies of patients succumbing from gangrenous wounds, Treille observed and reported the frequent presence of gastric erosions and superficial mucosal ulcers, probably the first mention of stress ulcers in surgical literature. The condition was augmented if such patients were given alcoholic drinks.[9]

The Crimean War

The English joined the French to support the Turks against Russian aggression in the Crimea. It is the story of hurried and inadequate preparation on all sides. The French had the advantage of light ambulances for transport of the wounded. It was one of the first major wars in which anesthesia was used, but as Larrey had insisted earlier, the shock and concern over acute injuries help dull a victim's sensitivity so that early amputation is almost painless — an argument several surgeons in the Crimean conflict urged against employing anesthesia.

The English surgeons in the Crimea avoided use of antiseptics in wounds. The French tried a number of local antiseptic agents. Salleron (1859) assessed ferric chloride and observed its effectiveness against hospital gangrene, affirmed also by Marie Bourot (1858). Suppuration of wounds in the hospitals was frightful.[10]

The reported mortalities for amputations of fingers and the forearm were only 0.5 to 1.8 percent; of the arm and shoulder joint, 22.9 to 27.2 percent. Amputations above the knee were attended by mortalities of 50 to 86.8 percent — the higher the level, the greater the mortality.[11]

The outstanding personality of the war was Florence Nightingale, whose capacity for organization and emphasis on sanitation readily won the approval of the English public, although many surgeons on the scene were slow to appreciate her innovations. Her solicitude for the ill and the wounded during her evening tours through several miles of barrack beds was readily communicated to every soldier. When amputations were in progress in the crowded wards, she provided an isolation screen about the bed so that those awaiting similar operations were spared the agony of watching. Although it has been intimated that Nightin-

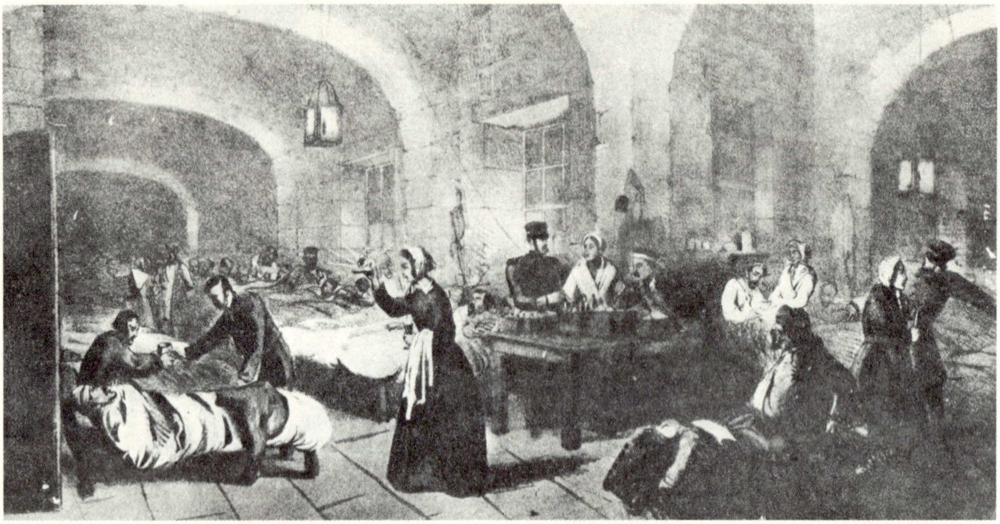

24.6 Florence Nightingale in the Crimea.

gale's nurses were mainly English noblewomen, such was not the case; they were a varied group of young women; for most of them, money was the inducement.[12]

Spencer Wells (1855), speaking at the Smyrna Hospital during the Crimean War, emphasized the great value of women nurses in the care of the wounded; he remarked that previously soldiers had been used for the purpose, and occasionally wives of soldiers in the area. He stated that both these methods had failed, that the trained and educated women coming to the Crimean hospitals had been a tremendous success, and that nurses were as important and helpful in military hospitals as in civilian hospitals. Wells favored isolation of patients with infectious fevers, a measure to which George Rolleston, a well-known physician, also at the Crimea, was opposed.[13] Lice, fleas, rats, cholera, and dysentery were constant companions of all combatants throughout the war, as they continued to be in more recent conflicts.

It is interesting that English surgeons had ready access to the thermometers for recording the temperatures of their patients. This contrasted with the experience of Billings and Keen during the American Civil War several years later; they reported that thermometers and syringes were rarely available.[14]

A few years after the end of the Crimean War, the French fought a bloody battle with the Austrians at Solferino, June 24, 1859. J. H. Dunant, a Swiss banker who was a witness, wrote an account of the battle and described the neglect of the wounded. His publication (1862) inspired the formation of the Red Cross and international agreements about caring for the wounded on the field of battle; in 1864 the Geneva Convention adopted the resolution he had urged. A century earlier Pringle and his patron, the Earl of Stair, had proposed that hospitals of opposing forces be considered sanctuaries for the sick and wounded, providing mutual protection to combatants of both forces; little notice was taken of this suggestion at the time.[15]

American Civil War

Perhaps never in the history of war have such detailed case accounts been kept of wounds and the wounded as in the Union reports published in a series of six volumes between 1870 and 1888, several years after the American Civil War was over. These large tomes, titled the *Medical and Surgical History of the War of the Rebellion*,[16] summarized the experience of the war and were greatly admired by many European authorities — pathologists and microbiologists, as well as military surgeons. In the surgical volumes are to be found pertinent historical citations to wound care dating back to John Hunter, Astley Cooper, Legouest, Macleod, and others.

Antiseptics

Probably the most notable achievement by Union medical officers in the war was the introduction of a number of antiseptic wound practices some years before Lister undertook his investigations. Antiseptics were not consistently employed in wound care by Union surgeons; however, several remarkable series of patients given antiseptic treatment for contaminated wounds and hospital gangrene were reported: Goldsmith's (1863) achievement with bromine has been alluded to — a mortality of only 2.6 percent among 308 patients with hospital gangrene, whereas it was 43.3 percent among 30 similar patients on whom the antiseptic was not used. Hachenberg (1864) advised the Surgeon General, on March 20, 1864, that he had found turpentine effective in the management of hospital gangrene; this was the antiseptic employed for wounds by Paré (1545) and Woodall (1617).[17]

Frequent applications of "strong nitric acid" were employed by North (1863) to treat sixty patients with hospital gangrene, four of whom died (6.6 percent mortality). He used wound debridement, cutting away dead tissue with scissors. North also injected dilute nitric acid into the tissues when the gangrene appeared to spread, obviously a procedure without merit. The *American Medical Times* (1863) published a series of nine short papers on military surgery, representing eleven lectures given by the New York surgeon Detmold. He too advised using nitric acid for hospital gangrene and postulated that "the disease may have its origin in the rapid generation of a destructive microscopic fungus." This statement evoked a reply from Assistant Surgeon General J. J. Woodward, who said that it was not borne out by facts, that high-power microscopic examination of pus from suppurating wounds had "utterly failed to demonstrate any cryptogamic organisms, except the ordinary vibrios, which are to be observed in every decomposing animal substance." The

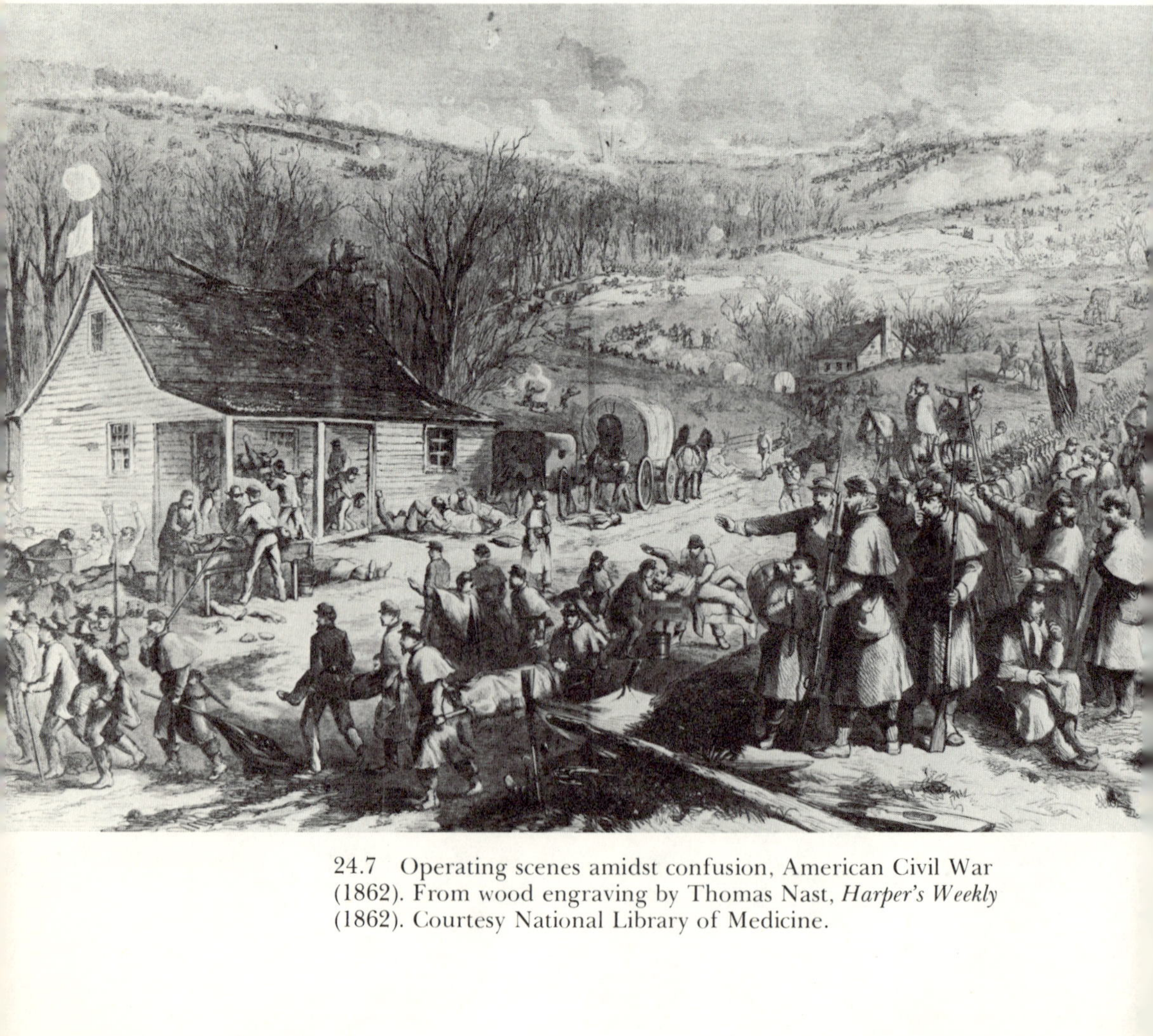

24.7 Operating scenes amidst confusion, American Civil War (1862). From wood engraving by Thomas Nast, *Harper's Weekly* (1862). Courtesy National Library of Medicine.

"ordinary vibrios" obviously were incorrectly regarded as harmless.[18]

Keen dilated on the great stores of alcohol — "400 dozen bottles of whiskey, brandy, sherry, etc.," in a smokehouse — confiscated by the Confederates after the Second Battle of Bull Run, and which the Union surgeons had no intention of using in wounds.[19]

Gunshot Wounds

In general hospital reports on the mortality from gunshot wounds (September through December 1862), Surgeon General W. A. Hammond noted that for flesh wounds of the upper extremity the mortality was only 1.2 percent, and of the lower extremity, 2 percent. The mortality for gunshot fractures of the humerus and upper arm was 30.7 percent; of the forearm, 21.9 percent; of the femur, 31.7 percent; and of the leg, 14.4 percent. These results in most categories were superior to those achieved in the Franco-Prussian War fought several years later. The relative harmlessness of bullet wounds of moderate velocity penetrating only the soft tissues of the extremities (1 to 2 percent mortality) contrasts with the greatly enhanced risk when similar missiles fracture bone. The greater susceptibility to infection of compound fracture wounds over soft tissue wounds obviously is inherent in this remarkable disparity, antedating prophylactic antiseptic practices. Whereas antiseptics and antibiotics have diminished the dissimilarity considerably, the difference has not been completely erased. A missile that breaks the bone obviously aggravates the risk considerably, an occurrence which still needs to be adequately explained.

In a summary of another series constituted by more than 87,000 gunshot injuries of the soft tissue of the upper extremity, the results favored conservative management — a mortality of 4 percent attended operative treatment and 2.2 percent conservative management. For the lower extremity these figures were 4.35 percent mortality for conservative management and 8.5 percent for operative. The low mortality in both series was owing to the high incidence of injuries limited to the soft parts, unattended by fracture.

Amputation

Amputation was performed on 29,980 patients, with an overall mortality of 26.3 percent. The lowest risk concerned hand and fingers, with a mortality of 2.9 percent. Amputation of the foot or toes took a toll of 5.7 percent; leg amputation, 33.2 percent; thigh amputation, 54.2 percent; and amputation at the hip joint, 83.3 percent. In most situations the mortality from excision was higher than from amputation. Toward the end of the war, most surgeons favored conservative management unless there were compelling indications for operation.[20]

Open Wound Treatment

In a directive to the Sanitary Commission of the United States Army, a group of well-known American surgeons acting as voluntary consultants to the Union Army indicated, "it is good practice to leave the wounds open to heal by granulation" in amputations and resections of the lower extremities.[21]

Dressings

Andrews (1861) of Chicago wrote that the same sponge should not be used upon successive patients because it was likely to carry contagion, adding, "Many military surgeons exclude sponges from the hospital entirely and use pledgets of tow and cotton in their place, throwing them away at each dressing." Commented Andrews further, "No probes or other instruments which have been used in a case of this disease [hospital gangrene] should ever be used on another patient, until they have been thoroughly cleansed by washing, and then dipped in boiling water. There is no doubt whatever, that some surgeons have carried death around their own hospitals, by their wont of care in cleansing their instruments." According to Andrews, the best local application was strong nitric acid. Erysipelas, said Andrews, is another scourge of war. "It falls like a pestilence upon the wounded, carrying off hundreds of men, who, in civil surgery, might have recovered with ease."[22]

Anesthesia

Anesthetics were used by Union military surgeons in no less than 80,000 patients: chloroform in 76.2 percent; ether in 14.7 percent; and a mixture of ether and chloroform in 9.1 percent. Chloroform, because of its simpler and shorter induction, was employed more than five times as often as ether. In the Union armies there were thirty-seven deaths from chloroform anesthesia. In the Confederate armies, only two deaths from chloroform were reported by Chisolm.[23]

Medical and Surgical Accomplishments

Had a policy been formulated to follow the antiseptic practices of Goldsmith, North, and Hachenberg, this could well have been the most important lesson of the war. What impressed most foreign students and critics was the detail of organization for which Surgeon General Hammond was largely responsible; unfortunately, he was deposed by the irascible Edwin Stanton, secretary of war, on August 6, 1864. The precipitating circumstance apparently was Hammond's withdrawal of calomel and tartar emetic from the army's pharmacopoeia. Hammond regarded them as poisons; his mistake was to outlaw the drugs, very popular with all physicians of the day. Before Hammond's removal, however, he had installed a system of pavilion hospitals, proper inspection of military medical units, and a trained ambulance corps.[24]

The German pathologist Virchow was unstinted in his praise of the medical organization of the Union Army in the war, and the microbiologist-pathologist Klebs was also much impressed with the published accounts. Their flattering expressions were probably manifestations of surprise that the American military forces were well organized and had the competence to develop a factual and detailed report. Hippolyte Larrey (1874), son of Napoleon's military surgeon, also had high praise for the intimate, factual, and minute reporting in the published volumes about the American Civil War. In no other war had the documentation of accumulated experience been reported so factually and in such detail.[25] It did much to improve the image of American medicine and surgery in the eyes of European critics.

The French military surgeon Legouest (1866) wrote very knowledgeably of the American Civil War, reporting that the military organization was strong and effective; even so, the mortality from disease and wounds, as summarized by Legouest, indicates definitely that achievements during the war left much to be desired. There were 359,528 deaths in the Union Army: 110,070 soldiers were killed in action or died of wounds, and more than twice as many died of disease. Among the Confederates, there were 133,783 deaths, of which number less than one-half were reported to have resulted from disease.[26]

Chisolm, professor of surgery in the Medical College of South Carolina and surgeon to the Confederate Army, in the third edition of his book on military surgery (1864) wrote with more perceptive understanding of the history of wound management than did most American surgeons of his day. He knew that Félix Hutin, from the Hôpital des Invalides, had insisted that bone sequestra be removed; he also was familiar with Baudens's experience with such fragments in the Crimean conflict. He wrote of Macleod, Roux, Guthrie, Dupuytren, Bégin, and Stromeyer. Chisolm related that cold water treatment of gunshot wounds was universally employed in the Confederate Army in both field and hospital practice and that it showed "great advantages over every other dressing, even in this hitherto fatal class of injuries [compound fracture of joints]." In joint injuries not operated upon, Chisolm stated that the survival rate was 50 percent. He advised rest, immobilization, cold water dressings, and irrigation of the wound, together with opium.

The mortality from femur amputations for compound fracture in all military hospitals was frightful, said Chisolm, concluding that conservative management probably was better. He related that in the Crimean War no amputations at the hip joint were successful; in the Confederate experience, one primary amputation of the hip joint had succeeded. Chisolm reported that in the Crimea the mortality from amputations of the thigh was 92 percent; it was 49 percent in thigh amputations in the hands of Confederate surgeons between June 1, 1862, and February 1, 1864. The amputating knife, said Chisolm, should immediately follow the decision to sacrifice the limb.[27]

Franco-Prussian War

Napoleon III of France was lured into war with Prussia when Bismarck was striving to achieve a confederated Germany that included the southern independent German states. France was totally unprepared militarily; Prussia, with assurances of nonintervention by Britain, Italy, and Russia, was ready and well prepared. France declared war on July 19, 1870; by September 1, Sedan fell and the emperor was captured and deposed.[28] The long Siege of Paris and its terrible famine began on September 19 and endured until January 28, 1871. A formal peace treaty was signed at Frankfurt on May 21, 1871, exacting an indemnity of 5 billion francs from France and the surrender of Alsace and most of Lorraine.

Lister (1870) wrote a special article on antiseptic treatment of war wounds for the instruction of field surgeons engaged in the Franco-Prussian War. His object was to encourage surgeons on both sides of the conflict to irrigate wounds with a 5 percent solution of phenol, to leave gunshot wounds open, and to let the long ligatures on blood vessels emerge from the lower angle of wounds. Such practices were observed by a few surgeons, but perhaps in no war of the second half of the nineteenth century were the results of wound treatment so poor. By contrast, in the

American Civil War, fought several years earlier, wounds fared better. More gunshot fractures were treated conservatively in the Franco-Prussian War than in the American conflict. Even so, in every category, there were more deaths in German hands, whether the fractures were treated conservatively, by excision, or by amputation. Mortality from gunshot fractures of the upper extremity at Metz and Gravelotte in the care of German-speaking surgeons totaled 41.2 percent; for the lower extremity, 50.6 percent. The mortality from thigh fractures was 65.8 percent; from fractures of the knee joint, 76.9 percent. In other series, mortalities varying from 54.2 percent to 91.7 percent were reported for gunshot fractures of the femur.[29]

Perhaps the worst results of amputation were reported by the French in the Siege of Paris. The ailing Nélaton emerged from retirement to assist at the Grand Hotel, which had been converted into a hospital, and experienced 70 deaths in 70 amputations — the same Nélaton who earlier (1864) had reported less than 4 percent mortality in elective operations. Several other French surgeons in the siege experienced similar results. Nélaton is quoted as having remarked that a statue of gold should be erected to the one who shows the way to conquer operative wound infection.[30]

Amputation continued to be the recommended remedy for compound fracture through the Franco-Prussian War and until Lister's work had found general acceptance. The Russian surgeon Reyher was the first to demonstrate in military conflict that early antiseptic wound management (1878), accompanied by debridement (1881), abolished the need for primary amputation.[31]

World War I

Blood transfusions were first used in military action during World War I and to good advantage. The toxic factor in shock was still debated, but the importance of blood loss in its genesis was suspected though not confirmed; it was to be firmly established by the work of Blalock (1930) well before the beginning of World War II.[32]

The open management of contaminated wounds with delayed closure was accepted at the Inter-Allied Surgical Conference in March 1917 before the United States entered the war. Moynihan crossed the Atlantic in 1917 and gave a number of lectures at the American College of Surgeons in Chicago. He subsequently went to Washington to meet President Wilson and address the

Cabinet and then spoke before large audiences in Philadelphia and New York. He was a talented orator who evoked ready emotional response from his large audiences and was invariably given enthusiastic rounds of applause wherever he appeared. In an address on treatment of gunshot wounds Moynihan favored primary closure of war wounds when seen early. He advised immediate debridement and recommended injection of brilliant green into the depths of the wound, allowing it to remain not less than two minutes. For wounds seen late, Moynihan endorsed open management followed by secondary closure. He also spoke on war injuries of knee joints and called for preliminary sterilization of the wound with the cautery. There was great although mixed enthusiasm for Dakin's solution in the control of wound infection among military leaders in World War I. Moynihan remarked, "The Carrel-Dakin method has achieved its greatest triumphs in cases where it need not in fact have been applied. . . . It is the primary mechanical cleansing . . . that is the supreme necessity."[33]

Dakin, working in the Herter laboratory in New York, had studied the bactericidal effects of a number of well-known antiseptic agents and concluded that a buffered sodium hypochlorite possessed satisfactory germicidal action and was the least toxic and irritating of antiseptic agents to wounds in the presence of blood serum. Carrel and G. Dehelly gave readers the impression that Dakin's solution, properly prepared, would control wound infection.[34] Keen and Halsted in exchanges of correspondence hailed the use of Dakin's solution as a return to Listerism. It came to be widely used by the Allies in World War I and, despite its ineffectiveness in dealing with cellulitic infections, retained its popularity in civil practice almost until the beginning of World War II.[35] Its special role apparently was to make a wound look healthy and to retard suppuration when the body's defenses already had the situation under control.

Most surgeons who acquired practical experience in World War I continued to implement this type of wound care throughout their professional careers. Those trained in the immediate post-World War I period, failing to find that Dakin's solution was a panacea for wound infections, were often told by their elders that failures were owing solely to technical errors with the method. Through the chastening influence of experience, many learned that Dakin's solution had no power to control cellulitic streptococcal infections.

In January 1934 the senior author observed the attempts of an experienced World War I surgeon to treat a female rural school-

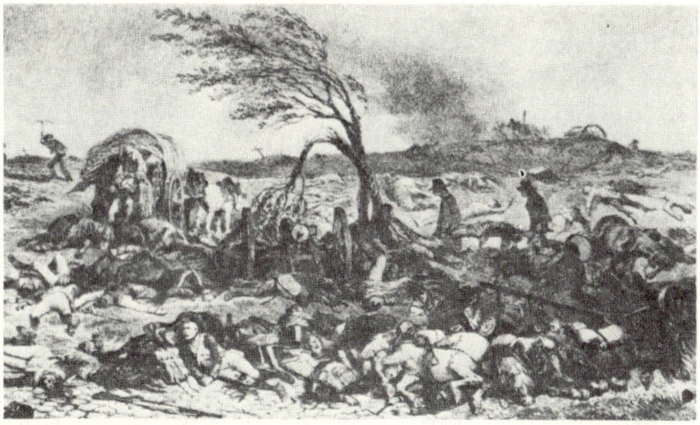

The day after

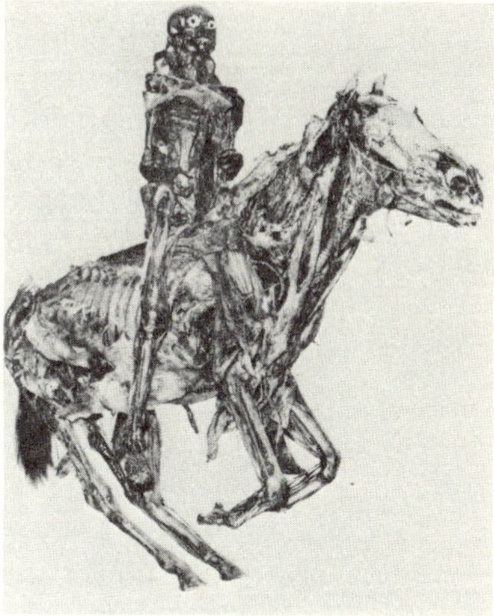

Fragonard's
Cavalryman

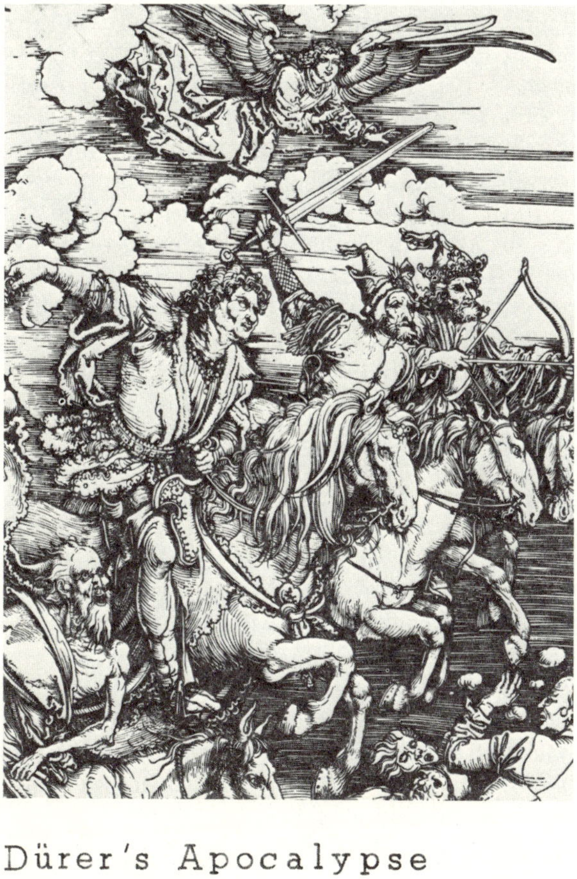

Dürer's Apocalypse

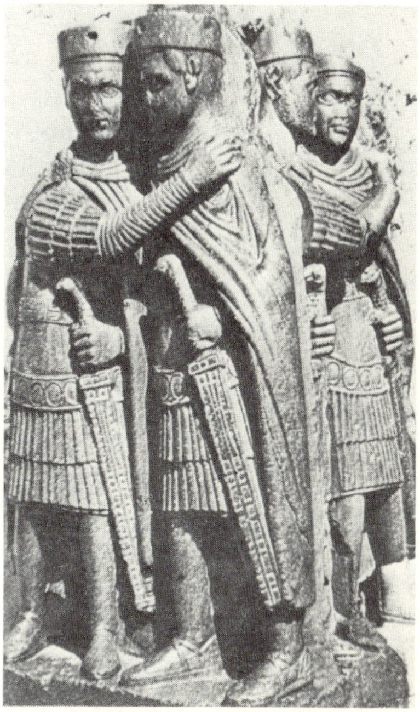

Why Peace Fails,
friendly hand on shoulder,
but other on dagger.

24.8 Aftermath of battle.

teacher twenty-three years of age who had a streptococcal phlegmon of the left lower extremity after a severe compound fracture of the femur. Mutiple long incisions were made in her thigh and leg in two operative sessions. Continuous irrigation of each resultant wound by the Carrell-Dakin treatment had not the slightest restraining influence upon the course of the infection nor upon the patient's picket-fence fever, often in excess of 104° F. A senior orthopedic surgeon, also with World War I experience, counseled amputation at the hip joint, advice the patient rejected. The senior author then applied a double spica body plaster cast extending from the toes of both feet to the axillary folds. The effect upon pain, fever, and the general course of the patient was immediate and dramatic; she made a satisfactory recovery from what appeared to be a hopeless situation. Later, an ankle stabilization was needed because foot drop developed from a common peroneal nerve paralysis, the result of prolapse of the sciatic nerve through one of the posterior thigh incisions. Thirty-three years later the patient is well and active; her only complaint is pain in the right "normal" hip. Before the arrival of sulfanilamide (1935–36), the device of complete immobilization in plaster, after drainage, was employed with satisfaction in a number of instances of cellulitic extremity infections in the University of Minnesota surgical clinic. The lesson of the above story is that an established infection cannot be excised, nor can a cellulitic infection be drained, nor is the Carrel-Dakin treatment of continuous irrigation with hypochlorite solution of the slightest value in controlling cellulitic infections. The role of the surgeon before sulfanilamide was essentially that of pus evacuator. The special role of debridement is excision of the dead tissue which accelerates peripheral spread of bacteria and infection.

Perhaps the most important lesson to emerge from World War I was the unavailability of any effective agent to deal with frequent cellulitic wound infections. Although surgeons were slow to admit the failure of Dakin's solution in such infections, Fleming at war's end boldly announced that antiseptics did more harm to tissues than to the bacteria in wounds.[36] The feature that distinguished the management of contaminated wounds in World War II from that in World War I was the omission of instillation of wound antiseptics in the latter.

Alexander Fleming (1881–1955)

Born on a farm south of Glasgow, Fleming was one of eight children in a closely knit family; sons and daughters worked for a living. When a bachelor uncle left each of the children an inheritance of £250, Fleming was able to study medicine at St. Mary's Medical School and Hospital in London, where he came under the tutelage of Wright, a voluble and dedicated microbiologist. Fleming had chosen surgery as a career and obtained the F.R.C.S., but under the guidance of Wright he turned to microbiology, following the example of Claude Bernard who chose physiology over surgery, two decisions that had important and enduring meaning for the advance of medicine. Fleming was a very astute observer and, like Bernard, a wise questioner of nature.

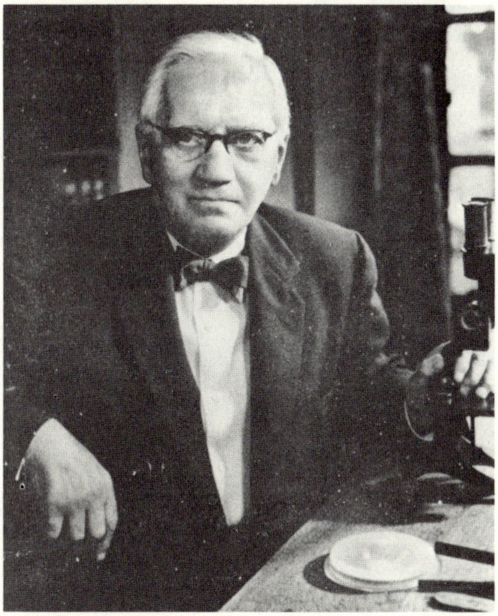

24.9 Fleming, Nobel Laureate, discoverer of penicillin (1929–45).

Fleming's critical and thoughtful studies in World War I, demonstrating the futility of wound antisepsis, led him to search for another agency to overcome infection. A decade later (1929) he observed the lytic effect upon staphylococcal and streptococcal cultures contaminated with the penicillium mold. Both Pasteur and Lister had been fascinated with the penicillium mold, but had not observed its lytic effect on micrococci. Fleming's experiments demonstrated the antibacterial role of the lytic agent, nicely shown on broth-agar pour plates; he called the lytic agent penicillin.[37]

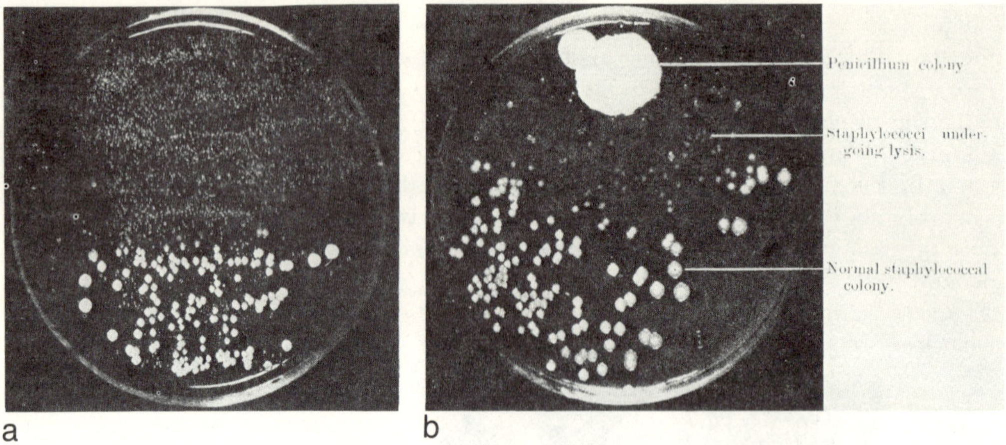

24.10 **a.** Staphylococcal culture before instillation of penicillium colony. **b.** Lytic action of the colony on staphylococcal culture.

Mobilized Forces in Two World Wars

The total mobilized belligerent forces in World War I numbered 65,038,810, of which 42,188,810 were members of the Allied forces and 22,850,000 of the Central Powers. A grand total of 8,538,315 were killed in action or died of wounds or disease. The United States military force numbered 4,734,991 men. The total American battle deaths of 53,402 were exceeded by deaths from disease in the number of 63,114, an occurrence in which influenza played an important role.

In World War II, there were almost 70 million combatants, of whom approximatedy 65 percent were fighting for the Allied cause, 35 percent for the Axis. The United States alone had 16,112,566 combatants and suffered 291,577 battle deaths and 113,842 deaths from disease and causes not primarily related to military action. The greatest losses in manpower were sustained by Russia and China. Of a peak strength of 12.5 million men, Russia sustained 7.5 million battle deaths; China, 2.2 million, of a total force of 5 million. Of Axis forces, Germany, with 10.2 million enlistments, lost 3.5 million; Japan's loss was 1,219,000, of a total force of 6,095,000. The fiscal cost to the United States has been placed in excess of $336 billion.

The most reliable source of information on American wars is probably the updated assessment issued by Roger Swanson and Robert Goldich, issued by the Library of Congress (1973). The Civil War, despite incomplete data on Confederate losses, emerges as the bloodiest of all wars in which American armies have participated; actually 62,933 more American enlisted personnel, Union and Confederate, were lost in this war than in World War II.[38]

World War II and Later Conflicts

World War II was the first war in which United States deaths from military action exceeded those from disease. It was also the first in which adjuvant chemotherapeutic and antibiotic measures were available to extend the effective reach of medical personnel in dealing with infections, especially cellulitic wound infections. Sulfanilamide became available to combat such infections in 1935–36. In the midst of World War II the work of Fleming was furthered through the cooperation of Howard Florey, Ernst Chain, John Fulton, and a number of pharmaceutical firms, including many in North America, to prepare penicillin for military use. It had a telling effect upon restraining the ravages of cellulitic infections.[39]

Smallpox had destroyed armies in the Napoleonic wars and typhoid fever took a larger toll than bullets in the Spanish-American War — these diseases no longer are serious threats for either military or civilian populations.

Major General Kirk (1943) issued a circular making it mandatory for military surgical personnel to leave all amputation wounds open, followed by delayed closure, confirming the 1917 action of the Inter-Allied Surgical Conference of World War I.[40] Blood banks were an innovation of World War II.

During World War II, 6 million people, largely Jews and Poles, were killed in gas chambers in three concentration camps; not included in that reckoning were Belsen, Buchenwald, and Dachau. It has been stated that Hitler and his henchmen were responsible for the torture, starvation, and outright murder resulting in the loss of 15 million people.

The bombing of large cities first by the Nazis and subsequently by the Allies in World War II took a large toll among noncombatants, women, and children. After the surrender of the Nazis in May 1945, the holocaust came to an abrupt end in August 1945, when a uranium bomb was exploded over Hiroshima by the American Air Force on August 6, with an explosive force of 20,000 tons of T.N.T., followed by a plutonium bomb dropped over Nagasaki on August 9; a few days later Japan capitulated; the worst of all wars was over. The casualties of these two atomic explosions were around 100,000 at Hiroshima and 50,000 at Nagasaki.

Availability of highly trained personnel and specialists in all medical disciplines has characterized our recent wars beginning with World War II. The development of sophisticated vascular surgery in the early 1950s made it possible to reconstruct severed blood vessels and save many extremities in the Korean War sacrificed under similar circumstances in World War II.[41]

Until World War I, the horse-drawn "flying ambulance" of Larrey was the standard method of conveying wounded to hospital facilities. Great advances have been made on this score. Helicopters and small aircraft transport wounded to the rear for definitive care, where quick action by trained personnel can salvage the lives of countless wounded. This feature of military organization played a significant role in the Vietnam War in which Surgeon General Heaton was able to report a mortality from wound infection that rivaled the achievement of civilian hospitals in elective surgery.[42]

The Vietnam War, our longest, endured from January 1, 1961 to January 27, 1973 — twelve long years. Our total armed forces numbered 8.4 million. There were 45,941 battle deaths; 10,306 died of disease and from other causes. Our troops sustained 303,648 nonmortal battle wounds. In retrospect, a costly war in every respect, in life, materiel, money, and loss of prestige. Despite utterances of our military that our objectives were attained, the world knows it was our first military defeat.

In a report upon wounds sustained in the October 1973 Egyptian-Israeli War, E. Simchen and T. Sacks identified three types of wounds inviting infection: burns exceeding 25 percent of the body surface, penetrating abdominal wounds with colon perforation, and compound femur fractures. The 420 patients were treated at Jerusalem's Hadassah Hospital: 8 of the wounded soldiers died of infection (1.9 percent), a low incidence for conditions of war. Nosocomial infections, especially *Pseudomonas, Klebsiella*, and bacteroides, were frequent environmental hazards of hospitalization; the authors stressed the need for potent specific chemotherapeutic and antibiotic agents.[43]

Some Reflections on Twentieth-Century Wars

With intercontinental ballistic power accessible to opposing world powers and atomic attack available to many nations, how can any political or military power dare risk another global conflict? Yet preparations go on, handicapping many nations with constant dread of war, accompanied by a tax burden exceeding all other costs.

How tragic and useless these struggles appear in retrospect. The sacrifice of its youth inevitably has a deteriorating and retarding influence upon any nation's future. The enemy is beaten to his knees, but the victor finds it necessary to reach out his hand and assist the vanquished to his feet, of which the unpaid war debts of many billions of dollars still owing the United States government provide dismal evidence. Russia emerged from World War II as a leading world power by shrewd political maneuvering in formulation of the peace treaty, apparently unrecognized, at least not fully appreciated by those who spoke for the other Allies. The British Commonwealth and France, for several centuries dominant nations in the world economy and affairs, although victorious, are now secondary powers, an inevitable consequence of their severe losses of manpower and dislocation of their nations' economies in two world wars.

What Substitute for War?

Wars at all periods have been fought for some advantage over the adversary, no matter what the stated cause. As long as governments and military leaders are willing to sacrifice hundreds of thousands, even millions, of innocent lives to achieve their objective, the future holds only faint hope for lasting peace. A better way must be found.

A fifth-century sculpture illustrates today's uncertain truces very well. The right hand of each combatant is upon the other's shoulders. But the hidden left hand of each is upon his dagger. Must it always be so?

During the twenty-second meeting of the International Surgical Society which convened in Moscow in August 1971, the authors of the present effort presented a paper on Reyher, a distinguished Russian military surgeon who was neglected and unappreciated even by his own countrymen. Boris Petrovsky, a well-known Russian surgeon and the minister of health, approached the podium and said, "I see you have a working wife too. Can you come to lunch?" It was a very relaxed occasion; ten of Petrovsky's sixteen deputy ministers of health were there and the fine Russian vodka flowed freely. The only protection against constant refilling of the glasses was quaffing the tasty liquor in miniscule sips. As the conversation, through interpreters, grew lively, the senior author addressed the minister saying, "We have no difficulty seeing eye to eye with the Russian people; how wonderful if only our governments could do that well." A moment of profound silence followed; the deputy minister of health from Minsk then spoke up and said "Doctor, we respect our government!" It was unnecessary to remind him that he had little choice.

Reduced to its simplest terms, such in essence is the situation: the people of adversary countries do not want war. Even so, their governments, having no faith in the sincerity of their opponents, arm themselves to the teeth as the only reliable protection against territorial aggression and disaster. Saber rattling in the world's pentagons intensifies the uncertainty urging on the need for endless military preparation. General Sherman wrote his wife (1864) that he had begun to "regard the death and mangling of a couple thousand men as a small affair, a kind of morning dash." There are probably very few, if any, lovable military leaders, however much they may be respected because of their victories. Robert E. Lee, great Confederate leader, much admired by both friend and foe, confessed that the love of victory, despite great sacrifice of men, was very attractive to all military leaders. Said he, "It is well that war is so terrible — we would grow too fond of it."[44] Immortality for military leaders can only be achieved on the field of battle. Are there not great threats to peace in taking their counsels too literally? How long can our great land continue its role of dominance as arbiter in world affairs? Despite the discouraging outlook, relentless search for an effective alternative to war must be continued.

In the midst of World War I, Gaston Bodart (1916), wrote on "Losses of Life in Modern Wars," in which he pointed out that in the seventeenth century, France had been at war 63 of the 100 years, at peace only 37. In the eighteenth century France was at war 55 years and enjoyed peace for 45. In the nineteenth century, the country was at war for 52 and enjoyed peace for 48 years.[45]

President Wilson believed, as did many of his fellow countrymen, that World War I was fought to end all wars. Neither the League of Nations nor the United Nations Assembly has had an effective influence on preventing international conflict.

May 14, 1948, marked the establishment of the Republic of Israel, fulfilling the Lord Balfour declaration of 1917. On May 13, the day before the ratification of the Republic of Israel, the senior author, at the request of the American Friends of Hebrew University in Palestine, gave a talk at their dinner meeting at the University of Minnesota on "International Universities and the Promotion of International Amity." On rereading that unpublished essay some three decades later, I confess that the travesties of the intervening years have diminished considerably the optimistic note sounded on that occasion, an admission made with great reluctance. The history of the past quarter-century offers little promise that wars can be avoided. Our defeat after twelve years of struggle in Vietnam, which terminated at the end of January 1973, taught us that we are not invincible. Our last military commander, General Frederick Weyand, announced on leaving, "Our mission has been accomplished — I have great pride in what our achievement represents" — certainly meaningless words we have come to expect from military leaders.[46]

In his Utopian *Looking Backward*, Bellamy (1888) conceived "the rosebush of humanity" gripping the peoples of the world in a warm glow of fraternity, such that by the year 2000, war would have ceased, making standing armies and navies unnecessary. La Fontaine's (1912) vision of a coordinated and harmonized world confederation and social structure still eludes us. America, the "Arsenal of Democracy," with great industrial might, must continue to explore avenues that can preserve international peace and tranquillity without global conflict. Will preparation and constant readiness for war continue to be the sole and sovereign deterrent?

The optimistic words of the aging Pasteur, read by his son on December 27, 1892, when Pasteur was honored at the Sorbonne for his life's work in creative and productive research, are worth recalling: "I am a man whose invincible belief is that science and peace will triumph over ignorance and war; that nations will unite, not to destroy but to build; and that the future belongs to him who has done most for suffering humanity," a prophecy of one of man's greatest benefactors, still awaiting fulfillment.[47]

Summary

The lessons of wars appear to be their utter futility. Military commanders, as long as successful, are glorified by their countrymen. Enduring peace is difficult to achieve, but ways of preventing war without world powers continuing to strain their economic resources to the utmost on military preparation must be sought and found. Pasteur's (1892) prediction that science and peace will triumph over war, and that nations will unite, not to destroy but to build, still awaits a feasible and workable proposal.

Larrey, Napoleon's celebrated military surgeon, established an enviable record as an amputationist, removing extremities as quickly as possible following injury when the syncope of shock permitted amputation without anesthesia. Florence Nightingale emerged a hero from the Crimean War. Her capacity for organization in care of the wounded was such that her very presence improved the morale of the soldiers to a degree that has become legend. Anesthesia was available in the Crimean conflict but not extensively used. Antiseptic wound care was used only by a few French military surgeons.

The American Civil War, one of the bloodiest in history, elevated American surgery considerably in the eyes of many European authorities and critics, who were astounded at the detailed factual accounts of the management of gunshot wounds appearing in six large volumes after the war. Actually, the results of wound management in that conflict were better in every respect than those of the Germans or the French in the Franco-Prussian War fought a few years later. Antiseptic wound management, although not routinely used, was employed to great advantage and with impressive reduction in mortality by a few Union military surgeons as well as by Confederate surgeons. There emerges in these accounts an important observation, overlooked by historians of surgery: the great disparity in mortality from penetrating gunshot extremity injuries of the soft parts contrasted with the heightened risk when the bone of the extremity is fractured too.

The Russian military surgeon Reyher was the first to project a controlled prospective study using Listerian principles (1878); in 1881 he conducted a similar study in which both antiseptic wound management and debridement were employed for gunshot extremity wounds, and to great advantage in two Russo-Turkish conflicts.

In March 1917, before the entry of the United States into World War I, the Allied surgeons had decided upon a policy of debridement and open wound management of all war injuries, a real advance, to which all military surgeons have since been committed. In World War I the mortality from disease exceeded deaths from military action for the last time in American wars of this century. At the end of that conflict Fleming announced that placement of any and all antiseptics into wounds did more harm to the tissues than to the bacteria in the wounds, an assertion that his demonstration of the lytic power of the penicillium mold (1929) substantiated. In the midst of World War II large-scale manufacture of penicillin augmented considerably the role of the surgeon in dealing with contaminated wounds and especially with cellulitic infections.

When the Korean conflict began in 1950, American surgeons were prepared to deal with vascular injuries and saved many extremities by arterial reconstruction. The Vietnam War demonstrated the tremendous effectiveness of transporting the injured by air to field stations behind the lines for early care.

(For notes, see pp. 707–11.)

CHAPTER 25

Surgical Specialization

MEDICAL SPECIALIZATION existed in antiquity. In Egypt, there were specialists for the eye, teeth, head, intestines, and other segments of the body. Medicine and surgery were treated as a unified body of knowledge in the Hippocratic writings, but apparently by the time of Celsus in the first century A.D. specialism had become well established in Greece.

During the Middle Ages a sharp separation developed between physicians and surgeons, with the physicians occupying a higher status in both the professional and the social hierarchy. There was additionally a third class composed of itinerant quacks and empirics who performed difficult and serious operations, and then went on their way. Only late in the nineteenth century did surgeons in our country begin to limit their practice to surgery, W. T. Bull and Arpad Gerster of New York being among the first to do so. Most surgeons, including professors of surgery, engaged in general medical practice.

Ophthalmology

The first among all surgical specialties, ophthalmology, has a long and distinguished history. Guy de Chauliac apparently was one of the earliest to undertake operations for cataract, largely theretofore in the hands of strolling mountebanks.[1] The story is told that King John of Bohemia in 1337, aged forty-two, visited a French physician in Breslau who attempted to cure him of an eye disorder. When the king became worse, he had the physician tossed into the Oder River. The king then consulted an Arab physician in Prague who wanted assurances that if he assumed treatment of the king he would not suffer the fate of the Breslau physician. The eye that the Prague physician treated became sightless. Finding that his vision in the remaining eye was diminishing, the king then went to see Guy de Chauliac, who told him that he had cataracts; presently he was completely blind. Guy wrote a treatise on the treatment of cataracts for the king, but no copies of this work are now in existence.[2] Surgery upon the eye in the eighteenth century offered far better chances of success.

Georg Bartisch of Dresden (1583) was the first to extirpate the human eye for cancer. Richard Banister of London (1622) noted the hardness of the eyeball in glaucoma. Michel Brisseau of Paris (1709) demonstrated that cataract was owing to opacity of the lens, which the studies of Maître-Jan had suggested (1707). Jacques Daviel of Paris (1753) originated extraction of the lens for cataract instead of couching, the old operation used by Brisseau and others, in which the lens was depressed and displaced out of the line of vision.[3]

It is surprising to note how many well-known general surgeons performed surgery on the eye, including Guillemeau (1585), Cheselden (1728), Samuel Sharp (1753), Scarpa (1801), Larrey (1802), Travers (1820), Guthrie (1823), Lawrence (1833), and Dieffenbach (1842).[4] In our country Edward Delafield, a gynecologist, was a founder of the American Ophthalmologic Society and its first president (1864). Physick, Samuel D. Gross, Alfred C. Post, Hayes Agnew, and others, best known to us as general surgeons, operated upon and wrote of the eye.[5]

The invention of the ophthalmoscope by Helmholtz (1851) perhaps more than any innovation furthered the development of ophthalmology as an independent surgical specialty.[6] The general surgeon who operated only upon the eye was superseded by the ophthalmologist whose interests concerned vision as much as remedial surgical measures. Koller's introduction of cocaine (1884) as a local anesthetic for ophthalmic operations also constituted a very important aid to the progress of the discipline. In England as well as in the United States there were special hospitals for the treatment of diseases of the eye before ophthalmology became a recognized specialty, a response within the profession to society's needs. In France diseases of the eye continued to be treated in general hospitals.

The elder Graefe, Carl Ferdinand (1787–1840), was professor

of surgery and ophthalmology at the University of Berlin from 1810 to 1840. He was a well-known military surgeon and wrote about many surgical disorders, including those of the eye.[7] It was his son Albrecht Graefe (1828–70) who gave ophthalmology everywhere a great forward thrust. He was only twelve when his father died at age fifty-three. A brilliant student, Albrecht entered the University of Berlin at age sixteen. Among his teachers were Ernst Brücke, Du Bois Reymond, Traube, Robert Remak, and Virchow, a truly remarkable faculty. The Graefes were a well-to-do family, and when Albrecht finished medical school he undertook a scientific study trip through several countries. He first visited Prague, where he was delighted with the teachers, and wrote, "What a heaven-wide difference between our arrogant, inhuman German professors and the lovable modest professors of Prague." It was the ophthalmologist Ferdinand Arlt at Prague who interested young Graefe in that discipline.

Later Graefe went to Paris and was fascinated with the teaching and wealth of clinical material and intrigued by the degree of specialization in Paris clinics. Albrecht was a keen observer and his notes concerning some of the professors are worth repeating: "The clinics of Bouillaud, Chomel, and Rostan were very instructive. Piorry is quite mad." Piorry, Bouillaud, Auguste Chomel, and Pierre Louis, whose clinics Graefe liked most of all, were advocates of anatomical diagnosis, a movement which brought important clinical advances. The young visitor was particularly attracted to the surgical clinics of Malgaigne. He found the eye clinics of Julius S. Sichel and Louis A. Desmarres, where two to three cataract extractions were done each week, interesting and very instructive. Graefe was charmed with Professor Philippe Ricord, who set aside the Hunterian thesis that gonorrhea and syphilis were the same disease. Graefe observed that Ricord's teachings were full of witticisms and that he never walked but half-danced and half-ran and always laughed; he lived like a king and was probably the most popular man in Paris.

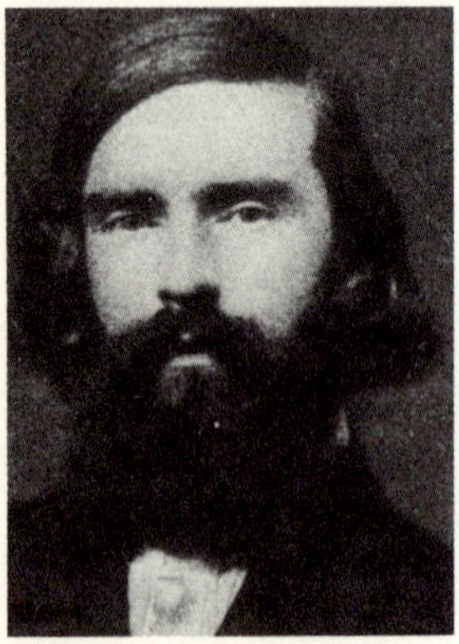
25.1 Albrecht Graefe (1828–70).

From Paris, Graefe went to Vienna in the winter of 1849–50 and was much impressed by the work of Rokitansky, Heschl, Skoda, Franz Schuh, Hebra, and others. Here he became acquainted with the teachings of the Beer-Jäger school of ophthalmology. In July 1850 he visited Bowman in London, went on to Edinburgh, and then traveled to see William Wilde in Dublin. He finally returned to Berlin, where he had twenty years of uninterrupted creative work ahead of him. Graefe was now twenty-two years of age and had, through his travels and contacts with outstanding teachers in several countries, eked out a very unusual education and training.

Graefe opened a private polyclinic in Berlin in November 1850, a year before Helmholtz perfected the ophthalmoscope. His unusual success with operations upon the eye soon attracted rich and poor alike — the latter he treated without fees. At age twenty-six he was appointed professor of ophthalmology at the University of Berlin (1857). Graefe came to be known as the "father of ophthalmology" and his achievement in a professional life of just twenty years is almost unbelievable. Garrison termed him "the creator of modern surgery of the eye, and indeed the greatest of all eye surgeons."[8] In 1854 Graefe founded *Archiv für Ophthalmology*, in which most of his papers were published. He introduced iridectomy for glaucoma and linear extraction of cataract, greatly reducing the incidence of loss of sight attending the operation; he established the thesis of sympathetic ophthalmia. Coronary occlusion and overwork terminated a brilliant career at age forty-two.[9]

Graefe's preparation for his life's work rested solely on observation and exposure to a large number of remarkable exponents of ophthalmology. Today the emphasis for surgeons, even in the finest university clinics, is on *doing* rather than on *observing*. Many great American surgeons in the last decades of the nineteenth century were trained primarily through observation in visits to recognized surgical teachers. There are probably no better examples of the benefit of such training than William and Charles Mayo.

The *power of appointment* is the finest possession of every institution of learning. What American university today would have the foresight and the courage to provide a promising young man, just twenty-six years old, with Graefe's background, to head and lead a department? Search committees obviously are attracted to trainees with more traditional training. And what of the Certifying Boards? Their regulations are not elastic enough to permit much deviation from prescribed procedure. Universities must continue to insist on more elasticity and greater latitude in their selection of people for important posts. Genuflection to convention fosters mediocrity.

Ophthalmology, the oldest of all surgical specialties, has come a long way since its sharp separation from general surgery some 125 years ago. Two of the most challenging problems of the discipline, retinal detachment and extraction of the opacified lens, are being met and dealt with today by new techniques in the hands of well-trained ophthalmologists the world over.

Laryngology

The development of the laryngoscope by Garcia (1854–55) helped establish laryngology as a separate surgical specialty, yet far into the twentieth century in American university clinics it was not unusual to find the specialties of ophthalmology, otology, laryngology, and rhinology listed as a unified department. General surgeons performed the operations of laryngo-fissure (splitting the thyroid cartilage) and laryngectomy for cancer of the larynx well into this century. The sad debacle over the management of Crown Prince Frederick's laryngeal cancer has already been related in chapter 8. For want of a histologic diagnosis of cancer, the highly trained surgical specialist Mackenzie refused to approve the thyro-fissure operation that Bergmann had scheduled. The endoscopist Chevalier Jackson (1865–1958) of Philadelphia made several refinements in the art of laryngoscopy that quickened its use for the detection and aspiration of lodged foreign bodies in the air passages and for the recognition of neoplasms.[10]

St. Clair Thomson (1859–1943), a house surgeon to Lister at King's College Hospital, received his training in laryngology and otology in Vienna, Paris, and Lausanne. His contribution to the laryngofissure procedure for early intrinsic cancer of the larynx marked a lessening of the mortality of the operation and has been recognized everywhere.[11]

Otology

Anton Troeltsch developed the otoscope (1860) and devised the operation of opening the mastoid for extensions of acute suppuration from the middle ear, a frequent procedure until the use of penicillin made its performance far less necessary.[12] Otolaryngologists today are gradually invading the field of the general surgeon in the management of oral and cervical lesions. In recent decades great progress has been made in the relief of deafness caused by otosclerosis. Ankylosis of the stapes was long known as an underlying factor in the genesis of otosclerosis. Genetic influences are significant too.

Julius Lempert (1938) in twenty-three sketches showed his one-stage procedure in which the bony capsule of the external semicircular canal is fenestrated, leaving a permanent window; it stayed open after operation in 22 of Lempert's 23 patients and was followed by substantial improvement of hearing in 19. Samuel Rosen (1953) substituted mobilization of the stapes for Lempert's fenestration technique.[13] Excision of the stapes is currently the procedure of choice for otosclerosis. Otologists were among the first to employ visual magnification, so helpful in bringing these small structures into clear view, facilitating the operative procedure. Important technical strides have been made with many intricate aural operations since the adoption of the operating microscope.

Prosper Menière (1861) described a disorder of the inner ear in which tinnitus, nystagmus, vertigo, deafness, and even convulsions are observed. The provoking causes apparently can be multiple.[14] Küttner, professor of surgery at Breslau, told the senior author in May 1928 that vigorous cannonade during the terminal months of World War I had provoked the Menière syndrome in him and some of his fellows. For long months, for fear of falling, he slept on a mattress on the floor. The troublesome symptoms often disappear spontaneously; there seems to be no consistently successful conservative treatment. For persistent cases, neurosurgeons occasionally divide the vestibular nerve on the affected side.

Plastic Surgery

Virtually every surgical specialty is involved in plastic surgery. Several professors in Berlin, the elder Graefe, Dieffenbach, among others, were professors of general surgery as well as of plastic and ophthalmic surgery. The earliest forms of reconstructive surgery involved plastic procedures about the face for restoration of a nose that had been struck off by a saber or bitten off by an assailant. The classical Indian method involved a narrow pedicle with its base situated directly above the eyebrow, the nose being reconstructed from a skin flap from the forehead extending to the hairline. Gaspare Tagliacozzi (1597) of Bologna employed a somewhat similar procedure, bringing a pedicled flap from the inner side of the upper arm after freshening the edges of the mutilated nose. Such nose operations were so successful in Tagliacozzi's hands that he became famous throughout Europe. The Sicilian Branca apparently had enjoyed successes with the method before Tagliacozzi.[15] Prolonged anchorage of the arm to the face was a trying ordeal for the patient and the Indian forehead flap has proved to be the more durable operation.

The French surgeon Garengeot reported that in 1724 almost the entire cartilaginous portion of a soldier's nose had been bitten off in a struggle with one of his comrades. The adversary spit the bit of flesh into the gutter and trampled upon it. The soldier picked it up and threw it into the shop of one of Garengeot's fellow practitioners, then pursued his attacker. The surgeon washed the piece of nose in a well and, when the soldier returned to have his wound dressed, cleaned the blood from the soldier's face, dipped the amputated portion into warm wine and put it back into place, retaining it with an agglutinating plaster and bandage. Garengeot dressed the wound with the attending surgeon on the fourth day and was convinced that the detached segment had united perfectly. J. S. Bushman, who again reported Garengeot's observation a century later (1833), added the instance of a patient who had lost an inch and a half of his index finger with the stroke of a hatchet. William Balfour, an Edinburgh surgeon, reapplied the severed segment and reported it healed in place with "a perfect recovery . . . of heat, and of sensation."[16]

J. Braid (1816), a surgeon, reported that a sixty-three-year-old miner cut off the forefinger of his left hand with a hatchet. Braid and the patient located the lost segment, covered with dust; Braid washed it off with warm water and reapplied it, fixing it in position with strips of adhesive tape. In seventeen days the transplanted finger looked all right; five weeks after the accident, the patient could use the finger when tying threads and weaving. Braid regarded it as a perfect result. Carlizze (1834) saw a woman whose nose was bitten off by an aggressive man whom she had no doubt resisted. Carlizze persuaded the woman to find the lost segment; two and a half hours later it was found, covered with filth; it was washed clean and put in place, held by a few sutures; the dressing was changed seven days later, when the nose was completely united; at thirty-seven days it was well consolidated. A patient visited John Mackenzie (1837) with the distal segment of his left thumb in his pocket. Mackenzie reapplied it. He dressed it three weeks later, when it was found to be "perfectly reunited." Seven years later the patient said hand and thumb were all right.[17] John Denny (1849) wrote of a laborer cutting grass with a sickle who severed part of his thumb, including a segment of the nail and distal phalanx and a portion of the forefinger. He sent the patient out to find the lost segments. Four hours later, Denny anchored the thumb in place with firm strapping and obtained a "perfect reunion"; the period of observation was not stated. Many of these evaluations of functional prognosis were undoubtedly made too soon after the accident to have a ring of authenticity, especially with reference to return of normal sensation. Eduard Zeis (1863) in his history of the literature of plastic surgery is quite skeptical of the validity of many such accounts.[18]

Skin Grafts

Jacques Reverdin (1870) from Félix Guyon's service at the Necker Hospital observed that occasionally little islets of epithelium appeared in the midst of granulating wounds, remote from the peripheral borders of the adjacent healthy skin, and that from these areas the epithelium proliferated to cover the raw areas. He thereupon applied small full-thickness free grafts of skin to granulation tissue. The method seemed to succeed. In explaining his technique before the Society of Surgery in Paris Reverdin had only one case to present; his teacher Guyon remarked that one case does not prove anything but that it did appear a practical method, an opinion voiced by many of the assembly. In a subsequent issue of the society's journal (1872) Reverdin is characterized as the "interne laureate," having won the Duval Prize in the *concours* with a thesis on studies of the internal urethra (1870). Ollier of Lyons (1872) cut skin grafts of intermediate thickness which he applied to fresh surfaces after cutting away the overlying scar tissue.[19]

Thiersch of Leipzig (1874) applied Reverdin skin grafts to a young boy's leg with an ulcer of four years' duration. The graft failed and the boy desired amputation. Thiersch regrafted eighteen hours before amputating, then injected the artery of the severed extremity with Gerlach's injection mass, and hardened the leg in alcohol. In microscopic sections, Thiersch was able to demonstrate dye in the capillaries of the transplanted skin and concluded that thinly cut grafts would be superior to the full-thickness grafts of Reverdin and that fresh raw surfaces would accept free grafts better than granulation tissue.[20] To reconstruct an eyelid John R. Wolfe (1875), a distinguished Glasgow ophthalmic surgeon, applied a free full-thickness skin graft with underlying fat, removed from the forearm, two inches long and one inch wide. A portion sloughed but enough survived to produce a good result. Professor Ceci of Genoa remarked that Wolfe replaced skin loss with healthy tissue whereas the epidermic grafts of Reverdin and Thiersch generated cicatricial tissue. As a young medical graduate Wolfe had studied in Paris with Nélaton and Desmarres.[21]

J. F. Esser (1917) of Holland, working in Julius Hochenegg's clinic in Vienna during World War I, wrote of pedicled well-vascularized grafts from the neck for replacement of facial defects, including those of the lips. The British plastic surgeon Harold Gillies (1920) converted pedicled skin grafts into tubes to enhance survival of the graft; V. P. Blair and Barrett Brown of

St. Louis (1929) introduced the split graft of intermediate thickness; Earl C. Padgett's dermatome (1939) made it practical to calibrate the thickness of skin grafts.[22]

Replantation of Extremities

The Harvard surgeons R. A. Malt and C. F. McKhann initiated replantation (1964) of completely severed extremities, restoring continuity of veins, arteries, and nerves to the severed segment after debridement and cleansing of both wounds. In 1972 Malt and associates reported five successful replacements of arms, functional at periods in time as late as five to ten years after the operation. Malt (1976) has had an experience with fifteen patients, in eleven of whom the replanted segment survived and became functional. The American Replantation Mission of eleven surgeons (1973) visited several hospitals in China, where there is great enthusiasm for such procedures. The severed extremity is cooled immediately to 4° C, thus extending its ability to withstand ischemia while the patient is transported to a replantation center. The bone is usually shortened to permit ready approximation of the severed segments; vein grafts are often necessary to permit restoration of blood vessels. These are time-consuming operations, often taking ten to twelve hours.[23]

Rejection of skin grafts between individuals has long been known. Zeis (1863) apparently was aware of such rejection. Lexer (1911) observed that all such transplants failed within four weeks, a phenomenon also recognized by Carrel about the same time. Peter B. Medawar, an ardent student of experimental skin transplantation, recognized that intolerance to foreign tissue was an immunologic reaction; by 1944 he had performed 802 skin grafts between paired rabbits, all of which failed.[24]

Padgett (1932) transferred skin successfully between two pairs of identical twins. Archibald McIndoe, a well-known London plastic surgeon, and A. Franceschetti employed this technique in a medico-legal case to establish the true identity of a pair of twins, one of whom had been inadvertently exchanged at the hospital where they were born. When the "twins" were six years old, their father noted that a boy in the area (place and names not identified) looked very much like one of his own. Questioning revealed that the strange boy was born the same night as his "twins" and in the same clinic. An inquiry was instituted. Blood group and subgroup factors pointed to the circumstance that one of the "twins" could not have been the mother's son. Fingerprints and teeth configuration also pointed that way. McIndoe made two full-thickness grafts between each of the three children. Those between the true twins took without any evidence of necrosis and were intact ten months later. Skin transfers between the mistaken twin failed in each instance. In 1948, a year after completion of the skin transfers, by court order, an exchange of the substituted children was effected, following which, said the authors, adaptation to the new environment was satisfactory, obviously not only an occurrence of great scientific interest, but one, no doubt, beset with severe emotional strain too.[25]

Orthopedic Surgery

The management of fractures and injuries of joints is one of the oldest concerns of surgery. The Australian-born G. Elliot Smith (1908), then professor of anatomy in the Egyptian Government Medical School of Cairo, a famous anatomist and anthropologist, conducted a considerable exploration of Egyptian tombs and mummies from the Fifth Dynasty of approximately 4,500 years ago. He indicated that the oldest medical instruments known are flint knives, used for circumcision. Smith found wooden splints of bark wrapped in linen about broken bones. The splints, usually two, were tied in place with linen around the fracture site. Smith believed that such splints constituted the oldest surviving evidence of how fractures were treated in antiquity. Fractures of the forearm apparently were frequent, as were those of the femur. The splints were only somewhat more than a foot long, obviously an inefficient device to hold broken bone ends in place; at best they limited motion, thereby reducing pain. Smith encountered healing fractures that displayed considerable shortening. He related (1924) that similar splints were still in use in the Sudan and Abyssinia. Apart from the splints, he found no evidence of surgical procedures on mummies.

Smith's anatomist colleague F. Wood Jones (1908) identified several recipients of splints for fractures without evidence of healing as having died, presumably of hemorrhage or infection, shortly after being injured. He stated that blood pigment cannot be identified in dead bodies after a lapse of more than 250 years; however, the red discoloration of the linen or palm leaf dressings served to indicate bloodstaining. Smith failed to observe any evidence of syphilitic bones in prehistoric Egyptian mummies.[26]

Fractures and their management were thoroughly discussed in the Hippocratic writings; the use of cerate bandages incorporating wooden splints for immobilization was standard practice. The role of exercise to prevent muscle atrophy during immobilization was emphasized, a thesis to which Lorenz Böhler (1929) of Vienna lent considerable emphasis, stressing exercise as an effective method of preventing stiffness of joints encased in plaster. In the spring of 1928 the senior author attended the clinics of Böhler, who was not then warmly accepted by Viennese surgeons for want of orthodox training in general surgery. Several instances of femur fracture were seen in which each patient had been urged to move his toes as well as his patella beneath a plaster cast encasing the limb from the lower abdomen to the toes. When patients had neglected this advice, on removal of the plaster, the injured knees were stiff. On the contrary, patients who had fully accepted Böhler's advice could move their knee joints freely and without pain immediately on removal of the cast. The late professor and his nephew Jörg Böhler in their 1966 supplement to fracture management were still ardent in the use of plaster casts, but they had accepted light metal splints and traction as an acceptable substitute for plaster, in suitable situations.[27] When applying plaster casts care must be taken that the plaster is snug but not so tight that it impedes the circulation. An occasional hazard is too snug application with ensuant ischemia. It is a good rule to examine the situation carefully within two hours after applying the plaster. If pinching of a protruding toe or finger produces a tingling sensation in a slightly cyanotic member, the cast obviously is too tight and immediate partial removal is in order.

William Eton (1801) related that whereas Turkish surgeons decried surgery, they had a special skill in treating fractures. After reduction, the extremity was placed "in a case of plaster of Paris (or gypsum) which takes exactly the form of the limb — and in a few minutes the mass is solid and strong."[28]

Antonius Mathijsen of the Netherlands is often credited with devising plaster of Paris bandages for immobilization of fractures (1852). At that time he wrote, "Although it is widely known that this material was already in use in earlier centuries . . . its use by no means found general application, it is not even spoken of anymore." In his introduction to the 1962 facsimile of Mathijsen's publication, G. J. Bremer reported that Arab physicians in the tenth century had employed plaster for the management of fractures, a practice that did not penetrate Europe until the end of the eighteenth century.[29] The advantage of Mathijsen's innovation was that the setting of the plaster took less than two hours, whereas plasters employed theretofore often required more than a day to solidify. In more recent developments plaster that sets in a few minutes has become available.

Cheselden related in his *Anatomy of the Human Body* (1741) that as a boy he was treated for an elbow fracture by Mr. Cowper, a "bone-setter" of Leicester, who, after reduction of the fracture, wrapped "it up in rags dip'd in the whites of eggs, and a little wheat flower mixed, this drying grew stiff, and kept the limb in a good posture." Added Cheselden, "there is no way better than this in [treating] fractures."[30]

A starch bandage, incorporating wooden splints, was a conventional manner of treating fractures before the plaster cast. Larrey (1824) used a bandage that incorporated wine, lead acetate, camphorated spirits, egg white, and styrax in the successful management of seven consecutive compound fractures; this antiseptic dressing hardened and immobilized the extremity, but was extremely heavy and therefore its use was limited to lower extremity fractures. Dieffenbach (1834) placed the fractured extremity in a wooden box that was well greased, as was the patient's skin; liquid plaster was then poured into the box and allowed to set and harden. The anterior surface of the fractured extremity was not covered by the plaster but left open for inspection. These methods, when a lower extremity was involved, kept the patient in bed.[31] Mathijsen's cast of rolled wet bandages containing the plaster made a much neater dressing.

William R. Beaumont (1831), an English surgeon, compared immobilization of fractures in rabbits, similarly treated except for the addition of complemental antiseptic management. Beaumont fractured a rabbit's tibia, compounding it such that the ends of the broken bone protruded through the skin; he then applied a plaster dressing to immobilize the extremity. He emphasized exclusion of air by the dressing. The plaster was removed after three weeks and four days; the wound was not quite healed and some inodorous pus was present. The bone seemed to have united firmly. A few days later, the rabbit was able to hop about upon the unsupported broken limb.

In a second experiment, the right radius and ulna of a rabbit were fractured and nitric acid was poured into the wound. An immobilizing plaster splint was then applied and also left in place for three weeks and four days. By then an abscess had formed, extending to the upper portion of the extremity, with rupture through the skin exposing the bone; osseous union had not occurred. The limb was immobilized in plaster as before. When the plaster dressing was removed after eight weeks, the wound was healed and the rabbit could bear weight upon the broken extremity. Nitric acid undoubtedly caused tissue necrosis and was not a proper antiseptic agent for the test. Beaumont apparently did not extend his observations and experiments to man, although he advised it. The editor of a journal in which Beaumont's experiments were reviewed opposed Beaumont's proposition, insisting that an unyielding bandage applied to the fractured extremity "must be precarious, if not decidedly injurious."[32]

Strong orthopedic groups developed in the United States, especially in Boston and New York, before they did in Germany. In fact, many German surgeons with a special interest in orthopedics came to our shores to visit American orthopedic clinics. Special orthopedic hospitals had appeared in Boston and New York in the first quarter of the nineteenth century; the American Orthopedic Association was formed in 1887. The German Orthopedic Association dates from 1902; it began as a splinter group from the German Surgical Congress, formed in 1872. Specialty groups prefer to hear papers related only to their own interests, unlike programs of general surgery that concern a far wider range of topics.

World War I lent great impetus to orthopedic surgery. Outstanding exponents were Robert Jones, Welsh orthopedic surgeon of Liverpool, and Vittorio Putti of Bologna, who worked in the Rizzoli Institute with its beautiful murals and frescoes. Jones preferred splints to plaster and is reported to have remarked, "nothing so barbarous as plaster of Paris is used any longer." He, like his uncle and predecessor Hugh Owen Thomas, was a master in designing light, efficient splints adaptable for specific uses. But wherever complete immobilization constitutes a significant advantage, a well-applied plaster of Paris cast best fills the need.[33]

Perhaps no surgical specialty in recent decades has extended its territory as broadly as has orthopedics. Concerned at first primarily with congenital osseous deformities, orthopedics has completely absorbed from general surgery the management of fractures, and in many clinics it has taken over surgery of the hand, including surgery for infections and tendon injuries. In this area today, it competes more often with plastic than with general surgery.

Arthroplasty

Ollier performed several resection arthroplasties on the elbow and other joints; by the time of his death in 1900 he had done a total of 270. Henri Comte (1926) sought out a number of these patients and obtained x-ray films of the elbows. Whereas the films often revealed a poor anatomic result, said Comte, functional results in the main were surprisingly good.[34]

Arbuthnot Lane (1903) employed metal plates and screws with considerable success in the operative management of human fractures of long bones. Hey Groves (1913) of Bristol in experiments upon rabbits observed that metal screws caused absorption of bone with lack of stable fixation; similarly circumferential wiring provided poor fixation. Arthur Zierold (1924) of the University of Minnesota implanted various metals into the marrow cavity of dogs; gold, aluminum, and "stellite" were well tolerated on implantation and offered least resistance to the osseous reparative process. He concluded that steel was the "least acceptable of all for bone prostheses."[35]

Gerhard Küntscher of Hamburg (1967) summarized his long experience dating back to 1940 with the use of long intramedullary nails, pins, and bolts for fixation of fractures and for arthrodesis. He favored immediate weight bearing, without support of external plaster, for lower extremity fractures. Leonard Peltier, now of Tucson, has experimented with intramedullary bars of plaster, which method has not yet enjoyed wide clinical trial. Küntscher's technique of fixation of fractures has enthusiastic advocates; in the main, however, the profession tends to prefer nonoperative means of reduction and fixation of broken bones.[36]

M. N. Smith-Petersen of Boston described vitallium arthroplasty of the hip. Charnley's complete prosthetic replacement of the upper femur and head for osteoarthritis of the hip, the most widely performed arthroplasty today, is followed by excellent functional results and relief of pain in most instances, constituting a major contribution to the advance of surgery. In the preface to his well-documented 1970 monograph, Charnley relates that he adapted from chemistry the use of an acrylic cement as a mechanical bond between the parts to be joined. The device enabled him to develop a method of total replacement of painful, fixed osteoarthritic hips, a technique which has proved eminently satisfactory.[37] His thoughtful address to maintenance of a bacteria-free atmosphere over the operative field came, no doubt, as a natural sequel to the hip replacement problem.

In their 1931 monograph on fundamentals of orthopedic surgery, R. B. Osgood and Nathaniel Allison wrote, "A surgical specialty should always be considered as part of general surgery, because it has no right to existence unless it is based upon, and strictly follows the principles which govern general surgery."

Obviously, the picture has changed. Representatives of most surgical specialties, including orthopedics, are not reticent in indicating that they believe they are well-enough oriented in the techniques of surgery to exist independently of general surgery.[38]

Neurosurgery

Before antiseptic practices were employed, neurosurgery was delimited to the elevation of depressed fractures of the skull. The first removal of a brain tumor was performed in 1884 by Godlee. The patient survived only a month. Macewen of Glasgow successfully removed a tumor involving the meninges in 1879, and Horsley, an extradural spinal cord tumor in 1888. England had its Horsley and Ballance, Germany its Krause; the real founder of neurosurgery, however, was Cushing. Yet many, because of Horsley's early exploits in the field, are willing to concede that Horsley deserves this title. Like Charles Frazier of Philadelphia, he never confined his practice to neurosurgery as Cushing did for several years before leaving The Hopkins in 1912 for Harvard's Peter Bent Brigham Hospital. Gilbert Horrax (1952), who at one time worked with Cushing at the Brigham, related that approximately 60 percent of Horsley's surgery concerned neurosurgery; the remaining 40 percent, general surgery. Horrax designated Horsley the founder of neurosurgery, a thesis with which Cushing apparently was in agreement.[39]

As early as 1905, Cushing favored considering neurosurgery as a surgical specialty. Cushing's silver clips and his development, with Bovie, of electrosurgery, providing cutting and coagulating currents, constituted very significant contributions to surgical hemostasis; they are used in surgery almost universally today. Probably more than any other individual Cushing developed techniques for the excision of all varieties of brain tumors that have served as models for neurosurgeons. His primary research interests concerned the hypophysis and the hypothalamus. One of Cushing's great contributions was the superb training he provided surgeons worldwide who were seeking careers in neurosurgery. Many of the famous neurosurgeons of the past four decades were trained by Cushing.[40]

Walter Dandy's imaginative work with air encephalograms, performed by spinal as well as by direct puncture of the cerebral ventricles, extended considerably the accuracy of diagnosing brain tumors. In sheer imaginative power and creative innova-

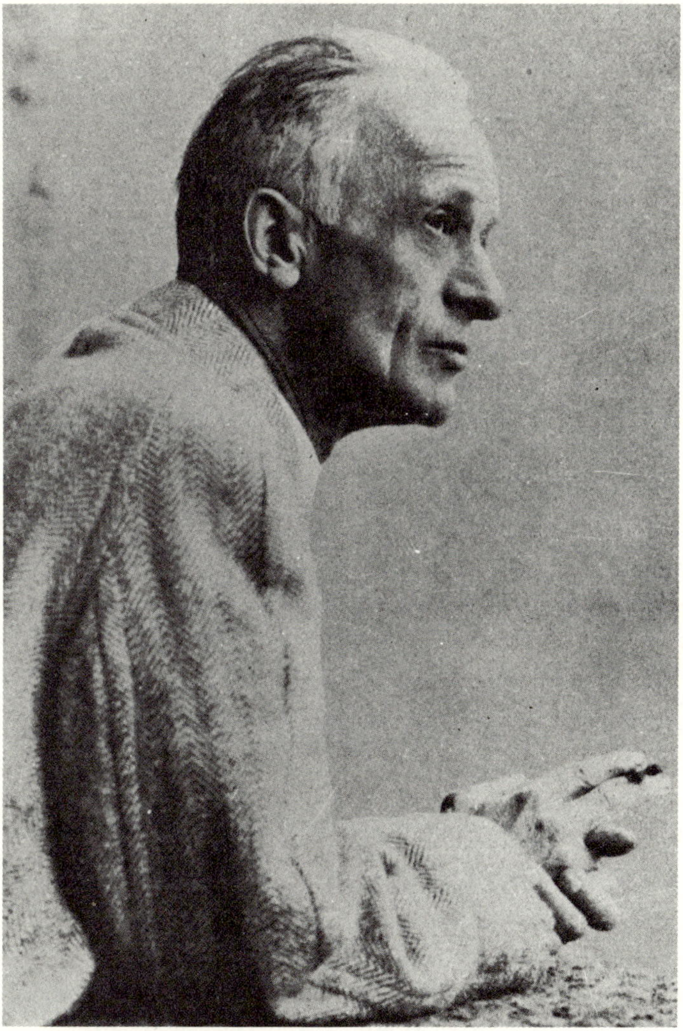

25.2 Harvey Cushing in 1929.

tions Dandy was probably Cushing's superior. It is tragic that two such great figures, both of whom originated in the Halsted Surgical School at The Hopkins, became bitter and lifelong enemies.[41]

The senior author has been witness to two bitter feuds between great American surgeons over the past dozen years; he suggested to the older, and presumptively the wiser, of the participants in the institutional struggles that they extend friendly handclasps to their opponents for the good of the great universities they were privileged to serve — a friendship can be carried unilaterally, making it easier for the other to resume it, when ready. Both attempts resulted in failure. Resentment and enmity beget bitterness which is not only self-defeating but which leaves a cloud over the departments and institutions involved that does not readily go away.

The first clinical objective evidence demonstrating the presence of brain tumors was provided by George Moore (1948), then a surgical intern at the University of Minnesota; he instituted cerebral roentgenography by adding radioactive iodine to fluorescein. On intravenous injection Moore observed an affinity of brain tumor tissue for radioactive iodine, eighty times the affinity of the adjacent normal tissue, making roentgenographic detection of neoplasms readily available.[42] With infiltrating gliomas, surgeons often had no way of ascertaining the limits of the tumor. Improved scanning techniques constitute one of the great advances in radiologic diagnosis, especially for neurosurgical lesions. More of these refined techniques are undoubtedly currently aborning.

When the senior author spent ten days in Cushing's clinic in September 1928, before the beginning of the fall school session, he was only one of two visitors at Cushing's operations. On completion of the visit, in thanking Dr. Cushing for his courtesy, the author asked how Cushing had recognized with such ease the limits of the several infiltrative brain tumors he had operated upon. Replied Cushing, "Experience." A more accurate statement undoubtedly would have been, "It is impossible," and is, in consequence, one of the real handicaps to achieving enduring cures in the management of such tumors. The greatest surgical accomplishment with brain tumors has been with well-circumscribed lesions, often benign in nature. Neurosurgery as a specialty undoubtedly owes more to Cushing than to any other individual. The demands upon neurosurgeons in skill and knowledge of minute anatomy are great, including a willingness to push on when the prospects appear unrewarding.

A few decades ago, neurosurgeons concerned themselves with division of the sympathetic nervous chain for a number of disorders including Raynaud's phenomenon and arterial hypertension. Today, with drugs that remove vasospastic factors, extensive operations for both those disorders are no longer performed. Reserpine, propranolol, and other vasodilating agents have replaced surgery. Neurosurgeons' development of techniques to deal with intracerebral aneurysm has been a nice achievement in recent decades, although Wilfred Trotter in 1924 successfully removed a correctly diagnosed intracerebral aneurysm and Norman Dott described a few successful cases more than four decades ago.[43]

Division of the sensory root of the fifth cranial for trigeminal neuralgia was introduced by W. G. Spiller and Frazier (1901). Cushing had extirpated the Gasserian ganglion for the same purpose a year earlier (1900), an operation that did not survive because of the frequency with which loss of sensation of the cornea was followed by keratitis. Division of the sensory root of the trigeminal nerve, sparing the ophthalmic fibers as well as the motor root, became standard procedure in the hands of Frazier and others. A. M. Dogliotti (1931) introduced subarachnoid alcohol injections for peripheral painful neuritis, a scheme subsequently adapted for injection of the root of the trigeminal nerve through the infraorbital foramen. Suture of peripheral motor nerves, such as the dorsal interosseous of the radial, has regularly produced excellent results; suture of mixed motor and sensory nerves is less likely to be accompanied by a perfect functional result. The success of Malt (1964) and others in restoring motor and sensory function in severed arms by careful replantation of the extremity, with resuture of nerves and reestablishment of the circulation, was mentioned earlier in this chapter.[44] Only time will determine whether the results of the procedure justify its adoption by the profession.

The important innovation of the Vienna otologist Oscar Hirsch, who dealt with acromegaly through the transnasal approach, deserves mention. When he presented his experience at the otological section of the Thirteenth International Congress of Medicine in London in 1913, Cushing came to hear him. Hirsch retold the story in 1959; the subtitle indicated he had followed thirty-three patients for twenty to thirty-seven years.[45]

The senior author had the privilege of seeing the talented and skillful surgeons Trotter and Percy Sargent perform several operations at London hospitals in August 1928. On one occasion, at the National Hospital for the Paralyzed and Epileptics at Queen Square, Sargent deftly removed an extradural tumor compressing the spinal cord at a high dorsal level. Charles Ballance, an impressive figure, then age sixty-three and still active in surgery, was present and remarked that he had successfully removed a very similar tumor at the identical thoracic level in the same hospital several years before.

One of the most frequently performed operations by

neurosurgeons is the removal of loose cartilage from a prolapsed intervertebral disk, a common cause of backache, a phenomenon described by Dandy in 1929.[46]

Urology

Max Nitze (1848–1906) of Vienna developed an electrically lighted cystoscope in 1877, which marked the beginnings of urology as a specialty of surgery.[47] Nevertheless, in many areas the urologist remained for long years essentially a diagnostician of urologic disorders. In his presidential address to the American Urological Association, Hugh Cabot (1911), then of Boston, asked: "Is urology entitled to be regarded as a specialty?" He answered in the affirmative but said, "until within the last few months there was not in New England a single large hospital making any separate or distinct provision for the study of urology except in the out-patient department, and no surgeon controlled any beds for the prosecution of this work." Cabot's plea was that urology should be regarded as a specialty, that those practicing it should be well versed in all the skills necessary for diagnosis and treatment of patients under their care. Cabot cited specifically prostatic disease, stone in the bladder, and renal disease.

Cabot said that almost universally surgeons with urologic training undertook all the diagnostic procedures, but when it came to operation the patient had to be turned over to a general surgeon. The time had come, insisted Cabot, when urologists should be sufficiently trained in operative techniques to undertake the entire care of the patient. J. Bentley Squier of New York reminded urologists that they first needed training in operative techniques, acquired on assignments in general surgery.[48]

Young's development of endovesical punch prostatectomy (1913) and Stern's (1926) creation of an instrument with an electrical current for removing prostatic obstructions finally brought operative urology out of the hands of the general surgeon, establishing urology as an independent discipline, represented by talented and skilled surgeons.[49]

Thomas Edison's invention of the incandescent lamp (1879), one of the great innovations of the final quarter of the nineteenth century, made it possible to place the light source at the distal end of endoscopes, dispensing with the need to reflect light by mirrors through the endoscopic tube.[50]

Gynecology and Obstetrics

Howard A. Kelly of The Hopkins viewed gynecology remaining as a surgical specialty independent of both obstetrics and general surgery. Said Kelly (1922), "Is she [gynecology] destined to live a spinster all her days? . . . on one hand courted by her obstetrical ancestor, who seeks to draw her once more into an unholy, unfruitful alliance . . . sucking the withered ancestral finger in the vain hope of nourishment . . . we see her wooed by a vigorous manly suitor, General Surgery, seeking to allure her from her autonomy into his own house, under his own name, obliterating her identity."[51]

Among American medical schools, there are, today, few arrangements in which obstetrics and gynecology are independent separate departments. Kelly very obviously underrated the great promise of obstetrics, which has had a flourishing record in recent decades in the reduction of both maternal and infant mortality during the perinatal period, and a viable interest in population control.

Obstetrics has had a long struggle for recognition in general hospitals, notably in England. Undoubtedly, one of the significant deterrents to recognition of obstetrics as a specialty deserving professional status in medical faculties in England was its close alignment with medicine rather than with surgery. Physicians tended to believe that midwives were quite adequate to deal with parturients. Henry Halford (1827), for twenty-four consecutive years president of the Royal College of Physicians, remarked, "Obstetrics is not for gentlemen" and wrote to Sir Robert Peel, "midwifery is an act foreign to the habits of gentlemen of enlarged academic education." Sir Anthony Carlisle (1834), president of the Royal College of Surgeons, advised Peel, "It is an imposture to pretend that a medical man is required at a labour."[52] Obstetrics was not granted a royal charter until 1942. The long delay and opposition came in part from the Royal College of Surgeons, which felt that obstetricians and gynecologists should have experience in general surgery. England today recognizes a Royal College of Obstetricians and Gynaecologists. The need for obstetricians to assume a posture as surgeons indicates that a closer affiliation with surgery rather than with medicine is definitely in order. Obstetricians like other surgical specialists obviously need exposure to acquire skill in surgical techniques.[53]

It does take time and practice for any surgeon to become

adept at surgical techniques reflecting obvious manifestations of expertise, accuracy, and delicacy of execution. The current-day obstetrician-gynecologist is emerging as a competent surgeon. The record of gynecologist-surgeons in dealing with vesico-vaginal fistula (1852), ovariotomy, ectopic pregnancy, and cesarean section in the twentieth century attests to their competence, as indicated in chapters 10 through 13 of this book.

Once Popular Operations

Abdominal organ suspension was a popular operation fifty years ago. In his widely read two-volume text on abdominal operations, Moynihan (1926) devoted twenty pages to the subject.[54] The two chief proponents of such operations were R. C. Coffey of Portland, Oregon, and Thorskild Rovsing of Copenhagen. The procedure that survived the longest was uterine suspension, which a number of American gynecologists enthusiastically endorsed for uterine prolapse. In the late 1920s the senior author was visited by a well-known Swedish general surgeon who wished to look in on operations in progress. On examining the morning's operating list, it was noted that five uterine suspensions were on the schedule. The author tried unsuccessfully to explain to his visitor what the gynecologists proposed to do. The visitor replied, "I have practiced surgery in Sweden for more than a quarter century and have never seen the operation performed." Uterine suspension died slowly in America.

In September 1927 the senior author had the privilege of spending an entire day with the chef de clinique, making ward rounds at the Rigshopitälet in Copenhagen. As we completed a very interesting day the author remarked to the senior resident, "You have not shown me a single instance of organ suspension." After a brief, thoughtful interlude, he replied, "Professor Rovsing has been dead six months." Even for acceptable operations, we still hear it said that indications for such procedures are often overused. Our profession is not inattentive to such criticisms. Tonsillectomy is a case in point, as is hysterectomy, each less frequently performed today than a decade ago.

Hemorrhoids: Return to Conservatism

Perusal of the management of hemorrhoids over many centuries indicates that treatment has been largely conservative. However, in the second half of the nineteenth century and during the first half of the twentieth, there emerged an attitude of aggressiveness among surgeons and proctologists in hemorrhoid therapy. Lesser numbers of patients with this ailment are scheduled for hemorrhoidectomy in our hospitals today than was customary in the first few decades of this century. Whether patients with hemorrhoids are being treated in the offices of proctologists by more conservative means is perhaps a good question. Certainly in recent times there has been a tendency to revert to the old Hippocratic method of ligating hemorrhoids.

One unfortunate effect of both clamp and cautery as well as excision is that normal rectal mucosa is destroyed; exposure of the hemorrhoidal veins attending incision of the mucosa, followed by ligature of submucosal vessels, is a more anatomical procedure. Two decades ago, the senior author suggested that many operations for hemorrhoids were unnecessary.[55] It is to be freely admitted that external thrombotic piles need emergency surgery for the relief of pain, that bleeding and prolapsing hemorrhoids require operative treatment. However, the very presence of hemorrhoids is not an indication for operation. Hemorrhoids are owing largely to the circumstance that the veins of the body cavities have no valves. In the sitting and standing postures, there is, therefore, a stagnant column of blood approximately 40 cms. in height, causing engorgement of the rectal mucosa; moreover, unlike the lower extremity where the same postural disadvantage obtains, the rectum is devoid of voluntary muscles that can urge on the venous column of blood. A day or two of recumbency in bed with the buttocks elevated on a few pillows beneath the groin, and the foot of the bed raised, often works miracles in reducing hemorrhoidal swelling.

Henry Smith (1823–94) of King's College Hospital, London, wrote in 1863 of three hundred operations for hemorrhoids in which the clamp and cautery were used. Smith had used the substance of these materials in his Lettsomian Lecture of 1855, when he had had experience with only thirty-eight cases; the results were so good that he was persuaded to continue. The operation, said Smith, could be done in five, ten, or fifteen minutes, depending on the magnitude of the problem. He had lost three patients following the treatment; one died with severe vomiting and intense jaundice on the fifth day, undoubtedly of sepsis — Smith raised the question of liver injury from chloroform.[56] Smith, a bluff and breezy man who retired from his professorship at King's in 1887, is quoted as saying, "hemorrhoids are a significant source of income." It would be unjust to attach his suggestion as a frequent indication for the procedure of hemorrhoidectomy, but a critical and periodic reassessment of indications for many operations is our profession's responsibility.[57]

Fragmentation of General Surgery

Specialization and the development of subspecialties have made great inroads upon the broad territories presided over by general surgeons in the first three decades of this century. The ophthalmoscope, the laryngoscope, and the otoscope created firm specialties in those areas in the nineteenth century. The first secessionists among disciplines still allied to general surgery were the classical specialties of plastic surgery, orthopedics, neurosurgery, urology, and gynecology; since then, splinter groups have formed within the very heart of the more recently acquired operative territory presided over by general surgeons. Such creations and extensions of general surgery as thoracic, peripheral vascular, and intracardiac surgery are now recognized specialties asserting their independence; some have established Certification Boards of their own. Thoracic surgery became a rising specialty in this country half a century ago; peripheral vascular and intracardiac surgery, in the early 1950s. All were once firmly rooted in the province of general surgery. Some still profess a loose attachment to the parent order. Transplantation surgery, still closely attached to general surgery, may presently elect to be known as a distinct specialty.

In consequence, general surgery, a contracting field, concerns itself primarily with abdominal surgery, and even therein a few subspecialties are staking out special provinces. Surgery of the thyroid, the endocrine system (including parathyroid, adrenal, and pancreatic tumors), and the breast and management of cancer of organs within the territorial areas of the neck, chest wall, and abdomen still claim the attention of general surgeons. Proctology, once a lowly branch of general surgery, today is beginning to assert claims to the entire colon and the rectum as its legitimate province. One dividend from this latter aggression will undoubtedly be fewer operations for hemorrhoids, in many instances an unnecessary operation, as King's College surgeon Henry Smith insisted more than a century ago.

Specialties and subspecialties no longer depend completely on general surgery for instruction and orientation in the principles of surgery for their own protégés, feeling they can do it about as well themselves. Obviously, the residual territory and functions of the general surgeon will need periodic redefinition. It, like its many offshoots, may also become a surgical specialty. Pushed upon from every side, general surgery aspires to be a comfortable colleague to its numerous progeny; it continues to have an important role in medical faculties and the curriculum. In Germany and Japan general surgeons often cultivate a collateral interest in another specialty such as urology, orthopedics, pathology, or radiology related to their primary professional interest.

General surgery has had a great seminal influence in generating ideas for progress and for the extension of the borders of surgery. Academician representatives of general surgery must continue to mount the watchtowers of scientific progress for signs and evidences of new approaches for the resolution of enigmatic problems. If general surgery can maintain its creative and innovative spirit, perhaps the spawning of new disciplines will become its most important function.

The senior author (1969) advocated development of a triennial American Congress of Surgery including all surgical specialties. The purpose of such sessions would be to exchange ideas; each specialty would have its representatives present two papers, one to emphasize problems peculiar to the specialty and the other to deal with advances within the disciplines.[58] As yet, there has been no suggestion of acceptance of the idea by prestigious surgical groups such as the American Surgical Association or the American College of Surgeons. Until his retirement from active surgery, Cushing continued to urge a closer alliance of physicians and surgeons. The more pressing problem for surgery today is, Can it survive as a unified body? Periodic free intercommunication could serve as a very useful device to ensure that survival. An annual meeting of family clans, widely separated geographically, does promote understanding and tolerance. Tight compartmentalization of disciplines stifles growth; cross-pollination, the true catalyst of life, emerging from such sessions could prove beneficial to all surgical specialties, ensuring their continued advance and growth. Surgery definitely needs fewer walls and more bridges between its many disciplines.

Summary

Therapeutic specialization by organ existed in ancient Egypt, for eyes, teeth, head, and other body segments. In the Hippocratic writings medicine and surgery were a unified body of knowledge. In America most physicians engaged in a general type of medical practice well into the twentieth century. Even professors of surgery did general or family practice in addition to surgery.

Ophthalmology, among the oldest of surgical specialties, emerged as a strict surgical specialty with the development of the ophthalmoscope by Helmholtz in 1851. Even so, several surgeons in universities held the rank of professor of surgery and ophthalmology well into this century, especially in Germany. Koller's introduction of cocaine as a local anesthetic for eye operations (1884) lent a strong forward thrust to the discipline. Special hospitals for diseases of the eye evolved in Britain and America. Albrecht Graefe, son of Carl Graefe, who had been professor of surgery and ophthalmology in Berlin from 1810 to 1840, emerged as probably the most innovative of all ophthalmologists. He became professor of ophthalmology in the University of Berlin at age twenty-six; he was trained largely by observing the work of distinguished ophthalmologists of Europe and Britain. His contributions to the discipline were various and significant. Today, well-trained ophthalmologists dot the geography of the world.

The laryngoscope devised by the Spanish singing master Garcia (1854–55) established laryngology as a specialty. Formidable operations upon the larynx, such as laryngectomy, were performed into this century by general surgeons in several countries including our own. In recent years laryngologists have been gradually acquiring the techniques of dealing with major laryngeal surgical problems, including radical cervical lymph node excision.

Troeltsch invented the otoscope (1860) and was the first to perform radical mastoidectomy in 1869, creating the specialty of otology. Great advances in the pathology and treatment of otosclerosis have come about in recent decades, bringing relief to many deaf and hard-of-hearing people. Otologists were among the first to adopt low-power magnification to facilitate their operations and to enhance the performance factor.

Plastic surgery shares with ophthalmology the distinction of being one of the oldest surgical specialties. Well-vascularized pedicled skin grafts are among the oldest operations of plastic surgery employed to repair cutaneous defects about the face. Free skin grafts were developments of the 1870s; autogenous grafts when well performed are almost uniformly successful; cutaneous allografts, on the contrary, invariably fail. Padgett demonstrated (1932) that skin grafts between identical twins succeed, a thesis put to the test by the London plastic surgeon McIndoe (1950) in a legal action involving confusion of babies born in the same hospital on the same day. The cutaneous grafts were successful only between the true identical twins. In renal and cardiac transplants the rejection phenomenon can be greatly ameliorated by treating the recipient of organ grafts with immunosuppressive agents. One of the striking developments in recent years has been autoreplantation of severed extremities by Malt (1964, 1972) and his Boston associates, an activity that has found wide application in several hospitals in China. The profession still awaits reports of restoration of motor power and sensation, the hallmarks of complete function.

No surgical specialty has extended its role of activity as widely as has orthopedic surgery since World War II. It has completely absorbed the management of fractures, infections, and injuries of the hand. The French orthopedist Ollier obtained satisfactory functional results with arthroplasty of the elbow in the final decades of the nineteenth century. Over the past ten years the British orthopedist Charnley has perfected a technique of arthroplasty for arthritic hips that has proved a great boon to many patients with painful stiff hip joints. The dependence of orthopedics upon general surgery admitted by keen representatives of the discipline half a century ago has completely disappeared.

Horsley of London is usually cited as the founder of neurosurgery, upon which he began concentrating in the last decade of the nineteenth century. He never did limit his work to that discipline as Cushing began to do in 1905. Because of his many significant contributions to the field as well as his influence on the lives of many of today's finest neurosurgeons the world over, many attribute to Cushing the greatest impact upon the discipline. Dandy, who like Cushing was a Halsted trainee, contributed important innovative diagnostic techniques to the specialty. Moore devised the first objective technological demonstration of cancer; employing an intravenous injection of radioactive fluorescein. Moore observed that cerebral neoplasms could readily be identified on roentgen examination owing to a significantly greater absorption of the agent by the tumor, contrasted with the adjacent normal tissue.

When Nitze of Vienna developed an electrically lighted cystoscope (1877), urology as a specialty had its beginnings. Edison's discovery of the incandescent lamp (1879) dispensed with the need for reflecting light to the distal end of the cystoscope by a system of mirrors. Yet leaders in urology remained essentially diagnosticians in their specialty for the first three decades of this century; general surgeons performed needed surgery upon bladder, ureter, and kidney. The development of the electrically operated resectoscope for prostatectomy gradually made urology a complete and independent discipline.

Obstetrics, long the province of the midwife and the family physician, has finally gained recognition as a specialty, even in England, where an independent royal charter for the discipline was first obtained in 1942. The striking accomplishments of obstetricians with cesarean section and ectopic gestation in recent decades are not surpassed in the field of surgery. One of the difficulties in England was that obstetrics was more closely identified with medicine than with surgery. In this country, too, in many areas gynecology remained a separate surgical specialty, distinctly apart from obstetrics. This arrangement is being changed, with a closer realignment of obstetrics and gynecology as a unified department. The profession has been slow to recognize the significant contributions of obstetricians to greater medicine, more important than the largely technical offerings of gynecologists in the management of malignancies of the female sex organs, in which areas radiologists and chemotherapists too have come to play increasingly important roles.

Half a century ago organ suspension was a popular operation. The last to be abandoned was uterine suspension, long defended by gynecologists. Tonsillectomy is performed far less often today than a decade ago. Hemorrhoidectomy, treated largely by conservative measures for centuries, in the last half of the nineteenth century and the first half of this century became a popular surgical procedure; today, performance of hemorrhoidectomy in our hospitals is being confined once more to strict indications.

The process of surgical fragmentation into specialties and subspecialties continues. Only free intercommunication of all surgical specialties can ensure the survival of surgery as a unified discipline.

(For notes, see pp. 712–16.)

CHAPTER 26

Retrospect and Prospect

Retrospect

THE HISTORY of advance in any discipline is the story of individuals of imagination and accomplishment who left their mark upon its development. The slow progress of surgery before the full acceptance of prophylactic antisepsis was owing in large measure to the reluctance of surgeons to subject suggested innovations to trial, preferring debate and argument.

Many surgeons of the eighteenth and nineteenth centuries were good anatomists and reasonably competent pathologists; a few were good physiologists, notably John Hunter and Bernard; several medical historians of the nineteenth century were surgeon-scholars, including Malgaigne, Gurlt, Sudhoff, J. S. Billings, and Pétrequin. Only a few surgeons in the mid-nineteenth century had training in research techniques, notably Lister in physiology and Billroth in surgical pathology. None of the early innovative microscopists was a surgeon. The first surgeon-microbiologist was Lister, whose entire professional career from 1858 to well beyond his 1893 retirement reflected an active participation in the practical aspects of microbiology. Billroth, primarily an innovative visceral surgeon and surgical pathologist, at one time in his career worked on microbiological problems and the nature of surgical fever, but he made no significant contribution to the advance of microbiology. Ogston (1881) of Aberdeen, a broadly trained surgeon, did accelerate surgeons' acceptance of the germ theory of infection by demonstration of the constant presence of staphylococci in abscesses and by quantitative studies on the number of bacteria in pus. Fortunately, in recent decades, there have been many surgeon-microbiologists in several countries, particularly in Britain and North America, helping to focus attention upon likely sources of wound infection, its prevention and management.

Only in the last fifty years have academic surgeons in this country been exposed to disciplines other than their own, especially during the past quarter century. The surgeon determined to stay in the academic arena obviously needs wide training in one or more of the basic medical disciplines if he hopes to contribute significantly to surgery's advance; in any case, his chances of adding to the patrimony of his discipline are enhanced thereby, including the replication of creative protégés. Nevertheless, we shall always expect to see occasionally the untutored novice with a perceptive and penetrating intuition discerning a way to resolve an enigmatic problem and acquiring the methodology to accomplish it. Unfortunately, such clairvoyance is not a daily phenomenon. Chance does favor the prepared mind, as Pasteur reminded us.

Paré, as early as 1536, had come to trust his own observations as the most reliable guideline for his surgical practice, abandoning traditional considerations that conflicted with his observations, accepting what he saw rather than seeing what he believed — the latter thesis unfortunately still dominated the thinking of many surgical leaders through the first three-quarters of the nineteenth century. Perusal of the early chapters in this text will suffice to indicate that consistent success with most operative procedures had to await prophylactic antisepsis.

This recital, assessing items contributing to the rise of surgery, began with an appraisal of the results of emergency surgery over the centuries and traced the long story of wound management in urgent situations, with primary emphasis upon the eighteenth and nineteenth centuries. Empiricism, without guidelines, was attended by chaotic confusion over the question of how best to deal with soft tissue wounds. The principles of treatment of simple fractures, on the contrary, have remained much the same, although the methods of achieving those ends have improved greatly. For centuries surgeons relied entirely on improvements in technical skills for advances in their discipline; their knowledge of anatomy, of the course of blood vessels and nerves, was of tremendous help in extremity surgery, enabling many a skilled surgeon to amputate an arm, leg, or thigh with record speed. Even so, such operations failed to reduce the overall mortality of amputation.

One of the impediments to progress was that general accountability came only with the emergence of microbiology, the demonstration of the pathogenicity of bacteria, and the development of elective surgery. To be certain, there were a few eighteenth-century surgeons with unusual accomplishments, able to report astounding results with amputation and lithotomy, unrivaled until prophylactic surgical antisepsis was generally adopted in the mid-1880s. In fact, a seventeenth-century surgeon, Woodall, author of *Surgeons Mate*, reported (1639) an amputation mortality of no greater than 20 percent in operations performed over a twenty-four-year period at St. Bartholomew's Hospital. Woodall, like Paré, was an early convert to the practice of placing turpentine in operative wounds and on wound dressings. The successes, it is to be noted, were solely with extracavitary surgery. Consistent good results with intraperitoneal operations would not be achieved until the arrival of elective surgery.

"Minute particulars" was a phrase used by Paré (1579) to account for his successes; Monro I credited "little circumstances." Monro's (1737, 1752) report of an 8 percent mortality from amputation at Edinburgh's Royal Infirmary was not exceeded until the acceptance of prophylactic surgical antisepsis more than 130 years later. Pouteau (1769) was an ardent advocate of cleanliness in surgery, including the hands. His achievement of a 2.5 percent mortality rate for perineal lithotomy was not equaled by the finest lithotomists of the nineteenth century. Delpech (1815), Ollivier (1822), and a few other surgeons insisted that communication of infection in wounds between surgical patients was owing to direct contact, a thesis proposed by Fracastoro (1546) more than two and a half centuries earlier.

Open management of contaminated wounds, tracing back to Guy de Chauliac (1363), produced results in the hands of a few surgeons in the first half of the nineteenth century, notably Kern (1826) of Vienna, Liston (1837, 1841) of London, and Burow (1859) of Königsberg, rivaling the achievements of the early proponents of antisepsis. This circumstance occasioned Billroth to insist, before giving Lister's antiseptic methods a trial, that open wound management was at least as good. Placement of antiseptics into wounds is of empirical origin and dates from antiquity.

Reyher, an accomplished but long neglected Russian military

surgeon, spent four weeks with Lister in Edinburgh early in 1874 and attended the German Surgical Congress in Berlin that April. There, Reyher, aged twenty-eight, announced his conviction of the value of Listerian practices, which more experienced surgeons throughout the world were condemning without benefit of trial. In 1876, Reyher demonstrated the superiority of Listerian wound methods over open wound management. The strong support of two well-known German professors of surgery, Volkmann (1874) of Halle and Nussbaum (1875) of Munich, provided Listerian practices the propellant thrust needed to convince other European surgeons.

The most significant observation to emerge from this historical quest is the primacy of the doctrine of Semmelweis (1847) in initiating prophylactic antisepsis. In fact, his practices constitute the very core of modern-day surgery. Semmelweis's emphasis was on precluding the entry of bacteria into wounds rather than on attempting to destroy them after they entered the wound, a salient feature of Lister's practices during his entire professional career. In 1919 Fleming, an ardent student of wound infections in World War I, urged rejection of placement of antiseptics into wounds, finding that all antiseptics did more harm to tissues than to bacteria. Whereas Lister's unique role in urging acceptance of antiseptic hospital practices was an important factor in improving the salubrity of hospitals, his wound techniques left much to be desired. Even so, the practice of irrigating wounds with Dakin's solution, a variant of Listerism, continued until specific antibacterial agents, the sulfonamides and antibiotics, became available to thwart infection in contaminated wounds.

One of the great surgical surprises of the early nineteenth century was McDowell's successful removal of a huge ovarian cyst (1809) in Danville, Kentucky, then an American outpost, at a time when the operation had not yet been tried by European surgeons. In fact, it was only after McDowell's report of three consecutive successes (1817) that ovariotomy was attempted by better-known surgeons in Britain, Europe, and North America.

Bloodletting after operations dates from antiquity. At the beginning of the nineteenth century Physick of Philadelphia employed extensive phlebotomy, up to two liters, as a device to provoke muscle relaxation and insensitivity to pain in the reduction of longstanding dislocations of extremities, a method that greatly facilitated its achievement and a procedure emulated by others before surgical anesthesia (1846). Physick's obstetrical colleague, Dewees, employed the method in difficult and protracted labor, holding that it quickened delivery and hurried relaxation of the perineal muscles and the uterine cervix.

The fruitful studies of the American army surgeon Beaumont (1833) on the nature of gastric secretion, pursued in the wilderness of Michigan and Wisconsin, will remain a great historic achievement. Anesthesia, however, was America's most important contribution to the progress of surgery;[1] ether was first employed for surgery by Long (1842) of Jefferson, Georgia, who failed to publish until 1849. The major credit for this significant innovation, in the judgment of contemporaries, was assigned to the Boston dentist Morton (1846). The very circumstance that ether and chloroform have been supplanted in current hospital practice by nitrous oxide, which Wells, another contender for the honor, had used successfully in 1844, definitely suggests that Wells deserved to be recognized in the partition of honors. His innovation has proved the more durable; perhaps in time it too will be replaced by an even more acceptable anesthetic agent.

Another important early American contribution to surgery's advance was the demonstration by Sims (1852) of Montgomery, Alabama, of a practical method of closing vesicovaginal fistulas, a crippling affliction of many parturients over the centuries. The repair of such a fistula, an extraperitoneal operation, could be done without great risk to life before the arrival of surgical antisepsis. A succession of failures had almost invariably attended attempts at closure by renowned plastic surgeons, notably Dieffenbach (1836) of Berlin. Sims's success was owing to use of the knee-chest posture that provided excellent exposure and of fine silver sutures that did not invite suppuration as did linen and silk in nonsterile operations antedating antiseptic practices.

The operation for aneurysm of the second-century Greek surgeon Antyllus was reborn in the hands of the American Matas (1888). The London surgeon Abernethy (1796) found it was safer to accompany ligature of large arteries for aneurysm by proximal division, a practice later adopted by Astley Cooper (1814) but completely overlooked by several generations of accomplished vascular surgeons, including Guthrie, Mott, and Halsted. Holman (1942) demonstrated experimentally that the great hazard of hemorrhage from ligature of large arteries could usually be avoided by concomitant division, not realizing that Abernethy had arrived at the same conclusion a century and a half earlier. Present-day achievements with aneurysm of the abdominal and thoracic aorta are astounding, reflecting surgery's growth since World War II.

An interesting fact turned up by this study was the Hippocratic admonition against external open drainage of empyema until the exudate acquired some density, about the fifteenth day; in the interval trocar drainage was employed. Sédillot (1841) rediscovered this Hippocratic doctrine as did the historian Littré (1861), after which the practice was completely forgotten. Graham and Bell (1918) established the validity and rationale of closed catheter or needle aspiration drainage for the serous exudates of streptococcal empyemas of World War I, followed by dependent open drainage when 50 percent of the exudate was thick cellular debris.

A primary concern of this effort has been to trace the development and role of microbiology in the evolution of surgery. It would be a serious oversight not to mention a few great scientists whose work in collateral fields influenced significantly the progress of medicine. A poignant lesson of history is how dependent advances in any discipline are upon the status of existing knowledge and achievement in related fields. How effective could the incisive thinking and creative experiments of Bernard have been had he lived a century earlier? Certainly not of the same order.

Bernard (1813–78), the first full-time professional physiologist in France, had seriously considered becoming a clinical surgeon. With Charles Huette he had written a nicely illustrated monograph on operative techniques of surgery (1848), a copy of which was put into the hands of every Union surgeon in the Civil War. At age forty Bernard (1853) decided on a career in physiology, a decision that left medicine the richer. In clarity of thinking and intuitive reasoning in pursuit of a problem, followed by the creation of critical experiments to test his hypotheses, Bernard has not been excelled. He also was a superb anatomist. Magendie had selected Bernard as his preparateur of physiologic experiments because of his unique skill in dissection. While a substitute lecturer for Magendie in 1847, Bernard said to his students, "Scientific medicine, which it is my duty to teach you, does not exist."[2] His insight and significant experiments helped establish medicine on a scientific basis. Great experimentalist that he was, he had not accepted surgical antisepsis, an innovation in experimental surgery invoked by Heidenhain in 1878.

The first controlled clinical experiment in the annals of medicine was probably Lind's (1753) observation that sailors affected with scurvy were cured and seaworthy within six days when given two oranges and a lemon each day. He took to sea

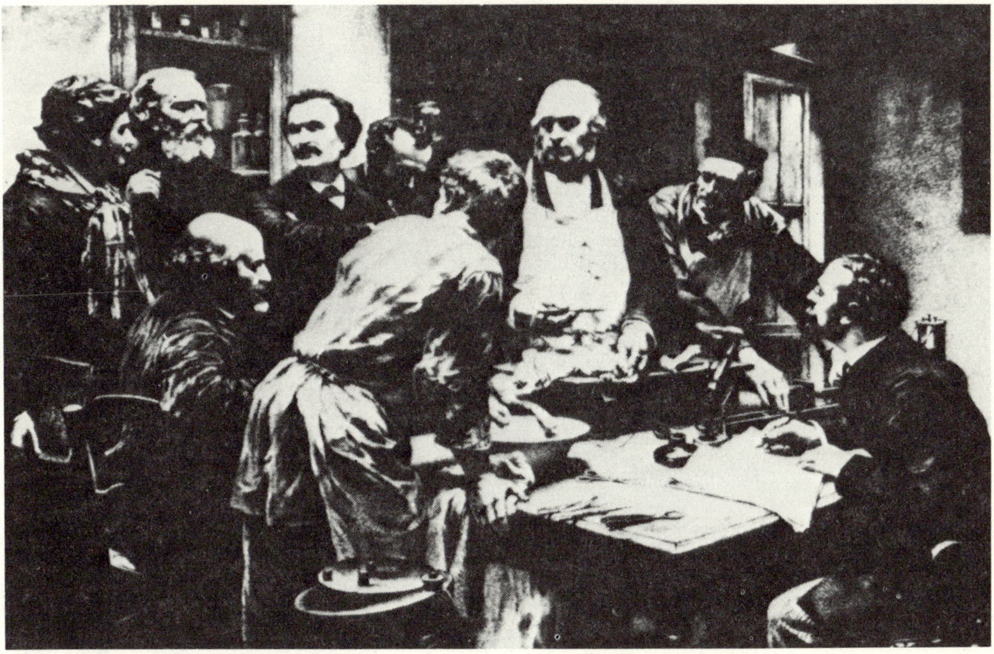

26.1 Claude Bernard, one of the first full-time professional physiologists, and his pupils. Photographed from the engraving by l'Hermite and presented to the authors by Franz Halbert, 1965.

twelve sailors with scurvy and divided them into six groups of two each. All received a very similar basic navy ration with specified additives. The sailors in the five groups not receiving citrus additives were unimproved. Balduinus Ronsseus (1564) and Woodall (1617) had made somewhat similar observations, but Lind proved his case with the aid of controls.[3] Even so, through the Napoleonic Wars and our own Civil War, scurvy remained prevalent.

Perhaps no discovery has influenced the fate of armies for the better so much as did Jenner's (1798) prophylactic inoculation against smallpox, an innovation Napoleon fully appreciated. "Anything Jenner wants shall be granted. He has been my most faithful servant in the European campaigns," said Napoleon when Jenner wrote to ask for the release of an imprisoned British officer.[4] The salvage of life, both military and civil, through smallpox inoculation has been tremendous. Smallpox once decimated populations; long prevalent in many countries of the world, it survives today only in Ethiopia, where through

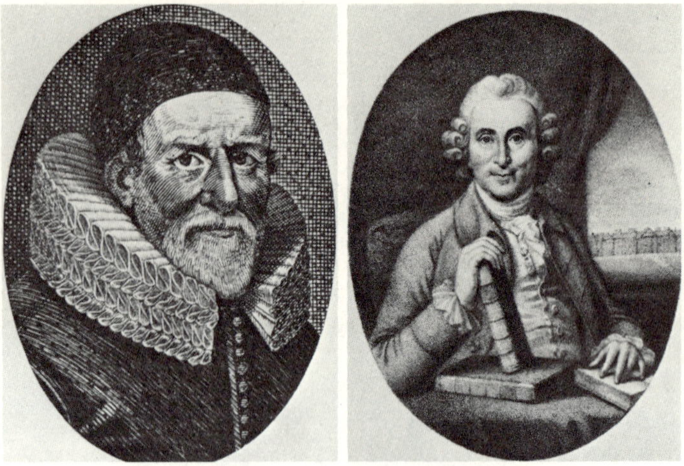

a b

26.2 **a.** John Woodall (1556–1643), great English military surgeon. **b.** James Lind in a simple controlled experiment established the role of lemon and lime juice in the prevention and cure of scurvy (1753).

public health measures it will presently be stamped out too.[5] Vaccination against smallpox is no longer compulsory in the United States. In many parts of the world, malaria continues to be the great crippler; it was an important contributing factor to the long delay in the completion of the Panama Canal.

In its struggle for advance, surgery has gained immeasurably by discoveries in other areas. The work of Heidenhain, Pavlov, Starling, and a host of more recent researchers has provided surgeons with unique physiologic guidelines to replace their empiric approaches to practical problems. What a lift to medicine's advance was the discovery of insulin by the orthopedic surgeon Frederick Banting (1922)! The first active parathyroid extract was the contribution of Adolph Hanson (1923),[6] a general surgeon of Faribault, Minnesota, reminiscent of the homespun accomplishments of McDowell in Kentucky, of Beaumont at Mackinac Island and at Fort Crawford in Prairie du Chien, of Long in Jefferson, of Sims in Montgomery, and of William and Charles Mayo in originating (1910–15) what has become one of the finest clinics in the world in Rochester, Minnesota. The pioneering innovative spirit of America stands out in each of these significant contributions. The experimental work of George Whipple with restoration of hemoglobin following hemorrhage through feeding with raw liver (1925), and similar management by George Minot and William Murphy of pernicious anemia (1926), led to the independent synthesis two decades later of vitamin B_{12} by E. L. Rickes and E. L. Smith (1948). William Castle's demonstration (1928–29) of the unique role of the gastric mucosa in sustaining normal hematopoiesis constituted an important link in understanding the genesis of pernicious anemia; it remains a classic in medical literature, underscoring the power of deductive reasoning verified by crucial experiments.[7]

Only surgeons who operated to relieve obstructive jaundice before 1940 can fully appreciate the protection afforded their patients by vitamin K, the discovery of the biochemists Carl Dam and E. A. Doisy (1939). Albert Szent-Györgyi (1928) identified vitamin C as a vital antiscorbutic agent and an important factor in wound healing. Cortisone (1936–39), the product of the Mayo Clinic investigators E. C. Kendall and P. S. Hench, and of the Swiss biochemist Tadeus Reichstein, has proved an invaluable agent in the success of organ transplantation, aided by azathioprine (imuran) and other suppressives in controlling rejection of foreign tissue.[8]

Since World War II, in academic medical centers almost worldwide, surgeons too have become far more research-minded, appreciating that it provides the surest means of advancing their discipline. The intimate cooperation of surgeons and physiologists since the mid-1930s at the University of Minnesota paid off handsomely in the 1950s, first in the use of the physicist Nier's mass spectrograph for the assessment of the concentration of inhaled anesthetic gases, subsequently in lending great impetus to the development of intracardiac surgery. Today the research-center multidisciplinary attack, crossing conventional departmental barriers, is being adopted as the most effective and reliable means of approaching enigmatic problems, such as the rejection of foreign tissue in transplantation, in which a host of compartmentalized segments of knowledge from anatomy to zoology are being applied. No one can predict which fusion of disciplines will ultimately contribute most to the solution of the riddle.

The surgeon's activity has been changed drastically by developments in other fields over the past several decades. His involvement in problems of bone and joint and lymph node tuberculosis has been completely suspended in Western countries by pasteurization of milk and elimination of bovine tuberculosis.[9] Similarly, pulmonary tuberculosis has been controlled in Western countries by isolation, streptomycin, and ancillary therapeutic agents, making pneumothorax, thoracoplasty, and excision of tuberculous lesions largely matters of past history. At the beginning of this century, tuberculosis was the leading cause of death in our country. The control of pneumonia has eliminated empyema, a few decades ago a challenging problem for surgeons. Bronchiectasis too has mysteriously disappeared, probably owing to the prevention of a number of childhood infections, especially measles and whooping cough.

The 1953–63 decade witnessed the elimination through research of that frightful crippler poliomyelitis, a truly great victory that put aside the once important commitment of orthopedic surgeons to the repair of incapacitating deformities. Immunization has made poliomyelitis in Western countries as rare as smallpox and typhoid fever,[10] achieving not only salvage of life but a great reduction in crippling disorders. The whole world applauds this achievement, a product of the research of John Enders and his associates, and of the vaccination programs of Albert Sabin and Jonas Salk.[11]

The definition by David Marine (1926, 1935) and others of the daily iodine requirements of man (0.04–0.08 mg.) has eliminated endemic goiter and changed materially the address of surgeons to thyroid disease.[12] In fact, prevention and prophylaxis more and more will become medicine's primary approach to challenging diseases.

John Hunter looked upon recourse to surgical operations as a recognition of defeat. Physicians and surgeons are often in disagreement about the management of several diseases, notably peptic ulcer and gallstones and other abdominal ills. Victory can come only when preventative measures eliminate the need for aggressive action. The events of the past quarter century indicate that whereas the need for surgical intervention has been eliminated in certain sectors, surgery has extended its range importantly and usefully in two previously unexplored areas, intracardiac surgery and organ transplantation. When homografts of skin can be effectively transferred between individuals, what a blessing it will be for persons who sustain extensive burns; it will certainly simplify significantly the surgeon's accomplishment with this defiant menace.

However important Lister's teachings and practices were in his day, the placement of antiseptics in wounds is definitely in eclipse. Moreover, in the minds of many surgeons and microbiologists, the role of the air in operating suites as a source of wound infection has been relegated to secondary considerations. At the 1971 meeting in Moscow of the International Surgical

Society, however, a number of distinguished British microbiologist-surgeons presented papers indicating their belief in the thesis that continued attack upon operating room and hospital air is important in the elimination of surgical wound infections.[13] These expressions are by no means universally accepted; even so, we must applaud efforts directed at eliminating all sources of infection during operation. The most likely source of wound infection is unquestionably the operating team. Surgeons' acceptance of mandated silence from all participants when operations are in progress may prove an important step in eliminating the operating room as a source of wound infection in elective surgery. The examples of Würtz (1563), Fergusson (1867), and Cushing (1928) and the experiments of Flügge and Mikulicz (1897) speak forcibly to the issue.

The two-stage elective operation for a number of surgical disorders was accepted practice through the first three decades of this century. Howard Lilienthal (1910) of New York stressed the advantage of such an attack for a host of conditions needing surgical relief.[14] With definition of the fluid and electrolyte requirements of patients, and greatly improved preoperative as well as postoperative treatment, the same situations today are almost invariably amenable to one-stage operative procedures, an occurrence that serves to emphasize the steady progress of surgery as its outlook has been guided increasingly by factual scientific data and the elimination of empiricism.

The science of microbiology emerged in the last quarter of the nineteenth century as mankind's greatest benefactor, owing primarily to the pioneer work of Pasteur and Koch, and their demonstration of the pathogenicity of bacteria. The significance of their labors for contemporary medicine and surgery is a continuing, beneficial influence manifest each day in every clinic of the world.

Research and technical advances have accelerated specialization in surgery. Ophthalmology and plastic surgery began to emerge as strong independent surgical specialties in the final decades of the nineteenth century. A new diagnostic tool, such as the ophthalmoscope, laryngoscope, otoscope, and cystoscope, often sounded the beginning of the separation of a special discipline from its parent, general surgery. Since World War II, newfound knowledge gained through research has accelerated the fission process, which obviously will continue endlessly into the future as research opens up new vistas.

Prospect

The vast array of individuals parading through the history of any scientific discipline over the centuries is impressive; many have contributed their mite to lessening the limitless area of the topography of ignorance. Then periodically there streaks across the firmament a person who sees far beyond the range of vision of the day the promise of a new approach for the resolution of unsettled problems. These men and women constitute the very substance and essence of history. These dreaming and discerning Josephs, sidestepping convention and tradition, unfortunately cross the horizon of time too infrequently and unpredictably. The penetrating discernment and capacity for synthesis of observations of a Semmelweis, the enthusiasm and originality of a Pasteur, the persistence of a Lister, the incisiveness of thought of a Bernard, the logical methodology of a Koch, and the simplicity in construction of a telling experiment of a Lind are among the qualities that enable the original thinker to prevail against the strong forces of tradition. Probably never are all those attributes of genius embraced by a single individual. We should be content and grateful for the harbinger carrying an important message, no matter what the source accountable for his imaginative and creative power.

Surgery's Needs

What has the future in store for surgical progress? Certainly the lessons of three decades following World War II speak emphatically for the important role of research in the advance of surgery. Until then surgery had been almost solely dependent upon discoveries and important advances in other disciplines for its own progress. Among innovations, long hoped for, the following are undoubtedly near the top of most surgeons' inventory of wishes: pharmacologic or antibacterial agents to eliminate or control pyogenic infection; techniques to ablate the antigenic properties of immune reactions which continue to retard development of organ transplantation; simpler and more effective hemostatic agents, as well as anticoagulants; even more efficient anesthetic agents than those now available; effective means of sustaining normal circulation during shock; mechanical devices to simplify operative procedures upon small tubular structures; and continued infusion from other scientific disciplines that will extend, augment, and simplify the role of the surgeon in both emergency and elective surgery.

It is to the interdisciplinary facets of biochemistry, biophysics, bioradiology, botany, experimental pathology, genetics, microbiology, pharmacology, physiology, and zoology that we must look for new ideas, tools, and techniques to realize these ends — and to yet unnamed interphase disciplines still in the making. The day is long past when surgeons are justified in defining surgical research as "investigation done by surgeons." Kidney transplantation and dialysis over the past three decades have extended the duration and quality of life of many individuals, well typified by the results obtained by the Harvard group at the Peter Bent Brigham Hospital and by John Najarian at the University of Minnesota.

The work of Shumway of Palo Alto and Barnard of Cape Town provides promise that worn-out and failing hearts can be replaced through cardiac transplantation, prolonging and improving the quality of life for a number of patients with terminal heart failure. When the phenomenon of rejection is better coped with, the results of cardiac transplantation will probably rival achievements with renal replacement. A few groups of investigators have placed their faith in the belief that mechanical hearts may also become a reality presently.

Many of these achievements of the post World War II period, products of research, present substantial evidence that long-hoped-for accomplishments do come about through that germinal and vitalizing agency. In the decades ahead, many recent innovations will be refined and greatly improved. It is, however, one of the demands and functions of periods of lull, while awaiting patiently the revelations of new ideas and discoveries, obviously not daily events, to assess critically current achievements in many areas. Recent decades have witnessed, particularly in obstetrics, how periodic critical reappraisal can greatly improve accomplishment by realigning indications for intervention. Recognizing the vulnerable areas and invoking prophylactic measures to preclude devastating complications will not only lend a new complexion to problems but often can provide the means of solution. Cesarean section, when employed as a last resort to terminate protracted and difficult delivery, was long followed by a formidable mortality; when it is used early for uterine fetal positions that portend difficult labor, the picture has changed so completely that a few obstetrical clinics in recent decades have been able to report large series of several thousand cesarean sections without a death. The pursuit and exposure of causes of maternal mortality in parturition by the New England group of obstetricians deserve emulation in every clinical discipline.

In his enthusiasm for early operation in appendicitis, McBurney (1889) expressed the hope that there would presently be no deaths from that disorder.[15] Achievement since the mid-1930s has been laudable, but the vital statistics for the United States in 1973 recorded 1066 deaths from appendicitis. Operation before perforation is the answer.

Massive gastric hemorrhage too is a case in point. Despite an abundance of research on the nature of the peptic ulcer diathesis since World War II, a significant imprint upon the mortality of hemorrhage, the chief lethal agent, remains to be achieved. A careful reassessment of the clinical situation may point the directional attack to accomplish what much recent laboratory research so far has failed to resolve; discovery of an effective antipeptic agent should prove helpful.

Special Research Areas

Since World War II, people everywhere have become deeply interested in many facets of research and its social implications. In consequence medicine is dealing with a continuously better informed public, as anxious to know that research is liberally supported as to learn the fruits of research. Today, the four great cripplers accounting for 75 percent of deaths in our country are diseases of the heart and blood vessels, cancer, trauma, and congenital deformities. Our leaders in government have directed the National Institutes of Health to funnel a large percentile of their allotted monies for research into the problems of heart disease, stroke, and cancer, believing that greater expenditures will quicken considerably the resolution of those scourges. Probably what is even more important would be a few good ten-cent ideas.

Will nutritional studies provide the needed information to prevent congenital cardiac and other birth anomalies? Can rheumatic heart disease be prevented? And what of cancer? Must early recognition and surgical excision continue to be our main resource? Or will the secrets of its genesis be ferreted out through research to the end that some cancers may be prevented? These are a few of the hopes and expectations that dominate the thinking of men and women of medicine everywhere. How long must we await their realization? Certainly the broad advance of medicine since World War II suggests that definite progress can be anticipated in many areas before the dawn of the twenty-first century.

Cancer

Early detection is still the *sine qua non* of success in the management of many malignancies, well documented for cancers of the cervix, breast, rectum, colon, and stomach.

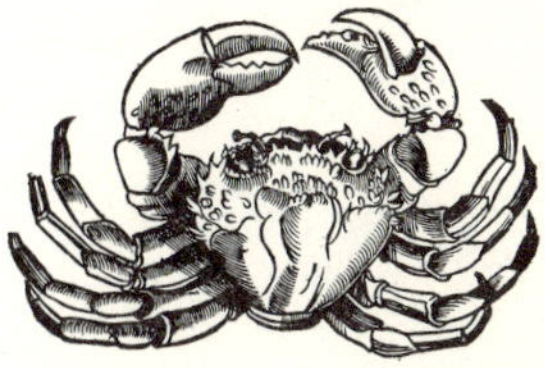

26.3 Paré's "*Crabb*, called Cancer *in Latine*. . . . A *cancer* is an hard Tumor . . . spred abroad to the similitude of the stretched out legs and clawes of a Crabb . . . therefore I . . . insert the Figure of the Crabb, that so the reason both of the name and thing might be more perspicuous." From Paré, *Workes*.

Radical mastectomy for cancer with total excision of the breast, excision of the axillary nodes, and removal of the pectoralis major muscle and fascia were interesting and successive developments after 1867, involving several contributions from distinguished surgeons. The procedure has come to be known in this country as the Halsted operation; he assembled the various components of the operation, invoked over the intervening years, when he wrote his essay upon breast cancer in 1894. Present-day cures in breast cancer are at least twice as great as in Halsted's day, owing largely to earlier recognition and adequate surgery. Currently in some quarters there appears to be less enthusiasm for the conventional radical mastectomy accompanied by axillary dissection than there was a decade ago, an admission that surgical achievement with involved axillary nodes has been disappointing and that early detection of breast cancer has yet to be achieved. On the latter score xerographic mammography appears promising. John N. Wolfe of Detroit (1976), its innovator, has studied the anatomy of the breast radiographically and observes that a rich duct system and abundant glandular tissue in the breast increase the susceptibility to cancer, as does a family history of breast cancer. He subscribes to the thesis that the silent interval in some types of breast cancer is surprisingly long; for these cases, when detected early, he favors complete subcutaneous excision.[16]

That breast cancer is hormone-dependent was shown by Beatson (1896, 1901), who invoked ovariectomy in advanced cases.[17] Because trials with adrenalectomy and hypophysectomy have not been too rewarding, greater dependence has been urged on chemotherapeutic agents and a large number have been employed, including cyclophosphamide, fluorouracil, methotrexate, vincristine, or a combination of two or more of these. Temporary favorable responses are frequent but suppression extending beyond a year apparently is not often seen. There is much testimony but yet not very convincing evidence of the efficacy of therapeutic agents in providing durable suppression of residuals and metastases attending operation for breast cancer. However, the current experience with several varieties of leukemia is reassuring on the score that protracted trials have produced a methodology that spells greater success.[18]

In 1958 Roy Hertz and his associates made the dramatic discovery that choriocarcinoma and related trophoblastic tumors responded favorably to methotrexate administered either by drip or by intramuscular injection; of 19 women with choriocarcinoma, complete remission was observed in 5 patients for eight to twenty-nine months; partial remission occurred in 7; death came in 6 after a temporary response. A subsequent study (1961) by the Hertz group reported favorable responses in metastatic choriocarcinoma with amethopterin and vincaleukoblastin; of 63 women, 30 had complete remission varying from six months to five years; 26 died.[19]

An area in which complementing aggressive surgery with irradiation and/or chemotherapy has greatly improved the achievement is in Wilms' tumor of the kidney in young children. Robert Gross (1953) reported a survival of 32.2 percent of such patients attending surgery, 47.3 percent when surgery was complemented by irradiation. In patients under one year of age, Gross and E. B. D. Neuhauser (1950) reported an 80 percent survival attending nephrectomy and postoperative irradiation. W. W. Sutow and associates reported in 1970 upon a nationwide survey on the results of the management of Wilms' tumor in young children. Between 1956 and 1962 they found marked frequency in use of chemotherapy for the neoplasm with a corresponding improvement in long survivals of all children without metastases. The drugs used were actinomycin D, vincristine, and cyclophosphamide.[20]

In a Harvey Lecture, Henry Kaplan (1969) summarized the experience of the Stanford University group with management of Hodgkin's disease by extensive radiation. Lymphangiography is employed to determine whether the para-aortic lymph nodes are involved. Routine abdominal exploration is performed and nodes in the para-aortic chains are excised to assess histologic involvement. The spleen, if enlarged, is excised. Prolonged survival attending this program has greatly extended the achievement with Hodgkin's disease. In Stages I and II, more than 50 percent of patients survive five years; thereafter relapses are rare. The relapse rate in Stages III and IV is higher, but after five years, recurrence is rarely observed, indeed a creditable accomplishment with a disorder believed to be almost uniformly fatal a few decades ago.

Sutow and R. G. Martin (1973) noted regression of metastases in Ewing's sarcoma of bone attending the administration of chemotherapeutic agents, including cyclophosphamide, actinomycin D, vincristine, uracil mustard, or combinations of these agents.[21]

The Mayo Clinic observers D. C. Dahlin and M. B. Coventry emphasize surgical management of osteogenic sarcoma (amputation). Since 1955 they have used x-ray treatment in several patients and in more recent years have also employed chemical oncolytic agents, but not as primary therapy. They were able to report a 25.4 percent five-year survival in patients with osteogenic sarcoma of humerus and femur, a tremendous improvement over results obtained by surgeons before World War II. The precise roles of radiotherapy and chemotherapy in the achievement were not spelled out. Henry J. Mankin and associates, orthopedists of the Massachusetts General Hospital, reported (1976) a follow-up study on nine massive resections for malignant osteogenic tumors, employing allografts of bone from patients newly dead, of the same sex and between the ages of fifteen and forty-five. Fifteen patients were followed for an average of twenty months. No metastases nor local recurrences were reported. Mankin and associates freeze the bone and articular surfaces of the epiphyses that have been removed en masse and detached from ligaments and muscle. The articular cartilage is immersed in dilute glycerol for fifteen minutes, and the entire preparation is frozen at −30° C and stored in a deep freeze unit until needed. The low temperature reduces the immunogenicity of the component parts of the allograft. They regard their trials as experimental, but satisfying function has been obtained in many cases. They note that Lexer reported functional joints obtained in this manner in publications of 1908 and 1925.[22]

CANCER DETECTION CENTERS

Experienced personnel can detect breast cancer in women who report to cancer detection centers annually sufficiently early so that the five-year survival in the group has been 90 percent — a 100 percent improvement over the situation obtaining for patients arriving at the outpatient clinic of most hospitals with a clinical diagnosis of breast cancer. Annual xerographic mammography has been extremely helpful in detecting nonpalpable lesions. Until major breakthroughs occur that will drastically change cancer management, cancer detection clinics must be looked to as a practical and very worthwhile direct attack upon the problem.

Application of the cervical Papanicolaou smear has diminished the mortality from cancer of the uterine cervix in the United States by 50 percent over the past two decades. Annual proctoscopic examinations similarly have lowered the death rate from cancer of the rectum by approximately 12 percent. Colonoscopy will undoubtedly heighten the chances of earlier recognition of small colic cancers. Routine use of Welin's (1955) air-contrast roentgenography of the colon could increase considerably the opportunity to recognize small lesions.[23] A high index of suspicion by the clinician is still invaluable in determining the direction of studies. It is to be remembered that a visceral cancer with symptoms may have been a cancer-in-situ for as long as two years, and even longer.

Following World War II when the senior author sought to establish a cancer detection center at the University of Minnesota, it took almost three years to overcome faculty disapproval and the objections of the Cancer Council of the Minnesota State Medical Society to such a project. Money for support of the center was unavailable from the National Cancer Institute and other large granting agencies. Its modest funding came from a few former patients and their friends. Today extremely generous support is available from the National Cancer Institute and the American Cancer Society for this activity that went begging three decades ago. Times are changing, adjudication committees also have been taught by experience. With liberal federal support, Victor Gilbertsen, director of the university's Cancer Detection Center, has pursued vigorously the study of patients found to have occult blood in the stool (Hemoccult evaluation). Of 475 patients examined, primary gastrointestinal cancer was found in 45 (9.4 percent). Endoscopy proved to be the most useful tool in the detection; 73 percent of the malignancies were mucosal Dukes' group A lesions, which should have a high cure rate.[24] All clinicians must be alert to the length (two or more years) of the silent asymptomatic interval in organ cancers.

The ability of Japanese clinicians, radiologists, gastroscopists, and surgeons (1966–68) to recognize mucosal gastric cancers, not penetrating beyond the submucosa, has renewed hope that the results of gastrectomy will presently demonstrate suggestions of definite improvement, as it apparently already has in the hands of Japanese surgeons.

Strangely enough, cancer of the esophagus is rarely recognized in the mucosal state. At a conference in Tokyo during the 1966 International Cancer Conference, Komei Nakayama said that in his 3,000 operations for esophageal cancer, he had observed the malignancy delimited to the mucosa in only four instances. It was conceded by Boris Petrov of Moscow and other well-known esophageal surgeons that penetration of the cancer through the entire esophageal wall with adherence to adjacent structures was the usual finding at operation. In that 1966 discussion, the senior author was able to report a patient with fixed esophageal cancer at the thoracic inlet who had survived esophagectomy (1945) for 21 years (and still survives without recurrence 33 years after excision).

Nakayama (1967) has reverted to staging esophageal excision into two or three operative sessions, with definite decrease in the mortality of the procedure, and uses preoperative irradiation, which has prolonged the four- and five-year survival rates. Dan Gavriliu of Bucarest (1975) also is optimistic over a better outlook in cases of esophageal cancer. He substitutes a long gastric tube, fashioned from the greater curvature of the stomach, swinging the distal antral end cephalad, to be anastomosed to either the cervical esophagus or the pharynx. One advantage of Gavriliu's method over the old Jianu, Lortat–Jacob gastric tube is that the antral esophageal anastomosis does not provoke stricture at the anastomotic site.[25]

THE SECOND LOOK

The length of the silent asymptomatic interval in many organ cancers persuaded the senior author (1948) to project a program of periodic second-look, or reentry, operations for patients with cancer of the colon presenting evidence of lymph-node metastases or involvement of the visceral peritoneum overlying the lesion.[26] Of patients in whom residual cancer was found on the first reentry and who were periodically subjected to the second-look procedure, 17.5 percent were alive and well and free from cancer five years after the last relook. The method had even better success rates when applied to ovarian cancers and to patients with retroperitoneal rhabdomyosarcomas, huge tumors in which often tiny fragments of the capsule may be left behind at operation. Obviously, if the same end can be achieved by noninvasive methods — chemotherapy or other — they are to be preferred.

This experience with the second-look procedure was a very reassuring one, not only on the score of additional salvage of life, but also because of the surprisingly hopeful attitude of the patients in the program. They uniformly welcomed the idea of being told they had cancer so that they could discuss the problem freely with their spouses, who did not appreciate that the patient knew she or he had cancer. The physician-guided and ill-conceived deception of not being frank with patients in this matter is finally disappearing, a story eloquently told in Tolstoi's powerful essay, *The Death of Ivan Ilyich* (1884), which should be required reading for every physician.

REALISTIC APPRAISAL OF THE CANCER MENACE (1928)

On the occasion of the London International Cancer Conference (August 1928), King George V's message to the congress was read by Lord Horder: "I note with interest that your object is research, both into the cure and causes of cancer. No doubt in the last resort the discovery of the cause is the only certain and absolute means of cure. But I am glad that you have not ignored the practical side of the problem. Remembering the thousands of sufferers from cancer I feel that if your discussions lead to advance in diagnosis, treatment or even palliation of the disease, this Conference will have justified itself and earned the gratitude of mankind."[27] Indeed, a prophetic statement made fifty years ago by King George V and his wise counselors, reflecting a more judicial appraisal than we are accustomed to hear from many modern-day visionary optimists who affect the role of prophet.

Surgery's Expanding Role

A. R. Dochez (1882–1964), a much respected New York physician in his day, described (1939) a case treated for heart failure at his hospital in 1908. The patient had dyspnea; physical examination of the chest was carefully done; hematological studies consisted of a blood count and urine examination; the blood pressure was taken frequently. There was no mention of any cardiac stimulants such as digitalis. The patient was bled immediately on admission to the hospital and actively purged by administration of calomel and saline cathartics! The author then related the situation of a similar patient in 1938. Following completion of the history and physical examination, the patient was immediately put on a salt-poor diet, with restriction of fluids, and given digitalis. The patient was weighed every day; the caloric intake was screened; a dyspneic patient was given oxygen.

Dochez dilated on the enlargement of scientific aspects of medicine in the intervening thirty years; he wondered whether every branch of medicine could mobilize resources for continued advancement of the discipline. He remarked that in his medical clinic sixteen different specialists were involved in the care of medical patients. He asked, "should we turn back to more simple techniques and leave the fundamentals to the underlying medical sciences of chemistry, biology, and physiology?" He queried whether medicine was the spoiled child of philanthropy and added, "It seems unlikely that resources ample to provide each branch with all the opportunities it may think desirable will be forthcoming" — obviously a gloomy prediction.[28] It took World War II to provide liberal federal monies to sponsor research in greater medicine.

A 1976 assessment of cardiac care serves to emphasize the current great stress on diagnostic laboratory data rather than on clinical acumen. Although a greater array of therapeutic pharmacologic agents is at the disposal of the physician, undoubtedly the most striking advance in the therapy of heart disease since World War II has been surgical. Operations for congenital heart disease and repair of valve defects today save large numbers of patients previously doomed to untimely demise, pointing up the increasing importance of surgery for broad current-day medical care. In endocrine disorders, gastrointestinal derangements, and other areas, the surgeon today is able to provide complemental help that augments significantly the overall achievement of medical care.

Renal transplantation probably represents interdisciplinary medicine at its very best, involving surgeons, urologists, renal physiologists, hematologists, geneticists, experimental pathologists, and pharmacologists. It is superior to other organ transplants because the patient can be maintained on dialysis if the transplanted kidney is rejected. Heart transplantation, surgery's boldest effort, yet in its early adolescence in the hands of its pioneers, promises, with resolution of the rejection phenomenon, to bring renewed and extended life to many with failing hearts. Thomas Starzl's work over a dozen years with liver transplantation, the most difficult of all organ grafts, deserves the admiration of the profession. Biliary atresia of infants and young children, hepatic neoplasms, hepatitis, and alcoholic cirrhosis in adults have been the most frequent indications for such replacement; 27 percent of Starzl's ninety-three patients with orthotopic liver transplants survived more than a year; one survived six years, and sixteen survive at thirteen to seventy-one months after transplantation. Unlike renal and cardiac transplanters, who attribute deaths of patients surviving operation for a few months to rejection and sepsis, Starzl (1976) tends to deemphasize rejection as the primary cause of late deaths in patients receiving liver transplants.[29]

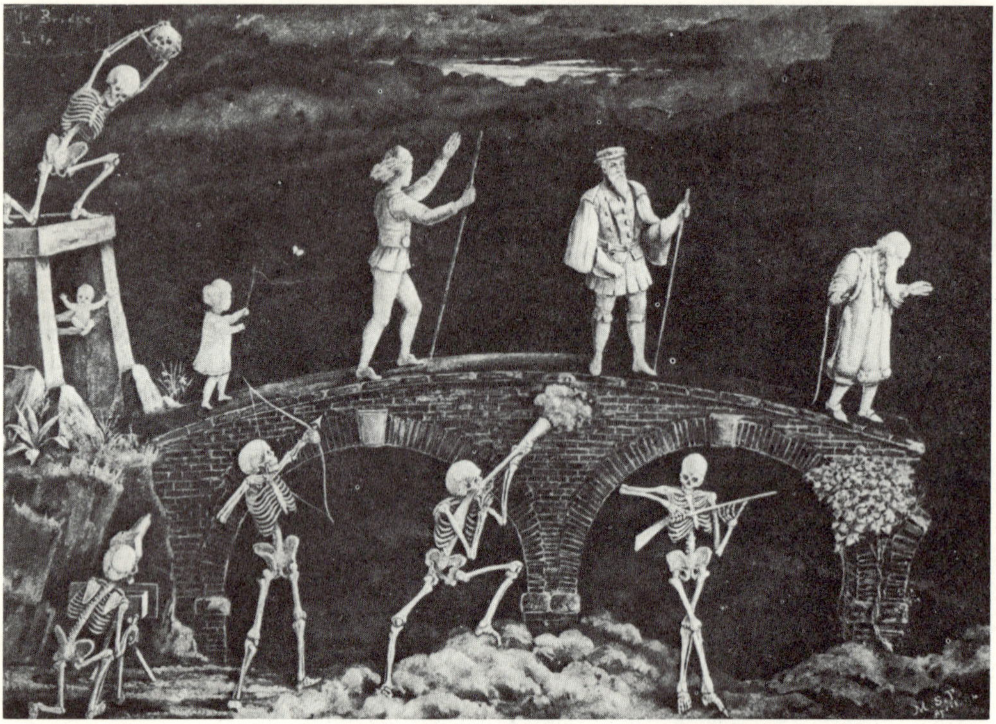

26.4 Karl Pearson's "Bridge of Life" (1897). The most impressive improvement has occurred in infant and child mortality from diarrhea and infectious diseases including tuberculosis. Frontispiece, Pearson, *Chances of death* (London and New York, 1897).

Heart Disease

The important role of the surgeon in dealing with congenital and valvular heart disease in recent decades constitutes a new venture for greater medicine — for centuries physicians held the field uncontested. Preventive measures to deal with nutritional deficiencies of the unborn and with rheumatic fever, the important causes of congenital and valvular disease, may lessen the role of the surgeon in those aspects of heart disease by the beginning of the twenty-first century. It would appear too that cardiac surgeons are improving both the length and the quality of life for many patients with occlusions of coronary arteries, an affliction which continues to take an enormous toll. Even here, however, the preventive role of a dietary regimen and regular exercise may provide more hope for the future than surgery. These tugs of war on the medical gridiron are constantly in motion. The ultimate victor is the discipline that can provide the greatest assurance with the simplest measures.

What Will Be the Nature of Future Medical Care?

Daniel Coit Gilman, first president of The Johns Hopkins, in intimate cooperation with Billings and Welch, selected a superb faculty that lent great impetus to upgrading medical education in America with emphasis upon research throughout the school, including the clinical departments. Over the past decade, interest in research among medical school faculties has declined, while primary emphasis has been upon adequate dispersion of medical care, with accentuation of the need for a large increase in medical graduates. The senior author is inclined to believe that William Mayo's thesis of geographically and strategically placed small clinics staffed largely with well-trained specialists and paramedical personnel will come before the dawn of the twenty-first century to supplant the wish, currently dominating the scene, of placing a physician in every hamlet of our great land; Mayo's scheme would provide superior professional care, requiring fewer physicians and at less cost to society in manpower and money.

Meanwhile, surgical academicians should strive to provide the first rather than the last word on the nature of surgical disorders and their management. The professor of surgery and his associates would do well to emulate the intimate teacher-student relationship reflected in the practices of Pierre Louis and Osler, cultivating a policy of the open door. A critical reassessment by professors of their teaching responsibilities should serve to indicate to medical students and their faculties that surgery has much important and useful information to impart, and that their professors are ready, prepared, and anxious to meet the challenge. In surgical clinics where the professor, by precept and example, reflects a spirit of inquiry and a love of learning there will be a rebirth of student interest in surgery as an important undergraduate discipline.

Longevity

And what of old age? The infirmities of increasing years are such that many welcome death. Many of the physical disabilities can be managed in the family home or in friendly and well-staffed nursing homes; mental and intellectual deterioration with complete loss of memory and total dependency on others is probably the most difficult for the patient and the family to support. The nursing home at best is not a pleasant substitute for family life in the eyes and experience of many; yet often for progressing disabilities there are no alternative choices. A continued unwilling existence, estranged from family and friends, has become the lot of many who survive into their late eighties and nineties. Society, in time, will undoubtedly need to take a second look at this feature of aging populations, acquiring in the appraisal greater respect for the wishes of those unhappy with complete dependency, and without hope for the future; may not such individuals be permitted to decline acceptance of a continued vegetable existence? There are fervid but unrealistic prophets among us who suggest that centenarians leading useful and productive lives will be numerous in future decades. Such seers cannot remain completely inattentive to the admonition of the Psalmist: "The days of our years are threescore and ten; and if . . . they be fourscore years, yet is their strength labor and sorrow." A useful life is a happy one and one of earth's greatest blessings. Why wish for more? To make maximal efforts to extend life into a period of cheerless gloom and regret appears to be at cross-purposes with societal designs for a meaningful and satisfying life for all.

Superannuation among Men and Women of Medicine

Morgagni was 79 when his *Seats and Causes of Disease* was published in 1761. He survived another decade. The surgeon-sanitarian Stephen Smith, who lived to be almost 100, was active and writing in his late nineties. Opie was publishing at 97; in fact, he indicated to the senior author he hoped to live to be 100 so that he could finish his work; six months later he was dead. George Whipple, Nobel Laureate, was active and productive in his early nineties and lived to be 97, spending his last years in hospital. Marine, of goiter fame, died at age 96, and had been under nursing care for several years. Lister died at age 85; his last two years were lived in total silence and darkness. Florence Nightingale, after her great work in the Crimea, lived a life of seclusion and inaccessiblity for almost fifty years but continued to be active and influential in hospital construction and sanitation until her death at age 90 in 1910.

Welch (1850–1934), one of the great men of American medicine, the first dean of the Hopkins faculty, was successively professor of pathology, public health, and the history of medicine and an influential member of many distinguished boards and committees on medical education. He remained active and productive into his eighties, publishing little in the last

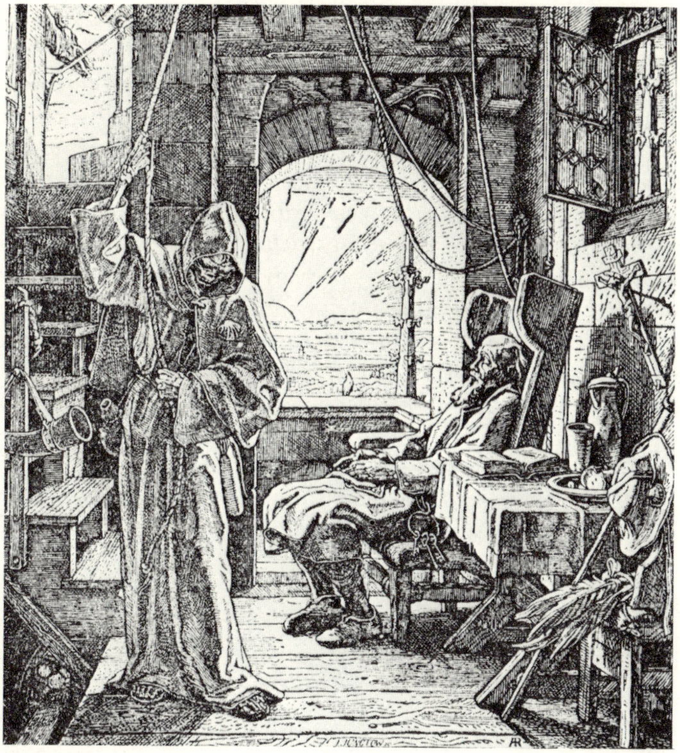

26.5 Friendly Death. "Come to thy grave in a full age." *Job* 5:26.

decade of his life. His eightieth birthday was celebrated worldwide for significant contributions to medicine's advance. Welch had been a zealous smoker throughout his adult years and died of a malignancy of the urinary bladder at age 84.

Alice Hamilton (1869–1970), who initiated studies on industrial poisons (1925), lived to be 101.[30] Allen Boyden (1885–1976), erstwhile distinguished anatomist at Minnesota, was active in productive research at the University of Washington (Seattle) in his ninety-first year, his investigations being still funded by the National Institutes of Health! These obviously are striking examples of extensions of activity to near the centenary mark, though rarely accompanied by evidences of the imaginative and viable creativity in earlier productive research that drew them originally into the scientific limelight.

Superannuation between the ages of 65 and 68 is the common procedure in our universities today. Retirement is looked upon by many, both the institutions of learning and the retirees, as a reward of idleness, a frosting on the cake, for prior years of devoted service. Undoubtedly there are those who look forward to a few years of truancy without daily obligations; but for those who from youth found inspiration and complete satisfaction in their work, retirement means only a search for another outlet providing similar rewards. Institutes of learning as well as big business regularly and arbitrarily supplant their aging men and women, who have had their opportunity, with younger persons of great promise to whom opportunity and the future rightly belong — a fully justifiable practice not likely to be set aside, at least in this century. Every species of creature appears to have an arbitrary limit on its life span, which apparently cannot be substantially lengthened by artificial means. The hope of keeping the body and mind of man forever young provides interesting contemplation for a few but is probably completely devoid of promise of fulfillment. The vibrancy of youth, pulsating with energy, is indeed an attractive quality, but it too, unfortunately, is a fleeting attribute.

American Centenaries

Assessed in the traditions of Europe, America is a relatively new land. In speaking of America's role in surgery at our first Centenary in Philadelphia (1876), S. D. Gross, great leader in American surgery, anxious to place its image in the best light, employed the opportunity to full advantage. We may smile with sympathetic and dutiful understanding at his swagger when we read, "It is not probable that America will ever again produce four surgeons of equal renown with Philip Syng Physick, John C. Warren, Valentine Mott, and Benjamin W. Dudley." Continued Gross, "in the treatment of fractures of the long bones, we are, it may fairly be assumed, decidedly in advance of every other nation"; and again, "in the treatment of affections of the joints, American surgeons stand preeminent." And "as lithotomists, American surgeons are not surpassed by any in the world."[31] This was America's Nestor of surgery, who had not accepted surgical antisepsis when his professional career terminated at Jefferson Medical College in 1882. He had been unpersuaded by Lister's visit to Philadelphia in 1876. There was a period in time, after Koch's (1878) demonstration of the pathogenicity of bacteria and before the almost universal acceptance of prophylactic surgical antisepsis (ca. 1885–86), when American elective surgery lagged for want of having given the practices of Semmelweis and Lister thorough clinical trial.

America is embarked upon the beginnings of its third centennial. World War II revealed to all the peoples of the globe their complete dependence upon scientific achievement for progress in the stream of time. Over the past three decades since that worldwide conflict terrorized peoples everywhere and threatened the very foundations of existence, the importance of research for the advance of medicine has become fully appreciated by the American public and its governmental leaders. These years have afforded American medicine the opportunity of repaying in part its debt to foreign lands, especially to Britain, France, and Germany, for the instruction, stimulation, and example they provided American men and women of medicine, not only during the period of our humble beginnings but well into this century too.

This study reaffirms the dependence for progress in all disciplines of medicine, including surgery, upon research; technical

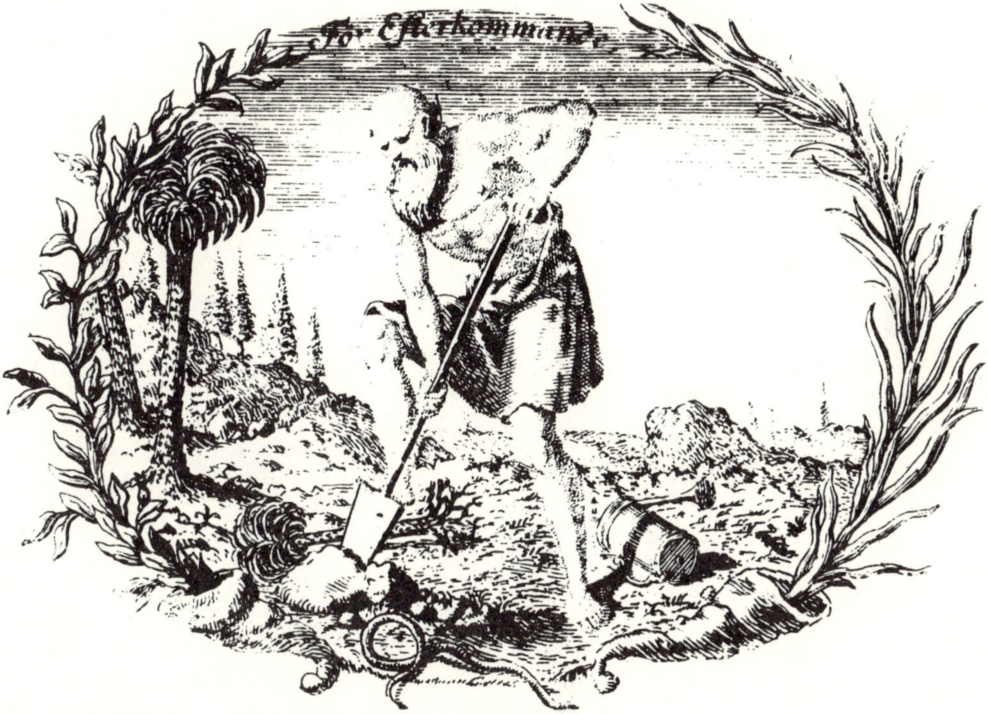

1739 Swenska Wetenskaps Acad.

26.6 Old man, not digging his grave, but planting a tree for posterity (1739), certainly every physician's great privilege.

improvements are not enough. Since the decline of the School of Surgery at Salerno and the rise of its illustrious successor Bologna, one city or nation after another has been the temporary host to a flourishing school of surgeons, and rarely for more than a generation or two. Successively, Montpellier, Paris, Edinburgh, London, Vienna, and Berlin enjoyed this great privilege in Europe; and in America sequentially Philadelphia, New York, Boston, and Baltimore showed the way.[32] Today splendid schools of surgery dot the geography of many lands and cities. None can lay claim to dominance in all the disciplines of surgery. A noticeable spirit of warm cooperation and reciprocation between institutions of learning is apparent today, accompanied by a strenuous but friendly competition for honors. The directional course of national aims and the status of the economy are significant factors in guiding the growth of all scientific disciplines. The zeal of motivation and sincerity of dedication of its votaries are powerful catalytic forces to be reckoned with in sustaining objectives and reaching goals, as the life and achievements of many of the heroes of greater medicine, recounted herein, attest.

(For notes, see pp. 717–20.)

NOTES AND FURTHER READINGS

Notes and Further Readings

Abbreviations follow those in the *Index-catalogue . . . of the Surgeon-General's Office* if the journal started publication before 1900. More recent publications are abbreviated according to the *World list of scientific periodicals published in the years 1900–1960* (London, 1962). Some obvious variations will be found. If the journal is obscure or if there is possibility of confusion, a fuller citation is provided. Publishers' names are supplied for books published in the twentieth century. For the assistance of readers, references in the notes, when feasible, provide the specific pages of the information cited, not necessarily the full pagination of the article.

Chapter 1. Overview

Notes

1. Maurice Maeterlinck, *Measure of the hours*, trans. Alexander Teixeira de Mattos (New York: Dodd, Mead, 1907), p. 97.

2. A. Puky, "Ueber Wundbehandlung mit besonderer Berücksichtigung der Lister'schen Methode," *Pester med.-chir. Presse* (1879), vol. 15, col. 194. A reprint appeared in Budapest in 1880.

3. Francis Bacon said (1605), "Cleanness of body was ever deemed to proceed from a due reverence to God," a suggestion traceable to the Hebrew fathers.

4. Fielding H. Garrison, *Introduction to the history of medicine*, 4th ed. (Philadelphia: W. B. Saunders, 1929), p. 280.

5. In 1787 one of the last of the old faculty, J. N. Corvisart, raised a bold argument with the grave question, "Should one drink pure wine while eating oysters?" His question is representative of the type posed to medical students in their examinations. A.-G. Maurice Raynaud, *Les médecins au temps de Molière*, 2d ed. (Paris, 1863), p. 67.

6. F. Campbell Stewart, *Hospitals and surgeons of Paris* (New York, 1843), p. 215. During the early nineteenth century human fat taken from dissection rooms was illicitly sold in Paris as horse or dog fat to grease wagon wheels. It was used to light the lamps of the Faculty of Medicine and the palace of Luxembourg for the marriage of Napoleon and Marie-Louise. Marie-José Imbault-Huart, *L'École Pratique de Dissection de Paris de 1750 à 1822*, Paris thesis, 1973, pp. 228–29.

7. Drewry Ottley, "Life of John Hunter," in John Hunter, *Works*, ed. James F. Palmer (London, 1835), 1:22; T. Clifford Allbutt, *The historical relations of medicine and surgery to the end of the sixteenth century* (London: Macmillan, 1905); Walter B. Cannon, *The way of an investigator* (New York: Hafner, 1945), p. 19. James was advising Cannon against choosing philosophy as a career.

8. Mme. de Maintenon, then Louis XIV's favorite mistress, had succeeded in getting the king's physician, Daquin, supplanted by her physician, Guy C. Fagon, who came to exert powerful influence at court. James R. Church, *Milit. Surg.* (1920), 47:706.

9. According to Alfred A.-L.-M. Velpeau, "Anus (fistules)," *Dict. de méd.*, Paris (1833), 3:329, Guy de Chauliac, like his master Henri de Mondeville, favored a grooved sound upon which he divided the fistulous tract with a heated bistoury. When James Syme of Edinburgh wrote on the surgery of fistula-in-ano in his *Principles of surgery* (Philadelphia, 1866), pp. 363–66, he could well have been describing the operation of Félix. Louis Le Monnier wrote a monograph on fistula-in-ano in 1689, three years after Louis XIV's operation. He indicated that Hippocrates felt that operations about the anus were not dangerous. Le Monnier stated that the sentiments of Hippocrates concerning the management of fistulas were supported by seventeenth-century surgeons. He added that Avicenna (980–1037) was conservative in his address to the problem.

10. Louis XIV died in 1715 at age seventy-seven, apparently of senile gangrene of the leg.

11. Serge Dos, an ardent student of the subject, provided much of the above material on the history of French surgery in a surgical seminar at the University of Minnesota in May 1967 and in letters to the authors of this volume (May 12, 1968, and August 28, 1974).

Further Readings

Averill, Charles. *A short treatise on operative surgery, describing the principal operations*. 2d ed. London, 1825.

Billings, John Shaw. The history and literature of surgery. In *System of surgery*, ed. Frederic S. Dennis, vol. 1, pp. 17–144. Philadelphia, 1895.

Billroth, Theodor. *Historical studies on the nature and treatment of gunshot wounds from the fifteenth century to the present time . . . Berlin, 1859*. Trans. C. P. Rhoads. New Haven, Conn.: Nathan Smith Medical Club, 1933.

Cumston, Charles Greene. *Introduction to the history of medicine, from the time of the pharaohs to the end of the XVIIIth century*. New York: Alfred A. Knopf, 1926.

Dana, Charles L. *The peaks of medical history: An outline of the evolution of medicine for the use of medical students and practitioners*. 2d ed. New York: Paul B. Hoeber, 1928.

Dionis, Pierre. *Cours d'operations de chirurgie, demontrées au Jardin royal*. Paris, 1707.

Fergusson, William. *Lectures on the progress of anatomy and surgery during the present century*. London, 1867.

Fischer, Georg. *Chirurgie vor 100 Jahren. Historische Studie*. Leipzig, 1876.

————. Handbuch der allgemeinen Operations- und Instrumentenlehre. *Dt. Chir.*, Stuttgart (1880), bk. 19.

Fourmestraux, J. de. *Histoire de la chirurgie française (1790–1920)*. Paris: Masson, 1934.

Fracastoro, Girolamo. *De contagione et contagiosis morbis et eorum curatione*. Venice, 1546. Translated with notes by Willmer C. Wright. New York: G. P. Putnam's Sons, 1930.

Garrison, Fielding H. *Notes on the history of military medicine*. Washington, D.C.: Association of Military Surgeons, 1922.

Gordon, Benjamin L. *Medicine throughout antiquity*. Philadelphia: F. A. Davis, 1949.

Gross, Samuel David. *A system of surgery*. 2 vols. Philadelphia, 1859.

Gründer, Johann W. L. *Geschichte der Chirurgie, von den Urzeiten bis zu Anfang des achtzehnten Jahrhunderts*. Breslau, 1859.

Gurlt, Ernst J. *Geschichte der Chirurgie.* 3 vols. Berlin, 1898. Reprint. Hildesheim: Georg Olms, 1964.

Guy de Chauliac. *La grande chirurgie de Guy de Chauliac, composée en l'an 1363.* Ed. Édouard Nicaise. Paris, 1890.

Haeser, Heinrich. Übersicht der geschichte der chirurgie und des chirurgischen standes. *Dt. Chir.*, Stuttgart (1879), bk. 1.

Haller, Albrecht. *Bibliotheca chirurgica.* 2 vols. Bern and Basel, 1774–75.

———. *Elementa physiologiae corporis humani.* Vol. 6. Lausanne, 1777.

Heister, Lorenz. *Chirurgie, in welcher alles, was zur Wund-Artzney gehöret, nach der neuesten und besten Art.* Nuremberg, 1719.

Helferich, Friedrich. Geschichte der Chirurgie. In *Handbuch der Geschichte der Medizin*, ed. Theodor Puschmann et al., vol. 3, pp. 1–306. Jena: Gustav Fischer, 1905.

Henri de Mondeville. *Chirurgie de maître Henri de Mondeville, composée de 1306 a 1320.* Ed. Édouard Nicaise. Paris, 1893.

Hippocrates. *The genuine works of Hippocrates.* Trans. Francis Adams. 2 vols. in 1. New York: William Wood, 1929.

Hippocrates. With English translations by W. H. S. Jones and E. T. Withington. 4 vols. Cambridge: Harvard Univ. Press, Loeb Classical Library, 1962–68.

Huard, Pierre Alphonse, and Grmek, Mirko Dražen. *Mille ans de chirurgie en Occident:* V^e-XVe *siècles.* Paris: Roger Dacosta, 1966.

Leonardo, Richard A. *History of surgery.* New York: Froben Press, 1943.

Lind, James. *A treatise of the scurvy.* Edinburgh, 1753.

Malgaigne, Joseph François. *Histoire de la chirurgie en Occident depuis le* VIe *jusqu'au* XVIe *siècle, et histoire de la vie et des travaux d'Ambroise Paré.* Paris [1840].

Meyer-Steineg, Theodor, and Sudhoff, Karl. *Geschichte der Medizin im Überblick mit Abbildungen.* 2d ed. Jena: Gustav Fischer, 1922.

Neuburger, Max. *History of medicine.* Trans. Ernest Playfair. 2 vols. London: Oxford Univ. Press, 1910.

Pagel, Julius L. *Einführung in die Geschichte der Medizin.* Ed. Karl Sudhoff. 2d ed. Berlin: S. Karger, 1915.

Paré, Ambroise. *The workes of that famous chirurgion Ambrose Parey.* Trans. Thomas Johnson. London, 1634. Facsimile. Pp. 1133–43. New York: Milford House, 1968.

Paul of Aegina. *The seven books of Paulus Aegineta.* Trans. Francis Adams. 3 vols. London: Sydenham Soc., 1844–47.

Pétrequin, Joseph P. E. *Chirurgie d'Hippocrate.* 2 vols. Paris, 1878.

Puschmann, Theodor; Neuburger, Max; and Pagel, Julius, eds. *Handbuch der Geschichte der Medizin.* Vol. 1. Jena: Gustav Fischer, 1902.

Quesnay, François. *Recherches critiques et historiques sur l'origine, sur les divers états, et sur les progrès de la chirurgie en France.* Paris, 1744.

Rochard, Jules E. *Histoire de la chirurgie française au* XIXe *siècle.* Paris, 1875.

Rohlfs, Heinrich. *Die chirurgischen Classiker Deutschlands.* 2 vols. Leipzig, 1883–85.

Scarpa, Antonio. *Tabulae nevrologicae, ad illustrandam historiam anatomicam cardiacorum nervorum, noni nervorum cerebri, glossopharyngaei et pharyngaei ex octavo cerebri.* Pavia, 1794.

Scultetus, Johannes. *Armamentarium chirurgicum.* Ulm, 1655.

Smith, Stephen. The evolution of American surgery. In *American practice of surgery*, ed. Joseph D. Bryant and Albert H. Buck, vol. 2, pp. 3-67. New York: William Wood, 1906.

South, John Flint. *Memorials of the craft of surgery in England.* Ed. D'Arcy Power. London, 1886.

Syme, James. *Contributions to the pathology and practice of surgery.* Edinburgh, 1848.

Theodoric, Bishop of Cervia. *The surgery of Theodoric, ca. A.D. 1267.* Trans. Eldridge Campbell and James Colton. 2 vols. New York: Appleton-Century-Crofts, 1955–60.

Tillmanns, Robert Hermann. Hundert Jahre Chirurgie. *Verh. Ges. dt. Naturf. Aerzte* (1898), 70 (1):36–60.

Vigo, Giovanni de. *Practica in arte chirurgica copiosa, continens novem libros.* Rome, 1514.
Young, Sidney. *The annals of the Barber-Surgeons of London, compiled from their records and other sources.* London, 1890.
Zimmerman, Leo M., and Veith, Ilza. *Great ideas in the history of surgery.* Baltimore: Williams and Wilkins, 1961.

Chapter 2. Wound Management in Amputation

Notes

1. Probably one of the earliest operations, still practiced by some primitive peoples, was ritual amputation. The so-called "mutilated hands" depicted by prehistoric man on the walls of the Gargas Cave in France may illustrate this custom, although recent studies suggest that the seemingly missing finger joints were merely bent under, perhaps to portray hunting signals. Henri Breuil, *Four hundred centuries of cave art,* trans. Mary E. Boyle (Montignac, France: Centres d'études et de documentation préhistoriques, 1952), p. 256; Walter Torbrugge, *Prehistoric European art,* trans. Norbert Guterman (New York: Abrams, 1968), p. 48.

2. Max Neuberger, *History of medicine,* trans. Ernest Playfair (London: Oxford Univ. Press, 1910), 1:21–32.

3. See W. H. S. Jones's introduction to his translation of *Hippocrates* (Cambridge: Harvard Univ. Press, Loeb Classical Library, 1962), 1:xx–xxi, xxx–xxxi.

4. Fielding H. Garrison, *Introduction to the history of medicine,* 4th ed. (Philadelphia: W. B. Saunders, 1929), pp. 92–100; Julius L. Pagel, "Wundbehandlung im Altertum und Mittelalter," *Dt. Med.-Ztg* (1891), 91:1036–40.

5. Though often attributed to Hippocrates, the passage giving this advice belongs to a period later than 400 B.C., according to Jones (n.3), 2:305.

6. Theodor Billroth, *Historical studies on the nature and treatment of gunshot wounds from the fifteenth century to the present time . . . Berlin, 1859,* trans. C. P. Rhoads (New Haven, Conn.: Nathan Smith Medical Club, 1933), pp. 2, 4. Heinrich Pfolspeundt's manuscript, *Buch der Bündth-Ertznei,* did not appear in print until 1868, some time after Billroth's publication came out. Hieronymus Brunschwig of Strasbourg, an army surgeon, promoted the belief that gunshot wounds were poisoned. He had little or no battlefield experience, according to Edmond Delorme in *Traité de chirurgie de guerre* (Paris, 1888), 1:2.

7. *Hippocrates,* with an English translation by E. T. Withington (Cambridge: Harvard Univ. Press, Loeb Classical Library, 1968), 3:361–63.

8. John Woodall, *The surgeons mate or military & domestic surgery* (London, 1639), pp. 156–59, 388–411; James Y. Simpson, "Our existing system of hospitalism and its effects," *Edinb. M. J.* (1869), 14:818. Woodall (1556–1643), a widely traveled barber-surgeon, wrote *Surgeon's mate* (1617) for navy surgeons after he became surgeon-general of the British East India Company. He was a surgeon of St. Bartholomew's Hospital, London, from 1616 until his death.

9. William R. LeFanu, April 20, 1966, personal communication; John Hunter, *Works* [from Hunter's lectures of 1786–87], ed. James F. Palmer (London, 1835), 1:538–39; Richard Wiseman, *Severall chirurgicall treatises* (London, 1676), p. 453. The *Treatises* were first published in 1672, the year Wiseman (ca. 1622–76) was appointed the principal surgeon to Charles II. They reflect the wide experience in combat emergencies of this leading British surgeon of his day. In 1683 the London *Philosophical Transactions* (vol. 8) ran a number of enthusiastic letters and reports concerning the royal styptic.

10. Pierre Dionis, *Cours d'operations de chirurgie, demontrées au Jardin royal* (Paris, 1707), pp. 617–28. A styptic button was a small piece of vitriol wrapped in a bit of cotton. Dionis (d. 1718) succeeded in making the Jardin-du-Roi a famous training ground for young surgical aspirants. Rabel's fiasco probably occurred around 1675, when the Marquis of Louvois and the

physician Duschesne, both mentioned by Dionis, were actively involved in Louis's newly established Hôtel des Invalides. Félix Hutin, *Fragmens historiques et médicaux sur l'Hôtel national des Invalides* (Paris, 1851), pp. 22–23.

11. Paul of Aegina, *The seven books of Paulus Aegineta,* trans. Francis Adams (London: Sydenham Soc., vol. 4:2, 1846), p. 409. Paul credits his technique of using the cautery to stop bleeding after amputation to Leonides (first century).

12. Avicenna, *Quarta fen primi libri de uniuersalieratione medendi,* trans. (into Latin) Iacob Mantini ([Venice], 1530), cap. 27, fols. 53–54; Albucasis, *On surgery and instruments*, a definitive edition of the Arabic text with English translation and commentary by M. S. Spink and G. L. Lewis (Berkeley: Univ. California Press, 1973), pp. 8–12, 162. Albucasis's text was the leading authority on surgery in the Middle Ages until superseded by Saliceto's writings. See Leslie T. Morton, *Medical bibliography (Garrison and Morton),* 3d ed. (Philadelphia: J. B. Lippincott, 1970), #5550. Albucasis lived in Spain.

13. Fabricius Hildanus, "De gangraena et sphacelo," in *Opera observationum et curationum medico-chirurgicarum* (Frankfurt, 1646), p. 804; "Sir Arbuthnot Lane's operative treatment of fractures at Guy's Hospital," *Br. J. Surg.* (1913), 1:314–16.

14. Dionis, *Cours d'operations* (n.10), pp. 704–5; Moublet, "Sur l'abus que les anciens ont fait du cautère," *J. de méd., chir., pharm.*, Paris (1761), 15:271.

15. *Recueil des pièces qui ont concouru pour le prix de l'Académie royale de chirurgie*, Paris (1786), 3:355–487. De la Bissière won the prize; Guillaume Louis, younger brother of the well-known Antoine Louis, was runner-up. In an 1854 Strasbourg thesis, *De l'emploi d'un nouveau mode de cauterisation* (pp. 1–2), C. Cochu-Dayème said that the *concours* had had no practical results and the cautery was then rarely in use in the great surgical clinics of Paris.

16. Albrecht T. Middeldorpf, *Die Galvanocaustik, ein Beitrag zur operativen Medicin* (Breslau, 1854); C. Pacquelin, "Sur un nouveau thermo-cautère instantané et permanent fonctionnant avec l'essence minérale," *Bull. gén. de thérap.* (1876), 90:433–40; Harvey Cushing, "Electro-surgery as an aid to the removal of intracranial tumors with a preliminary note on a new surgical-current generator by W. T. Bovie," *Surg. Gynec. Obstet.* (1928), 47:751–84. Howard A. Kelly and Grant E. Ward gave a good account of origins in *Electrosurgery* (Philadelphia: W. B. Saunders, 1932), pp. 1–9.

17. Celsus, *De medicina,* with an English translation by W. G. Spencer (Cambridge: Harvard Univ. Press, Loeb Classical Library, 1961), 2:105, 127–29. Aetius of Amida provides an excellent account of Leonides' operation. See *Aetios of Amida: The gynaecology and obstetrics of the VIth century, A.D.*, ed. and trans. James V. Ricci (Philadelphia: Blakiston, 1950), p. 50.

18. Henri de Mondeville, *Chirurgie, composée de 1306 à 1320*, ed. Édouard Nicaise (Paris, 1893), p. 564 n.; Guy de Chauliac, *La grande chirurgie de Guy de Chauliac, composée en l'an 1363*, ed. Édouard Nicaise (Paris, 1890), pp. 436, 592. The writings of these two great Frenchmen are magnificent sources for the historian of the practices and doctrines of pre-Renaissance surgery in Europe. Mondeville (ca. 1260–1320) studied under Theodoric in Bologna and Pitard in Paris. He taught in Montpellier and Paris and was surgeon to two French kings. His treatise on surgery, composed between 1306 and 1320, remained in manuscript form until 1890 and never had the impact of Guy's popular *Grande chirurgie* (1363), which appeared in many editions and became the authoritative text on surgery for the two hundred years before Paré. Mondeville, like Guy, was both cleric and physician. Guy de Chauliac (ca. 1298–1368) pursued his medical education in Montpellier, Toulouse, and Paris and studied anatomy under Bertuccio of Bologna. His final residence was Avignon, then the seat of the Papacy and a famous center of learning, where he served a succession of popes.

19. Giovanni de Vigo, *The most excelent worckes of chirurgery*, trans. ([London], 1550), fol. 115 verso. Guy de Chauliac used either cautery or boiling oil on the healthy flesh after amputation. *Grande chirurgie* (n.18), p. 436. Both Brunschwig and Hans Gersdorff (ca. 1456–1517) used boiling oil to check hemorrhage after amputation. Garrison, *History of medicine* (n.4), p. 202.

20. The usually accepted date of Ambroise Paré's birth is 1510, although dates varying from 1509 to 1517 have been suggested. In the strictest sense Paré cannot be labeled a military surgeon; there was then no organized medical service in the French army. However, most of his professional life was spent in wars. His was primarily a personal commitment to a succession of kings whom he served over a period of more than three decades. The autobiographical version of his rejection of boiling oil was related by the sixty-five-year-old Paré in 1575 and appears in *The workes of that famous chirurgion Ambrose Parey*, trans. Thomas Johnson (London, 1634), pp. 408–9, 1143. The anecdote was not mentioned in Paré's *La méthode de traicter les playes faictes par hacquebutes et aultres bastons à feu* (Paris, 1545). Oil of roses was a filtered mixture of rose petals and olive oil.

21. Paré, *Workes* (n.20), pp. 457–64, 1064.

22. Peter Lowe, *The whole course of chirurgie* (London, 1597), treatise 4, chap. 6; Wiseman, *Treatises* (n.9), p. 453; Woodall, *Surgeons mate* (n.8), p. 388. Lowe (ca. 1550–1612) practiced for many years on the Continent. Returning to Scotland, he established the Faculty of Physicians and Surgeons of Glasgow (1599). His book was the first comprehensive text on surgery published in Great Britain.

23. John Bell, *The principles of surgery*, ed. Charles Bell, new ed. (London, 1826), 1:136; Claude Pouteau, *Oeuvres posthumes* (Paris, 1783), 3:252–55. André Dussaussoy also recommended cauterization when hospital gangrene made rapid progress, saying that boiling oil was no substitute. See his *Dissertation et observations sur la gangrène des hôpitaux* (Geneva, 1787), pp. 40–43. Pouteau (1724–75), whose skill as a lithotomist and whose wisdom in discerning the nature of infection will be discussed later, became chief surgeon at the Hôtel-Dieu in Lyons in 1747. It was said that "his genius disdained the routine and opened new paths for the art." J. E. Pétrequin, *J. de méd. de Lyon* (1844), 7:427–30.

24. Jacques Delpech, *Mémoire sur la complication des plaies et des ulcères, connue sous le nom de pourriture d'hôpital* (Paris, 1815), pp. i-viii, 89–92, 101–2. In a visit to Montpellier in 1968, the authors found Delpech's statue in the courtyard of the reconstructed hospital of Saint-Éloi. The memory of this forthright and innovative surgeon is still treasured in the city where he contributed so forcefully to the upgrading of surgery. Delpech was assassinated by a deranged former patient in 1832. Louis Dulieu, *Essai historique sur l'hôpital Saint-Éloi de Montpellier, 1183–1950* (Montpellier: Déhan, 1953), pp. 151, 207–8, 238.

25. Johann Nussbaum, *Die chirurgische Klinik zu München im Jahre 1875* (Stuttgart, 1875), pp. 3–5; Amédée Bonnet, "Mémoire sur la cautérisation considérée comme moyen de combattre les accidents . . . a la suite des opérations." *Bull. gén. de thérap.* (1848), 34:119–30. Bonnet also used such caustics as nitrate of silver, which was then becoming popular; these materials will be discussed in chapter 17 on antiseptics. Paul Trudeau in *Traitement du phlegmon diffuse par le fer rouge*, a Paris thesis of 1878, remarks that in using incision with cautery, Bonnet and Léon Labbé combined the advantages of debridement and cauterization (p. 7). He gives a number of case histories from their two services.

26. Berkeley Moynihan, *American addresses* (Philadelphia: W. B. Saunders, 1917), p. 76; Bodo-Heinz Wiebeck, *Über die Kauterisation akzidenteller Wunden der Hand und Finger*, Berlin thesis, 1935, pp. 8–17. Moynihan, essentially an abdominal surgeon, was a deft operator, probably the finest surgical orator of his day, and a keen student of surgical literature. He helped found the *British Journal of Surgery*. The provincial Chirurgical Club now bears his name, and the British Association of Surgeons, which has had an important influence upon British surgery, owes much to Moynihan. He was knighted in 1912 and became Lord Moynihan in 1929. He has said of himself: "I have gathered a posie of other men's flowers, nothing but the thread that binds them is mine own," a very unpretentious statement of a man not always so modest.

27. Albucasis, *On surgery and instruments* (n.12), pp. 138, 800.

28. Pierre-François Percy, *Pyrotechnie chirurgicale-pratique; ou, l'art d'appliquer le feu en*

chirurgie (Paris, 1811); Dominique-J. Larrey, *Observations on wounds, and their complications by erysipelas, gangrene and tetanus*, trans. E. F. Rivinus (Philadelphia, 1832), pp. 45–46.

29. Joseph Lister, "Report of some cases of articular disease occurring in Mr. Syme's practice, illustrating the advantages of the actual cautery," *Month. J. M. Sc.*, London & Edinb. (1854), 19:134–37; E. Mitchell Banks, "On the neglect of the actual cautery," *Liverpool M.-Chir. J.* (1892), 12:96–97.

30. Ambroise Paré, *Dix livres de la chirurgie* (Paris, 1564), fols. 111–12 recto; Paré, *Workes* (n.20), pp. 1134, 1148; John Thomson, *Lectures on inflammation*, 2d Am. ed. (Philadelphia, 1831), p. 219.

31. Whereas Celsus does not specifically say he employed the ligature in amputation, he used it to staunch brisk bleeding, with the cautery as a last resort. See *De medicina* (n.17), 3:405. Lister, a profound student of amputation as well as of inflammation, expressed the belief, in all three editions of his monograph on amputation in Timothy Holmes's *System of surgery* (1862, 1871, 1883) that Celsus probably employed the ligature in amputations, a view shared by the authors of this volume. Leo M. Zimmerman and Ilza Veith in *Great ideas in the history of surgery* (Baltimore: Williams and Wilkins, 1961), pp. 130–34, make it quite clear that the Flemish surgeon Jean Yperman (thirteenth century) used the ligature and therefore probably applied it in amputations. He ligated arteries much as did Brunschwig and Paré. Albucasis was pessimistic about the control of arterial hemorrhage in wounds by ligature, undoubtedly because of the danger of infection. Albucasis, *On surgery and instruments* (n.12), pp. 162–64.

32. William Clowes, *A prooved practice for all young chirurgions, concerning burnings with gunpowder, and wounds made with gunshot* (London, 1588), pp. 28–33; Fabricius, *Opera* (n.13), p. 802.

33. Paré, *Workes* (n.20), pp. 327, 458–60; Hieronymous Brunschwig, *Das Buch der Cirurgia* (Strasbourg, 1497; facsimile, with a study on Brunschwig by Henry E. Sigerist, Milan: Lier, 1923), fol. 25 verso. See Joseph-François Malgaigne's discussion in his excellent edition of the *Oeuvres complètes d'Ambroise Paré* (Paris, 1840), 2:224–25.

34. M. Roman and J. Klopfer, "Zur Amputations-Statistik," *Beitr. klin. Chir.* (1890), 6:409.

35. Paré, *Workes* (n.20), p. 460; Dionis, *Cours d'operations* (n.10), p. 620.

36. Woodall, *Surgeons mate* (n.8), p. 157; Dionis, *Cours d'operations* (n.10), p. 620; Hugues Ravaton, *Chirurgie d'armée ou traité des plaies d'armes a feu et d'armes blanches* (Paris, 1768), p. 263. For a field hospital serving an army of 20,000 men, Ravaton states that a day's major military engagement may produce 2,000 injured, requiring the services of one competent surgeon, 10 intelligent surgical aides, and 30 students of surgery (pp. 636–37).

37. William Fergusson, *A system of practical surgery*, 3d Am. ed. (Philadelphia, 1848), p. 395; John [G.] Cross[e], *Sketches of the medical schools of Paris* (London, 1815), pp. 70–71.

38. This spirited version appears in a translation by "N. C." of Fabricius Hildanus, *Lithotomia vesicae* (London, 1640), p. 93. N. C. erroneously translated "leg" as "thigh."

39. Thomson, *Lectures on inflammation* (n.30), p. 219; Jacques Guillemeau, *The Frenche chirurgerye*, trans. A. M. (Dort [Dordrecht], 1597), fol. 38.

40. This view is expressed by Thomson in *Lectures on inflammation* (n.30), p. 220, and by Gustav Wolzendorff in "Die locale Behandlung frischer Wunden im 15., 16. und 17. Jahrhundert," *Dt. Z. Chir.* (1877), 8:264–65.

41. Guy de Chauliac, *Ars chirurgica* (Venice, 1546), fol. 63 verso. Allen O. Whipple credits Gersdorff with the first use of a tourniquet (1517) in amputation. Our reading of Gersdorff and of Ernst Gurlt's commentary persuades us that Gersdorff's device was essentially the same as the tight bands Guy used. See Whipple, *The story of wound healing and wound repair* (Springfield, Ill.: Charles C Thomas, 1963), p. 57; Hans Gersdorff, *Feldtbůch der Wundartzney* (Strasbourg, 1526), fols. 25 recto, 80–81 verso; and Gurlt, *Geschichte der Chirurgie* (Berlin, 1898; reprint, Hildesheim: Georg Olms, 1964), 2:232.

42. Leonardo Botallo, "De curandis vulneribus sclopettorum," pp. 612–14 in his *Commen-*

tarioli duo, alter de medici, alter de aegroti munere (Leyden, 1565); Fabricius, *Opera* (n.13), p. 808; Johannes Scultetus (Schultes), *Armamentarium chirurgicum* (Ulm, 1655), table 18; Dionis, *Cours d'operations* (n.10), p. [606], fig. 47; p. 621. *Armamentarium chirurgicum* of Scultetus (1595–1645) was first published at Ulm in 1653 after his death. Botallo (b. 1530), an Italian physician-surgeon, practiced in Paris.

43. Jean-Louis Petit, "D'un nouvel instrument de chirurgie," *Mém. Acad. roy. sci.* (1718), pp. 252–55; Ravaton, *Chirurgie d'armée* (n.36), pp. 109–11. Petit (1674–1750), a child prodigy with keen interest in anatomy, became the most distinguished French surgeon of his time.

44. Hunter, *Works* (n.9), 1:538; Irving F. Enquist, Karl E. Karlson, Clarence Dennis, et al., "Statistically valid ten-year comparative evaluation . . . of management of massive gastroduodenal hemorrhage," *Trans. Am. Surg. Assoc.* (1965), 83:237. Reinfusion of the dog's lost blood without occlusion of the bleeding vessel, however, pyramided blood loss considerably. A British consul in Abyssinia (1848–60) wrote that when criminals there were punished by amputation at wrist, ankle, knee, or elbow, all assistance was sometimes denied, scarce any means of stopping bleeding was known, yet few died. Walter C. Plowden, *Travels in Abyssinia and the Galla Country* (London, 1868), p. 97. A harrowing account of three such amputations in Abyssinia, with survival of the victims, is described by Antoine Petit, *Gaz. hôp.*, Paris (1840), 2:481–82, 489–90.

45. Johann L. Schmucker, *Chirurgische Wahrnehmungen* (Berlin and Stettin, 1774), 2:498–99; J. C. Rougemont, ed., *Bibliothèque de chirurgie du nord* (Bonn, 1788), 1:41–42.

46. Jean Faure's winning answer (1756) to the questions posed by the subject "l'amputation étant absolument nécessaire dans les plaies compliquées de fracas des os," appears in *Pièces qui ont concouru pour le prix* (n.15), 3:488–520. Boucher, "Observations sur des plaies d'armes à feu, compliquées de fracture," *Mém. Acad. roy. chir.* (1753), 2:287–307, 461–83. The French defeated the Anglo-Allied forces at Fontenoy, Belgium, May 11, 1745, during the Austrian War of Succession.

47. Dominique-J. Larrey, *Mémoire sur les amputations des membres à la suite des coups de feu* (Paris, 1797); Larrey, *Mémoires de chirurgie militaire, et campagnes* (Paris, 1817), 4:57, 176–77. A recent excellent study, *Larrey: Surgeon to Napoleon's Imperial Guard* by Robert G. Richardson (London: Murray, 1974), explains the advantages of immediate amputation after gunshot wounds, especially those caused by cannon-fire, as follows: During the first hours, the limb was numb and the muscles were relaxed a few inches above the injury; the low blood pressure in shock helped to stop bleeding. Moreover, a soldier with a surgical stump was safer and easier to transport than one whose unattended wound was a "bloody, dirty mess" (p. 23).

48. Joseph-F. Malgaigne, "Études statistiques sur les résultats des grandes opérations dans les hôpitaux de Paris," *Arch. gén. de méd.* (1842), 13:399; William MacCormac, "Operation rooms, past and present," *Bristol M.-Chir. J.* (1898), 16:304.

49. John Thomson, *Report of observations made in the British military hospitals in Belgium after the Battle of Waterloo* (Edinburgh, 1816), pp. 247–52; H. Home Blackadder, *Observations of Phagedaena gangraenosa* (Edinburgh, 1818), p. 124. One hundred years earlier Dionis (1707) found it necessary to defend the king's chirurgeons against the charge of being so eager for amputation that "they reckoned up their exploits in a campaign by the number of legs and arms they had cut off." *Cours d'operations* (n.10), p. 608.

50. Pierre-F. Percy and Deschamps, *Rapport fait à l'Institut . . . dans la séance de 25 juillet, 1814*, p. 61, in P.-J. Roux, *Mémoire et observations sur la réunion immédiate* (Paris, 1814). John Hennen added a list of "most melancholy" mortality estimates for compound fracture to the second edition of his *Principles of military surgery* (Edinburgh, 1820), pp. 108–9.

51. George J. Guthrie, *Treatise on gunshot wounds*, 3d ed. (London, 1827), pp. 227–28; Guthrie, *Clinical lectures on compound fractures of the extremities* (Philadelphia, 1839), p. 50; Joseph-F. Malgaigne, *Traité des fractures et des luxations* (Paris, 1847), 1:739.

52. Larrey: *Mémoire sur les amputations* (n.47), and *Mémoires de chirurgie militaire* (n.47), 4:25.

53. F. A. Ammon, *Parallele der französischen und deutschen Chirurgie* (Leipzig, 1823), pp. 37–38; Charles Averill, *A short treatise on operative surgery*, 2d ed. (London, 1825), p. 154; Amédée Forget, "De l'opportunité et des lois générales des amputations dans la continuité," *Gaz. hôp.*, Paris (1840), 13:325; John T. Morse, Jr., *Life and letters of Oliver Wendell Holmes* (Boston, 1896), 1:92. Holmes (1809–94) spent two years studying medicine in Paris hospitals following three years in Harvard Medical School. His fame as a poet began at Harvard.

54. Benjamin Bell, *A system of surgery* (Edinburgh, 1788), 6:361; Larrey, *Mémoires de chirurgie militaire* (n.47), 3:161–62; D'Arcy Power, "Robert Liston (1794–1847)," *Dictionary of national biography* (1909), 11:1236.

55. Fergusson, *Practical surgery* (n.37), pp. 164, 395; Frederic S. Dennis, "Memoir of Dr. James R. Wood," *N. York M. J.* (1884), 39:31.

56. Samuel W. Francis, *Memoir of the life and character of Valentine Mott*, 2d ed. (New York, 1865), pp. 19–20. Valentine Mott (1785–1865) was then professor of surgery at New York University Medical College.

57. Paré, *Workes* (n.20), p. 459; Malgaigne, *Oeuvres de Paré* (n.33), 2:225. The spring was first illustrated in the 1585 edition of Paré's *Oeuvres*, which was not the source of Johnson's 1634 translation. The enlarged second edition of Paré's collected works, published in French in 1579, was translated into Latin in 1582, reaching a wide audience. Johnson's English translation of 1634, the *Workes*, with which we are chiefly concerned in this discussion, was from the 1582 Latin version. A good account of the many editions of Paré's publications is given in Janet Doe, *Bibliography of the works of Ambroise Paré* (Chicago: Univ. Chicago Press, 1937).

58. Malgaigne, *Oeuvres de Paré* (n.33), 1:389. This illustration had appeared in 1564 in Paré's *Dix livres* (fol. 225 verso), so we may be certain it was his own choice. The design, however, apparently has a more ancient history. Nicaise, who did considerable research on the instruments available to Henri de Mondeville and Guy de Chauliac, included a similar knife in his illustrations of their works. Unfortunately Nicaise did not provide the source of his information. Guy de Chauliac, *Grande chirurgie* (n.18), p. 703, fig. 3, #53.

59. Alfred A. L. M. Velpeau, *New elements of operative surgery*, trans. P. S. Townsend (New York, 1847), 2:473–74; Jacques Bourakhowitch, *Contribution à la bio-bibliographie d'Antoine Louis*, Rennes thesis, 1958, p. 20.

60. The relative order of sensitivity of tissues was established by K. G. Lennander by operating under light anesthesia or local anesthesia in the early decades of the twentieth century. "Beobachtungen über die Sensibilität in der Bauchhöhle," *Mitt. Grenzgeb. Med. Chir.* (1902), 10:38–104. Pierre Huard and M. D. Grmek illustrate a variety of instruments in use from the period before the Napoleonic Wars into the midnineteenth century, in *Sciences, médecine, pharmacie, de la Révolution à l'Empire (1789–1815)* (Paris: Roger Dacosta, 1970).

61. James Yonge, *Currus triumphalis è terebinthô* (London, 1679), p. 110. Gurlt reminds us, in *Geschichte der Chirurgie* (n.41), 1:541, that Oribasius (325–403) employed skin flaps in amputation considerably earlier. Samuel C. Harvey, in his footnotes to Billroth's *Historical studies of gunshot wounds* (n.6), p. 27, credits Pierre Sabouris with the use of skin flaps in finger amputation in 1696 and Pierre A. Verduin with the same procedure in 1697. In the *Journal of James Yonge [1647–1721]*, ed. F. N. L. Poynter (Hamden, Conn.: Archon Books, 1963), Yonge mentions a surgeon friend, Caleb Lowdham of Chudleigh (p. 152), undoubtedly the surgeon referred to in *Currus triumphalis*. G. E. Larks, a Plymouth surgeon, has recently found an unpublished manuscript by Yonge, "An account of many secrets in art & nature," in which the flap amputation is mentioned, seven years before the published account, and credited to "Smith, a surgeon at Exeter." Personal communication, May 20, 1974.

62. Celsus, *De medicina* (n.17), 3:405, 467, 471. The quotation is from L. E. Parmentier, *Quelques recherches sur la cicatrisation des plaies exposées au contact de l'air* (Paris, 1854), p. 8. See Alexis Carrel, "The treatment of wounds," *JAMA* (1910), 55:2148–50.

63. Galen, *Opera omnia*, ed. C. G. Kühn (Leipzig, 1829), 18:718. Galen remained a

peripatetic, migrating from place to place as interests and opportunities took him. His great skill in treating wounds of trauma was acquired as surgeon to the gladiators in Pergamon and Rome. He also performed some elective operations in several sectors of surgery. He wrote extensively and was the author of many books; these became the undisputed authority for generations of practitioners. As theorist and practical man of medicine, Galen deservedly commanded the respect and admiration of successive generations of men of medicine. See Garrison, *History of medicine* (n.4), pp. 113–17; Louis H. Toledo-Pereyra, "Galen's contribution to surgery," *J. Hist. Med.* (1973), 28:357–75.

64. Paré, *Workes* (n.20), p. 378.

65. Theodoric, "Chirurgia," in Guy de Chauliac, *Ars chirurgica* (n.41), fol. 140 recto; Henry Sigerist, ed., *Ambroise Paré, die Behandlung der Schusswunden (1545)* (Leipzig: Barth, 1923), p. 10. See also Zimmerman and Veith, *Great ideas* (n.31), p. 101.

66. Guy de Chauliac, *Ars chirurgica* (n.41), tract 3, doc. 1, cap. 1; cap. 2, fol. 31 recto.

67. T. Clifford Allbutt, *Historical relations of medicine and surgery to the end of the sixteenth century* (London: Macmillan, 1905), p. 52; Garrison, *History of medicine* (n.4), p. 157. The same critiques have been echoed more recently by Eldridge Campbell and James Colton in "Theodoric on wounds," *Surg. Gynec. Obstet.* (1951), 93:373, and by Frank B. Berry in his foreword to Campbell and Colton's translation of *The surgery of Theodoric, ca. A.D. 1267* (New York: Appleton-Century-Crofts, 1955), 1:xxxciii. See also Malgaigne, *Oeuvres de Paré* (n.33), I:lxvi, and Nicaise's preface to Guy's *Grande chirurgie* (n.18), pp. iii–viii.

68. For a more general appreciation of Guy's contribution to wound management, including current reappraisals, see Pagel (n.4), p. 1039; Walter Brunn, "Die Stellung des Guy de Chauliac in der Chirurgie des Mittelalters," *Arch. Gesch. Med.* (1920), 12:85–100, (1921), 13:65–106; Zimmerman and Veith, *Great ideas* (n.31), pp. 152–54; Jordan D. Haller, "Guy de Chauliac and his Chirurgia Magna," *Surgery* (1964), 55:337–43; and Edward D. Churchill, "Healing by first intention and with suppuration," *J. Hist. Med.* (1964), 19:200–202.

69. Paré, *Workes* (n.20), p. 460, and *Dix livres* (n.30), fol. 112 verso.

70. Brunschwig, *Cirurgia* (n.33), fol. 21.

71. Philibert-J. Roux, *Relation d'un voyage fait à Londres en 1814* (Paris, 1815), pp. 96, 116. See also chapter 3, note 6.

72. Philibert-J. Roux, in Lucien Baudens et al., *Plaies d'armes à feu, communications faites a l'Académie nationale de médecine* (Paris, 1849), pp. 36–37.

73. Theodor Billroth, "Beobachtungs-Studien über Wundfieber und accidentelle Wundkrankheiten," *Arch. klin. Chir.* (1865), 6:444.

74. Edward Alanson, *Practical observations on amputation, and the after-treatment,* 2d ed. (London, 1782), pp. xv, 22–24, 87–103. Alanson mentions the thirty-five consecutive ("such as promiscuously occurred") successful operations in the preface. He devotes a chapter to the importance of hospital sanitation, observing that "Many hospitals are so tainted by unwholesome effluvia, that they are rather a pest, than a relief, to the objects they contain." His recommendations included special rooms for surgery patients and a special house for convalescents, periodic whitewashing of wards, frequent changes of bedding, iron bedsteads, baking of infected clothing, and isolation of patients with gangrenous sores.

75. Vincenz Kern, *Ueber die Handlungsweise bey Absetzung der Glieder* (Vienna, 1826), pp. 30–35; Carl A. Burow, "Ueber die Ursache der häufigen Todesfälle nach Amputationen," *Dt. Klinik,* Berlin (1859), 11:207–17; Burow, "Offene Wundbehandlung," *Dt. Z. Chir.* (1873), 2:425–37.

76. Jacques Lisfranc, "Eine neue Verfahrungsart zur Exarticulation des Oberschenkels," *Froriep Notizen* (1823), 5:159; J. P. Maunoir, *Mémoires sur les amputations* (Geneva, 1825), pp. 17, 44; Guillaume Dupuytren, *Leçons orales de clinique chirurgicale* (Paris, 1834), 4:413–14; Alcide-A. Gronnier, *Essaie sur la réunion immédiate à la suite des amputations,* Montpellier thesis, 1835; Voison, "Revue des blessés du 5 et 6 juin, admis a l'hôpital Saint-Louis," *Gaz. méd. Paris* (1832), 3:430–35; Maximilian J. Chelius, *Handbuch der Chirurgie* (Heidelberg, 1844), 2:766.

77. Robert Liston, "Four cases of amputation," *Br. Ann. Med., Pharm.* (1837), 1:518–22, and "Results of amputations at University College Hospital, London," *Med.-Chir. Trans.* (1841), 24:155–76; John E. Erichsen, "Liston and water-dressing," letter to the editor, *Lancet* (1879), 1:65; Joseph Lister, "Effects of the antiseptic system upon the salubrity of a surgical hospital," *Lancet* (1870), 1:40. Lister began his antiseptic treatment in 1865; however, in the assessment of mortality he unfortunately placed the experiences of 1866, for which the mortality among his patients was 50 percent, in the preantiseptic period.

78. "Heroes of medicine: Robert Liston," unsigned article, *Practitioner*, London (1899), 10:548; Erichsen (n.77); [discussion], *Congrès méd. internat. de Paris, 1867* (Paris, 1868), p. 301; George M. Humphry, "On the treatment of wounds and patients after operations," *Br. M. J.* (1860), 2:841. Humphry said that in nearly all operations, "The integuments are united by sutures placed at intervals of about an inch; and the wound, as well as adjacent surface is left quite exposed to the air . . . no dressing of any kind" was used.

79. The 1861 report, perhaps the first military directive urging open management of amputation wounds, was made by the Medical Commission of the State of Massachusetts, headed by George Hayward, to the U.S. Sanitary Commission (Sanitary Commission F. Report . . . on the subject of amputations, Boston, 1861). S. D. Townsend and J. M. Warren were among the signers. Signatories of the second document were Mott, Gurdon Buck, John Watson, Alfred C. Post, Willard Parker, Ernest Krackowizer, and W. H. Van Buren, a roster of prominent New York surgeons. Sanitary Commission G. Report . . . on amputations through the foot (New York, 1862).

80. Frederic S. Dennis, "On the treatment of amputations by the open method," *N. York M. J.* (1876), 23:11, 15–17. Halsted wrote William H. Welch in 1922 concerning his intern days at Bellevue: "Lister had just visited this country and his methods were enthusiastically adopted by Stephen Smith and Sabine — not by any other surgeon at Bellevue." Since Dennis's report concerns patients operated upon in 1875, more than a year before Lister's visit to the International Medical Congress in Philadelphia, it would appear that Halsted, in his exchange with Welch many years later, overlooked Dennis's acceptance of at least some of Lister's practices. See W. G. MacCallum, *William Stewart Halsted, surgeon* (Baltimore: Johns Hopkins Press, 1930), p. 17.

81. R. R. Kendrick, "Below-knee amputation in arteriosclerotic gangrene," *Br. J. Surg.* (1956), 44:13–17; LeRoy H. Stahlgren and Merlin Otteman, "Review of criteria for the selection of the level for lower extremity amputation for arteriosclerosis," *Ann. Surg.* (1965), 162:886–92.

82. Gersdorff, *Feldtbůch* (n.41), fols. 80–81. Fabricius (1646) also used adhesive tape and disapproved of sutures (n.13), p. 815. Paré, *Dix livres* (n.30), fol. 112 verso. A good illustration of the dry suture appears in Paré, *Workes* (n.20), p. 383.

83. Antoine Louis, "Mémoire sur la saillie de l'os après l'amputation des membres," *Mém. Acad. roy. chir.* (1753), 2:269–70.

84. G. B. P. Pibrac, "Mémoire sur l'abus des sutures," *Mém. Acad. roy. chir.* (1757), 3:408–30. Delpech used the adhesive method of suture with brilliant success for nineteen years, says Antonio do luz Pitta of Madeira in a Paris thesis (*De la réunion immédiate et de ses advantages*, 1831, p. 11). Chelius (1844) considered sutures injurious in uniting an amputation stump; see *Handbuch* (n.76), 2:768.

85. William H. Welch, "Conditions underlying the infection of wounds," in Congress of American Physicians and Surgeons, *Transactions* (1891), 2:1–28; Welch, "Some considerations concerning antiseptic surgery," *Maryland M. J.* (1891), 26:45–57; Welch, "General bacteriology of surgical infections," pp. 249–334, in Frederic S. Dennis, ed., *System of surgery* (Philadelphia, 1895). 1:250–52, 272; William S. Halsted, "The radical cure of hernia," *Johns Hopkins Hosp. Bull.* (1889), 1:13; Halsted, "The treatment of wounds: The management of the dead spaces," *Johns Hopkins Hosp. Rep.* (1891), 2:304–5. See also fig. 6 in Halsted, "Ligature and suture material," *JAMA* (1913), 60:1123.

86. Stephen D. Elek, "Experimental staphylococcal infections in the skin of man," *Ann. N.Y. Acad. Sci.* (1956), 65:85–90. In a subsequent paper Elek and P. E. Conen dealt additionally with the susceptibility of the host and the virulence of the organism. *Br. J. Exp. Path.* (1957), 38:573–86.

87. M. T. F. Carpendale and W. Sereda, "The role of the percutaneous suture in surgical wound infection," *Surgery* (1965), 58:672–77; Richard F. Edlich, Ming-Shiung Tsung, Waid Rogers, Palmer Rogers, and O. H. Wangensteen, "Studies in management of the contaminated wound. I. Technique of closure," *J. Surg. Res.* (1968), 8:585–92. B. Bell, *System of surgery* (n.54), 1:3–4. Samuel Young, who favored closing wounds by adhesive tape, disapproved strongly of Bell's treatment. Young, *An attempt at a systematic reform of . . . adhesion: especially . . . the use and abuse of the thread suture* (London, 1808).

88. P. J. Morris, B. A. Barnes, and J. F. Burke, "The nature of the 'irreducible minimum' rate of incisional sepsis," *Arch. Surg.* (1966), 92:367–70; John M. Howard, chairman, "Postoperative wound infections . . . Report of an *ad hoc* committee," *Ann. Surg.* (1964), vol. 160, (August) supplement. See chapter 3.

89. See n.46.

90. Woodall, *Surgeons mate* (n.8), p. 388. Woodall added that he could produce more than twenty witnesses to confirm that his results in amputation had been good (p. 391).

91. Alexander Monro I, "Remarks on the amputations of the larger extremities," *Med. Essays & Obs.* Edinburgh (1737), 4:342; ibid., 4th ed. (1752), 4:276. The 1970 edition of *Garrison and Morton* (n.12) fails to mention Monro I (1697–1767), stating "Alexander *secundus* was the greatest of the three famous Monros" — probably a debatable issue.

92. James Y. Simpson, "On surgical fever," *Med. Times & Gaz.* (1859), 39:412; Thomas B. Peacock, *Statistical tables of the Royal Infirmary of Edinburgh . . . for the year 1843* (Edinburgh, 1843), p. 19.

93. J. P. Maunoir, *Mémoires sur les amputations* (n.76), p. 17, 42; Paul Dubois, letter, *J. hebd. de méd.* (1830), 7:27–32; Stephen L. Hammick, *Practical remarks on amputations* (London, 1830), p. 39; Liston, "Results of amputations" (n.77); Paul F. Eve, "Remarks on the statistics of amputation," *South. M. & S. J.* (1846), 2:468. C. Maunoir, reports his brother, had no deaths in 30 major amputations performed since 1801. Dubois reported 3 in 28, including 13 thighs; Hammick, 2 in 49; Liston, 6 in 52; Eve, who included some minor amputations, no deaths in 51.

94. Malgaigne (n.48), 13:389–418; 14:50–81. Whereas the mortality from amputation through fingers and toes, in which the soft tissue covering is relatively slight, was considerably less than for major extremities, J. F. W. Nevermann, Velpeau, and a number of others have indicated the great threat to life which even the sacrifice of a finger commanded. Nevermann, "Ueber die Vorzüge der Lappenamputation vor dem Cirkelschnitte, nebst Bermerkungen," *Klin. Ztschr. f. Chir. u. Augenh.* (1836–37), 1:437; Velpeau, *Operative surgery* (n.59), 2:461.

95. Dupuytren's opinion is reported in Malgaigne's "Revue de la clinique de M. le professeur Dupuytren," *Gaz. méd. Paris* (1832), 3:392–95, L.-J. Sanson believed that better results were obtained among military personnel (contrasted with civilian amputations) because the former were steeled to accept stoically whatever the attending surgeon recommended. Sanson, "Remarques sur la différence dans le résultats des amputations practiquées dans les hôpitaux civils ou sur le champ de bataille," *Répert. gén. d'anat. et physiol. path.* (1827), 3:226–28.

96. *The life of Sir Robert Christison, Bart.*, ed. by his sons (Edinburgh, 1885), 1:229.

97. Guillaume Dupuytren, *Leçons orales de clinique chirurgicale . . . recueillies par A. Paillard et Marx* (Paris, 1839), 6:108–15; Thomson, *Lectures on inflammation* (n.30), p. 392; Blackadder, *Phagedaena gangraenosa* (n.49), pp. 46–47.

98. Nicolai I. Pirogoff: *Klinische Chirurgie: Eine Sammlung von Monographien über die wichtigsten Gegenstände der praktischen Chirurgie* (Leipzig, 1854), 1:22–47, and *Grundzüge der allgemeinen Kriegschirurgie* (Leipzig, 1864), pp. 2, 947–53. That a surgeon plagued with intractable diarrhea prior to the advent of rubber gloves had trouble with wound infection occasions no surprise.

99. William D. Hodges, "Massachusetts General Hospital — surgical cases — antiseptic

treatment," *Physicians' Mag.*, Philadelphia (1885–86), 1:188–91; Richard Volkmann, "Ueber den antiseptischen Occlusivverband und seinen Einfluss auf den Heilungsprocess der Wunden," *Samml. klin. Vortr.* (1874), Chir. no. 30, pp. 759–812.

Further Readings

Ballu, André. *L'arsenal chirurgical ancien.* Paris thesis, 1905.

Bartholinus, Casper. *Syntagma medicum & chirurgicum de cauteriis.* Copenhagen, 1624.

Bigg, H. R. H. *Artificial limbs.* London, 1885.

Committee on Prosthetics Research. *Conference on the geriatric amputee.* Washington, D.C.: National Academy of Sciences–National Research Council, 1961.

Fandre, A. *Le catgut, les ligatures, et les sutures chirurgicales à travers les âges.* Paris: Masson, 1944.

Fee, H. J.; Friedman, B. H.; and Siegel, M. E. Selection of an amputation level with radioactive microspheres. *Surg. Gynec. Obstet.* (1977), 144:89–90.

Gillis, Leon. *Amputations*, 1954. New York: Grune and Stratton, 1954.

Girard, Charles. Désarticulation de l'os iliaque pour sarcome. *Congrès français de chirurgie* (1895), 9:823–27.

Gordon-Taylor, Sir Gordon, and Wiles, Philip. Interinnomino-abdominal (hind-quarter) amputation. *Br. J. Surg.* (1935), 22:671–95.

Gritti, Rocco. Dell'amputazione del femore al terzo inferiore e della disarticulazione del ginocchio. *Ann. univ. di med.*, Milan (1857), 161:5–32.

Harvey, Samuel C. *The history of hemostasis.* New York: Paul B. Hoeber, 1929.

Heyfelder, Johann Ferdinand Martin. *Ueber Resectionen und Amputationen.* Breslau and Bonn, 1854.

Jaboulay, Mathieu. La désarticulation interilio-abdominale. *Lyon méd.* (1894), 75:507–10.

Kershaw, Alister. *A history of the guillotine.* London: John Calder, 1958.

Kirk, Norman T. Development of amputation. *Bull. Med. Libr. Assoc.* (1944), 32:132–63.

Krukenberg, Hermann. Eine neue osteoplastische Amputationsmethode des Oberschenkels. *Zentbl. Chir.* (1917), 44:578.

Little, J. M. *Major amputations for vascular disease.* Edinburgh and New York: Churchill Livingstone, 1975.

Magnus, Peter P. *Discorso sopra il modo di fare i cauteri.* Brescia, 1618.

Milne, John Stewart. *Surgical instruments in Greek and Roman times.* Oxford: Clarendon Press, 1907.

Mital, Mohinder A., and Pierce, Donald S. *Amputees and their prostheses.* Boston: Little, Brown, 1971.

Møller-Christensen, Vilhelm. *History of the forceps.* Trans. W. E. Calvert. Copenhagen: Levin and Munksgaard, 1938.

Nicholas, Gary G., and DeMuth, William E., Jr. Evaluation of use of the rigid dressing in amputation of the lower extremity. *Surg. Gynec. Obstet.* (1976), 143:398–400.

Nissen, Rudolf, and Bergmann, Ernst. *Cineplastic operations on stumps of the upper extremity.* New York: Grune and Stratton, 1942.

Putti, Vittori. The utilization of the muscles of a stump to actuate artificial limbs: cinematic amputations. *Br. M. J.* (1918), 1:635–38.

Rochard, Jules E. *Histoire de la chirurgie française au XIXe siècle.* Paris, 1875.

Rosenbach, Anton J. F. Der hospitalbrand. *Dt. Chir.*, Stuttgart (1888), vol. 15, bk. 6.

Scultetus, Johannes. *L'arcenal de chirurgie.* Lyons, 1675.

Severin, Marc A. *De la médecine efficace, ou la manière de guerir les plus grandes & dangereuses maladies . . . par le fer & par le feu.* Geneva, 1668.

Syme, James. Amputation at the ankle-joint. *Month. J. M. Sc.* (1843), 3:93–96.

Thompson, Charles J. S. *The history and evolution of surgical instruments.* New York: Schuman, 1942.

Wangensteen, O. H.; Smith, Jacqueline; and Wangensteen, S. D. Some highlights in the history of amputation reflecting lessons in wound healing. *Bull. Hist. Med.* (1967), 41:97-131.

Chapter 3. Debridement

NOTES

1. The extraction of arrows and missiles, including lead balls and pebbles, in Roman warfare was meticulously described by Celsus. As Spencer points out, his treatment was followed by well-known surgeons as late as Paré in the Renaissance period, although gunpowder had altered the type of wounds in warfare. Celsus, *De medicina*, with an English translation by W. G. Spencer (Cambridge: Harvard Univ. Press, Loeb Classical Library, 1961), 3:214–23.

2. See discussion of cautery in chapter 2. Servier spoke of the actual cautery as a means of debridement, in "Débridement," *Dict. ency. sc. méd.* (1882), 26:121.

3. Ambroise Paré, *The workes of that famous chirurgion Ambrose Parey*, trans. Thomas Johnson (London, 1634), pp. 324, 429. Johnson's translation was from the 1582 Latin edition of Paré's 1579 collected works, the second French edition.

4. Guy de Chauliac, *La grande chirurgie de Guy de Chauliac, composée en l'an 1363*, ed. Édouard Nicaise (Paris, 1890), p. 213 (traité 3, doc. 1, chap. 1); Hans Gersdorff, *Feldt bůch der wundtartzney* (Strasbourg, 1517; facsimile, New York: Editions Medicina Rara [1971]), fol. 25 recto; Paré, *Workes* (n.3), p. 419; Laurens Joubert, *Traitté des arcbusades* (Lyons, 1574), pp. 52–55, 95–98. Said Joubert, "De vray les playes sont les mieux ouuertes, sont de meilleure guerison: dont ne faut espargner les orifices, où l'incision n'est autrement suspecte." Delorme says that Joubert opposed debridement, that Paré was partial to preventive or incisional debridement. *Traité de chirurgie de guerre* (Paris, 1888), 1:11, 27. We have not found that either Paré or Joubert employed the term "débridement" in their discussions.

5. The French originally identified *preventive debridement* as free incision of fascial aponeurosis to obviate necrosis of underlying tissue by swelling or strangulation from arrest of arterial flow or venous egress. Hence the term "unbridling." In fact, division of a constricting band in a strangulating hernia was looked upon as a form of debridement. See also John Homer Woolsey, "Débridement," *Am. J. Surg.* (1951), 82:179–82.

6. Henri de Mondeville, *Chirurgie, composée de 1306 à 1320*, ed. Édouard Nicaise (Paris, 1893), pp. 192–93, 209; Guy de Chauliac, *Grande chirurgie* (n.4), p. 213. George[s] de La Faye, *Principes de chirurgie*, 6th ed. (Paris, 1777), pp. 226–27, defines a *charpie* as linen cut into small bits. He says that *tentes* were made by rolling a *charpie* between the hands to form a rather stiff tampon with a head at one end, shaped like a nail. Besides linen, *tentes* were sometimes made of sponge or root of gentian. Their purpose was to dilate the wound or at least to hold it open.

7. Ambroise Paré, *Oeuvres complètes*, ed. J.-F. Malgaigne (Paris, 1840), 1:435. Malgaigne characterized this as a new doctrine.

8. Augustin Belloste, *Le chirurgien d'hôpital* (Paris, 1696), pp. 1–43. Belloste (1654–1730) believed that exclusion of air from wounds was important for healing. This theory he attributed to Cesare Magati, who also wrote against *tentes* (1616).

9. Jean-Louis Petit, *Traité des maladies chirurgicales*, posthumous, new ed. (Paris, 1790), 1:69–70. Petit died in 1750. Hugues Ravaton, *Chirurgie d'armée ou traité des plaies d'armes a feu et d'armes blanches* (Paris, 1768), pp. 573–74.

10. Henry St. John Neale, *Chirurgical institutes, drawn from practice, on the knowledge & treatment of gun-shot wounds* (London, 1804), pp. 24, 104–6; John Hunter, *Treatise on the blood, inflammation, and gun-shot wounds* (Philadelphia, 1796), 1:192–98; 2:253–62.

11. Pierre-F. Percy, *Manuel du chirurgien-d'armée* (Paris, 1792), p. 186. See also Percy's article on debridement in *Dict. d. sc. méd.* (1814), 8:109–17, and *Réponses du citoyen Percy, chirurgien en chef de l'armée de la Moselle, aux questions épuratoires . . . , première série* [n.d.], pp. 3, 11–12.

12. Dominique-J. Larrey, *Mémoires de chirurgie militaire, et campagnes* (Paris, 1812), 1:50. Another French military surgeon of the Napoleonic period who favored debridement was A. M. Martial (*Sur la nécessité des débridemens instantanés dans les plaies d'armes à feu aux extrémités*, a Paris thesis, 1814).

13. Pierre-J. Desault was born in 1738, although his birth date is often incorrectly given

as 1744, following an error in Xavier Bichat's account. See C. Jean Prat, *Un chirurgien au XVIIIe siècle, J. P. Desault (1738–1795)*, a Paris thesis, 1929 (p. 11). Desault studied under Antoine Louis and S.-F. Morand. After some years at La Charité he was named first surgeon at the Hôtel-Dieu where, under his brief leadership, there emerged an impressive school of surgeons trained in anatomy and techniques of operation. From among the more than six hundred students inscribed in his service came the finest Paris surgeons of that day. François Chopart, Percy, A. Dubois, Bichat, Larrey, and Dupuytren all received their stimulus from his teachings. His influence continued through a second generation of great French surgeons: Roux, Lisfranc, Velpeau, Malgaigne, and Nélaton. The physicians Corvisart, Broussais, and Cruveilhier drew their inspiration also from Desault's surgical school. Larrey says of his instruction concerning debridement: "*Desault nous apprit qu-il ne suffit pas de rendre une plaie saignante pour la faire passer de l'état compliqué a l'état simple; que le seul moyen d'y parvenir est de rafraîcher avec l'instrument tranchant les bords contus.*" Larrey, *Mémoires de chirurgie militaire* (n.12), 1:50.

14. Guillaume Dupuytren, *Traité theorique et pratique des blessures par armes de guerre . . . publié sous sa direction par . . . Paillard et Marx* (Paris, 1834), 2:444–46.

15. Philippe-Frédéric Blandin, "Plaies par armes a feu: thérapeutique qui leur est applicable — du débridement," *Gaz. hôp.*, Paris (1839), 12:398. Blandin (1798–1849) was chief of a service at the Hôtel-Dieu (1842–58). Louis Stromeyer (1804–76) is quoted in Jules Rochard, *Histoire de la chirurgie française au XIXe siècle* (Paris, 1875), pp. 857–58.

16. Lucien Baudens, *Clinique des plaies d'armes à feu* (Paris, 1836), pp. x–xi, 30–38.

17. For discussion of debridement, see Lucien Baudens et al., *Plaies d'armes à feu, communications faites a l'Académie nationale de médecine* (Paris, 1849), pp. 21, 70–71, 86, 136, 147, 163, 175. Louis-Jacques Bégin (1793–1859) was one of the "last survivors of the great imperial phalange," said Rochard, *Histoire* (n.15), p. 301. Pierre Charles Huguier (1804–73), a civilian surgeon, served with distinction during the Siege of Paris, 1870.

18. All were panelists except Lisfranc (d. 1847), who was referred to by Velpeau (p. 86).

19. George J. Guthrie, "Remarks on the practice of 'debridement,' " *Lancet* (1848), 2:521–22. Guthrie said the principle no longer prevailed "that it was necessary a man should be cut, because he had been shot." Antoine Jobert (de Lamballe) is discussed in several later chapters.

20. Léon Legouest, "La chirurgie militaire contemporaine," *Arch. gén. de méd.*, Paris (1859), 13:90, and *Traité de chirurgie d'armée* (Paris, 1863), p. 181; Thomas Longmore, *Treatise on gunshot wounds* (Philadelphia, 1862), pp. 54–55; Nicolai I. Pirogoff, *Grundzüge der allgemeinen Kriegschirurgie* (Leipzig, 1864), p. 621.

21. Rickman Godlee in *Lord Lister* (London: Macmillan, 1917), p. 350, relates that Reyher spent four weeks at the Edinburgh clinic in 1874. At the German Surgical Congress in 1874, Reyher reported favorably upon Lister's phenol management of wounds. "Ueber die Lister'sche Wundbehandlung," *Verh. dt. Ges. Chir.* (1874), 3(2):165–84. In 1876 he published on antiseptic and open wound management, finding better results with the former. "Antiseptische und offene Wundbehandlung," *Arch. klin. Chir.* (1876), 19:712–27.

22. Carl Reyher, "Die antiseptische Wundbehandlung in der Kriegschirurgie," *Samml. klin. Vortr.* (1878), Chir. no. 45, pp. 1207–62. This study was based on Reyher's experience in the Serbian-Turko-Russian conflict in the Caucasus (1876), where, under the aegis of the Red Cross, a field hospital of 150 beds and a flying camp of 50 additional beds were placed under his supervision, according to I. P. Usharenko, "Karl Karlovich Reyher and his role in Russian surgery," *Vestnik Khirurgii*, Leningrad (1939), 58:55–66, translated for the authors by Mark Graubard in 1971. Here Reyher established the superiority of antiseptic management in a detailed analysis and comparison of wounds not treated by antiseptics. For patients treated by Listerian antisepsis, Reyher's mortality was 10.5 percent, contrasted with 62.9 percent using conservative management but without antiseptics. Reyher had not then come to appreciate the role of debridement in war wounds.

23. Shortly thereafter Bergmann also went to war. Usharenko (n.22) states that

Bergmann, not utilizing debridement, had little success with the management of war wounds in the Russo-Turkish conflict. Nor was Bergmann then persuaded that Listerism had a useful role. At this time he developed the plaster cast method of dealing with compound fractures from gunshot wounds.

24. Tatiana Petrova Petrov, October 6, 1970, personal communication; N. N. Ivanov's biography of Reyher, *Chir. Vestnik*, St. Petersburg (1893), vol. 9, January–April.

25. Carl Reyher, "Ueber primäres Debridement der Schusswunden," 7th International Medical Congress, *Transactions*, London (1881), 2:587–97. See also Reyher's comments, p. 497.

26. H. F. L. Melladew, "What did the late Russo-Turkish campaign teach us concerning the antiseptic treatment of wounds in war?" 7th International Medical Congress, *Transactions*, London (1881), 2:486–88; Friedrich Esmarch, discussion, ibid., pp. 495–96.

27. [Abstract of Reyher's address], *Br. M. J.* (1881), 2:557.

28. Petrov (n.24).

29. Max Salomon, "Der internationale medicinische Congress," *Dt. med. Wschr.* (1881), 7:522–23; Ernst J. Gurlt, "Kriegschirurgie," *Jahresb. ü. d. Leistung. d. ges. Med.* (1882), 16:323.

30. Congrès français de chirurgie, Paris 1885, *Procès-verbaux* (Paris, 1886), 1:199; Delorme, *Chirurgie de guerre* (n. 4), 1:368. Eugène Audet, in his *Manuel de chirurgie d'armée* (Paris, 1886), pp. 2, 9–10, 12, described Reyher's good results with antiseptic treatment of wounds, but ignored the subject of debridement.

31. One control, however, is missing in Reyher's significant contribution. Whereas he collected data with and without antisepsis in intermediate and delayed debridement, in the primary debridement group he always employed wound antisepsis.

32. Petrov (n.24); Usharenko (n.22); O. H. Wangensteen and S. D. Wangensteen, "Carl Reyher . . . : His demonstration of the role of debridement in gunshot wounds and fractures," *Surgery* (1973), 74:641–49.

33. Paul L. Friedrich, "Die aseptische Versorgung frischer Wunden," *Arch. klin. Chir.* (1898), 57:288–310. Friedrich later was professor of surgery at Greifswald. Curt Schimmelbusch (1893) found that a mouse could not be saved by amputation of its tail 2 cms. proximal to the site of injection of anthrax organisms if the amputation was delayed beyond ten minutes. *Verh. dt. Ges. Chir.* (1893), 22(1):111–14.

34. H. Wagner, "Die Behandlung von granulierenden Hautwunden," *Zentbl. Chir.* (1903), 50:1361–65.

35. Carl Hueter, "Ein Fall von Heilung bei Gangraena septica acutissima (Gangrène foudroyante)," *Zentbl. Chir.* (1879), 6:521–25; Louis Ferraton, "Trois cas de gangrène gazeuse terminés par guérison," *Arch. de méd. et pharm. mil.* (1902), 40:64–71; Alex van Emden, "Traitement de la gangrène gazeuse," *Rev. méd. Suisse Rom.* (1915), no. 1, abstr. in *Zentbl. Chir.* (1915), 42:709; Jacques G. T. Maisonneuve, "Sur la gangrène foudroyante," abstr. in *Bull. Acad. imp. de méd.* (1853), 18:1174–75; Fielding H. Garrison, *Notes on the history of military medicine* (Washington, D.C.: Association of Military Surgeons, 1922), p. 201; Thomas S. Cullen, "A progressively enlarging ulcer of the abdominal wall involving the skin and fat," *Surg. Gynec. Obstet.* (1924), 38:579–82; H. Home Blackadder, *Observations of Phagedaena gangraenosa* (Edinburgh, 1818); F. L. Meleney, "Bacterial synergism in disease processes, with a confirmation of the synergistic bacterial etiology of a certain type of progressive gangrene of the abdominal wall," *Ann. Surg.* (1931), 94:961–81. Use of the cautery by Pouteau and Delpech for treatment of hospital gangrene is discussed in chapter 2.

36. H. M. W. Gray, "Treatment of gunshot wounds by excision and primary suture," *Br. M. J.* (1915), 2:317; Théodore Tuffier, "Traitement des plaies de guerre," Société de chirurgie, *Bull. et mém.* (1916), 42:2458.

37. "General principles of the treatment of wounds of war," *Br. M. J.* (1917), 2:838. The conference was attended by delegates from England, Belgium, France, Italy, Japan, Portugal, and Serbia. At subsequent conferences the United States and Russia were also represented.

38. *General principles guiding the treatment of wounds of war, conclusions adopted by the Inter-Allied Surgical Conference held in Paris, March and May, 1917* (London: H. M. Stationery Office, [n.d.]), pp. 4, 16. A studied effort obviously was made to avoid the term "debridement" in the English report of the conference as well as in the American translation of French papers presented before the research committee of the American Red Cross Society in 1919 (*Med. Bull.*, Paris, vol. 1, suppl., March 1918). "Excision of devitalized tissue" was apparently the preferred designation. French surgeons have clung to the term *débridement*, and it has become a familiar and accepted word in all languages, synonymous with wound revision. The word appeared in an English lexicon by Mayne in 1854, some twelve years after the American Dunglison had included it in his dictionary. Guthrie used it as a French term in 1848 (*Lancet*, 2:521). *Gould's medical dictionary* first listed debridement in the 1911 edition.

39. René Lemaitre, "A-propos de 2537 cas de sutures primitives pour plaies de guerre," *Lyon chir.* (1918), 15:107. See also his "Suture of war wounds," *Med. Bull.*, Paris (1918), 1:292–329.

40. Norman T. Kirk, U.S. War Department, Army Service Forces. Office of the Surgeon General, Circular Letter 91, April 26, 1943; subject: amputations. Use of the word "guillotine" is unfortunate. A well-performed circular amputation envisages cutting skin, muscle, and bone at desired levels providing adequate soft tissue coverage. See also Kirk, "Development of amputation," *Bull. Med. Libr. Assoc.* (1944), 32:162.

41. Elliot C. Cutler, Paul C. Morton, and William R. Sandusky, "Observations on the prophylactic use of penicillin in the wounds of aerial warfare," *Br. J. Surg.* (1944), 32:210–11.

42. Leonard D. Heaton et al., "Military surgical practices of the United States Army in Viet Nam," *Curr. Probl. Surg.*, November 1966, p. 19. John M. Howard, chairman, "Postoperative wound infections . . . Report of an *ad hoc* committee," *Ann. Surg.* (1964), vol. 160 (August) supplement.

43. David Patey, "Debridement," and Owen H. Wangensteen, "The role of debridement — reply to Mr. Patey's interrogatory," letters to the editor, *Surgery* (1974), 76:347–50; Surindar N. Bhaskar, Duane E. Cutright, Ervin E. Hunsuck, and Arthur Gross, "Pulsating water jet devices in debridement of combat wounds," *Milit. Med.* (1971), 136:264–66; Usha Dhingra, Robert R. Schauerhamer, and Wangensteen, "Peripheral dissemination of bacteria in contaminated wounds; role of devitalized tissue: Evaluation of therapeutic measures," *Surgery* (1976), 80:535–43.

Further Readings

Dennis, Clarence. Disaster following femoral vein ligation for thrombophlebitis; relief by fasciotomy. *Surgery* (1945), 17:264–69.

Gustilo, Ramon B., and Anderson, John T. Prevention of infection in treatment of one thousand and twenty-five open fractures of long bones. *J. Bone Jt. Surg.* (1976), 58A:453–58.

Jepson, Paul N. Ischemic contracture; experimental study. *Ann. Surg.* (1926), 84:785–95.

Monroe, Clarence W. Débridement — when and how much? A comparative study of battle casualties. *Surg. Gynec. Obstet.* (1944), 79:478–81.

Patman, R. Don, and Thompson, Jesse E. Fasciotomy in peripheral vascular surgery. *Arch. Surg.* (1970), 101:663–72.

Trueta, José. *Principles and practice of war surgery.* St. Louis: C. V. Mosby, 1943.

Wangensteen, O. H. Boris Petrov, great Russian surgeon, and the Sklifosovsky Institute of Emergency Surgery. *Surgery* (1974), 76:204–8.

Whipple, Allen O. *The story of wound healing and wound repair.* Springfield, Ill.: Charles C Thomas [1963].

Chapter 4. Lithotomy and Lithotomists

Notes

1. Ernest Desnos, "Histoire de l'urologie," in *Encyclopédie française d'urologie* (Paris: Doin, 1914), 1:146; Constant Saucerotte, "Lunéville et sa division de cavalerie," *Rec. de mém. de méd. . . . mil.*, Paris (1857), 20:203–4. Stanislas was the exiled king of Poland.

2. William Wadd, surgeon extraordinary to the king in 1827, quoted in John Langdon-Davies, *Westminster Hospital, two centuries of voluntary service, 1719–1948* (London: John Murray, 1952), p. 44; Alexander Marcet, *An essay on the chemical history and medical treatment of calculous disorders* (London, 1817), pp. 23–25, 28. Marcet, a London physician who took these figures from the hospital records in 1817, was startled to find that "the largest hospitals of London, St. Bartholomew's, St. Thomas's, Guy's and the London" had preserved "no ostensible records" of their cases of lithotomy. For excerpts from the hospital minute-book records, see Peter Eade, *The Norfolk & Norwich Hospital, 1770 to 1900* (London, 1900), pp. 54, 60, 70, 91. The old minute books are still to be seen in the hospital's library. Thompson is quoted in A. Batty Shaw's excellent review, "The Norwich school of lithotomy," *Med. Hist.* (1970), 14:222.

3. Eric Riches, "The history of lithotomy and lithotrity," *Ann. R. Coll. Surg.* (1968), 43:185; S. G. Shattock, "A prehistoric or predynastic Egyptian calculus," *Trans. Path. Soc. London* (1905), 56:278. G. Elliot Smith and Warren R. Dawson found urinary calculi extremely rare in thirty thousand mummies of early Egyptian dynasties. *Egyptian mummies* (London: G. Allen and Unwin, 1924), p. 156.

4. Mahmoud Ghanem, September 1973, personal communication. T. B. Osborne and L. B. Mendel (1917) produced vesical stones in rats by diets deficient in vitamin A (*JAMA*, 69:32–33). R. McCarrison (1927–28) extended these observations in India (*Indian J. Med. Res.*, Calcutta, 14:895–99; 15:801–6). The relationship of inadequate fluid intake to the causation of bladder stone is reemphasized in a recent review by Asser H. Østergaard of Copenhagen, *Calculus vesicae hos børn* (Copenhagen: Fadl, 1976), who postulates that the condition is prevalent in newborns when breast feeding is replaced by diets low in liquid (pp. 158–59).

5. Kathleen Lonsdale and Phoebe Mason, "Uric acid dihydrate, and urates in urinary calculi," *Science* (1966), 152:1511–12; Lonsdale, "Human stones," *Science* (1968), 159:1199–1207; D. June Sutor, "Growth studies of calcium oxalate," *Br. J. Urol.* (1969), 41:171–78. X-ray diffraction and chemical studies indicate significant differences in composition of urinary calculi. The vesical stones of boys in Thailand are pure urate with an admixture of calcium oxalate. Today the most common urinary calculi of adults in countries of Western culture are renal stones, predominantly uric acid, oxalate, and phosphate in composition. Indolence, lack of exercise, and a high-protein diet in adults appear to be contributing factors. Body immobilization in plaster for injuries of the spine and pelvis has been responsible for many instances of renal calculi. They are extremely frequent in hyperparathyroidism, owing to disordered reabsorption in the kidney.

6. George Corner and Willard Goodwin, "Benjamin Franklin's bladder stone," *J. Hist. Med.* (1953), 8:359–77; Catherine Drinker Bowen, *Miracle at Philadelphia: The story of the Constitutional Convention, May to September 1787* (Boston: Little, Brown, 1966), p. 34.

7. Félix Vicq d'Azyr, "Observations sur la taille latérale de Cheselden," *Hist. Soc. roy. de méd. . . . 1777–78*, Paris (1780), 2(2):579. Vicq d'Azyr was paraphrasing an earlier remark by Buffon about botany.

8. Celsus, *De medicina*, with an English translation by W. G. Spencer (Cambridge: Harvard Univ. Press, Loeb Classical Library, 1961), 3:427–47. There are those who insist that Celsus was not a surgeon, but the experienced surgeon is readily persuaded that only someone with a firsthand acquaintance with the procedure could have written Celsus's description of perineal lithotomy, for it reflects knowledge of how to avoid opening the rectum on incising the bladder.

9. Guy de Chauliac, *La grande chirurgie de Guy de Chauliac, composée en l'an 1363*, ed. Édouard Nicaise (Paris, 1890), pp. 544–45; Ambroise Paré, *The workes of that famous chirurgion*

Ambrose Parey, trans. Thomas Johnson (London, 1634), pp. 672–81. Guy ends his brief description of the operation: "Dieu nous soit en ayde." Malgaigne reaffirms the opinion that Paré did not do lithotomy, in his introduction to *Oeuvres complètes d'Ambroise Paré* (Paris, 1840), 1:lxvi, cclxxi. Jean Falcon in a thousand-page monograph, *Remarques sur la chirurgie de M. Guy de Chauliac* (Lyons, 1649), makes no mention of Guy's cutting for stone.

10. Édouard Nicaise, ed., *Chirurgie de Pierre Franco . . . composée en 1561* (Paris, 1895), pp. ii–iii; Pierre Bail, *Un chirurgien urologiste du XVIe siècle*, Paris thesis, 1932. In a short essay on Franco in *Investigative Urology* (1965), 2:405–7, Ronnie B. Bush and Irving M. Bush comment on his high ethical standards.

11. Pierre Franco: *Petit traite* (Lyons, 1556), pp. 78–94, and *Traité des hernies* (Lyons, 1561), pp. 121–40.

12. Johannes Scultetus, *Armamentarium chirurgicum bipartitum* (Frankfort, 1666).

13. Marianus Sanctus, *De lapide renum* (Venice, 1535).

14. This is the estimate of Jean B. Senac in his anonymous preface to François Colot, *Traité de l'opération de la taille* (Paris, 1727), pp. xii, xliii.

15. Laurent Colot, founder of the dynasty, became court lithotomist to Henry II of France in 1556. Philippe Colot, François's father, was the most famous. He claimed to have an annual income of 13,000 to 14,000 *livres* from his practice. He agreed in 1674 to take pupils at the Hôtel-Dieu if alloted 30,000 *livres* and an assured annual income of 2,000 during his life and his wife's. The offer was refused. See Leon Briele, ed., *Collection de documents pour servir a l'histoire des hôpitaux de Paris* (Paris, 1881), 1:201–10.

16. Colot, *Traité de l'opération* (n.14), p. 205.

17. Jean Mery, *Observations sur la manière de tailler . . . pratiquée par Frère Jacques* (Paris, 1700), pp. 73–75. Jean Mery (1645–1722), then the chief surgeon of the Hôtel-Dieu, was particularly engrossed in problems of anatomy. Marie-José Imbault-Huart, *L'École Pratique de Dissection de Paris de 1750 à 1822*, Paris thesis, 1973, p. 18.

18. "Part of the letter from Mr. Bussiere . . . wherein he gives an account of the new way of cutting for the stone by the Hermit," *Phil. Trans.* (1700), pp. 100–6.

19. Charles Bell, "On lithotomy," *Lancet* (1827), 12:773–74. Bell credits this description to Claude-Nicolas Le Cat (1700–68), but Le Cat was not born until 1700 and probably never saw Jacques operate.

20. Martin Lister, *A journey to Paris in the year 1698* (London, 1698), pp. 233–36; Mery, *Sur la manière de tailler* (n.17), p. 74. Martin Lister (1638–1711), a physician, is best known for his contributions to natural history, especially in conchology. Mery states that 25 of 60 patients who had lithotomies done by Jacques in Paris died (41.6 percent). Mery's report was only an impression, says J.-F. Malgaigne in a *concours* thesis, *Parallèle des diverses espèces de taille* (Paris, 1850), p. 23. See also Desnos (n.1), pp. 153–59.

21. Benjamin Bell, *A system of surgery*, 2d Am. ed. (Troy, N.Y., 1804), 3:183.

22. C. Bell (n.19), p. 774; Desnos (n.1), p. 157. Fagon suffered from vesical calculus and debated having Frère Jacques as his lithotomist, but decided in favor of Georges Mareschal. The operation was successful. Later, the maréchal de Lorges placed twenty-two patients with vesical calculus under Jacques's care, all of whom he operated upon successfully. Jacques was then asked to operate upon the maréchal for vesical calculus. The maréchal died. Gabriel Mareschal de Bièvre, *Georges Mareschal . . . (1658–1736)* (Paris: Plon-Nourrit, 1906), pp. 122–23.

23. B. S. Albinus, "Abregé de la vie de seu M. Rau," trans., in René-J.-C. de Garengeot, *Traité des operations de chirurgie*, 2d ed. (Paris, 1731), 2:93; Pieter Camper, *Demonstrationum anatomico-pathologicarum. Liber secundus. Pelvis humanae fabricam et morbos* (Amsterdam, 1762), p. 14.

24. Colot, *Traité de l'operation* (n.14), p. 29.

25. John Bell, *The principles of surgery* (London, 1806), 2:128–44. John Bell (1763–1820) of Edinburgh was Charles's elder brother, less brilliant and original, but an impressive teacher whose writings deserve the attention of today's surgeons. See chapter 12 on ovariotomy.

C. Bell, although aware of Rau's deception, characterized Rau as "the greatest lithotomist that ever lived"! (n.19), p. 774. Bell obviously did not know of Camper's evaluation.

26. Jean Baseilhac: *Receuil de pièces importantes concernant la taille par le lithotome caché*, 2 vols. (Paris, 1751), and *Nouvelle méthode d'extraire la pierre de la vessie urinaire par-dessus le pubis* (Paris, 1779).

27. Joseph C. Carpue, *A history of the high operation for the stone, by incision above the pubis* (London, 1819), p. 143. C. D. Creevy gave a modern appraisal of Carpue's history in the University of Minnesota's *Bio-Med. Libr. Bull.*, no. 12, February 1970, pp. 3–7. Creevy mentioned the difficulty of diagnosis in Carpue's era and the likelihood of diagnostic error.

28. Carpue, *History of the high operation* (n.27), pp. 52–53.

29. William Cheselden, *Treatise on the high operation for the stone* (London, 1723).

30. Claude Pouteau, *Oeuvres posthumes* (Paris, 1783), 3:219.

31. Peter Le Mercier, "Sur la taille," *J. de méd., chir., pharm.* (1767), 26:264.

32. Lister, *Journey to Paris* (n.20), p. 232; J. Bell, *Principles of surgery* (n.25), p. 144; James Douglas, *Appendix to the history of the lateral operation for the stone, containing Mr. Cheselden's present method* (London, 1731), p. 16. The *Lancet* estimate appeared April 5, 1828 (p. 20), in a series of polemics directed by the editor, Thomas Wakley, against Sir Astley's nephew, Bransby Cooper, following a fatal lithotomy in which Cooper took fifty-five minutes to remove a stone. A notorious lawsuit ensued between Cooper and Wakley. Cooper came off the victor but with permanent injury to his professional reputation. It is interesting that he became an accomplished lithotomist, reporting in 1852 a mortality of 6.7 percent in 134 lithotomies. Bransby B. Cooper, *Lectures on the principles and practice of surgery* (Philadelphia, 1852), p. 494.

33. Charles Bell, *Surgical observations* (London, 1816), p. 123. Bell (1774–1842) is best known for his work on the functions of the nerves.

34. Pouteau: *Oeuvres posthumes* (n.30), 3:214, 227–38, and *Mélanges de chirurgie* (Lyons, 1760), pp. 198–99, 206–11.

35. John G. Crosse, *Treatise on the formation, constituents, and extraction of the urinary calculus* (London, 1835), p. 78. Crosse misinterpreted his source somewhat. Le Cat lost six out of nine patients, each cut in about two minutes. However, in defense of Le Cat it must be said that he was attempting a new technique which, on reassessment, he altered. In the previous 1732–34 period he lost no patients. See Claude-Nicolas Le Cat, *Pièces concernant l'operation de la taille* (Rouen, 1749), recueil 1, pp. 78–79; Johann J. Hartenkeil, *De vesicae urinariae calculo* (Würzburg, 1785), pp. 95–98, a doctoral thesis.

36. Henri-François Le Dran: *Operations in surgery*, trans. Thomas Gataker, 3d ed. (London, 1757), pp. 232–44, and *Parallele des differentes manières de tirer la pierre hors de la vessie* (Paris, 1730), p. 151. Le Dran (1685–1770) was chief of surgery at La Charité and consultant to the army.

37. John Shaw, "Inquiry into the present methods of performing the operation of lithotomy," *Quart. J. For. M. & S.*, London (1821), 3:45; Nicolas Saucerotte, *Mélanges de chirurgie* (Paris, 1801), 2:552. Shaw had the report from someone who had witnessed Dupuytren's cases.

38. A. B. Shaw (n.2), pp. 221–22, 234, 248–49; Francis Avery Jones, "The Norwich schools of surgery," *Ann. R. Coll. Surg.* (1976), 58:203–21; Crosse, *Treatise on urinary calculus* (n.35).

39. Believing anesthesia was hazardous, Frederick Le Gros Clark, a well-known St. Thomas's surgeon, left the option of its usage to his patients. If anesthesia was chosen, the surgeon was thus absolved of cross-examination before a coroner's jury in case of death or accident, said a reporter in *Med. Circ.*, London (1858), 13:70.

40. Frederick J. Brown, "Report of a case of operation for stone, on Allarton's principle," *Lancet* (1855), 2:321–22.

41. William Cheselden, *Anatomy of the human body*, 5th ed. (London, 1740), pp. 333–34. A century later the physician John Yelloly of Norwich, in describing perineal lithotomy by

Cheselden, James Douglas, Morand, and others, succeeded in showing how confused the situation was. *Med.-Chir. Trans.*, London (1829), 15:339–68.

42. No question of Pouteau's credibility has come to our notice, although Desnos sounds somewhat cynical in stating that Pouteau "sur cent vingt calculeux prétend n'en avoir perdu que 3." Desnos (n.1), p. 172. An anonymous polemicist, sometimes identified as L. Vitet, made a savage attack upon Pouteau for using the cautery in suppurating wounds, but spoke in highest terms of Pouteau's accomplishment as a lithotomist and urged him to confine his skill to this activity. See *Avis d'un serviteur d'Esculape* (1761), pp. 1–17, 48–50.

43. George Allarton, *Treatise on modern median lithotomy* (London, 1863), pp. 5, 499–504.

44. Reported by W. J. Penny, *Br. M. J.* (1882), 1:87.

45. John Hunter's unpublished case books transcribed by William Clift (1825), p. 59. The case books may be seen at the Royal College of Surgeons Library in London. Mullineux related several instances and presented sketches of vesical calculi extruded without lithotomy in *Phil. Trans.* (1693), 17:817–24. He indicated that Thomas Bartholinus, Daniel Angelus, Petrus Borellus, and Nicolaus Tulpius had made similar observations. The Reverend Dr. Wallis reported removal of a vesical calculus, 5½ inches in circumference, from a woman of sixty-three by her husband; thereafter she was incontinent. *Phil. Trans.* (1685), 15:1271.

46. Jean-J.-L. Hoin, "Sur l'opération de la taille," *Mém. Acad. d. sci. Dijon* (1769), 1:193, 200–15, 218–19. Hoin related that when his friend J.-P. Maret was visiting him, a little girl of eight was brought in. Maret sounded the child's bladder and confirmed the diagnosis of vesical calculus, which he extracted without effort after dilating the urethra. The patient got off the table, curtsied, and left with the woman who brought her, neither of them speaking a word.

47. Miley B. Wesson, "Fasciae of the urogenital triangle," *JAMA* (1923), 81(2):2024–29; Thomas M. Oelrich, "Anatomy of the urogenital diaphragm," *Anat. Rec.* (1964), 148:318.

48. Jack Lapides, "Structure and function of the internal vesical sphincter," *J. Urol.* (1958), 80:341–53; Russell T. Woodburne, *Essentials of human anatomy*, 3d ed. (New York: Oxford Univ. Press, 1965), pp. 520–21, and "The sphincter mechanism of the urinary bladder and the urethra," *Anat. Rec.* (1961), 141:11–20. Dr. Morris Smithberg, professor of anatomy, University of Minnesota, directed the authors' attention to Woodburne's studies.

49. Otto Kalischer, a pupil of Heinrich Waldeyer, in a comprehensive monograph, emphasized the role of the longitudinal smooth muscle extending the entire length of the urethra in providing sphincteric control. *Die Urogenitalmuskulatur des Dammes* (Berlin: Karger, 1900), pp. 146, 180.

50. G. S. Pattison, "Experimental observations on the operation of lithotomy, with the description of a fascia of the prostate gland which appears to explain anatomically the cause of urinal infiltrations and consequent death," *Am. M. Recorder*, Philadelphia (1820), 3:1–24; Pattison, "A reply to certain oral and written criticisms, delivered against an essay on lithotomy," ibid., pp. 351–71; William Gibson, *Strictures on "Mr. Pattison's reply to certain oral and written criticisms"* (Philadelphia, 1820), pp. 4–7; Abraham Colles, *Treatise on surgical anatomy* (Dublin, 1811), pp. 189–90. A number of accounts deal with Pattison's tempestuous career. See William Snow Miller, "Granville Sharp Pattison," *Johns Hopkins Hosp. Bull.* (1919), 30:98–104; Frank H. J. Figge, "Granville Sharp Pattison, the dueling anatomist," *Bull. Md Univ. Sch. Med.* (1938), 23:81–92; W. R. Merrington, *University College Hospital and its medical school: A history* (London: William Heinemann, 1976), pp. 5, 11–12; and letters and editorials in *Lancet*, 1830–32. Episodes of Pattison's personal life, including use of his name, perhaps falsely, in a divorce case and a duel in Delaware in which his antagonist General Thomas Cadwalader was severely wounded, were repeatedly recalled by opponents seeking to damage his advancement. Pattison became the target of *Lancet's* editor Wakley and was dismissed from the London faculty — from which Charles Bell and others had resigned. It is hard to separate truth from prejudiced insinuations. Perhaps it was dislike of Pattison as a Scotsman and a fox-hunting sportsman that proved his downfall in London. One tale is that he sometimes lectured in his pink riding coat, wearing boots. On his return to America he taught anatomy at Jeffer-

son Medical College (1831–40), resigning to become professor at the new University of New York in 1841.

51. Garengeot, *Traité des operations* (n.23), 2:204.

52. Charles-Pierre Denonvilliers: "Anatomie du périnée," abstract in *Bull. Soc. anat. de Paris* (1836), 1:105–7, and *Propositions et observations d'anatomie, de physiologie et de pathologie,* Paris thesis, 1837.

53. Samuel D. Gross, *Practical treatise on the . . . urinary bladder*, 2d ed. (Philadelphia, 1855), pp. 603–4; Claude Pouteau, *La taille au niveau* (Avignon, 1765), pp. 5–10.

54. Johann N. Hunczovsky, *Medicinisch-chirurgische Beobachtungen* (Vienna, 1783), pp. 11–17. Young Hawkins told Hunczovsky that his father, Caesar Hawkins (1711–86), hesitated to publish because William Hunter, far better known, had used a very similar instrument and Hunter's friends might accuse him of plagiarism. Although William Hunter did surgery early in his practice, neither the titles of his publications nor his biographers reveal an interest in lithotomy. Hawkins and his son operated at St. George's. Hunczovsky's tour of French and British hospitals is discussed in chapter 18 on hospital practices.

55. C. Bell, *Surgical observations* (n.33), p. 121; Astley Cooper, *Lectures on the principles and practice of surgery*, 2d ed. (London, 1830), p. 326; J. Bell, *Principles of surgery* (n.25), p. 173.

56. Antonio Scarpa, *Traité de l'opération de la taille*, trans. C. P. Ollivier (Paris, 1826), p. 16. Malgaigne, *Diverses espèces de taille* (n.20), considered Scarpa's arithmetic not entirely accurate (pp. 29–30).

57. Celsus, *De medecina* (n.8), 3:439; Franco, *Petit traite* (n.11), pp. 88–90.

58. J. P. Maret, "Sur les avantages de différer l'extraction de la pierre," *Mém. Acad. d. sci. Dijon* (1769), 1:95–118. Fabricius Hildanus declared that if all lithotomists and rupture-cutters used Franco's two-stage method many patients would escape death. *Lithotoma vesicae: That is an accurate description of the stone in the bladder*, trans. N. C. (London, 1640), p. 109. In 1784 François Chaussier advocated that a two-stage operation, so successful in lithotomy, be used in cataract removal (*Mém. Acad. d. sci. Dijon*, 19:206–7).

59. Pieter Camper, "Brief . . . over het Steensnyden in Twee Reizen," September 13, 1777. An abstract of his account of two-stage lithotomy from an Amsterdam journal appears in *London M. J.* (1789), 10(2):162–77. See a pamphlet by ten Haaff and Gerrit Jan van Wy, *Vorschriften des Celsus, Albucasis, Le Dran and Louis* (1784), and a review of van Wy's *Heelkundige Mengelstoffen* (Amsterdam, 1784), in *Chir. Biblioth.*, Göttingen (1785), 8(2):46–66; Hunczovsky, *Beobachtungen* (n.54), pp. 317, 324–25.

60. Adrianus Maret, *An calculi vesicae extractio sit aliquando procrastinanda?*, Paris thesis, 1776; Joseph Covillard, *Observations iatrochirurgiques . . . augmentée de . . . observations par Jean-Franç. Thomassin* (Strasbourg, 1791), p. 52. We were encouraged by Maret's thesis and the suggestion of ten Haaff and van Wy that Louis had published a discussion of the two-stage operation in a *précis* in 1770. After a futile search, we asked Professor Pierre Huard for assistance in February 1968. He and his associate Mme. Marie-Josę Imbault-Huart took a keen interest in hunting down the missing paper, but were unable to find it. Their conclusion is that Louis gave his paper on April 26, 1770, but did not publish the memoir. It is not to be found in the Archives of the Royal Academy of Surgeons nor among Louis's manuscripts preserved by the municipal library in Metz. Huard and Imbault-Huart, "La taille en deux temps et ses avantages," *Episteme*, Milan (1970), 4:91–98.

61. F. J. Deschamps, *Traité historique et dogmatique de l'opération de la taille* (Paris, 1796), 4:59.

62. J. A. Treyeran, *le jeune*, said the patient's spirit suffers with the knowledge that the stone is still in him and his morale gradually fails. *Parallèle des diverses méthodes proposées pour l'extraction des calculs vésicaux* (Paris, 1802), p. 181.

63. J.-P. Maret (n.58), pp. 98, 115–17.

64. John Thomson, *Appendix to a proposal for a new manner of cutting for the stone* (Edinburgh, 1810), pp. vii–ix.

65. Ralph Fletcher, *Medico-chirurgical notes and illustrations* (London, 1831), pp. 85–86.

66. Colot, *Traité de l'operation de la taille* (n.14), pp. 167–91, 275–78; François Tolet, *Traité de la lithotomie*, 5th ed. (Paris, 1708), pp. 139, 157–65, 203, 246–50, 253–56; Deschamps, *Traité historique* (n.61), pp. 29–36; John Freind, *History of physick* (London, 1725), 2:182. François Colot did 7, the most reported by one surgeon, and without a death. His mortality for the one-stage procedure was 21.2 percent. F. Tolet and Deschamps each describe 4, with no deaths. Freind states that Cyprian frequently practiced two-stage lithotomy when he was in London. Huard and Imbault-Huart mention that Pierre Guérin, following the first operation, dilated the perineal wound progressively with a dry carrot while awaiting the second stage. Obviously, such a procedure vitiates the advantage of the two-stage operation as conceived by Franco and disqualifies the cases as bona fide two-stage operations. Among his 20 cases Guérin had 2 deaths (n.60), p. 95.

67. J. L. Schmucker, *Vermischte chirurgische Schriften* (Berlin, 1782), 3:44–56.

68. O. H. Wangensteen, S. D. Wangensteen, and John Wiita, "Lithotomy and lithotomists," *Surgery* (1969), 66:936–37.

69. Theodor Billroth, "Beobachtungs-Studien über Wundfieber und accidentelle Wundkrankheiten," *Arch. klin. Chir.* (1865), 6:444.

70. See discussion of open wound management in chapter 2.

71. Franco, *Petit traite* (n.11), pp. 93–94. The 1561 edition (p. 139) gives the patient's age as about two years. According to some accounts, the first suprapubic cystostomy was performed in 1474 on a thief reprieved from hanging when he submitted to having his bladder opened by the suprapubic route for experimental examination. The man had suffered from vesical calculus and Louis XI was much concerned over the frequency of stone in France. The peritoneal cavity was opened as well as the bladder and the "entrails were placed back again"! The patient survived. Charles G. Cumston discusses the operation in "A short account of the early history of suprapubic cystotomy," *Boston M. & S. J.* (1912), 166:516–18.

72. François Rousset, *Traitte nouveau de l'hysterotomotokie ou enfantement caesarien* (Paris, 1581), pp. 77–79, and *Hysterotomotokias (id est) caesarei partus assertio historiologica* (Paris, 1590), pp. 270–75. These books are discussed more fully in the chapter on cesarean section. Rousset's 1590 account is the more detailed. Rousset relates that Henry II promised to let him perform the high operation on four criminals, but the king died before Rousset took advantage of his promise.

73. Le Mercier's 1635 proposal is reprinted in Cheselden's *Treatise on the high operation* (n.29), pp. 141–49. Fabricius Hildanus (1628) approved of the high operation in children, but thought the surgeon's fingers were not long enough to elevate the stone from the depths of the bladder to the level of the abdominal wall in adults. He recommended that the surgeon insert the fingers of his left hand through the anus to bring the stone within reach of his free hand through the suprapubic bladder incision. *Lithotomia vesicae: hoc est, accurata descriptio calculi vesicae* (Basel, 1628), pp. 114–16.

74. Pierre Dionis, *Cours d'operations de chirurgie, demontrées au Jardin royal* (Paris, 1707), pp. 193–96. Dionis probably referred to Jean Bonnet. Among 100 males and females undergoing suprapubic lithotomy, Frère Côme lost 19. Pascal Baseilhac, *De la taille latérale par le périnée, et celle de l'hypogastre ou haut appareil* (Paris, 1804), pp. 332–33.

75. The autopsy findings in Cheselden's two fatalities failed to indicate the cause of death (pp. 11–21).

76. John Douglas, *Lithotomia Douglassiana or a new method of cutting for stone* (London, 1720). The controversy is recounted in Cumston (n.71), p. 522; F. H. Garrison, *Introduction to the history of medicine*, 4th ed. (Philadelphia: W. B. Saunders, 1929), p. 343; Deschamps, *Traité historique* (n.61), 2:196–203. James Douglas's anatomical description of the peritoneum appeared in 1730.

77. See James Douglas, *History of the lateral operation* (London, 1726), and the preface to his *Appendix to the history of the lateral operation* (London, 1731).

78. The French surgeons were probably thinking of priority.

79. Carpue, *History of the high operation* (n.27), pp. 2–7; Joseph Souberbielle, "Sur l'opération de la taille," *Mém. Acad. roy. méd.*, Paris (1840), 8:56–99. One patient said to Carpue: "Sir, for many years the Countess [his daughter] used to come to console her father; now she comes to rejoice with him, as I am now free from pain, after having suffered for a period of upwards of twenty years" (p. 6).

80. Joseph O. Thomson, "Urinary calculus at the Canton Hospital, Canton, China," *Surg. Gynec. Obstet.* (1921), 32:44–55. The technique is not given for 2 percent of the operations.

81. Good historical accounts of lithotrity are provided by L. J. Bégin, "Sur la lithotritie," *J. compl. d. sc. méd.*, Paris (1826), 24:3–16, and by J. Civiale, *Lettres sur la lithotritie, ou broiement de la pierre dans la vessie* (Paris, 1827). R. J. Willan presents a brief but more recent account of the evolution of lithotrity in *Br. J. Surg.* (1913), 1:406–18. Ammonius' technique is described by Ernst Gurlt, *Geschichte der Chirurgie* (Berlin, 1898), 3:779.

82. In a retrospective consideration, *Lithotripsie, l'art de broyer les pierres dans la vessie* (Paris, 1857), Charles L. S. Heurteloup assigned the German Gruithuisen the major credit for devising lithotrity and avoided discussing the long bitter quarrel between Civiale and Leroy-d'Étiolles over priority. The major contestants for priority presented their claims before the Royal Academy of Medicine in 1835. See P. Doubovitzki, *Reproduction fidèle des discussions qui ont lieu sur la lithotripsie et la taille* (Paris, 1835).

83. Henry Earle, "Remarks on the danger of extracting large calculi," *Med.-Chir. Trans.* (1820), 11:77–79; Paré, *Workes* (n.9), p. 679. Every surgeon who has tried to crush a large fresh wet stone, whether vesical or biliary, knows it can resist a great force. The senior author of this volume has seen a large Payr gastric clamp sprung in an attempt to crush a large gallstone through the intact bowel wall over gauze and has observed the jaws of the powerful Bigelow lithotrite similarly sprung when the surgeon persisted in trying to crush a large vesical calculus. A few days after removal, when evaporation has dried the stones, a very small force suffices to crush them. Today direct vision can be employed to complement litholapaxy.

84. J. E. Pétrequin, "Considérations sur la méthode à suivre . . . en combinant la taille et la lithotritie," *Bull. gén. de thérap.*, Paris (1851), 41:442–50.

85. Martin's instrument is illustrated by Marcet in the second edition of his *Essay on calculous disorders* (1819), p. 21. (See n.2.) Marcet said the original instrument was then in the possession of Monro, the Edinburgh anatomist. Bégin (n.81), p. 5, and Civiale, *Lettres* (n.81), p. 14, were both familiar with this unusual case. Here should be mentioned Albucasis's use of a fine drill to perforate and break a small calculus impacted in the urethra; the pieces were washed out with the urine. *On surgery and instruments*, trans. and ed. M. S. Spink and G. L. Lewis (Berkeley: Univ. California Press, 1973), pp. 416–18.

86. Henry Jacob Bigelow, "Lithotrity by a single operation," *Am. J. Med. Sci.* (1878), 75:117–34.

87. Albert Vander Veer surveyed the surgical literature for the period 1878–86 and observed an overall mortality of 12.5 percent among 64 patients operated upon by the suprapubic route by about as many surgeons, the majority of whom had capitulated to acceptance of antisepsis. Among 16 patients over fifty years, the mortality was 21.2 percent. *Trans. Am. Surg. Assoc.* (1887), 5:79–124.

88. Henry Thompson: "Account of 500 cases of operation for stone in the bladder of the male adult," *Med.-Chir. Trans.* (1878), 61:167, and "The suprapubic operation for opening the bladder," *Br. M. J.* (1886), 2:617.

89. Joanna Stephens, "A full discovery of the medicines given by me," *Gentleman's Mag.* (1739), 9:298–99; C. J. S. Thompson, *The quacks of old London* (New York: Brentano, 1928), pp. 294–97; E. Lee Strohl, "Parliament hoodwinked by Joanna Stephens," *Surg. Gynec. Obstet.* (1963), 116:509–11.

90. William Falconer, *An account of the efficacy of the aqua mephitica alkalina . . . in calculous disorders*, 4th ed. (London, 1792). The first edition appeared in 1787.

91. *Am. J. Med. Sci.* (1831), 9:263, 537–38; Samuel D. Gross, *Lives of eminent American physicians and surgeons* (Philadelphia, 1861), pp. 221–22.

92. D'Arcy Power, "An historical lithotomy, Mr. Samuel Pepys," *Br. J. Surg.* (1931), 18:541–45; J. H. Kiefer, "Lithotomy set to music: An historical interlude," *Urol. Surv.* (1964), 14:2–7.

93. John Ranby, "*Narrative of the last illness of . . . The Earl of Orford*," 2d ed. (London, 1745), appendix, p. 40.

94. R. Scott Stevenson, *Famous illnesses in history* (London: Eyre and Spottiswoode, 1962), pp. 103–15; *Lancet* (1873), 1:111–12. Several other famous cases are described by Harold Ellis in his interesting monograph, *History of bladder stone* (Oxford and Edinburgh: Blackwell, 1969), pp. 44–71.

Further Readings

Camper, Pieter. *Observationes circa mutationes quas subeunt calculi in vesica.* Pest, 1784.

Groenveldt, Jan. *A compleat treatise of the stones and gravel.* London, 1710.

Gurlt, Ernst. Der Stein- und Bruchschnitt im Mittelalter und der Renaissance. In *Geschichte der Chirurgie*, vol. 1, pp. 100–101. Berlin, 1898.

Heller, Johann F. *Die Harnconcretionen.* Vienna, 1860.

Heurteloup, Charles L. S. *Mémoire sur la lithotripsie par percussion.* Paris, 1833.

The John A. Benjamin Collection of Medical History: Catalogue & first supplement. Compiled by C. D. O'Malley and Martha Teach Gnudi. Los Angeles: Univ. California Library, 1968.

————. *Second supplement.* Complied by Martha Teach Gnudi. Los Angeles: Univ. California Library, 1968.

Prien, Edwin L., Sr. The riddle of urinary stone disease. *JAMA* (1971), 216:503–7.

Reid, Alexander. A remarkable case of a person cut for the stone in the new way, commonly called the lateral, by Wm. Cheselden. *Phil. Trans.* [for 1746] (1748), 44:33–35.

Wollaston, William H. On gouty and urinary concretions. *Phil. Trans.* (1797), 87:386–400.

Chapter 5. Prostatic Obstruction

Notes

1. Eccles. 12:5

2. Henry Thompson, *Lectures on . . . surgery of the urinary organs* (Philadelphia, 1884), p. 102.

3. In their monograph *Studien zur Anatomie und Klinik der Prostatahypertrophie* (Berlin: Springer, 1922), Julius Tandler and Otto Zuckerkandl describe and illustrate the development of the prostate (pp. 4–14). It surrounds the proximal urethra and lies between the urinary bladder above and the bulbous urethra below. They describe five lobes: the anterior lobe, which remains rudimentary; the two lateral lobes; the mid-lobe; and the posterior lobe. Complete prostatectomy is probably very rarely done. The so-called complete prostatectomy is usually constituted by a fairly complete excision of the two lateral lobes and the mid-lobe.

4. John Adams, *Anatomy and diseases of the prostate gland* (London, 1851), p. 1.

5. John Baptist Morgagni, *The seats and causes of diseases investigated by anatomy*, trans. Benjamin Alexander (London, 1769; facsimile, New York: New York Academy of Medicine, Hafner, 1960), 2:454, 467. In a monograph, *Traek af prostatahypertrofiens historie* (Copenhagen: Munksgaard, 1968), pp. 224–25, Laurits Lauridsen, a Danish urologist, substantiates the view that Morgagni identified and delineated the role of prostatic hypertrophy in urinary retention.

6. Jean Z. Amussat, *Lectures on retention of urine, caused by strictures of the urethra*, ed. A. Petit, trans. James P. Jervey (Philadelphia, 1840), p. 88.

7. Everard Home, *Practical observations on the treatment of the diseases of the prostate gland* (London, 1811), pp. 1–14, 74–94. Home's remarks before the Royal Society, "An account of a

small lobe of the human prostate gland, which has not been taken notice of by anatomists," appeared in *Phil. Trans.* (1806), 96:195–204. Garrison says that Home "consigned himself to oblivion by burning Hunter's manuscripts after using them as the groundwork for sundry Croonian lectures and other alleged scientific contributions of his own devising." Garrison, *Introduction to the history of medicine*, 4th ed. (Philadelphia: W. B. Saunders, 1929), p. 346. See also Jessie Dobson, *William Clift* (London: Heinemann, 1954), pp. 62–69. Brian Livesly and Gillian M. Pentelow have come forward with a very novel thesis to account for Home's burning of the manuscripts. They believe that not Hunter himself but young Home, then eleven years old, was the subject of Hunter's inoculation experiments on the nature of venereal disease and may have contracted luetic general paresis despite early liberal treatment with mercury inunctions. In confiscating and burning many of Hunter's unpublished papers, Home may have been attempting to destroy evidence of his identity in the experiments. Home, the authors say, was also known to have been a chronic alcoholic. "The burning of John Hunter's papers: A new explanation," *Ann. R. Coll. Surg.* (1978), 60:79–84.

8. John Hunter: *Observations on certain parts of the animal oeconomy* (London, 1786), pp. 36–41, and *Treatise on the venereal disease* (London, 1786), pp. 171–75.

9. Joseph Griffiths, "Observations on the function of the prostate gland in man and the lower animals," *J. Anat. Physiol.* (1890), 24:27–41. Griffiths alludes to Wenzel Gruber's report of a man castrated in early youth, who died at the age of sixty-five. The prostate was very small. Griffiths adds that Alfonsus Bilharz examined the prostate in two castrated men, confirming Gruber's observations (Berlin thesis, 1859). Griffiths also quotes Eugenii Pelikan, who, in a Russian publication in 1876, wrote of a sect in Russia that fostered castration. Pelikan related that the prostate in eunuchs is of the size found in a child.

10. Robert A. Moore, "The evolution and involution of the prostate gland," *Am. J. Path.* (1936), 12(2):620. Moore was then pathologist at Washington University, St. Louis.

11. Related by a physician member of the Russian Embassy in Peking, W. Korsakow, *Dt. med. Wschr.* (1898), 24:338–40.

12. Tivadar Duka, "A case of emasculation . . . among the Mahomedans in East India," *Trans. Path. Soc. London* (1866), 17:184–85. Duka (1866) sent St. George's Hospital Pathological Museum, London, a specimen of the pubic area of a sixty-year-old eunuch who died in a Bengal prison. H. Ebden wrote from India that the mortality from the operation was said to be only 1 in 1,000 castrated children and that the operation was usually done on slaves or orphans. See *Indian Ann. M. Sc.*, Calcutta (1856), 3:520–25. Eunuchs were still being sold in North Central Africa in 1915, according to John J. Abel, *Science* (1915), 42:165.

13. Edmund Andrews, "The Oriental eunuchs," *JAMA* (1898), 30:175–76. Origen, famous Christian philosopher and scholar of the third century, out of zeal for purity, castrated himself, a sacrifice he subsequently regretted.

14. Samuel D. Gross, *Practical treatise on the diseases, injuries, and malformations of the urinary bladder, the prostate gland, and the urethra*, 2d ed. (Philadelphia, 1855), pp. 377, 704–5. Gross concedes (p. 712) that excision of the middle lobe might have a "fair prospect of success."

15. Benjamin C. Brodie, *Lectures on the diseases of the urinary organs* (London, 1842), pp. 175–85; Maximilian J. Chelius, *Handbuch der Chirurgie* (Heidelberg, 1844), 2:156, #1807; Frederick J. Gant, *Diseases of the bladder, prostate gland, and urethra*, 5th ed. (New York, 1884), pp. 282–84.

16. W. F. Teevan, "Treatment of strictures of the urethra, enlarged prostate, and stone in the bladder," *Lancet* (1880), 1:592; James Paget, *Clinical lectures and essays* (London, 1875), p. 69. Teevan, surgeon to St. Peter's Hospital, stated that many a prostatic in London used to have a mahogany case containing seven gum elastic catheters, one for each day of the week, but that "all this cumbersome appliance" had been eliminated. A French contemporary claimed that the elastic gum catheter represented perfection in modern surgery and was one of the finest instruments of the nineteenth century. J. J. Cazenave, *Histoire abrégée des sondes et des bougies uréthro-vésicales* (Paris, 1875), p. 49.

17. Historical accounts of the catheter may be found in François Chopart, *Traité des*

maladies des voies urinaires, 2 vols. (Paris, 1791–92); Ernst Gurlt, *Geschichte der Chirurgie* (Berlin, 1898), 2:303, 358; and Ernest Desnos, "Histoire de l'urologie" in *Encyclopédie française d'urologie* (Paris: Doin, 1914), 1:108–15. See W. G. Spencer's translation of Celsus, *De medicina* (Cambridge: Harvard Univ. Press, Loeb Classical Library, 1961), 3:425, and the Spink and Lewis translation of Albucasis, *On surgery and instruments* (Berkeley: Univ. California Press, 1973), pp. 402–3.

18. Ambroise Paré, *The workes of that famous chirurgion Ambrose Parey*, trans. Thomas Johnson (London, 1634), pp. 121, 665; Fabricius Hildanus, *Lithotomia vesicae: hoc est, accurata descriptio calculi vesicae* (Basel, 1628), pp. 43–45; Joannes B. van Helmont, "De lithiasi," in *Opuscula medica inaudita*, 5th ed. (Lyons, 1655), chap. 7, p. 44.

19. Poulletier de la Salle, Macquer, and Vicq d'Azyr, "Sondes de gomme élastique pour les rétentions d'urine . . . l'invention du sieur Bernard, orfevre [goldsmith] méchanicien pour les instruments de chirurgie," *J. de méd., chir., pharm.*, Paris (1782), 58:85–94. John Syng Dorsey, *Elements of surgery*, 2d ed. (Philadelphia, 1818), 2:158–59. John W. S. Gouley wrote that until 1875 catheters and bougies used in America had largely come from France, Germany, and England but that recently American manufacturers had increasingly met local needs for these instruments. *N. York M. J.* (1893), 58:85–88.

20. George J. Guthrie, *On the anatomy and diseases of the neck of the bladder and of the urethra* (London, 1834), pp. 271–77; L.-Auguste Mercier, "Nouvelles observations sur le traitement des valvules du col de la vessie," *Rev. méd.-chir. de Paris* (1847), 2:210–23; John W. S. Gouley, "Some points in the surgery of the hypertrophied prostate," *Trans. Am. Surg. Assoc.* (1885), 3:183–84.

21. Jean Cruveilhier, *Anatomie pathologique du corps humain* (Paris, 1829), 1(2), fasc. 17, pl. 2, p. 4; P. Huard and M. J. Imbault-Huart, "La vie et l'oeuvre de Jean Astruc (1684–1766)," *Clio med.* (1969), 4:85. Astruc was on the faculty of the University of Paris from 1731 until his death in 1766 at age eighty-two.

22. Reginald Harrison, "On the treatment of certain cases of prostatic obstruction by a section of the gland," in Congrès périodique international des sci. méd., 8th session, Copenhagen 1884, *Compte-rendu* (1886), vol. 2, sect. de chir., pp. 42–46; Thomas Annandale, "Clinical remarks upon the operative surgery of the male bladder," *Edinb. Med. J.* (1888), 33:1065–68.

23. Enrico Bottini, "Di un nuovo cauterizzatore ed incisore termo-galvanico contro le iscurie da ipertrofia prostatica," *Galvani* (1874), 2:437–52; "Thermo-electric prostatotomy," editorial, *Lancet* (1885), 1:582–83. A. A. Hoehling, surgeon, United States Navy, Naval Dispensary, Washington, D.C., wrote the editor of the *Medical Record* (1882), 21:306, suggesting that electrolysis be given a trial in cases of prostatic obstruction. These were apparently the first suggestions for relief of prostatic obstruction by the galvanocautery. In 1910 Edwin Beer of New York developed transurethral fulguration by an electric current, the forerunner of transurethral prostatectomy with an electric knife. *JAMA* (1910), 54:1768–69.

24. Bernard Lytton, *Catheters and sounds* (Nutley, N.J.: Roche Laboratories, 1975).

25. Frederic E. B. Foley, "A self-retaining bag catheter for use as indwelling catheter for constant drainage of the bladder," *J. Urol.* (1937), 38:140–43.

26. At the Baragwanath Hospital near Johannesburg in 1964 the senior author of this volume saw a large ward of paraplegics apparently doing very well and without evidence of bedsores, owing to superb nursing care. Most of the patients were victims of a mode of recrimination among the Bantus in that area of South Africa in which a bicycle spoke is the weapon. The opponent is grasped by the nape of the neck and bent forward. The spoke is thrust into the spinal column, frequently causing irreparable damage to the spinal cord with ensuant paraplegic bladder, a terrible price to pay for what often began as friendly sport.

27. V. H. K. Moorhouse, "Observations on the spinal integration of standing," *Am. J. Physiol.* (1930), 92:716–27. Carl Credé also employed his maneuver to encourage contraction of the uterus and expulsion of the placenta.

28. Henry Thompson, *Diseases of the prostate: Their pathology and treatment*, 3d ed. (London,

1868), p. 243; Gant, *Diseases of the bladder* (n.15), p. 283; Cornelius Van Zwalenburg, "Emptying a chronically distended bladder: Description of a simple device," *JAMA* (1920), 75:1711–12.

29. C. D. Creevy, "Sudden decompression of the chronically distended urinary bladder," *Arch. Surg.* (1932), 25:356–85; Stephen D. Elek, "Experimental staphylococcal infections in the skin of man," *Ann. N.Y. Acad. Sc.* (1956), 65:85–90. Paul B. Beeson warned against indiscriminate use of urinary catheters which invite cystitis and pyelonephritis. *Am. J. Med.* (1958), 24:1–3.

30. Leopold Dittel, Professor of Surgery, University of Vienna, wrote a 258-page monograph on *Die Stricturen der Harnröhre* (Stuttgart, 1880). For urinary retention occasioned by prostatic hypertrophy, he recommended suprapubic drainage. He mentioned electrolysis but offered no suggestion of a direct surgical attack upon the prostate. However, in 1885, Dittel excised the middle lobe of the prostate. The patient died of infection in six days. *Wien. med. Bl.* (1885), 8:270–72, 301–2.

31. A. F. McGill, "On suprapubic prostatectomy, with three cases in which the operation was successfully performed for chronic prostatic hypertrophy. Read November 11, 1887," *Trans. Clin. Soc. London*, 21:52–57, abstracted, *Lancet* (1887), 2:1016–17; McGill, "Hypertrophy of the prostate, and its relief by operation," *Lancet* (1888), 1:216; William T. Belfield, "Prostatic myoma — a so-called 'middle lobe' of the hypertrophied prostate — removed by suprapubic prostatectomy," *JAMA* (1887), 8:303. Later Belfield (1890) summarized his personal experience with prostatectomy by both the suprapubic and perineal routes. In 133 operations, he lost 17 patients, a mortality of 12.7 percent. *Am. J. Med. Sci.*, 100:451.

32. Eugene Fuller, "Six successful and successive cases of prostatectomy," *J. Cutan. & Genito-Urin. Dis.* (1895), 13:229–39. Inasmuch as the approach and general conduct of the operation is the same whether by excision with knife or scissors or by finger enucleations, it would appear that McGill's (1887) publication eight years earlier deserves recognition.

33. Peter J. Freyer, "Total extirpation of the prostate for radical cure of enlargement of that organ," *Br. M. J.* (1901), 2:125–29; Freyer, *Clinical lectures on enlargement of the prostate*, 3d ed. (New York: Wood, 1906), pp. 6–9, 37–45, 139. Belfield, McGill, Fuller, and Freyer each claimed priority for originating prostatectomy; each had his band of faithful supporters. Moynihan (1904) too claimed discovery of total suprapubic prostatectomy (*Ann. Surg.*, 39:1). The McGill operation was essentially a limited prostatectomy; the Fuller and Freyer prostatectomies were far more complete. The literature on the controversy is voluminous. See especially Fuller, *Ann. Surg.* (1905), 41:520–34, and Freyer, *Enlargement of prostate*, pp. 144–54.

34. Terence Millin, "Retropubic prostatectomy, a new extravesical technique, report on 20 cases," *Lancet* (1945), 2:693–96.

35. Hugh H. Young, "A new procedure (punch operation) for small prostatic bars and contracture of the prostatic orifice," *JAMA* (1913), 60:253–57, a paper presented at a meeting of the American Medical Association in 1912; William F. Braasch, "Median bar excisor," *JAMA* (1918), 70:758–59.

36. Maximilian Stern, "Resection of obstructions at the vesical orifice, new instruments and a new method," *JAMA* (1926), 87(2):1726–29; Joseph F. McCarthy, "A new apparatus for endoscopic plastic surgery of the prostate, diathermia and excision of vesical growths," *J. Urol.* (1931), 26:695–96.

37. C. D. Creevy informed the authors, January 4, 1975, that the hospital mortality in his last 500 transurethral resections was 0.6 percent.

38. J. William White, "The present position of the hypertrophied prostate," *Trans. Am. Surg. Assoc.* (1893), 11:167–204, 209–10, and "The present position of the surgery of the hypertrophied prostate," *Ann. Surg.* (1904), 40:788–92. Controversial editorials and letters by Arthur T. Cabot and White appear in *Ann. Surg.* (1896–97), 24:265–85, 388–98; 25:107–12, 121–27.

39. George T. Beatson, "On the treatment of inoperable cases of carcinoma of the mamma," *Lancet* (1896), 2:104–7, 162–65. The history of oophorectomy for breast cancer,

including Albert S. Schinzinger's 1889 proposal of the therapy, is given by H. H. Simmer, *Clio med.* (1969), 4:227–49.

40. Charles Huggins and Clarence V. Hodges, "Studies on prostatic cancer. 1. The effect of castration, of estrogen and of androgen injection on serum phosphatases in metastatic carcinoma of the prostate," *Cancer Res.* (1941), 1:293–97. For this work Huggins shared the Nobel Prize, in 1966, with Peyton Rous of New York.

41. An interesting discussion of these diverse views by George R. Prout, Jr., and David F. Paulson is to be found in *Med. Wld News* (1974), vol. 15, no. 42, pp. 27–35.

42. A rich vascular plexus of blood vessels underlies the prostatic fascia. G. S. Pattison (1820) pointed out its importance for the safety of perineal lithotomy. Ignoring it was the nemesis of many an eighteenth-century lithotomist. See chapter 4.

43. John Simon's operation was considered so significant by the editors of *Lancet* that a full description was delayed until results were known. On the death of the patient, the case history was supplied by the journal, the editors remarking, "The case is highly important, for it will show how well-directed surgical efforts may effectually change and modify the natural relation and function of parts." *Lancet* (1851), 2:370; (1852), 2:568–70.

Further Readings

Ballenger, Edgar Garrison, ed. *History of urology*. Prepared under the auspices of the American Urological Association. 2 vols. Baltimore: Williams and Wilkins, 1933.

Briggs, James E. A method of controlling the bleeding after suprapubic prostatectomy. *New Engl. M. Gaz.* (1906), 41:391–93.

Murphy, Leonard J. T. *The history of urology; incorporating in pt. I, L'histoire de l'urologie by Ernest Desnos* [trans. Murphy]. Springfield, Ill.: Charles C Thomas, 1972.

Randall, Alexander. *Surgical pathology of prostatic obstructions*. Baltimore: Williams and Wilkins, 1931.

Weyrauch, Henry M. *Life after fifty; the prostatic age*. Los Angeles: W. Ritchie, 1967.

Chapter 6. Intestinal Obstructions

Notes

1. Sir Frederick Treves's manuscript, written in his clear hand, can be seen at the Royal College of Surgeons Library in London. It is in two volumes: the descriptive section in volume 1 is 384 pages; volume 2 has approximately one hundred original illustrations, apparently executed by the author. Professor Robert Milnes Walker told the authors that Treves received £15 for the Jacksonian Prize Essay, which is still the financial reward attending the much coveted honor. It was published with the title *Intestinal obstruction, its varieties, with their pathology, diagnosis, and treatment: The Jacksonian Prize Essay of the Royal College of Surgeons of England, 1883* (London, 1884). The revised edition appeared in 1899. The Clifton Bridge, which is 250 to 275 feet above the Avon River, is mentioned in the revised edition (p. 476).

2. Jonathan Hutchinson, "Notes on intestinal obstruction: Its diagnosis and treatment," *Br. M. J.* (1878), 2:305–7; Caspar Stromayr, *Die Handschrift des Schnitt- und Augenarztes* (1559), ed. Walter Brunn (Berlin: Selle, 1925), pp. 196, 266; Percivall Pott, *Chirurgical works* (London, 1771), 1:62–63. Harold Speert gives a good historical account in "Friedrich Trendelenburg and the Trendelenburg position," *Surg. Gynec. Obstet.* (1957), 105:114–19. See also chapter 13 on vesicovaginal fistula.

3. Astley Cooper, *The anatomy and surgical treatment of inguinal and congenital hernia* (London, 1804), p. 23; S. Monrad, "Acute invagination of the intestine in small children," *Acta paediat.* (1926), 6:31–52; C. P. B. Clubbe, *The diagnosis and treatment of intussusception*, 2d ed. (London: Oxford Univ. Press, 1921); P. L. Hipsley, "Intussusception and its treatment by hydrostatic pressure," *Med. J. Australia* (1926), 2:201; Yngve Olsson and Gustaf Pallin, "Über

das Bild der akuten Darminvagination bei Röntgenuntersuchung und über Desinvagination mit Hilfe von Kontrastlavements," *Acta chir. scand.* (1926–27), 61:371–83.

4. Thomas Sydenham, *Works,* trans. R. G. Latham (London: Sydenham Society, vol. 15:1, 1848–50), pp. 68, 194–97. Kenneth Dewhurst relates that Sydenham regarded research as totally irrelevant to the physician's main task of alleviating sickness, believing that medical progress could best be achieved by studying the natural histories of the diseases under his care, of which Sydenham's writings provided good evidence. *Br. M. J.* (1963), 2:859.

5. Hugh Owen Thomas, *Diet and opium: The past and present treatment of intestinal obstructions* (London, 1879), pp. 2–5.

6. William Brinton, *Intestinal obstruction*, ed. Thomas Buzzard (London, 1867), p. 110.

7. Treves, *Intestinal obstruction* (n.1), p. 554.

8. Otto Leichtenstern, "Constrictions, occlusions, and displacements of the intestines," trans. Lewis A. Stimson, pp. 477–666 in H. von Ziemssen, ed., *Cyclopaedia of the practice of medicine* (New York, 1876), 7:644.

9. Successful issue following the administration of 7 pounds of metallic mercury was recorded by Benjamin W. Brown, *Assoc. M. J.*, London (1853), 1:121. Auguste Matignon provided a full account of the role of metallic mercury in intestinal obstruction in a Paris thesis of 1879, *Du traitement de l'occlusion intestinale par le mercure métallique à haute dose.*

10. Pillore de Rouen, "Opération d'anus artificiel, par la méthode de Littre," pp. 85–88 in Jean-Z. Amussat, *Mémoire sur la possibilité d'établir un anus artificiel dans la région lombaire sans pénétrer dans le péritoine* (Paris, 1839).

11. Jean-J. Leroy-d'Etiolles, "Sur l'emploi du galvanisme dans les hernies étranglées et les étranglemens internes," *Arch. gén. de méd.*, Paris (1826), 12:270–77; L. Biett, "Histoire de la maladie de Talma," *Répert. gén. d'anat. et physiol. path.* (1827), 3:99–118; Herbert F. Collins, *Talma: A biography of an actor* (London: Faber and Faber, 1964), pp. 359–71. Biett was put in charge of Talma's case on June 4, 1826, and presents a fairly detailed account of the progression from that date to Talma's death on October 19, 1826, including opinions and suggestions of the consultants called by him and the family. Collins says Biett summoned Robert-Fleury to make the well-known painting of the deathbed scene.

12. Guillaume B. Duchenne de Boulogne, *De l'électrisation localisée et de son application* (Paris, 1855).

13. George M. Beard and Alphonso D. Rockwell, *Practical treatise on the medical & surgical uses of electricity,* 2d ed. (New York, 1878), pp. 579–84; Jean-B. Ballouhey, *De l'électricité appliquée au traitement de l'occlusion intestinale*, Paris thesis, 1880.

14. A. M. Bilgutay, Robert Wingrove, Ward O. Griffen, Jr., Raymond C. Bonnabeau, and C. Walton Lillehei, "Gastrointestinal pacing, a new concept in the treatment of ileus," *Biomedical Sciences Instrumentation* (1963), 1:377–83.

15. A. Cahn, "Heilung von Ileus durch Magenausspülung: Unter Benutzung eines Vortrages des Herrn Geheimrath Dr. Kussmaul," *Berl. klin. Wschr.* (1884), 21:669–72, 685–87; Heinrich Curschmann, "Der heutige Standpunkt und die nächsten Ziele der Behandlung des Ileus," *Therap. Monatsh.*, Berlin (1889), 3:201; Edward Martin and H. A. Hare, *Surgical treatment of wounds and obstruction of the intestines* (Philadelphia, 1891), p. 91. Instances of death from lavage are recorded by Cahn and in R. Peters, "Magenausspülung bei Ileus: Casuistischer Beitrag," *St. Petersb. med. Wschr.* (1885), 10:63–64. Franz Mahnert of Graz provides a series of early trials with gastric lavage in *Memorabilien*, Heilbron (1888), 33:257–71, 321–35, 385–98.

16. Fridericus D. W. Mensching, *De operationibus quibusdam chirurgicis temere institutis*, Rostock thesis, 1756; Leichtenstern (n.8), p. 658; John G. Blake, "A case of intestinal obstruction of eighteen weeks' duration," *Boston M. & S. J.* (1876), 95:601–8. The article includes a letter from Henry J. Bigelow, consultant in the case.

17. John W. Ogle, *On the relief of excessive and dangerous tympanites by puncture of the abdomen* (London, 1888); Martin and Hare, *Surgical treatment of wounds* (n.15), pp. 107–8.

18. See chapter 7.

19. *The genuine works of Hippocrates* (1929), trans. Francis Adams (New York: William Wood, 1929), 1:71. Adams notes that this treatise is "not one of the genuine productions of Hippocrates."

20. As pointed out by Daniel Le Clerc, *The history of physick*, trans. Drake and Baden (London, 1699), pp. 330–37.

21. Caelius Aurelianus, *On acute diseases and on chronic diseases*, ed. and trans. I. E. Drabkin (Chicago: Univ. Chicago Press, 1950), p. 403; Christian G. Gruner, *Bibliothek der alten aertze, Nachfolger des Hippokrates* (Leipzig, 1782), pp. 634–35; Ernst J. Gurlt, *Geschichte der Chirurgie* (Berlin, 1898), 1:304; Karl Sudhoff, "Zur operativen Ileusbehandlung des Praxagoras," *Quell. Stud. Gesch. Naturw. Med.* (1933), 3:151–54. Aurelianus (fifth century) regarded the Praxagoras operation as authentic, as did Gruner, Gurlt, and Sudhoff. But, adds Sudhoff, Praxagoras had no followers in antiquity. The terms *iliac passion, miserere mei*, and *dolore iliaco* were used indiscriminately in the early literature for volvulus, strangulated hernia, intussusception, or other condition causing acute pain in the upper abdomen.

22. *Sushruta Samhita, Chowkhamba Sanskrit studies*, trans. K. K. Bhishagratna, 2d ed. (Varanasi: Vidya Vilas Press, 1963), 2:80, 442. Sushruta, an innovative surgeon, taught at Benares in India sometime between 800 and 600 B.C. His remarkable accomplishments deserve greater recognition in Western medical history. See Udaya B. S. Prakash, "Shushruta of ancient India," *Surg. Gynec. Obstet.* (1978), 146:262–72.

23. Gurlt, *Geschichte der Chirurgie* (n.21), 1:703, 716–54, 765. The "Four Masters" — Archymatheus, Petronsellus, Platearius, and Ferrarius — lived in the thirteenth century and are often cited by Guy de Chauliac.

24. Gurlt, *Geschichte der Chirurgie* (n.21), 2:652; Pierre Franco, *Petit traite* (Lyons, 1556), pp. 46–49; *Chirurgie de Pierre Franco*, ed. Édouard Nicaise (Paris, 1895), pp. 30, 56–58; Ambroise Paré, *The workes of that famous chirurgion Ambrose Parey*, trans. Thomas Johnson (London, 1634), p. 308. This passage first appeared in Paré's collected works of 1575, according to Janet Doe, *Bibliography of the works of Ambroise Paré* (Chicago: Univ. Chicago Press, 1937), p. 106. See also J.-F. Malgaigne, *Oeuvres complètes d'Ambroise Paré* (Paris, 1840), 1:410–11, and T. Clifford Allbutt, *The historical relations of medicine and surgery* (London: Macmillan, 1905), pp. 74–76.

25. Pierre Franco, *Traité des hernies* (Lyons, 1561), pp. 59–68; John Woodall, *The surgeons mate or military & domestique surgery* (London, 1655), pp. 196–99.

26. Pierre Pigray, *Epitome des preceptes de médecine et chirurgie* (Rouen, 1615), pp. 257–89.

27. Paul Barbette, *Opera chirurgico-anatomica* (Leyden, 1672), pp. 381–82; Laurenz [Lorenz] Heister, *Medical, chirurgical, and anatomical cases and observations*, trans. George Wirgman (London, 1755), pp. 39–40. Rau is best known as a lithotomist.

28. Cornelius H. Velse, *De mutuo intestinorum ingressu*, Leyden doctorate thesis, 1742, in Albrecht Haller, *Disputationum anatomicarum selectarum* (Göttingen, 1751), 7:126–27. We have been unable to locate Nuck's own account of the operation.

29. Theophilus Bonet, *Sepulchretum, sive anatomia practica ex cadaveribus morbo denatis* (Geneva, 1679), p. 912. Prudent Hévin retells this case history but with some reservation, inasmuch as Bonet came by the report secondhand. "Récherches historiques sur la gastrotomie," *Mém. Acad. roy. chir.* (1768), 4:206–7.

30. François de La Peyronie (1678–1747) of Montpellier became Louis XV's surgeon in 1736, succeeding Mareschal. Much of the success of the Royal Academy and the rising status of the French surgeon may be credited to La Peyronie's wise leadership. He left his entire fortune to the advancement of surgical education. A fine account of the emergence of French surgery after the "grande opération" of Louis XIV and the creation of the Royal Academy of Surgery is given by Marie-José Imbault-Huart in a Paris thesis of 1973, *L'École Pratique de Dissection de Paris de 1750 à 1822*, pp. 1–80.

31. Jean Mery, "Observations sur les hernies," *Hist. Acad. roy. d. sc.* [*de Paris*] *1701* (1707), pp. 356–80.

32. See Observation 8 in "Diverses observations anatomiques," *Hist. Acad. roy. d. sc.* [*de Paris*] *1723* (1725), pp. 32–33. La Peyronie's name is strangely withheld in this early account of

his exploit in 1723; the unnamed narrator states only that the surgery was performed by "a famous surgeon of the highest attainable position." However, Antoine Louis refers to the operation as La Peyronie's in *Mém. Acad. roy. chir.* (1757), 3:169–71. La Peyronie reviews his earlier operation and that of 1743 in "Observations avec des réflexions sur la cure des hernies avec gangrène," *Mém. Acad. roy. chir.* (1743), 1:337–42.

33. Subsequent hospital reentry for recurrent obstruction of a few patients after spontaneous closure of an artificial anus in the small bowel suggests persistence of a spur at the site of union. Dupuytren's spur divider was illustrated and apparently used by Astley Cooper.

34. Alfred A. L. M. Velpeau, *New elements of operative surgery*, trans. P. S. Townsend (New York, 1851), 3:624.

35. Antoine Louis, "Sur la cure des hernies intestinales avec gangrène," *Mèm. Acad. roy. chir.* (1757), 3:145–201, and "Réflexions sur l'opération de la hernie," ibid. (1768), 4:281–322; [Claude] Pipelet *l'aîné*, "Sur la réunion de l'intestin qui a souffert déperdition de substance, dans une hernie avec gangrène," *Mém. Acad. roy. chir.* (1768), 4:164–72.

36. Regnauld's case is reviewed in *J. de méd., chir., pharm.*, Paris (1787), 71:546–51. A British case merits mention with the French reports of the eighteenth century. In 1731 William Cookesley, a surgeon in Credition, Devonshire, attended a chimneysweep of about thirty who had a large strangulated inguinal hernia as a result of "overheaving himself" carrying water to a fire. The surgeon cut away the involved portion of the scrotum and gangrenous bowel with scissors, establishing a fecal fistula in the wound. During convalescence an additional 6 inches of bowel was removed. Eventually, the wound healed and the patient recovered; intestinal continuity was reestablished spontaneously. Cookesley's report, "A considerable share of the intestines cut off after a mortification in a hernia," appeared in *Med. Essays & Obs.*, Edinburgh, 4th ed. (1752), 5(1):351–54.

37. Jean-Louis Petit, *Traité des maladies chirurgicale et des opérations qui leur conviennent, ouvrage posthume* (Paris, 1790), 2:273-358.

38. L. J. Maunoury, *Considérations sur l'étranglement interne du canal intestinal*, Paris thesis, 1819. Maunoury's proposed operation was attempted unsuccessfully by Monod in 1838, according to Armand Trousseau, *Clinique médicale de l'Hôtel-Dieu de Paris*, 2d ed. (Paris, 1865), 3:205. In 1857 L. Veillard quoted Maunoury's thesis in conjunction with Auguste Nélaton's enterotomy, *Union méd.* (1857), 11:371–73.

39. John Hunter, *Works*, ed. James F. Palmer (London, 1835), 1:448, 3:587; Pott, *Chirurgical works* (1771–75), vols. 1 and 4. As treatment for intussusception Hunter suggested emetics and purgatives. Lord Brock has written a sensitive appreciation of Astley Paston Cooper and his work, which reveals him as a kindly, courteous, industrious surgeon with a huge surgical practice — bold in some matters and timid in others — and a great surgical anatomist. Cooper (1768–1843), the son of a Norfolk clergyman, was sent to London to study surgery under the guardianship of his uncle, William Cooper, Surgeon to Guy's Hospital, the position to which Astley eventually succeeded. Young Astley chose to be apprenticed to Henry Cline, an ardent admirer of John Hunter, and audited Hunter's lectures. His uncle found these sessions less inspiring, stating that he never could understand Hunter and usually went to sleep in his classes. See Charters J. Symonds, "Astley Cooper," *Guy's Hosp. Rep.* (1922), 72:1–3; Russell C. Brock, *The life and work of Astley Cooper* (Edinburgh: Livingstone, 1952).

40. Charles Williams Jones, *A series of lectures on . . . surgery, principally derived from the lectures delivered by Astley Cooper*, ed. Charles Mingay Syder, 1st Am. ed. (Boston, 1823), pp. 281–85.

41. Charles Bell uses an almost identical statement in writing of strangulated hernia in his *Illustrations of the great operations of surgery* (London, 1831), p. 50.

42. Astley Cooper, *The anatomy and surgical treatment of crural and umbilical hernia* (London, 1807), p. 18.

43. John Bland-Sutton, *Tumours innocent and malignant, their clinical characters and appropriate treatment*, 7th ed. (New York: Hoeber, 1922), p. 302.

44. Astley Cooper, *The anatomy and surgical treatment of abdominal hernia*, from 2d London

ed., ed. C. Aston Key (Philadelphia, 1844). [The first London edition appeared in two volumes, 1804 and 1807.] These results are to be found in case histories scattered between pages 11 and 307.

45. Pott, *Treatise on ruptures* (1756); A. G. Richter, *Abhandlung von den Brüchen* (Göttingen, 1778–79); Pieter Camper, *Icones herniarum* (Frankfurt-am-Main, 1801); Antonio Scarpa, *Sull'ernie, memorie anatomico-chirurgiche* (Milan, 1809); Benjamin Travers, *An inquiry into the process of nature in repairing injuries of the intestines* (London, 1812), p. 225; William Hey, *Practical observations in surgery* (London, 1803), p. 143. Shortly after the Cooper era, Paul Broca, a famous French neurologist-surgeon, used for his Paris *concours* thesis (1853) a treatise on strangulated hernia (*De l'étranglement dans les hernies abdominales et des affections qui peuvent le simuler*). He reports (p. 154) that Kajetan Textor of Würzburg between 1816 and 1842 reduced 114 strangulated hernias by taxis with a mortality of 7.9 percent. In 56 patients subjected to operation, the mortality was 42.8 percent. Broca's monograph reflects a conservative surgical attitude. It provides, however, an excellent bibliography of the early surgical literature of strangulated hernia. Obviously the boldness of the French surgeons of the past century had mellowed.

46. Louis (n.35), pp. 188–90; Cooper, *Inguinal and congenital hernia* (n.3), pp. 35–40. Lancelot Haire, "Remarks on Mr. Lucas's practical observations on amputation," *London M. J.* (1786), 7:390; P. D. Gordon Pugh, *Nelson and his surgeons* (Edinburgh and London: Livingstone, 1968), p. 15. Little is known of Duverger (or Duvergé). He was surgeon in the hospital of Mauberge, inspector of military hospitals, and lived at Tours in 1763, according to L. Hahn, *Dict. encycl. d. sc. méd.* (1884), 30:729. Cutting on the knot is sometimes attributed to William Lawrence (1815). See his "New method of tying the arteries in aneurism, amputation, and other surgical operations," *Med.-Chir. Trans.* (1815), 6:156–208.

47. Johann F. Moebius, *Observationes medicae miscellaneae theoreticae et practicae*, in Haller (n.28), 6:745–46; A. J. Jobert, "Récherches sur l'opération de l'invagination des intestins," *Arch. gén. de méd.* (1824), 4:71–80. Jobert (de Lamballe) (1799–1867) subsequently wrote a two-volume work on hernia (1829). In a 1938 Paris thesis on Jobert, Robert Le Sage described him as "un grand chirurgien Breton," stating that in the 1850s Jobert had the first surgical practice in Paris. His operation for vesicovaginal fistula is described in chapter 13.

48. Antoine Lembert, "Mémoire sur l'entéroraphie, avec la description d'un procédé nouveau pour pratiquer cette opération chirurgicale," *Répert. gén. d'anat. et physiol. path.* (1826), 2:100–7. Lembert's paper was translated into English in 1960 and is available through the John Crerar Library Translation Center in Chicago.

49. William S. Halsted, "Circular suture of the intestine," *Am. J. Med. Sci.* (1887), 94:436–61; Peter D. Olch, personal communication.

50. J. B. Murphy, "Cholecysto-intestinal, gastro-intestinal, entero-intestinal anastomosis," *Med. Record* (1892), 42:665–76; W. S. Halsted, "Blind-end circular suture of the intestine," *Ann. Surg.* (1922), 75:356–64.

51. C. Duret, "Observation sur un enfant né sans anus," *Rec. périod. Soc. de méd. de Paris* (1798), 4:45–50. Alexis Littre (1658–1725) made the suggestion in a pathologic anatomical presentation, reported in *Hist. Acad. roy. d. sc.* (1710), pp. 47–48.

52. Henric Callisen, *Systema chirurgiae hodiernae* (Copenhagen, 1798), 1:469–70, 711; J.-Z. Amussat, "Quelques réflexions pratiques sur les obstructions du rectum," *Gaz. méd. Paris* (1839), 7:1–8; Thomas Bryant, *On the mode of death from acute intestinal obstruction* (London, 1885).

53. Erskine Mason, "Six cases of lumbar colotomy," *Am. J. Med. Sci.* (1873), 66:354–92.

54. Auguste Nélaton [discussion], *Union méd.* (1851), 5:344; Nélaton and L. Veillard, "Une observation de rétrécissement et d'oblitération du colon ascendant . . . autres observations d'entrérotomie," *Union méd.* (1857), 11:363–64, 371–73, 379–80; Armand Trousseau, *Lectures on clinical medicine*, trans. John R. Cormack (London: New Sydenham Soc., vol. 51:4, 1871), pp. 219–25.

55. Walter F. Atlee, *Clinical lectures on surgery by M. Nélaton* (Philadelphia, 1855), pp.

570–88; Auguste Nélaton, *Exposé des titres et des travaux scientifiques de M. A. Nélaton* (Paris, 1867), pp. 16–17. Trousseau (1801–67) performed operations and occasionally spoke of himself as a surgeon. From his own narrative it would appear that in some operations he actively participated with the surgeon, a practice now frowned upon by most surgical bodies. It is possible, therefore, that Trousseau and Nélaton are independently reporting the same cases!

56. Theodor Kocher, *Text-book of operative surgery*, trans. Harold J. Stiles and C. Balfour Paul, 3d ed. (New York: Macmillan, 1911), 2:613; Victor Bonney, "Faecal and intestinal vomiting and jejunostomy," *Br. M. J.* (1916), 1:583–85. In some sections of Minnesota in the mid-1920s, following the publications of Bonney (1916) and W. Sampson Handley (1925), it became standard practice to perform a high jejunostomy employing the Nélaton or Stamm-Kader techniques of enterostomy for a miscellany of acute abdominal conditions including peritonitis. This "triumph of Sampson Handley," as A. L. McGregor termed it, fortunately was short lived. This surgeon's first exposure to intestinal surgery in the mid-1920s was the repair of residual fistula resulting from such operative procedures. See Handley, *Br. J. Surg.* (1925), 12:417; and McGregor, *Med. Jl. S. Afr.* (1925), 20:292.

57. Oscar Witzel, "Zur Technik der Magenfistelanlegung," *Centralbl. f. Chir.* (1891), 18:601–4, and "Zur Indikation und Technik der Kolostomie und Enterostomie," ibid. (1894), 21:937–41. It has been this surgeon's practice when performing enterostomy to employ a catheter with a diameter no larger than 14 French, thus ensuring prompt closure of the tunnel on withdrawal of the catheter.

58. Alexandre Savopoulo, *De l'étranglement interne et des divers modes de son traitement* (1854), pp. 60–63, Paris thesis; [Félix Guyon and Léon Labbé], *Rapport sur les progrès de la chirurgie par Mm. Denonvilliers, Nélaton, Velpeau, Félix Guyon, Léon Labbé* (Paris, 1867), pp. 688–89.

59. Barthélemi Saviard, *Nouveau recueil d'observations chirurgicales* (Paris, 1702), p. 110–11; Louis (n.35), pp. 188–90.

60. Thomas Annandale, "Case in which an intestinal obstruction was removed by the operation of gastrotomy," *Edinb. M. J.* (1870–71), 16:700–4; George Buchanan, "On gastrotomy; with a case of intestinal obstruction," *Lancet*, June 10, 1871, pp. 776–79.

61. Hutchinson (n.2), pp. 305–7, 316; T. Clifford Allbutt, "Some remarks on obstruction of the bowels," *Br. M. J.* (1879), 1:40–41; T. P. Teale, "On exploration of the abdomen in obstruction of the bowels," ibid., pp. 41–43. Allbutt concluded his retraction by saying. "To deny operation to a case of internal hernia is, in my opinion, to deny to the patient some fair chance of life."

62. Rushton Parker, "Intestinal obstruction" [and discussion], *Br. M. J.* (1883), 2:669–71.

63. E. H. Greves, "On a case of acute intestinal obstruction in a boy," *Liverp. M.-Chir. J.* (1885), 5:118–30. Pughe's remarks follow (pp. 130–35).

64. *Liverp. M.-Chir. J.* (1885), 5:137–38; Hugh Owen Thomas, *The collegian of 1666 and the collegians of 1885; or what is recognised treatment?* (London, 1885).

65. John Ashhurst, Jr.: "On laparotomy, or abdominal section, as a remedy for intussusception," *Am. J. Med. Sci.* (1874), 68:48–64; *The principles and practice of surgery* (Philadelphia, 1886), p. 790; and "Treatment of intestinal obstruction," in *International encyclopaedia of surgery*, rev. ed. (New York, 1887), 6:60–79. It was largely owing to Ashhurst that the designation "gastrostomy" for abdominal section was given up in favor of "laparotomy," a term which several German-speaking surgeons had long employed. If the bowel was opened, the earlier appellation was "gastroenterostomy."

66. Otto W. Madelung, "Zur Frage der operativen Behandlung der inneren Darmeinklemmungen," *Verh. dt. Ges. Chir.* (1887), 16(2):63–64; discussion by Mikulicz reported, 16(1):67. The presentations of Reginald H. Fitz and Nicholas Senn on intestinal obstruction run consecutively in the *Transactions* of the Congress of American Physicians and Surgeons (1888), 1:1–42, 43–167. T. G. Morton's discussion appears 1:172–73.

67. Two years later at the Berlin International Medical Congress (1890), Senn was given an hour in which to demonstrate the effectiveness of his method of detecting leaks or wounds

in the intestine by insufflation of hydrogen through the rectum. He had brought his equipment for the purpose as well as an assistant to aid with the demonstration. The dog was shot through the abdomen and laid out on the table. The hour went by, but no evidence of inflation of the dog's abdomen was observed, and the experiment had to be abandoned. Senn had been outwitted by his assistant's deficient knowledge of comparative anatomy: there were two orifices beneath the dog's tail! The *Transactions* of the Berlin conference made no mention of this frustrating mishap, which has been related by G. W. Broome. *Med. Pickwick* (1915), 1:430–31.

68. See the discussions by Leichtenstern (pp. 21–58), Curschmann (pp. 58–85), and Paul Fürbringer (pp. 97–99) in *Verhandlungen des Congres für innere Medicin*, 8th Congress, April 1889. Leichtenstern's large monograph on bowel obstruction (n.8) contains an extensive critique on conventional surgical measures. He alludes (p. 660) to the Paris debates of the waning years of the eighteenth century in which Boinet summed up the prevailing attitude of the session, "it was better to leave the patient affected with ileus to Providence, even if the case was hopeless, than to endanger the profession and the authority of physicians by performing laparotomy."

69. Since 1934 this surgeon has been at pains to point out that feculent vomiting in his experience has been observed only in obstructions of the small intestine. Vomiting in colic obstructions is usually not a prominent symptom and may be absent; feculent vomiting is not observed. This circumstance reflects the competency of the ileocecal valve and sphincter, whose presence and activity were known to Caspar Bauhin in 1579 three centuries before Richard Heschl (1880), a University of Vienna pathologist, recognized the importance of the ileocecal valve in the genesis of diastatic perforation of the cecum. See Bauhin, "Valvula in intestino colo, anno 1579, à me reperta," in Israel Spach's compilation, *Gynaeciorum, sive de mulierum* (Strasbourg, 1597), pp. 490–91; Richard Heschl, "Mechanik der diastätischen Darmperforationen," *Wien. med. Wschr.* (1880), 30:1–6.

70. John O'Reilly, *Hints on the treatment of strangulated hernia* (New York, 1863), p. 20.

71. Treves, *Intestinal obstruction* (n.1), p. 320; Gottwald Schwarz, "Die Erkennung der tieferen Dünndarmstenose mittels des Röntgenverfahrens," *Wien. klin. Wschr.* (1911), 24:1386–90; Hans Kloiber, "Die Roentgendiagnose des Ileus ohne Kontrastmittel," *Arch. klin. Chir.* (1919), 112:513–91; J. T. Case, "A new aid in the early recognition of post-operative ileus," *J. Mich. St. Med. Soc.* (1920), 19:151–54.

72. W. B. O'Shaughnessy, "Proposal of a new method of treating the blue epidemic cholera by the injection of highly-oxygenised salts into the venous system," *Lancet* (1831–32), 1:366–71. O'Shaughnessy's analyses of the electrolyte content of watery diarrheal stools of patients with cholera were his guidelines. See his monograph with a very modern ring, *Report on the chemical pathology of the malignant cholera* (London, 1832).

73. Carl Schmidt, *Characteristik der epidemischen Cholera gegenüber verwandten Transsudationsanomalieen* (Leipzig, 1850); Sidney Ringer, "Regarding the action of hydrate of soda, hydrate of ammonia, and hydrate of potash on the ventricle of the frog's heart," *J. Physiol.* (1880–82), 3:195–202; Rudolph Matas, "Clinical report on intravenous saline infusion in the wards of the New Orleans Charity Hospital from June 1, 1888, to June 1891," *N. Orleans M. & S. J.* (1891), 14:1–32, 81–93. Matas used 0.7 percent saline solution intravenously in surgical emergencies. The effect, he observed, was often evanescent (pp. 31–32). Even though blood was transfused by vein, surgeons in the early 1920s rarely administered fluid other than under the skin.

74. J. Bottin, *Les causes de la mort au cours de l'occlusion intestinale haute expérimentale* (Louvain: Ceuterick, 1938), pp. 2–3; Amussat (n.52).

75. George H. Whipple, H. B. Stone, and B. M. Bernheim, "Intestinal obstruction . . . Study of a toxic substance produced by the mucosa of closed duodenal loops," *J. Exp. Med.* (1913), 17:307–23; John A. Hartwell and J. P. Hoguet, "Experimental intestinal obstruction in dogs with special reference to the cause of death and the treatment by large amounts of normal saline solution," *JAMA* (1912), 59:82–85; Russell L. Haden and Thomas G.

Orr, "Chemical changes in the blood of man after acute intestinal obstruction," *Surg. Gynec. Obstet.* (1923), 37:465–68; and three studies on chemical changes in the blood of the dog after intestinal obstruction in *J. Exp. Med.* (1923–24), 37:365–75; 38:55–71; 39:321–30; James L. Gamble and Monroe A. McIver, "A study of the effects of pyloric obstruction in rabbits," *J. Clin. Invest.* (1925), 1:531–45.

76. Louis Sperling and O. H. Wangensteen, "Transperitoneal absorption. VI. Significance of impaired viability and influence of distention on its occurrence," *Proc. Soc. Exp. Biol. Med.* (1935), 32:1385–89; Wangensteen and Charles E. Rea, "The distention factor in simple intestinal obstruction: An experimental study with exclusion of swallowed air by cervical esophagostomy," *Surgery* (1939), 5:327–39. Bernhard Breslau of Zürich (1866) related that he submitted the intestinal gas of a child who had lived eighteen hours to analysis. The chemist found it had the composition of atmospheric air. The presence of gas in the gastrointestinal tract, Breslau insisted, was proof that a child had lived after birth. (*Mschr. Geburtsch. Frauenkr.*, 28:11).

77. Horace G. Scott and O. H. Wangensteen, "Length of life following various types of strangulation obstruction in dogs," *Proc. Soc. Exp. Biol. Med.* (1932), 29:424–27; idem, "Blood losses in experimental intestinal strangulations and their relationship to degree of shock and death," ibid., pp. 748–51; John F. Perry, Jr., Stanley C. Von Drashek, and Wangensteen, "Studies in the recognition of strangulating intestinal obstructions with special reference to the value of pneumoperitoneography," *Surgery* (1956), 39:725–35.

78. C. Jeff Miller, "A study of three hundred forty-three surgical cases of intestinal obstruction," *Ann. Surg.* (1929), 89:91–107. High-pitched sounds with a metallic tinkling quality at the acme of the gas pain characterize early acute obstruction; gurgling, like that occasioned by the inrush of air when a partially filled bottle is inverted, denotes fluid accumulation and diminished absorption found in obstruction of several days' duration.

79. See F. T. van Beuren and Beverly C. Smith, *Arch. Surg.* (1927), 15:288–97; van Beuren, *Ann. Surg.* (1929), 90:387–93; John Scudder, R. L. Zwemer, and Allen O. Whipple, *Ann. Surg.* (1938), 107:161–97; Kocher, *Operative surgery* (n.56); Berkeley Moynihan, *Abdominal operations*, 4th ed. (Philadelphia: W. B. Saunders, 1926), 1:489; O. H. Wangensteen, *Intestinal obstructions*, 3d ed. (Springfield, Ill.: Charles C Thomas, 1955), pp. 270–71.

80. Astley Cooper's record concerns only patients operated upon. How many died without operation is not known.

81. Paul Nemir, Jr., "Intestinal obstruction: Ten-year statistical survey at the Hospital of the University of Pennsylvania," *Ann. Surg.* (1952), 135:367–75; Leonard D. Miller, Julius A. Mackie, and Jonathan E. Rhoads, "The pathophysiology and management of intestinal obstruction," *Surg. Clins N. Am.* (1962), 42(5):1304.

82. J. Parran Jarboe and Joseph H. Pratt, "Strangulated femoral hernia: Surgical management," *Surg. Gynec. Obstet.* (1947), 85:185–94; John Y. Brown, "Primary bowel resection versus artificial anus in the treatment of strangulated hernia," *Surg. Gynec. Obstet.* (1905), 1:364–65; Edward C. Saltzstein, William J. Marshall, and Robert J. Freeark, "Gangrenous intestinal obstruction," *Surg. Gynec. Obstet.* (1962), 114:695.

83. Clinical Research Committee of the Public Health Department of the London County Council, "Viability of strangulated bowel," *Br. M. J.* (1948), 1:43–46.

84. Claude Frankau, "Strangulated hernia: A review of 1487 cases," *Br. J. Surg.* (1931), 19:176–91; J. Englebert Dunphy, "The diagnosis and surgical management of strangulated femoral hernia," *JAMA* (1940), 114:394–96.

85. Clarence Dennis and Richard L. Varco, "Femoral hernia with gangrenous bowel," *Surgery* (1947), 22:312–23; Pipelet (n.35).

86. Leland S. McKittrick and S. Peter Sarris, "Acute mechanical obstruction of the small bowel; its diagnosis and treatment," *New Engl. J. Med.* (1940), 222:611–22; Charles L. Scudder, "Principles underlying treatment of acute intestinal obstruction; study of 121 cases . . . from Massachusetts General Hospital Clinic," *Trans. New Hamps. Med. Soc.* (1908), pp. 234–76; Edward P. Richardson, "Acute intestinal obstruction . . . second series of cases from Mas-

sachusetts General Hospital," *Boston M. & S. J.* (1920), 183:288; M. A. McIver, "Acute intestinal obstruction," *Arch. Surg.* (1932), 25:1099.

87. Arnold S. Leonard, Demetre M. Nicoloff, Ward O. Griffen, Jr., Harlan D. Root, Peter A. Salmon, and O. H. Wangensteen, "Intestinal decompression: Use of a long tube with a coiled spring for relief of distension," *Surgery* (1961), 49:440–49; Leonard, Nicoloff, Griffen, E. T. Peter, Wangensteen, "Long coiled-spring tube for operative intestinal decompression," *Am. J. Surg.* (1962), 104:427–32; Leonard and Wangensteen, "Operative intestinal decompression by means of a long coiled-spring intestinal tube," *Surgery* (1965), 57:491–94; Richard F. Edlich, Eugene Gedgaudas, Leonard, and Wangensteen, "New long intestinal tube for rapid nonoperative intubation," *Arch. Surg.* (1967), 95:443–50; F. W. Johnson, Robert L. Goodale, Leonard, R. L. Varco, "Rapid long tube intubation of the jejunum by a new endoscopic device," *Am. J. Surg.* (1976), 131:91–93.

88. J. H. Louw, "Resection and end-to-end anastomosis in the management of atresia and stenosis of the small bowel," *Surgery* (1967), 62:940–50.

89. Robert M. Zollinger and David L. Kinsey, "Diagnosis and management of intestinal obstruction," *Am. Surg.* (1964), 30:3; LaSalle D. Leffall, Jr., Joseph Quander, and Burke Syphax, "Strangulation intestinal obstruction: A clinical appraisal," *Arch. Surg.* (1965), 91:592–96.

90. J.-F. Malgaigne, "Examen des doctrines reçues jusqu'à ce jour sur l'étranglement des hernies," *Gaz. méd. Paris* (1840), 8:577–82, 609–15, 641–46.

91. James C. Ellis and Lester R. Dragstedt, "Liver autolysis in vivo," *Arch. Surg.* (1930), 20:8–16.

92. John Baptist Morgagni, *The seats and causes of diseases*, trans. Benjamin Alexander (London, 1769; facsimile edition, New York: Hafner, 1960), vol. 2, book 3, letter 35, article 5, pp. 167–68.

93. H. D. Root, Charles W. Hauser, C. Richard McKinley, James W. LaFave, and Ramon P. Mendiola, Jr., "Diagnostic peritoneal lavage," *Surgery* (1965), 57:633.

94. M. Ghanem, R. L. Goodale, P. Spanos, M. S. Tsung, and O. H. Wangensteen, "Value of leukocyte counts in the recognition of mesenteric infarction and strangulation of shorter intestinal lengths," *Surgery* (1970), 68:635–45; Conrad B. Jenson and Grafton A. Smith, "Clinical study of 51 cases of mesenteric infarction," *Surgery* (1956), 40:933; Egil Amundsen and B. E. Gustafsson, "Results of experimental intestinal strangulation obstruction in germfree rats," *J. Exp. Med.* (1963), 117:823–32; William O. Barnett, James C. Griffin, and James D. Hardy, "The efficacy of antibiotics combined with irrigation in experimental strangulated intestinal obstruction," *Surg. Gynec. Obstet.* (1958), 106:38–40; Isidore Cohn, Jr., *Strangulation obstruction* (Springfield, Ill.: Charles C Thomas, 1961); C. E. Yale and W. R. Culbertson, "Technique for the isolation and visualization of intestinal segments for study of closed loop strangulation," *J. Surg. Res.* (1963), 3:471–74.

95. John Parkinson, "Case of diseased appendix vermiformis," communicated by James Parkinson, *Med.-Chir. Trans.* (1812), 3:57–58; Adolph Volz, *Die durch Kothsteine bedingte Durchbohrung des Wurmfortsatzes* (Carlsruhe, 1846); Reginald H. Fitz, "Perforating inflammation of the vermiform appendix; with special reference to its early diagnosis and treatment," *Trans. Ass. Am. Physns* (1886), 1:107–44.

96. Ludwig Aschoff, *Der appendicitische Anfall, seine Aetiologie und Pathogenese* (Berlin: Springer, 1930), pp. 70, 109.

97. O. H. Wangensteen, "The genesis of appendicitis in the light of the functional behavior of the vermiform appendix," *Proc. Inst. Med. Chicago* (1939), 12:266–90; O. H. Wangensteen and Clarence Dennis, "Experimental proof of the obstructive origin of appendicitis in man," *Ann. Surg.* (1939), 110:629–47; and "Production of experimental acute appendicitis (with rupture) in higher apes by luminal obstruction," *Surg. Gynec. Obstet.* (1940), 70:799–806.

98. Claudius Amyand, "Of an inguinal rupture, with a pin in the appendix caeci, incrusted with stone," *Phil. Trans.* (1736), 39:329–42; F. F. Mestivier, "Observation sur une

tumeur située proche la région ombilicale, du côté droit, occasionée par une grosse epingle trouvée dans l'appendice vermiculaire du caecum," *J. de méd., chir., pharm.*, Paris (1759), 10:441–42.

99. Willard Parker, "An operation for abscess of the appendix vermiformis caeci," *Med. Record*, N. Y. (1867), 2:25–27.

100. Charles McBurney, "Experience with early operative interference in cases of disease of the vermiform appendix," *N. York M. J.* (1889), 50:676–84; Frederick Treves, "Some phases of inflammation of the appendix" [a lecture delivered on June 20, 1902, to the West London Medico-Chirurgical Society], *Br. M. J.* (1902), 1:1593–94; Treves developed an enormous private surgical practice and abandoned his hospital appointment at the London at age forty-five. At age fifty-five he withdrew completely from surgery to devote himself to travel. He died from peritonitis at age seventy-two in a Lausanne nursing home. Unfortunately a postmortem examination prior to cremation was not performed. Could incomplete cecal descent, a clinical entity identified by Treves, attended by appendical obstruction have accounted for the peritonitis that took his life? It has been suggested that the peritonitis was biliary in origin. But certainly rupture of the appendix is a far more frequent cause of peritonitis than is cholecystitis. Treves died December 7, 1923. Data relative to his final illness and death certificate were supplied by A. M. A. Moore, Honorary Consultant to the London Hospital, February 1, 1977.

101. Vital statistics of the United States for 1935, 1950, 1972, 1973, Government Printing Office, Washington, D.C.

102. Robert W. Toon and O. H. Wangensteen, "Effect of antibiotics on obstructive appendicitis in rabbits," *Proc. Soc. Exp. Biol. Med.* (1952), 80:578–80.

Further Readings

Barbee, Charles L., and Gilsdorf, Robert B. Diagnostic peritoneal lavage in evaluating acute abdominal pain. *Ann. Surg.* (1975), 181:853–56.

Boley, Scott J. *Vascular disorders of the intestine.* New York: Appleton-Century-Crofts, 1971.

Boley, Scott; Brandt, Lawrence; and Veith, Frank J. Ischemic disorders of the intestine. *Curr. Probl. Surg.* (1978), vol. 15, no. 4.

Braun, W., and Wortmann, W. *Der Darmverschluss und die sonstigen Wegstörungen des Darmes.* Berlin: Springer, 1924.

Friedenwald, Julius, and Morrison, Samuel. History of the development of the stomach tube with notes on the duodenal tube. *Bull. Hist. Med.* (1936), 4:425–54.

Frimann-Dahl, Johan. *Roentgen examinations in acute abdominal diseases.* Springfield, Ill.: Charles C Thomas, 1951.

Getzen, Lindsay C. Intestinal suturing. 2 pts. *Curr. Probl. Surg.* (August-September 1969).

Lawrence, William. *Treatise on ruptures.* 2d ed. London, 1810.

McIver, Monroe A. *Acute intestinal obstruction.* New York: Paul B. Hoeber, 1934.

Olivier, Claude. *Radio-diagnostic des occlusions intestinales aiguës.* Paris: Masson, 1955.

Paine, John R. History of the invention and development of the stomach and duodenal tubes. *Ann. Intern. Med.* (1934), 8:752–63.

Smith, Rodney. *Acute intestinal obstruction.* London: E. Arnold, 1948.

Wangensteen, O. H. Historical aspects of the management of acute intestinal obstruction. *Surgery* (1969), 65:363–83.

Welch, Claude E. *Intestinal obstruction.* Chicago: Year Book Publishers, 1958.

Wilms, Max. Der Ileus; Pathologie und Klinik des Darmverschlusses. *Dt. Chir.*, Stuttgart (1906), vol. 46.

Chapter 7. Gastric Surgery

Notes

1. See chapter 12.

2. Johann G. Schenck, *Observationum medicarum, rararum, novarum, admirabilium*

monstrosarum (Frankfurt, 1600), p. 622; Nolleson *le fils*, "Sur une plaie d'estomac, guérie par la suture de pelletier," *J. de méd., chir., pharm.* (1767), 27:595–98. Schenck's observations 121 and 122 showing "the possibility of healing gastric wounds" are mentioned in Rudolf Maier, *Johannes Schenck von Grafenberg, seine Zeit, sein Leben, seine Werke* (Freiburg, 1878), p. 124.

3. Oswald Croll, *Basilica chymica* (Frankfurt, 1609), pp. 64–65.

4. Daniel Becker, *Cultrivori prussiaci curatio singularis* (Leyden, 1640), pp. 19–20, 122; David Charles Schechter and Henry Swan, "A seventeenth century gastrotomy," *Surgery* (1962), 51:814–18.

5. Pierre Huard and Marie-José Imbault-Huart, "A propos de la taille gastrique pour corps étrangers au XIXème siècle," *Episteme* (1971), 5:45–50.

6. Benno Credé, "Gastrotomie wegen Fremdkörper," *Arch. klin. Chir.* (1886), 33:574–89.

7. Jacob Helm, *Zwey Krankengeschichten . . . nebst Untersuchung der Verdaulichkeit der Nahrungsmittel* (Vienna, 1803).

8. William Beaumont, *Experiments and observations on the gastric juice, and the physiology of digestion* (Plattsburgh, N.Y., 1833); Jesse S. Myer, *Life and letters of Dr. William Beaumont* (St. Louis: C. V. Mosby, 1939), pp. 212–14.

9. Johannes Müller and Theodor Schwann, "Versuche über die künstliche Verdauung des geronnenen Eiweisses," *Arch. f. Anat. Physiol. u. wissensch. Med.* (1836), pp. 66–89; Schwann, "Ueber das Wesen des Verdauungsprocesses," ibid., pp. 90–138.

10. Lester R. Dragstedt, "Acid ulcer," *Surg. Gynec. Obstet.* (1936), 62:118; Donald J. Ferguson, Enrique Sanchez-Palomera, Yoshio Sako, H. William Clatworthy, Robert W. Toon, and O. H. Wangensteen, "Studies on experimental esophagitis," *Surgery* (1950), 28:1022–39; Wangensteen, Harlan D. Root, Conrad B. Jenson, Kamil Imamoglu, and Peter A. Salmon, "Depression of gastric secretion and digestion by gastric hypothermia: Its clinical use in massive hematemesis," *Surgery* (1958), 44:265–74.

11. Otto Gruenewaldt, *Succi gastrici humani indoles physica et chemica, ope fistulae stomachalis indagata*, Dorpat dissertation, 1853; A. J. Carlson, "Contributions to the physiology of the stomach," *Am. J. Physiol.* (1912–15), vols. 31–38; Stewart G. Wolf and Harold G. Wolff, *Human gastric function, an experimental study of a man and his stomach* (New York: Oxford Univ. Press, 1943).

12. Pierre Flourens, "Expériences sur le mécanisme de la rumination," *Ann. d. sci. nat.*, Paris (1832), 27:34–57, 291–309.

13. Henri Braconnot, "Expériences chimiques sur le suc gastrique," *Ann. de chim. et phys.*, Paris (1835), 59:348–58; Nicolas Blondlot, *Traité analytique de la digestion considérée particulièrement dans l'homme et dans les animaux vertébrés* (Paris, 1843). In his introductory lecture to Harvard medical students (1861) entitled "Border lines in medical science," Oliver Wendell Holmes, anatomist and poet, said "the long-agitated question of the nature of the acid of the gastric juice is becoming settled in favor of the lactic." The quotation appears in *Medical essays, 1842–1882*, vol. 9, p. 237, of *Writings of Oliver Wendell Holmes* (Boston, 1892).

14. Wassili Bassow, "Voie artificielle dans l'éstomac des animaux," *Bull. Soc. imp. d. nat. de Moscou* (1843), 16:315–19; Heinrich Adolf Bardeleben, "Beiträge zur Lehre von der Verdauung," *Arch. f. physiol. Heilk.* (1849), 8:1–9; Christian A. Egeberg, "Om behandlingen af impenetrable Stricturer i Madröret (Oesophagus)," *Norsk Mag. Laegevidensk.* (1841), 2:97–106; Charles Sédillot, "Operation de gastro-stomie, pratiquée pour la première fois le 13 novembre 1849," *Gaz. méd. Strasbourg* (1849), vol. 9, cols. 366–78. The date usually listed for this operation (*Garrison-Morton* #3451) is 1846, but in the 1846 paper (*Compt. rend. Acad. d. sci.*, 23:222–27) Sédillot merely described "gastrotomie" as a feasible operation.

15. Aristide A. S. Verneuil, "Sur une opération de gastrostomie," *Bull. Acad. de méd.* (1876), 5:1016–17; Charles R. Richet, "Résumé des observations faites sur Marcelin R . . . atteint de fistule gastrique," *J. de l'anat. et physiol.* [*etc.*], Paris (1878), 14:326–33; K. G. Lennander, "Temporäre Gastrostomie bei Magen- oder Duodenalgeschwüren, besonders bei perforierten Geschwüren," *Dt. Z. Chir.* (1908), 92:297–311.

16. The first full-length biography of Billroth, by Karel B. Absolon, is in press (two volumes).

17. Carl Gussenbauer and Alexander Winiwarter, "Die partielle Magenresection: Eine experimentelle, operative Studie," *Arch. klin. Chir.* (1876), 19:347–80.

18. Jules Emile Péan, "De l'ablation des tumeurs de l'estomac par la gastrectomie," *Gaz. hôp.*, Paris (1879), 52:473–75; Ludwik Rydygier, "Wyciecie raka odźwiernika zoladkowego, smieré w 12 godzinach," *Przegl. lek.* (1880), 19:637–39; Theodor Billroth, "Offenes Schreiben an Herrn Dr. L. Wittelshöfer," *Wien. med. Wschr.* (1881), 31:161–65.

19. Herbert Ziegler, "Billroths erste Magenresektion," *Krebsarzt* (1949), 4:49–59; Hans Haberkant, "Ueber die bis jetzt erzielten unmittelbaren und weiteren Erfolge der verschiedenen Operationen am Magen," *Arch. klin. Chir.* (1896), 51:546.

20. Carl Schlatter, "Ueber Ernährung und Verdauung nach vollständiger Entfernung des Magens, Oesophagoenterostomie, beim Menschen," *Beitr. klin. Chir.* (1897), 19:757–76; Charles B. Brigham, "Case of removal of the entire stomach for carcinoma, successful esophago-duodenostomy, recovery," *Boston M. & S. J.* (1898), 138:415–19; J. Lynwood Herrington, Jr., "Remedial operations following gastric resection," in Henry N. Harkins and Lloyd M. Nyhus, eds., *Surgery of the stomach and duodenum*, 2d ed. (Boston: Little, Brown, 1969), p. 751.

21. Daniel Merrem, *Animadversiones quaedam chirurgicae experimentis in animalibus factis illustratae* (Giessen, 1810); John M. T. Finney, "The influence of John Hunter upon American surgery," *Lancet* (1927), 1:471; Owsei Temkin, "Merrem's youthful dream," *Bull. Hist. Med.* (1957), 31:29–43, and postscript, ibid. (1960), 34:74–75.

22. William H. Welch, "Cancer of the stomach," in William Pepper, *System of practical medicine by American authors* (Philadelphia, 1885), 2:575.

23. O. H. Wangensteen, "The problem of gastric cancer," *JAMA* (1947), 134:1161–69; Stanley R. Friesen, "The silent interval in gastric cancer," *J. Natl Cancer Inst.* (1949), 10:545–49; Walter B. Cannon, "The movements of the stomach studied by means of the Roentgen rays," *Am. J. Physiol.* (1898), 1:359–82.

24. David W. Gelfand, "The double-contrast upper gastrointestinal examination in the Japanese style," *Am. J. Gastroent.* (1975), 63:216–20; Masaru Kuru, ed., *Atlas of early carcinoma of the stomach* (Tokyo: Nakayama-Shoten, 1967); Hikoo-Skirakabe and associates, *Atlas of x-ray diagnosis of early gastric cancer* (Tokyo: Igaku Shoin, 1966); Komei Nakayama, *Atlas of gastrointestinal surgery* (Tokyo: Igaku Shoin, 1968); O. H. Wangensteen and Henry Sosin, "How can the outlook in alimentary tract cancer be improved?" *Am. J. Surg.* (1968), 115:6–16.

25. Benjamin Brodie, "Experiments and observations on the influence of the nerves of the eighth pair on the secretions of the stomach," *Phil. Trans.* (1814), 104:102–6; Friedrich H. Bidder and Carl Schmidt, *Die Verdauungssäfte und der Stoffwechsel* (Leipzig, 1852); Moritz Schiff, *Leçons sur la physiologie de la digestion* (Florence and Turin, 1867), 1:36.

26. Rudolf Heidenhain, "Ueber die Pepsinbildung in den Pylorusdrüsen," *Pflüg. Arch. ges. Physiol.* (1878), 18:169–71. Claude Bernard's important experiments on the pancreas (1849) would have benefited considerably had he been aware of the protection provided by the prophylactic antisepsis of Semmelweis.

27. Ivan P. Pavlov and E. Schumova-Simanovskaja, "Innervation der Magendrüsen beim Hunde," *Zentbl. Physiol.* (1889), 3:113–14; N. P. Jurgens, "Sur la sécrétion stomacale chez les chiens ayant subi la section sous-diaphragmatique des nerfs pneumogastriques," *Arch. d. sc. biol.*, St. Petersburg (1892), 1:323–49.

28. Karl Schwarz, "Ueber penetrierende Magen- und Jejunalgeschwüre," *Beitr. klin. Chir.* (1910), 67:111.

29. Eugen Bircher: "Die Resektion von Aesten der N. vagus zur Behandlung gastrischer Affektionen," *Schweiz. med. Wschr.* (1920), 50(1):519–28, and *Die Technik der Magen chirurgie auf Grund von 1500 Operationen* (Stuttgart: Enke, 1925).

30. André Latarjet, "Résection des nerfs de l'estomac. Technique opératoire. Résultats cliniques," *Bull. Acad. de méd.* (1922), 87:681–91; Latarjet and P. Wertheimer, "Quelques résultats de l'énervation gastrique," *Presse méd.* (1923), 2:993–95.

31. Lester R. Dragstedt and Frederick M. Owens, "Supra-diaphragmatic section of the vagus nerves in treatment of duodenal ulcer," *Proc. Soc. Exp. Biol. Med.* (1943), 53:152–54.

32. American Gastroenterological Association, Committee on Study of Vagotomy and Gastric Resection for Peptic Ulcer; Sara M. Jordan, chairman; Report; *Gastroenterol.* (1952), 22:297–499; A. V. Pollock, "Vagotomy in the treatment of peptic ulceration, review of 1524 cases," *Lancet* (1952), 2:795–800.

33. P. J. Lyndon, J. Greenall, R. B. Smith, John C. Goligher, and D. Johnston, "Serial insulin tests over a five-year period after highly selective vagotomy for duodenal ulcer," *Gastroenterol.* (1975), 69:1188–95.

34. Alton Ochsner, Paul R. Zehnder, and Shirley W. Trammell, "The surgical treatment of peptic ulcer — a critical analysis of results from subtotal gastrectomy and from vagotomy plus partial gastrectomy," *Surgery* (1970), 67:1017–28; Leslie Wise and Walter F. Ballinger, "The elective surgical treatment of chronic duodenal ulcer: A critical review," *Surgery* (1974), 76:811–26.

35. Max Madlener, "Über Pylorektomie bei pylorusfernem Magengeschwür," *Zentbl. Chir.* (1923), 50(2):1313–17.

36. Richard Lewisohn, "The frequency of gastrojejunal ulcers," *Surg. Gynec. Obstet.* (1925), 40:70–76; Berkeley G. A. Moynihan, "The prognosis of gastric and duodenal ulcer," *Br. M. J.* (1932), 1:1–3.

37. H. Schmilinsky, "Die Einleitung der gesamten Duodenalsäfte in den Magen (innere Apotheke)," *Zentbl. Chir.* (1918), 45:416–18.

38. Hans Haberer, "Meine Korrekturoperationen bei voraufgegangenen Eingriffen am Magen und Duodenum," *Arch. klin. Chir.* (1939), 196:304–22; Norman B. Ordahl, Frederick P. Ross, and Donald V. Baker, Jr., "The failure of partial gastrectomy with gastroduodenostomy in the treatment of duodenal ulcer." *Surgery* (1955), 38:158–68; J. C. Goligher, P. J. Moir, and J. H. Wrigley, "Billroth I and Polya operations for duodenal ulcer — a comparison," *Lancet* (1956), 1:220-22; Sten Wallensten, "Gastric resection for peptic ulcer; Billroth I versus Billroth II," *Surgery* (1957), 41:341–44. Haberer (1875–1958), a Viennese by birth, was professor of surgery at Innsbruck (1911–24) and subsequently at several German-speaking universities. His last assignment was Cologne.

39. D. H. Stern and J. H. Walsh, "Gastrin release in postoperative ulcer patients: Evidence for release of duodenal gastrin," *Gastroenterol.* (1973), 64:363–69.

40. W. G. Rhea, Jr., D. A. Killen, and H. W. Scott, Jr., "Long-term results of partial gastric resection without vagotomy in duodenal ulcer disease," *Surg. Gynec. Obstet.* (1965), 120:970–74.

41. J. Mikulicz, "Chirurgische Behandlung des chronischen Magengeschwürs," *Dt. Ges. Chir.* (1897), 26(2):31; Bernard Riedel, "Entfernung des mittleren Abschnittes vom Magen wegen Geschwür," *Dt. med. Wschr.* (1909), 35:17–21, 54–57; Erwin Payr, "Erfahrungen über Excision und Resection bei Magengeschwüren," *Arch. klin. Chir.* (1909), 90:989–1024; O. H. Wangensteen, "Segmental gastric resection for peptic ulcer; method permitting restoration of anatomic continuity," *JAMA* (1952), 149:18–23; O. H. Wangensteen, Henry Sosin, and Victor A. Gilbertsen, "Segmental resection in surgery of peptic ulcer with special reference to duodenal ulcer," pp. 529–39, in Harkins and Nyhus, *Surgery of stomach and duodenum* (n.20).

42. Tetsuo Maki and associates, "Pylorus-preserving gastrectomy as an improved operation for gastric ulcer," *Surgery* (1967), 61:838–45; Takeshi Sekine, Toshio Sato, Tetsuo Maki, and Tsuneo Shiratori, "Pylorus-preserving gastrectomy for gastric ulcer — one- to nine-year follow-up study," *Surgery* (1975), 77:92–99.

43. Hermann Kriege, "Ein Fall von einen frei in die Bauchhöhle perforirten Magengeschwür. Laparotomie. Naht der Perforationsstelle. Heilung," *Berl. klin. Wschr.* (1892), 29:1244–47, 1280–84; H. P. Dean, "A case of perforation of a chronic ulcer of the duodenum successfully treated by excision," *Br. M. J.* (1894), 1:1014–15.

44. Hans Haberer, "Zur Therapie akuter Geschwürsperforationen des Magens und

Duodenums in die freie Bauchhöhle," *Wien. klin. Wschr.* (1919), 32:415; Axel Odelberg, "Primary resection of the stomach in perforating gastric and duodenal ulcers," *Acta chir. scand.* (1927), 62 (suppl. 8:159–66); Serge Yudin, "A propos du traitement des ulcères perforés de l'estomac et du duodenum," *Bull. Soc. de Chir.* (1929), 55(2):1233–43; Yudin, "Étude sur les ulcères gastriques et duodénaux perforés," *J. int. chir.* (1939), 4:219–338.

45. Michael E. DeBakey, "Acute perforated gastroduodenal ulceration," *Surgery* (1940), 8:852–84, 1028–76; DeBakey and George L. Jordan, Jr., "Gastrectomy for perforated ulcer," pp. 834–35, in Harkins and Nyhus, *Surgery of stomach and duodenum* (n.20).

46. Not published until 1937. See George S. Bergh, Warner F. Bowers, and O. H. Wangensteen, "Perforation of the gastro-intestinal tract," *Surgery* (1937), 2:196–210.

47. O. H. Wangensteen, "Nonoperative treatment of localized perforations of the duodenum," *Minn. Med.* (1935), 18:477–80; Hermon Taylor, "Perforated peptic ulcer treated without operation," *Lancet* (1946), 2:441–44; Taylor, "The nonsurgical treatment of perforated peptic ulcer," *Gastroenterol.* (1957), 33:353–68; Sam F. Seeley and Donald Campbell, "Nonoperative treatment of perforated peptic ulcer," *Int. Abstr. Surg.* (1956), 102 (suppl.):435–46.

48. Anton Eiselsberg, "Über Ausschaltung inoperabler Pylorus-strikturen nebst Bemerkungen über die Jejunostomie," *Arch. klin. Chir.* (1895), 50:919–39; Hans Haberer, "Zur Radicaloperation des ulcus pepticum jejuni postoperativum," *Dt. Ges. Chir.* (1913), 42:68–95; Haberer, "Die Bedeutung des Pylorus für das Zustandekommen des Postoperative Jejunalulcus," *Arch. klin. Chir.* (1921), 117:50–67; Hans W. Smidt, "Über Magenresektionen und Magenchemismus," *Arch. klin. Chir.* (1924), 130:307–22; Eugen Enderlen and L. Zukschwerdt, "Erregung der Magensaftsekretion nach Resektion des Antrum," *Dt. Z. Chir.* (1931), 232:290–98; Lester R. Dragstedt and associates, "Experimental hyperfunction of gastric antrum with ulcer formation," *Ann. Surg.* (1951), 134:332–45.

49. W. Heneage Ogilvie, "Physiology and the surgeon," *Edinb. Med. J.* (1936), 43:61–83; Ogilvie, "The approach to gastric surgery," *Lancet* (1938), 2:295–99; R. Wilmanns, "Resectio praepylorica bei ulcus duodeni," *Zentbl. Chir.* (1926), 53:1874–75; William R. Waddell and Marshall K. Bartlett, "Antral exclusion with vagotomy for duodenal ulcer," *Ann. Surg.* (1957), 146:3–11; Lester R. Sauvage, Henry N. Harkins, and associates, "The relation between physiologic stimulatory mechanisms of gastric secretion and . . . peptic ulceration," *Surg. Gynec. Obstet.* (1953), 96:127–42; William D. Kelly, Frederick S. Cross, and O. H. Wangensteen, "The importance of the spatial relationship of the gastric antrum in the development of gastrojejunal ulcer in the dog," *Surg. Forum* (1953), 4:339–45.

50. Edward Mason, April 9, 1976, personal communication; Hugh Devine, "Treatment of peptic ulcer," *Med. J. Australia* (1937), 2:952–58.

51. Vital statistics of the United States for 1935, 1950, 1972, Government Printing Office, Washington, D.C.; Meredith P. Smith, "Decline in duodenal surgery," *JAMA* (1977), 237:987–88.

52. Robert M. Zollinger and Edwin H. Ellison, "Primary peptic ulcerations of the jejunum associated with islet cell tumors of the pancreas," *Ann. Surg.* (1955), 142:709–28; R. A. Strøm, "Case of peptic ulcer and insuloma," *Acta chir. scand.* (1952), 104:252–60; Frank Forty and Geoffrey M. Barrett, "Peptic ulceration of third part of the duodenum associated with islet-cell tumors of the pancreas," *Br. J. Surg.* (1952), 40:60–63; R. A. Gregory, "Gastric secretion," in Adam N. Smith, ed., *Symposium on the surgical physiology of the gastro-intestinal tract, Edinburgh, 1962* (Edinburgh: Morrison and Gibb, 1962), pp. 57–70; Gregory and Hilda J. Tracy, "Constitution and properties of two gastrins extracted from hog antral mucosa," *J. Physiol.*, London (1963), 169:18P–19P; Ellison and Stuart D. Wilson, "Zollinger-Ellison syndrome: Reappraisal and evaluation of 260 registered cases," *Ann. Surg.* (1964), 160:512–30. Everett J. Schmitz presented a good summary of the disorder in Harkins and Nyhus, *Surgery of stomach and duodenum* (n.20), pp. 315–29.

53. Stanley R. Friesen, "Effect of total gastrectomy on the Zollinger-Ellison tumor: Observations by second-look procedures," *Surgery* (1967), 62:609–13.

54. James C. Thompson, ed., *Gastrointestinal hormones, a symposium* (Austin and London: Univ. Texas Press, 1975).

55. A preliminary report by Ivan D. Baronofsky, David State, Stanley R. Friesen, Minnie Finn, and O. H. Wangensteen appeared in *Ann. Surg.* (1950), 131:31–43.

56. Conrad Rammstedt [Ramstedt], "Zur Operation der angeborenen Pylorusstenose," *Medsche Klin.* (1912), 8:1702–5; W. Weber, "Ueber eine technische Neuerung bei der Operation der Pylorus stenose des Säuglings," *Berl. klin. Wschr.* (1910), 47(1):763–65; Henri Dufour and Pierre Fredet, "La sténose hypertrophique du pylore . . . et son traitement chirurgicale," Rev. de chir. (1908), 37:208–53.

57. Edward J. Donovan, "Congenital hypertrophic pyloric stenosis in infancy," *JAMA* (1937), 109:558–60; Robert E. Gross, *Surgery of infancy and childhood* (Philadelphia: W. B. Saunders, 1953), p. 143.

58. J. Marion Sims, "Remarks on the treatment of gunshot wounds of the abdomen in relation to modern peritoneal surgery," *Br. M. J.* (1881), 2:925–26, 971–73; (1882), 1:184–86, 222–23, 260–62, 302–4.

59. D. W. Bliss, "Report of the case of President Garfield, accompanied with a detailed account of the autopsy," *Med. Record* (1881), 20:393–402; *Excerpts from opinions of distinguished medical men in this and other countries justifying the treatment of the late President Garfield* (Washington, D.C., 1882); Friedrich Esmarch, "Concerning the treatment of the wound of President Garfield, an address before the Physiological Society of Kiel, delivered February 2, 1882," trans. R. Stansbury Sutton, *Boston M. & S. J.* (1882), 107:234–37. Esmarch concluded that sepsis from the multiple probing of the president's wound with fingers, catheters, and instruments was the chief causative factor in his death, a thesis with which the authors are in complete agreement. The wound was potentially serious. The bullet shattered the body of the twelfth thoracic vertebra, but the spinal cord was spared; the left genitofemoral nerve was injured, accounting for the scrotal pain; the bullet came to lodge in juxtaposition to the splenic artery. Fatal hemorrhage occasioned by sepsis occurred eleven weeks later from the splenic artery. Professional fees submitted by the seven major consultants totaled $91,000, of which $27,500 was allowed, according to Joseph H. Miller, *Surg. Gynec. Obstet.* (1958), 107:116.

60. Charles T. Parkes, "Gun-shot wounds of the small intestines," *JAMA* (1884), 2:589–608.

61. George H. Makins, *Surgical experiences in South Africa, 1899–1900* (Philadelphia: Blakiston, 1901), pp. 446–86; Nicholas Senn, *Medico-surgical aspects of the Spanish American War* (Chicago: AMA Press, 1900), pp. 97–132.

62. "The case of President McKinley . . . report by . . . the medical staff attending the late President," *Am. Gynaec. Obstet. J.* (1901), 19:289–318; Nelson W. Wilson, "Details of President McKinley's case, narrated by the recorder at the operation," *Buffalo Med. J.* (1901), 41:207–25. Neither Garfield nor McKinley was hospitalized. Garfield was brought to the "family room" in the White House; on completion of McKinley's operation he was transferred to the home of John G. Milburn, with whom he had been staying. Nurses were constantly in attendance. Gaylord's findings at autopsy on McKinley of a 4.5 cm. necrotic area in the middle of the pancreas, from which *B. welchii* was isolated, seem to account adequately for the unhappy sequence of events.

63. P. Lockhart Mummery, "Injuries to the bowel from shell and bullet wounds," *Br. M. J.* (1914), 2:914–15. Eugen Enderlen and F. Sauerbruch, "Die Operative Behandlung der Darmschüsse im Krieg," *Medsche Klin.* (1915), 11:823–28.

64. Frederick F. Cartwright, *The development of modern surgery* (London: Arthur Barker, 1967), p. 109. Boris V. Petrovsky, July 17, 1978, personal communication. Petrovsky wrote that "Gedroyts" became chairman of surgery in the Kiev Medical School in 1929 and died in 1930 from cancer of the uterus. She was also a poet and author under the pen name "Sergey Gedroyts."

65. Gerald W. Shaftan, "Indications for operation in abdominal trauma," *Am. J. Surg.* (1960), 99:657–64.

Further Readings

Bernard, Claude. *Leçons de physiologie expérimentale appliquée à la médecine*. Vol. 2, pp. 260–67. Paris, 1855–56.

__________. *Leçons de pathologie expérimentale*. P. 456. Paris, 1872.

Eiseman, Ben, and Heyman, Robert L. Stress ulcers; a continuing challenge. *N. Engl. J. Med.* (1970), 282:372–74.

Friesen, Stanley R., and Wangensteen, O. H. Role of hemoconcentration in production of gastric and duodenal ulcer following experimental burns. *Proc. Soc. Exp. Biol. Med.* (1947), 64:81–85.

Kamegashira, Masaki; Goodale, R. L., Jr.; Borner, J. W.; Dhingra, Usha; and Wangensteen, O. H. Role of pepsin in species differences in erosive gastritis. *Arch. Surg.* (1977), 112:193–97.

Pavlov, Ivan P. *The work of the digestive glands.* Trans. W. H. Thompson. Pp. 177–83. London: Griffin, 1902.

Réaumur, R. A. F. de. Sur la digestion des oiseaux. *Mém. Acad. roy. d. sci.*, Paris (1752), 2:395–457; 3:701–52.

Samloff, I. Michael; Secrist, Donald M.; and Passaro, Edward. Effect of betazole on serum group I. pepsinogen levels: Studies in symptomatic patients. *Gastroenterol.* (1976), 70:1007–13.

Simonian, Simon J., and Curtis, Lon E. Treatment of hemorrhagic gastritis by antacid. *Ann. Surg.* (1976), 184:429–34.

Verneuil, Aristide S. [Discussion]. In Association française pour l'avancement des sciences, *Compte rendu de la 2me session, Lyon, 1873*, p. 817. Paris, 1874.

Wangensteen, O. H. *Cancer of the esophagus and the stomach.* 2d ed. New York: American Cancer Soc., 1956.

Welbourn, R. B. Current status of the Apudomas. *Ann. Surg.* (1977), 185:1–11.

Chapter 8. Tracheostomy and Respiratory Obstruction

Notes

1. James Craik and Elisha C. Dick [account of the death of George Washington], *Med. Reposit.*, New York (1800), 3:311–12; J. H. Mason Knox, Jr., "The medical history of George Washington, his physicians, friends and advisers," *Bull. Hist. Med.* (1933), 1:174–91. See also chapter 14 on phlebotomy.

2. A number of historical studies of tracheostomy have appeared within the past fifty years. Particularly useful is that of E. W. Goodall, "The story of tracheotomy," *Br. J. Child. Dis.* (1934), 31:167–76, 253–72. Goodall's survey was extended by F. J. Collet of Lyons in "Notes sur l'histoire de la trachéotomie," *Lyon méd.* (1936), 157:235–43, 263–71, and "Les premières trachéotomies," *Annals Otolar.* (1945), 12:365–70. See also R. Scott Stevenson and Douglas Guthrie, *History of oto-laryngology* (Edinburgh: Livingstone, 1949), and Thomas G. Nelson, *Tracheotomy: A clinical and experimental study* (Baltimore: Williams and Wilkins, 1958), pp. 1–13. Ottokar Chiari provides an excellent account in his *Chirurgie des Kehlkopfes und der Luftröhre* (Stuttgart: Enke, 1916). Earlier historical surveys are those of Bernhard Schuchardt, "Zur Geschichte der Tracheotomie bei Croup und Diphtherie, besonders in Deutschland," *Arch. klin. Chir.* (1887), 36:527–604; William Lawrence, "On some affections of the larynx which require . . . bronchotomy," *Med.-Chir. Trans.* (1815), 6:221–62; and Antoine Louis, "Sur la bronchotomie," *Mém. Acad. roy. chir.* (1784), 12:201–90.

3. The information on Asclepiades performing tracheostomy appears in the introduction to "Medicus," in Galen, *Opera omnia*, ed. C. G. Kühn (Leipzig, 1827), 14:734. Galen used the word "artery" to designate the windpipe; Hieronymus Fabricius ab Aquapendente (1617) was among the first to employ the term "trachea." Aretaeus of Cappadocia in Asia Minor (first

century) mentioned the use of tracheostomy to prevent suffocation in cases of quinsy, but he opposed the operation. He said that the wound increased the inflammation, thereby augmenting suffocation and cough, and that the cartilaginous wound would not heal. See Aretaeus, *Extant works*, ed. and trans. Francis Adams (London: Sydenham Soc., vol. 28, 1856), pp. 406–7.

4. Caelius Aurelianus, *On acute diseases and on chronic diseases*, ed. and trans. I. E. Drabkin (Chicago: Univ. Chicago Press, 1950), p. 323. Antyllus is quoted by Paul of Aegina in *The seven books of Paulus Aegineta*, trans. Francis Adams (London: Sydenham Soc., vol. 4:2, 1846), pp. 301–2.

5. Albucasis, *On surgery and instruments*, trans. and ed. M. S. Spink and G. L. Lewis (Berkeley: Univ. California Press, 1973), p. 338.

6. Antonio Musa Brasavola (1500–55) gave his account in comments to his 1546 edition of Hippocrates, "De ratione victus in morbis acutis," bk. 4, sect. 35, col. 2, p. 114.

7. Hieronymus Fabricius ab Aquapendente, *Opera chirurgica* (Frankfurt, 1620), pt. 1, chap. 44, pp. 155–66 (the first edition appeared in 1617); Julius Casserius, *De vocis auditusque organis historia anatomica* (Ferrara, 1601), bk. 1, chap. 20, pp. 119–21.

8. Nicolas Habicot, *Question chirurgicale par laquelle il est démontré que le chirurgien doit assurément pratiquer l'opération de la bronchotomie, vulgairement dicte laryngotomie* (Paris, 1620), pp. 73–86. One patient, suffocating from accumulation of blood in the larynx after twenty-two knife wounds, had been left for dead. He recovered when Habicot opened the trachea, perhaps the first recorded use of tracheostomy for removal of a foreign body, says Goodall (n.2), p. 225. The wound was kept open by a cannula. In another case a boy fearing robbery swallowed a package of coins, which lodged in his upper esophagus. Habicot opened the trachea to prevent suffocation and, using a leaden sound per orem, pushed the package into the stomach. The mass passed through the anus.

9. Including Brasavola's case and Habicot's four cases, Goodall (n. 2) could find only twenty-eight successful cases in the literature before Bretonneau's of 1825.

10. George Martin[e], "Postscript of a letter . . . giving an account of the operation of bronchotome," *Phil. Trans.* (1730), 36:448–55. Martine (1702–43) was a Scot, a graduate of Leyden. The minister had undoubtedly observed the problems in care of Martine's patient, a boy with "angina" of the throat. Coincidentally, a double tube was also suggested by another layman, a general in the artillery, who had watched his little girl's distress during frequent cleanings of a single tube after a tracheostomy performed by Trousseau in 1842. His idea was implemented by Trousseau. See Albert Sanné, *Traité de la diphthérie* (Paris, 1877), pp. 505–6.

11. Xavier Bichat, *Oeuvres chirurgicales ou exposé de la doctrine et de la practique de P. J. Desault* (Paris, 1801), 2:275.

12. Lawrence (n.2), pp. 249–50.

13. Nelson, *Tracheotomy* (n.2), p. 7; Lyman Richards and Frank Glenn, "The histopathologic reactions of the tracheotomic wound," *Archs Otolar.* (1932), 15:394.

14. Pierre Bretonneau, *Des inflammations spéciales du tissu muqueux, et en particulier de la diphthérite* (Paris, 1826). Included are two memoirs which Bretonneau presented to the Royal Academy of Medicine in Paris in 1821, describing the two unsuccessful tracheostomies (pp. 95–103, 220–22) and his experiments on dogs. *Garrison-Morton* (#5053) credits Bretonneau with the first successful tracheostomy for croup, probably an error. John Andree of London performed a "most happy" operation for "cynanche trachealis" on a boy of five in 1782; a silver cannula was inserted in the opening but was removed almost immediately because of violent coughing. The case is reported in Thomas White's 1786 Leyden thesis, *De cynanche tracheali* (pp. 25–27), in Giambattista Borsieri de Kanilfeld's *Institutionum medicinae practicae* (Leipzig, 1787), 3:404, and by J. R. Farre, *Med.-Chir. Trans.* (1812), 3:335–37, who adds a description of the operation supplied by Astley Cooper. Another early tracheostomy for croup was that of P. Hume, "Case of cynanche trachealis, for which tracheotomy was performed," *London M. Reposit.* (1824), 22:30–32. Andree's case was the subject of much controversy, said Trousseau in *Lectures on clinical medicine*, trans. John Rose Cormack (London: New Sydenham Soc., vol. 42:2, 1869), p. 594.

15. Bretonneau's unique personality and consuming absorption in his research and patients were affectionately portrayed in the orations of his distinguished pupils Velpeau and Trousseau at his funeral services in 1862 (*Union méd.*, Paris, 14:273–76, 289–92). Both spent some of their early years under his tutelage at Tours. Trousseau said that all his life he was treated by Bretonneau as his son. Velpeau said that Bretonneau and he performed thirty-six autopsies in a few months, thanks to their practice of scaling cemetery walls at 2:00 A.M. Bretonneau forgot engagements and rarely attended meetings. He had to be persuaded to announce his successes, and he did not bother to bill his patients; gifts were quickly given away. Through his former professor's unsolicited generosity, Velpeau was able to continue his studies in Paris.

16. Bretonneau, *De la diphthérite* (n.14), pp. 299–323. The date of the tracheostomy would be June 21, 1825, according to the tabulation in Bretonneau's case history; it is often listed as a July operation. In an earlier case Bretonneau improvised a quill as a tube until a rubber sound could be obtained; he later found a double tube superior (pp. 96, 326). Bretonneau reported that he had seen two horses with tin tracheostomy tubes to overcome their wheezing from the fumes in a red-lead manufacturing plant (p. 219).

17. Armand Trousseau, *Clinique médicale de l'Hôtel-Dieu de Paris* (Paris, 1865), 1:439–40.

18. The designation "tracheotomia" appears in a posthumous 1649 (MDCIL) Frankfurt publication, *Libri chirurgici XII* (p. 35), by Thomas Fienus (Feyens), professor of medicine at the University of Louvain. Napoleon's military surgeon Percy (1792) alluded to use of *trachéotomie* in his *Manuel du chirurgien-d'armée* (Paris, 1792), p. 119.

19. Antoine Louis (n.2), pp. 231–33. Louis credits the tale to Rodericus a Fonseca (1619). In a sequel (pp. 292–99) Louis tells of a seven-year-old girl who died when a bean became lodged in her trachea; the parents refused to let him do a tracheostomy. Louis related no instance in which he had performed tracheostomy.

20. Paul Brouardel, *La pendaison, la strangulation, la suffocation, la submersion* (Paris, 1897), pp. 36–55; Ezra Dyer, "Fracture of the crystalline lens in persons executed by hanging," *Trans. Am. Ophthal. Soc.* (1869), 1(6):72–75.

21. E. Schweninger of Munich observed that when the carotid arteries were tied after tracheostomies had been done in cats and rabbits, the animals survived hanging. *Aerztl. Int.-Bl.*, Munich (1876), 23:324–25. Body weight and the height of the drop may have been important factors.

22. Ernest W. White, "Resuscitation and recovery after apparent death by hanging," *Lancet* (1884), 2:401–2; Sir Clifford Naunton Morgan, "Surgery and surgeons in 18th century London," *Ann. R. Coll. Surg.* (1968), 42:7. Hanging was the most common method of suicide for men and women in Middlesex County, England, 1819–42, according to coroners' inquests reviewed by Thomas R. Forbes. Hanging accounted for 51 percent of the 469 male suicides and 36.4 percent of the 214 female suicides. *J. Hist. Med.* (1977), 32:390.

23. Armand Trousseau, "De la trachéotomie dans le cas de croup," *Dict. de méd.* (Paris, 1835), 9:382. Trousseau added that neither Velpeau, Paul-L.-B. Guersent, Sanson, nor Blandin had any survivors from tracheostomy. Alfred A. L. M. Velpeau, *New elements of operative surgery*, trans. P. S. Townsend (New York, 1851), 3:469.

24. Sanné, *La diphthérie* (n.10), pp. 464–70; Rudolf Krönlein, "Diphtheritis und Tracheotomie," *Arch. klin. Chir.* (1877), 21:287–92.

25. Ch. Hardy, "Recherches sur l'opération de la trachéotomie," *Bull. gén. de thérap.*, Paris (1858), 55:310–19, 345–53; W. E. Steavenson, "Some notes on tracheotomy," *St. Barth. Hosp. Rep.* (1882), 18:309–31. Steavenson presents a table of 57 patients subjected to tracheostomy with 14 recoveries (75.4 percent mortality). Of the 44 patients upon whom tracheostomy was performed for diphtheria, 36 died (81.8 percent mortality).

26. Theodor Billroth, *Clinical surgery . . . between the years 1860–1876*, trans. and ed. C. T. Dent (London: New Sydenham Soc., vol. 94, 1881), pp. 141–42. Of Billroth's 22 cases tracheostomy was performed in 13 for edema of the glottis from various causes; in 8, laryngotomy was done for great dyspnea caused by a goiter that compressed the trachea.

27. Charles M. Maingault's first presentation, "Quelques considérations sur la trachéotomie," and discussion following are reviewed in *Arch. gén. de méd.* (1832), 30:419. His address at the Académie des sciences on July 1, 1833, "De l'urgence de la trachéotomie dans le croup," is abstracted in *Rev. méd. franç. et étrang.*, Paris (1833), 51:141–42. Maingault, the author of several surgical texts, died in 1840. He opposed the common practice of instilling or insufflating astringents and caustics through the tracheostomy tube.

28. Whereas Emil Behring received the Nobel Prize in 1901 for clearing up the nature of diphtheria, several years intervened before a protective antiserum became generally available. In 1913 Behring described an effective toxin-antitoxin immunization; efficient initiation of such programs has eliminated this dreaded disease that continued to exact a heavy toll into the early decades of the twentieth century. *Dt. med. Wschr.* (1893), 19:543–47; (1894), 20:645–6; (1913), 39:873–76; (1914), 40:1139.

29. O. H. Wangensteen, "The surgeon's approach to the problem of alimentary tract malignancy," *J.-Lancet* (1950), 70:415. See also Thomas E. Starzl, William H. Meyer, and John J. Farrell, "Prophylactic tracheostomy in aged and poor risk general surgical patients," *JAMA* (1959), 169:691–95.

30. Stuart W. Arhelger, September 27, 1975, personal communication; Arhelger, "Study of the use of tracheotomy in the management of respiratory complications after extensive abdominal or thoracic surgery and development of a new tracheal tube," Master's thesis, University of Minnesota, 1951.

31. Nils G. Toremalm, "Postoperative care and complications after tracheotomy in infants and children," *Acta anaesth. scand.* (1960), 4:105–24; J. McK. Watts, "Tracheostomy in modern practice," *Br. J. Surg.* (1963), 50:954–75.

32. Peter Oliver, John R. Richardson, Robert W. Clubb, and Carlyle G. Flake, "Tracheotomy in children," *New Engl. J. Med.* (1962), 267:631–37.

33. Nelson, *Tracheotomy* (n.2), p. 67; R. M. A. McClelland, "Tracheostomy, a retrospective study of the value," *Anaesthesia* (1965), 20:88–89.

34. Chevalier Jackson, "Tracheotomy," *Trans. Am. Lar. Rhinol. Otol. Soc.* (1909), p. 337. Chevalier Jackson simultaneously filled five medical chairs in the five medical colleges of Philadelphia. See *The life of Chevalier Jackson, an autobiography* (New York: Macmillan, 1938), p. 207.

35. Friedrich Trendelenburg, "Beiträge zu den Operationen an den Luftwegen," *Arch. klin. Chir.* (1871), 12:112–33.

36. Victor R. VerMeulen and Herbert Birck, "Prolonged intubation vs. tracheotomy in children," *Archs Otolar.* (1968), 87:152–54; Blair Fearon, Robert E. MacDonald, Code Smith, and David Mitchell, "Airway problems in children following prolonged endotracheal intubation," *Ann. Otol. Rhinol. Lar.* (1966), 75:975–86.

37. Carl-Eric Lindholm, "Prolonged endotracheal intubation," *Acta anaesth. scand.* (1969), suppl. 33, pp. 16–25.

38. See discussion of surgical accountability in chapter 19.

39. Michael M. Paparella, November 20, 1974, personal communication.

40. W. J. Glover, "Artificial ventilation, tracheostomy and prolonged intubation in infancy," in Stanley A. Feldman and Brian E. Browley, eds., *Tracheostomy and artificial ventilation in the treatment of respiratory failure*, 2d ed. (Baltimore: Williams and Wilkins, 1972), p. 129.

41. Raphaël-B. Sabatier, *De la médecine opératoire,* 2d ed. (Paris, 1810), 3:51–52; Félix Vicq d'Azyr, "Laringotomie," *Hist. Soc. roy. de méd., 1776* (1779), 1(1):311.

42. Henry J. Heimlich, "A life-saving maneuver to prevent food-choking," *JAMA* (1975), 234:398–401. Such an emergency occurred at a black-tie dinner of surgeons in St. Paul many years ago before it was appreciated that a sudden thrust to the epigastrium could dislodge an aspirated piece of steak. At one of the tables a large middle-aged surgeon suddenly had what seemed to be a severe heart attack; fortunately, at that table a wise young surgeon had a pocketknife; he extended his dying colleague's head over his knee, opened the trachea and inserted his fountain pen into the tracheal opening to provide an airway. Meanwhile, the

meat, lodged in the larynx, was ejected. The evening's program continued as though nothing unusual had happened, but many present that evening have carried pocketknives ever since.

43. Horace Green, *On the surgical treatment of polypi of the larynx, and oedema of the glottis* (New York, 1852), pp. 14–27, 62–69.

44. Manuel Garcia, "Observations on the human voice," *Proc. R. Soc.*, London (1854–55), 7:399–410; Stevenson and Guthrie, *History of oto-laryngology* (n.2), pp. 98–103.

45. Carl Gussenbauer, "Ueber die erste durch Th. Billroth am Menschen ausgeführte Kehlkopf-Exstirpation," *Arch. klin. Chir.* (1874), 17:343–56 (a harrowing account); Fritz Salzer, "Larynxoperationen in der Klinik Billroth, 1870–1884," *Arch. klin. Chir.* (1885), 31:848–88.

46. Gurdon Buck, "On the surgical treatment of morbid growths within the larynx," *Trans. AMA* (1853), 6:509–35. The operation was done with the patient in a sitting position and apparently without anesthesia. Afterward she was fitted with a tracheal cannula with an orifice making it possible for her to converse, which gave her much pleasure. Three months later when breathing again became difficult, a more aggressive operation was done; the section was extended to the hyoid bone. Halsted was listed among the witnesses of this operation. After a third attempt to remove all the tumor, the patient's condition rapidly deteriorated.

47. Bernhard Fränkel, "Erste Heilung eines Larynx-Cancroids vermittelst Ausrottung per vias naturales," *Arch. klin. Chir.* (1887), 34:281–86. At the conclusion Fränkel tells of an instance in which Bergmann did a laryngofissure for him on another patient with cancer of the larynx, with a completely satisfactory result. Actually, it was more than a laryngofissure; it was a partial laryngectomy.

48. The following sources cover the story of Frederick III's illness and the ensuing controversy over its management: Felix Semon, "Die Krankheit Kaiser Friedrich des Dritten und die Laryngologie," *Internat. Centralbl. Laryngol. Rhinol.* (1888), 5:49–55, 243–304; *La maladie de l'Empereur Fréderic III, rapports officiels des médecins allemands*, trans. Luc (Paris, 1888); "Medical protocol concerning the result of the examination of the body of . . . Frederick the Third," *Br. M. J.* (1888), 2:141; Morell Mackenzie, *The fatal illness of Frederick the Noble* (London, 1888); "The case of the late Emperor Frederick," *Br. M. J.* (1888), 2:836–41; "Obituary, Sir Morell Mackenzie," *Br. M. J.* (1892), 1:362–63; Arend Buchholtz, *Ernst von Bergmann* (Leipzig: Vogel, 1911), pp. 460–504; R. Scott Stevenson, *Morell Mackenzie: The story of a Victorian tragedy* (London: Heinemann, 1946); Terence Cawthorne, "Two historical tracheostomies," *Proc. R. Soc. Med.* (1968), 61:1169–76.

49. The crown princess, a confirmed Liberal, was unalterably opposed to Bismarck's political views. When this surgeon attended lectures in Freiburg forty years later (1928), he heard Erich Lexer review the whole story in a lecture on cancer of the larynx.

50. In September 1887 Queen Victoria conferred a knighthood upon Mackenzie. When Prince Frederick acceded to the throne on his father's death, he promptly conferred upon Mackenzie the Grand Cross and Star of the Royal Order of Hohenzollern. See Mackenzie's obituary, *Br. M. J.* (1892), 31:362–63. Mackenzie obviously had qualities that endeared him to his royal patient, despite his misdirected management of the situation. Had the operation proposed by Bergmann been carried out, the history of the first quarter of the twentieth century might have been different. Frederick III was loved and trusted by the German people. When he succumbed to cancer of the larynx, his impulsive and militarily aggressive son, Wilhelm II, became emperor at age twenty-nine.

51. Basil C. Morson and I. M. P. Dawson, *Gastrointestinal pathology* (Oxford: Blackwell Scientific Publications, 1972), pp. 522–29; Victor A. Gilbertsen, Genell L. Knatterud, Paul H. Lober, and O. H. Wangensteen, "Invasive carcinoma of the large intestine: A preventable disease?" *Surgery* (1965), 57:363–65. Years of experience with the fate of adenomatous polyps of the rectum in the senior author's clinic have suggested that many cancers of the colon and rectum are probably preventable if adenomatous polyps are excised or fulgurated, a point of view currently gaining acceptance.

52. Fritz De Quervain of Bern, Switzerland, loved to tell his students (1927) about one of his patients, a farmer's wife with a large goiter. Her operation was so long delayed that a permanent tracheostomy had to be made to maintain an adequate airway. In the hospital she wore a tube without an aperture admitting air to the larynx; on dismissal she was given a tube with an aperture on the upper convex border enabling her to speak. A week later her husband brought her back demanding that the former tube be reinserted.

53. "Passages from the notebooks of Sir Frederick Treves, Bt.," *Ann. R. Coll. Surg.* (1961), 28:384–88; Cawthorne (n.48), pp. 1173–76. Hearing of Millais's plight, Queen Victoria sent Princess Louise to inquire whether there was anything she could do to help. Millais replied, "Yes, let her receive my wife," and Victoria obliged, despite the scandal involving Effie, Millais's wife. Effie was married to Ruskin in 1848 but had left him after six years of marriage during which Ruskin made no effort to consummate the union. According to Mary Lutyens in *Millais and the Ruskins* (London: John Murray, 1967), Ruskin suffered a traumatic shock on his wedding night when he discovered that Effie had pubic hair (pp. 156, 196). It is a reasonable inference that he was impotent. Edmund Berger wrote in the psychoanalytic journal *Am. Imago* (1948), 5:182–201, that the judge (1854) declared the marriage null and void because of Ruskin's "incurable impotency." Effie married Millais a year later, by whom she had eight children; he survived the tracheostomy only briefly.

54. Rudolf Link and Wolfgang Pascher, "Klinische Gesichtspunkte zum Stimmbandkarzinom," pp. 92–103, in Josef Becker and Friedrich Gauwerky, eds., *Tumoren der Mundhöhle, des Rachens und des Kehlkopfes, interdisziplinäre Diskussionen Deutscher Röntgenkongress, 1968* (Munich: Urban and Schwarzenberg, 1969). Th. Gluck and J. Soerensen (1920) gave the results of a series of 100 total extirpations of the larynx. The first 75 operations were done without mortality. Two patients died among the last 25, both corpulent men between sixty and seventy with emphysema and shortness of breath; they died of heart failure. *Arch. f. Lar. u. Rhinol.* 33:84–102.

55. Chevalier L. Jackson and Charles M. Norris, *Cancer of the larynx* ([New York]: American Cancer Soc., 1963), p. 37. Chevalier L. Jackson is the son of Chevalier Jackson, who is mentioned earlier in this chapter.

Further Readings

Arhelger, Stuart W. Advantages of tracheostomy and use of a new tracheal tube in the management of intratracheal aspiration. *Surgery* (1951), 29:260–66.

Behring, Emil. *Die Geschichte der Diphtherie, mit besonderer Berücksichtigung der Immunitätslehre.* Leipzig, 1893.

Chauveau, C. *Histoire des maladies du pharynx.* 2 vols. Paris: Baillière, 1901.

Löffler, Friedrich. Untersuchungen über die Bedeutung der Mikroorganismen für die Entstehung der Diphtherie beim Menschen, bei der Taube und beim Kalbe. *Mitt. k. Gesundh. Amte.* (1884), 2:421–99.

O'Dwyer, Joseph P. Intubation of the larnyx. *N. York M. J.* (1885), 42:145–47.

Roux, Pierre Paul Emile, and Yersin, Alexandre Emil Jean. Contribution à l'étude de la diphthérie. *Ann. de l'Inst. Pasteur* (1888), 2:629–61; (1889), 3:273–88; (1890), 4:385–426.

Semon, Felix. *The autobiography of Sir Felix Semon.* Ed. Henry C. Semon and Thomas A. McIntyre. Pp. 146–70. London: Jarrolds, 1926.

Stevenson, R. Scott, and Guthrie, Douglas. *A history of oto-laryngology.* Edinburgh: E. and S. Livingstone, 1949.

Virgili, Pedro. Sur une bronchotomie faite avec succès. *Mém. Acad. roy. chir.* (1743), 1:581–83.

Chapter 9. Empyema

Notes

1. Dupuytren (1777–1835) had an occurrence of slight facial paralysis while lecturing, November 15, 1833. After a vacation in Italy he tried to resume his duties at the Hôtel-Dieu in the spring of 1834, but he could not continue long beyond his opening lecture. Following an attack of pleurisy Dupuytren's condition progressively worsened over the next six months; empyema developed. He died on February 8, 1835. See Jules Rochard, *Histoire de la chirurgie française au XIXe siècle* (Paris, 1875), p. 161; Henri Mondor, *Anatomistes et chirurgiens* (Paris: Editions Fragrance, 1949), pp. 314–17. During a session of the Royal Academy of Medicine in 1836, H. M. Husson of the Hôtel-Dieu quoted Dupuytren's rejection of the operation. Husson had been one of Dupuytren's physicians in his final illness. Sanson also gave his version of the incident, saying that he went to get his instruments for the operation. When he returned Dupuytren "was no more." See *Arch. gén. de méd.* (1836), 12:252, and *Bull. Acad. roy. de méd.* (1836), 1:64–65.

2. James R. Church, "Medicine in the time of Louis XIV of France," *Milit. Surg.* (1920), 47:707.

3. The discussions arose from a report by Sanson and J. B. Bouillaud on a paper by R. Faure of Strasbourg who had urged early puncture when other measures failed to clear thoracic collections. The discussions are abstracted in *Bull. Acad. roy. de méd.* (1836), 1:62–67, 103–4, 120–26, 138–48, 159–60, 164–69, 180–91, and in *Arch. gén. de méd.* (1836), 12:252–54, 356–63, 491–98.

4. Charles E. Sédillot, *De l'opération de l'empyèma,* Paris, 1841. The thesis was 141 pages in length. The *concours* competition was for a chair of operative surgery in the Faculty of Medicine. A *concours* in Paris faculties and hospitals until quite recently was the accepted method of advancement. Sédillot (1804–83) was appointed professor of surgery at Strasbourg in 1841. He was director of the school of military medicine there from 1860 to 1868. At a meeting of the French Academy of Medicine in 1872 he once again urged return to the Hippocratic traditions of treatment of empyema. See Léon Bouveret, *Traité de l'empyème* (Paris, 1888), pp. 127–28.

5. *Oeuvres complètes d'Hippocrate; traduction nouvelle avec le texte grec en regard,* trans. Émile Littré (Paris, 1851), 7:71; Guido Majno, *The healing hand* (Cambridge: Harvard Univ. Press, 1975), pp. 156–58; C. D. O'Malley, *Andreas Vesalius of Brussels, 1514–1564,* (Berkeley: Univ. California Press, 1964), p. 230.

6. Armand Trousseau, "De la paracentèse du thorax dans certains cas de pleurésie aiguë," *J. de méd.*, Paris (1843), 1:321–30; Trousseau, "Deux nouveaux cas de paracentèse du thorax," ibid. (1844), 2:225–32; Henry I. Bowditch, *Thoracentesis, and its general results during twenty years of professional life* (New York, 1870), p. 4; H. M. Hughes and Edward Cock, "Paracentesis thoracis; with cases," *Guy's Hosp. Rep.* (1844), 2:48–104, 355–66. In commenting upon the method of Hughes and Cock more than thirty years later, James F. Goodhart stated that unless a better method were found the mortality of empyema would continue high. Among 77 cases treated by various methods, including external drainage, since 1866 at Guy's and Evelina hospitals, Goodhart observed a mortality of 44.1 percent. *Guy's Hosp. Rep.* (1877), 22:179–257.

7. Georges Dieulafoy, *De l'aspiration pneumatique sous-cutanée* (Paris, 1870). A subcutaneous aspirator was presented to the Imperial Academy of Medicine collections in the name of Dieulafoy of Paris on November 2, 1869, according to a note in the Academy's *Bulletin,* 34:1016.

8. F. Cresswell Hewett, "Thoracenteses: The plan of continuous aspiration," *Br. M. J.* (1876), 1:317; Pierre K. E. Potain, "Pleurésie purulente, ponction ou [sic] empyème," *Gaz. hôp.*, Paris (1886), 59:281–82; G. Bülau, "Für die Heber-Drainage bei Behandlung des Empyems," *Zt. klin. Med.* (1891), 18:31–45. Potain (1825–1901), a distinguished professor of

medicine at the University of Paris, had an enormous consulting practice but wrote little. Obituaries of Potain appear in *Dt. med. Wschr.* (1901), 27:63, and *Br. M. J.* (1901), 1:121.

9. Henry I. Bowditch, "On pleuritic effusions, and the necessity of paracentesis for their removal," *Am. J. Med. Sci.* (1852), 23:320–50; Bowditch, *Thoracentesis* (n.6). Bowditch was professor of clinical medicine at Harvard (1859–68). For the obituary of Morrill Wyman (1812–1903), see *Boston M. & S. J.* (1903), 148:164–65.

10. William Osler, "A clinical lecture on empyema and its antiseptic treatment," *Med. News*, Philadelphia (1882), 41:113–15.

11. Rickman J. Godlee, "Surgical treatment of empyema," *Lancet* (1886), 1:51–54, 95–97, 143–54, 189–91.

12. Ernst Küster, "Ueber die Grundsätze der Behandlung von Eiterungen in starrwandigen Höhlen, mit besonderer Berücksichtigung des Empyems der Pleura," *Dt. med. Wschr.* (1889), 15:185–87, 213–15, 233–36, 254–57. Küster advocated rib resection. The presentations by Karl F. H. Immermann (pp. 19–40) and Max Schede (pp. 41–100) and the ensuing discussions on "Die Behandlung der Empyeme," April 15–18, 1890, appear in *Verh. d. Cong. f. innere Med.*, 9th Congress (1890), 9:19–141.

13. *Garrison-Morton* (1970, #3171) erroneously credited Jacob A. Estlander (1879) with originating the operation to ensure collapse of empyema cavities in "Resektion af refben vid kroniskt empyem," *Nord. med. Ark.*, vol. 11, no. 21, pp. 1–4, also *Rev. mens. méd., chir.*, Paris, 3:157–70, 885–88. Schede (n.12), who did devise the operation, is not mentioned.

14. Emanuel A. Aufrecht, "Die Heilung des Empyems," *Dt. Arch. klin. Med.* (1894), 52:1–20. Iodine injections employed in France in the mid-nineteenth century are discussed in detail by one of the innovators, F.-A. Aran, a Paris physician, in *Union méd.*, Paris (1853), 7:385–86 et seq.

15. Ordinary pleural exudate does not have a foul odor.

16. William F. Whitney (1875) analyzed a group of patients treated for empyema at Massachusetts General Hospital. Patients drained surgically did the best, but the mortality was high, around 50 percent for adults, lower in children. In several instances, because of deferred treatment, external drainage occurred spontaneously. There was hazard too from anesthesia. Local anesthesia was not yet available, which compounded the problem. *Boston M. & S. J.*, 93:153–58.

17. Evarts A. Graham and Richard D. Bell, "Open pneumothorax: Its relation to the treatment of empyema," *Am. J. Med. Sci.* (1918), 156:839–71; "Empyema in base hospitals," unsigned editorial, *Am. J. Med. Sci.* (1918), 156:899–900, summary of a report in *Review of war surgery and medicine* (Washington, D.C., 1918), 1:1. For an account of Dakin's solution, see chapter 24 on the surgery of war.

18. George J. Heuer, "Acute empyema," *J. Thorac. Surg.* (1932), 1:461–84; Alexander Fleming, "The action of chemical and physiological antiseptics in a septic wound," *Br. J. Surg.* (1919), 7:99–129; Joseph A. Danna, "Treatment of empyema by aspiration and air replacement without drainage," *JAMA* (1931), 96:1453–56.

19. Osler himself had empyema following pneumonia, and it has been said that intercostal hemorrhage from a wound of a subcostal blood vessel was an unfortunate complication. In his *Life of Sir William Osler* (Oxford: Clarendon Press, 1925), 2:684, Harvey Cushing wrote, "The end came at 4:30 on the afternoon of December 29th, after a haemorrhage from his [chest] wound." Every surgeon of experience knows, however, that an intercostal tap should be directly over the superior margin of the rib, as far away from the subcostal vessels of the rib as possible, thereby precluding injury to the subcostal blood vessels.

20. O. H. Wangensteen, "Observations on the treatment of empyema with special reference to drainage and expansion of the lung," *J. Thorac. Surg.* (1935), 4:399–413.

21. Edmond Delorme, "Nouveau traitement des empyèmes chroniques," *Gaz. hôp.*, Paris (1894), 67:94–96; Alex. Hugh Ferguson, "Thoracoplasty in America and visceral pleurectomy, with report of a case," *JAMA* (1897), 28:56–62; George R. Fowler, "A case of thoracoplasty for the removal of a large cicatricial fibrous growth from the interior of the chest, the result of an

old empyema," *Med. Record* (1893), 44:838–39; Paul Reclus, "Traitement des pleurésies purulentes: Extirpation des néo-membranes enserrant le poumon," *Presse méd.*, March 31, 1894, pp. 97–98.

22. O. H. Wangensteen, discussion, *J. Thorac. Surg.* (1932), 2:180.

23. Carl Eggers, "Radical operation for chronic empyema," *Ann. Surg.* (1923), 77:327–53.

24. O. H. Wangensteen, "The pedicled muscle flap in the closure of persistent bronchopleural fistula with employment of the intercostal muscle bundles by a process of ribboning in the obliteration of large chronic empyema cavities," *J. Thorac. Surg.* (1935), 5:27–53.

25. Pierre Duval, *War wounds of the lung: Notes on their surgical treatment at the Front*, English translation (Bristol: Wright, 1918), pp. 3–4; Duval, "Gunshot wounds of the lung and their treatment at the Front," *Surg. Gynec. Obstet.* (1919), 28:1–4. The sucking of thoracic wounds by means of a tin or silver syringe is described in a little book, *L'art de succer les plaies*, published in Amsterdam in 1707. The author, Dominique Anel, says that in sword cuts of the lung when the surface of the lung is not adherent to the parietal pleura the application of suction can expand the lung, bringing healing sometimes "in less than two days." The sucking of wounds was apparently an occasional ancient form of therapy — in fact, there were professional wound suckers. Anel's syringe was to provide protection from infection caused by mouth sucking.

26. Ferdinand Sauerbruch, "Die Behandlung der Brustfelleiterung," *Arch. klin. Chir.* (1929), 157:237. Sauerbruch made this statement at the German Surgical Congress of 1929.

Further Readings

Gooch, George P. *Maria Theresa, and other studies.* New York: Longmans, Green, 1951.

Keller, William L. Treatment of chronic empyema where the recognized surgical procedures have failed to produce obliteration. *Ann. Surg.* (1922), 76:549–80.

Kirschner, Martin. Zur Radicalbehandlung des chronischen Pleuraempyems. *Arch. klin. Chir.* (1921), 117:205–31.

Mayo, Charles, and Beckman, E. H. Visceral pleurectomy for chronic empyema. *Boston M. & S. J.* (1914), 171:424–26.

Meade, Richard H. Empyema. In *History of thoracic surgery*, pp. 234–56. Springfield, Ill.: Charles C Thomas, 1961.

Tuffier, Théodore. Treatment of chronic empyema. *Ann. Surg.* (1920), 72:266–87.

Chapter 10. Cesarean Section

Notes

1. Friedrich B. Osiander, *Handbuch der Entbindungskunst*, 2d ed. (Tübingen, 1830), 2:450; J. H. Young, *Caesarean section, the history and development of the operation from earliest times* (London: H. K. Lewis, 1944), p. 2. Aurelia was alive when Caesar invaded Britain. A plausible explanation of the term "cesarean section" is that it was so named "because the Roman or Caesarean law demanded that when a pregnant woman died, her body should not be buried until the child had been removed." Douglas Guthrie, *Janus in the doorway* (London: Pitman, 1963), p. 82.

2. Several of these quaint and often beautiful pictures of Caesar's birth, by Arabian and Ethiopian as well as European artists, are reproduced in J. Paul Pundel, *Histoire de l'opération césarienne* (Brussels: Presses académiques européenes, 1969). The traditional stork is occasionally included as a spectator.

3. Guy de Chauliac, *La grande chirurgie de Guy de Chauliac, composée en l'an 1363*, ed. Édouard Nicaise (Paris, 1890), pp. 549–50.

4. How like Shakespeare's Macduff (*Macbeth*, act 5, scene 8, printed 1623 but probably finished by 1606). The quotation appeared also in *Holinshed's chronicle*, Macduff saying he "was

never borne of my mother, but ripped out of her wombe." Josephine Nicoll and Allardyce Nicoll, *Holinshed's chronicle as used in Shakespeare's plays* (London: J. M. Dent, 1927), p. 223.

5. Jacques Guillemeau, *Child-birth or, the happy deliverie of women* (London, 1612; facsimile, New York: Da Capo Press, 1972), pp. 185–88. The original French edition appeared in 1609. Théophile Raynaud (1583–1663), a French Jesuit priest, is sometimes given credit for initiating (1637) the term "cesarean section" as opposed to "cesarean birth" or other appellation. However, Guillemeau's translator used the words "cesarean section" in 1612. Raynaud maintained that the term "cesarean birth" was incorrect because a child so delivered was not, strictly speaking, born. He was writing primarily of the morality of performing cesarean section on dead mothers, but he did allow that, as a last resort, the operation could be done on living women who could not be delivered otherwise. *De ortu infantium contra naturam, per sectionem Caesaream* (Lyons, 1637), pp. 5, 45.

6. Guy and Guillemeau endorsed these old precautions, Guy's excuse being that it was what the women wanted. Guillemeau admitted that the child did not breathe in the womb, but apparently he hated to revoke a time-honored custom. Paré's discussion of cesarean section and extraction of a dead child appears in his *Workes*, trans. Thomas Johnson (London, 1634), pp. 914–17, 923.

7. Edward L. Duer, "Post-mortem delivery," *Am. J. Obst.* (1879), 12:1–22; John V. Kelly and Hebert G. Winston, "Successful postmortem cesarean section," *Am. J. Obstet. Gynec.* (1956), 72(1):203–7. For a sampling of the miraculous in obstetrical history, see Johann H. Finn's 1839 inaugural thesis, University of Würzburg, *Der Kaiserschnitt nach seiner geschichtlichen Entwicklung aus den Quellen dargestellt*, pp. 9–18. Extraction of living babies from dead mothers, says Finn, was well known in Egypt, Greece, and Rome 715 years before Christ. Attendants who failed to observe this practice were looked upon as murderers.

8. François Rousset, *Traitte nouveau de l'hysterotomotokie ou enfantement caesarien* (Paris, 1581), called one of the finest books of the sixteenth century by J.-F. Malgaigne in his edition of Paré's *Oeuvres* (1840), 2:718. Kenneth L. Pickerell pointed out that Paré could not have entirely opposed cesarean operations, for Paré signed his approval to the first edition of Rousset's book. See Pickerell, "Inquiry into the history of cesarean section," *Bull. Soc. Med. Hist.*, Chicago (1935), 4:419–20. Rousset's account of suprapubic lithotomy is mentioned in chapter 4.

9. The case of the woman with six cesarean sections was not reported by an eyewitness. According to the account, she succumbed during her seventh pregnancy, unable to be delivered because her surgeon, Guillet, a barber of Milly, had died. Two hundred years later, in a defense of cesarean section, J.-L. Baudelocque censured Paré and Guillemeau for not determining the accuracy or otherwise of Rousset's accounts. Young, *Caesarean section* (n.1), p. 67.

10. François Rousset, *Foetus vivi ex matre viva sine alterutrius vite periculo*, trans. (to Latin) Caspar Bauhin (Basel, 1591). Bauhin (1560–1624) was a professor of anatomy, botany, medicine, and Greek at Basel, later the city physician and the rector of the university.

11. Probably through-and-through sutures were used to close the abdominal wall.

12. Skeptics include the German obstetrician Caspar Siebold, *Versuch einer Geschichte der Geburtshülfe* (Berlin, 1845), 2:97; Pickerell (n.8), pp. 416–18; and Franklin S. Newell, *Caesarean section* (New York: Appleton, 1921), p. 4. Fielding H. Garrison credits the story in *Introduction to the history of medicine*, 4th ed. (Philadelphia: W. B. Saunders, 1929), p. 228, as does Piero Gall, "L'operazione di Giacome Nuffer," *Rass. clin.-scient.*, Milan (1935), 13:365–66.

13. Walter Oswald, "Bericht aus dem Jahre 1411 über eine Hebamme, die angeblich 7 Kaiserschnitte mit gutem Erfolg für Mutter und Kind ausgeführt hat," *Arch. Gesch. Med.* (1933), 26:340–43.

14. Robert W. Felkin, "Notes on labour in Central Africa," *Edinb. M. J.* (1884), 29 (2):922–30. Felkin was allowed to intervene before the knife was used in another case and delivered the parturient without difficulty.

15. Walter C. Plowden (British Consul to Abyssinia), *Travels in Abyssinia and the Galla*

Country, ed. Trevor C. Plowden (London, 1868), p. 115. According to Plowden, the Gallas are Muhammadans who conquered parts of Abyssinia (p. 2).

16. Daniel Sennert, *Institutionum medicinae libri V* (Wittenberg, 1611), pp. 160–62. In the 1619 Paris edition Sennert reports the child's death (p. 161).

17. Geronimo Scipione Mercurio, *La commare o riccoglitrice* (Venice, 1621), pp. 188–89, first published in 1596. Dr. George E. Merino translated the text for the authors, remarking that Mercurio's postpartum drink is a popular cocktail recipe in Northern Italy today. Mercurio (1550–1616) was a Dominican monk who had studied anatomy and obstetrics at Bologna and practiced as a physician.

18. Jean Ruleau, *Traité de l'opération césarienne, et des accouchemens difficiles & laborieux* (Paris, 1704), pp. 71–82. According to P.-H. Nysten, *Dictionnaire de médecine* (Paris, 1824), *baume d'Arcaeus* was an ointment composed of fat, turpentine, and resin.

19. Lawson Tait, "Address on the surgical aspect of impacted labour," *Br. M. J.* (1890), 1:659. A list of publications on cattle-horn deliveries is given in the National Library of Medicine, *Index catalogue* (1898), s. 2, vol. 3, p. 34.

20. Pierre Dionis, *A general treatise of midwifery*, trans. (London, 1719), p. 252.

21. Percival Willughby's *Observations in midwifery, as also the country midwifes opusculum or vade mecum*, found in manuscript form by Henry Blenkinsop, was edited and published by him at Warwick in 1863 (p. 340). James Primrose was a well-known physician and writer of the day who attempted to refute William Harvey's theory of the circulation of the blood. The term "obstetrician" was not invented until 1828, according to Thomas R. Forbes, *Yale J. Biol. & M.* (1976), 49:173.

22. Duncan Stewart, "The caesarean operation done with success by a midwife," *Med. Essays & Obs.*, Edinburgh (1752), 5(1):360–62.

23. John Hull, *A defence of the cesarean operation . . . addressed to W. Simmons* (Manchester [1799]), pp. 66–68, 229. In his zeal for reporting successful cesarean operations Hull (pp. 12–14) credits the belief that Jane Seymour, Henry VIII's third wife, was delivered by cesarean of the child who became Edward VI. Hull quotes the French Dionis and François Mauriceau in support of this view. Their story was that when the queen was in labor the king was asked whether her life or the child's should be saved, for it seemed unlikely both could be saved. The king said, "The child's, for I shall be able to find mothers enough." The queen survived the ordeal twelve days. Hull (p. 15) quotes from John Aikin's biographic memoirs and says "He (Dr. G. Owen) was a witness to the will of King Henry VIII, who left him a legacy of a hundred pounds." Adds Aikin, "Edward VI, was brought into the world by Dr. Owen's means, who performed the Caesarean operation on his mother." It seems more likely that the cause of the queen's death was puerperal fever.

24. Young, *Caesarean section* (n.1), pp. 65–69. Jean-L. Baudelocque (1746–1810) was also instrumental in forwarding instruction of midwives. Irving S. Cutter and Henry R. Viets, *A short history of midwifery* (Philadelphia: W. B. Saunders, 1964), pp. 92–93.

25. Paul Dubois, in a supplement to "Césarienne," *Dict. de méd.*, Paris, 2d ed. (1834), 7:152. The figures he quoted are from Gustav Adolph Michaelis, *Abhandlungen aus dem Gebiete der Geburtshülfe* (Kiel, 1833). Paul Dubois (1795–1871), accoucheur to the Empress Eugénie, was the son of one of Desault's famous pupils, Baron Antoine Dubois. P. Dubois' amputation record has been mentioned (chapter 2).

26. Edward W. Murphy, *Lectures on the principles and practice of midwifery* (London, 1852), pp. 202–3; Joseph Späth, "Erfahrungen über Sectio cäsarea; Aüsführung dieser Operation mit Exstirpation des Uterus (Methode nach Porro)," *Wien. med. Wschr.* (1878), 28:324.

27. Marie-A. Desormeaux, "Césarienne," *Dict. de méd.*, Paris (1822), 4:542. Osiander, *Handbuch der Entbindungskunst* (n.1), 2:478.

28. Benjamin Moseley, *A treatise on tropical diseases, on military operations, and on the climate of the West Indies*, 4th ed. (London, 1804), pp. 108–9. The account is retold in a letter by "A.B.," *Boston M. & S. J.* (1835), 12:398–99.

29. E. Rosenzweig, "Auto-sectio caesarea," *Zentbl. Gynäk.* (1960), 82(2):1787–90. Rosenzweig depicts the razor, needle, and thread and the appearance of the uterus at autopsy.

30. The celebrated case of "Mrs. R." [Reybold] was reviewed many times in *American Journal of Medical Sciences*; see especially Joseph G. Nancrede (1835), 16:343–54; William Gibson (1835), 17:264–68; and Robert P. Harris (1879), 77:59. Charles D. Meigs devoted over 20 pages to her four confinements in the 1842 edition of his *Philadelphia practice of midwifery*. A detailed account of the craniotomy controversy appears in Young, *Caesarean section* (n.1), pp. 73–92.

31. Herbert R. Spencer, *Caesarean section* (New York: William Wood, 1925), pp. 12, 25. Louyse Bourgeois *dite* Boursier (1563–1636), accoucheuse to French royalty and pioneer of scientific midwifery, practiced induced labor in cases of contracted pelvis, according to *Garrison-Morton*, #6145.

32. Rousset, *Hysterotomotokie* (n.8), pp. 223–24. Probably the earliest report of Lebas's case is contained in a letter from Gallot to Bougourd, physicians of the Montpellier faculty. Gallot interviewed patient and participants a month after the operation. The letter may be found in the supplement to the year 1770, *J. de méd., chir., pharm.*, Paris, 34:177–86, cahier 1. See also Théodore E. Lauverjat, *Nouvelle méthode de pratiquer l'opération césarienne* (Paris, 1788), pp. 150–51; Stéphane Tarnier, "Opération césarienne" [and discussion], *Bull. Soc. imp. de chir.*, Paris (1871), 11:29, 43. Lebas (also Le Bas) is sometimes erroneously identified as Jean Le Bas, notorious for his publications on retarded birth to defend the legitimacy of a child born to a marquis's widow 319 days after her husband's death.

33. Max Sänger, "Zur Rehabilitirung des classischen Kaiserschnittes," *Arch. Gynaek.* (1882), 19:370–99; Nicholson J. Eastman, "The role of frontier America in the development of cesarean section," *Am. J. Obstet. Gynec.* (1932), 24:922–23. Young, *Caesarean section* (n.1), pp. 123–46, gives a full account of the acceptance of sutures in uterine wounds.

34. Sänger (n.33), p. 372; F. A. Kehrer, "Ueber ein modificirtes Verfahren beim Kaiserschnitt," *Arch. Gynaek.* (1882), 19:177–78; Young, *Caesarean section* (n.1), pp. 114–16.

35. Fritz Frank, "Die suprasymphysäre Entbindung . . . bei engen Becken," *Arch. Gynaek.* (1907), 81:46–94.

36. F. A. Ritgen, "Geschichte eines mit ungünstigem Erfolge verrichteten Bauchscheidenschnittes und Folgerungen daraus," *Heidelb. klin. Ann.* (1825), 1:266–71.

37. William E. Horner to William P. Dewees, September 28, 1824, in Dewees, *A compendious system of midwifery* (Philadelphia, 1824), pp. 580–81. The book is dedicated to Philip Syng Physick, "the splendour of whose professional reputation is only exceeded by the purity of his private character." Physick had studied with John Hunter and received a degree at Edinburgh in 1792. He and Horner were members of the faculty of the University of Pennsylvania.

38. T. Gaillard Thomas, "Laparo-elytrotomy, a substitute for the caesarean section," *Am. J. Obst.* (1878), 11:230–41. Thomas coined the unusual term "gastro-elytrotomy" for extraperitoneal cesarean section in which he extended the uterine incision into the vagina, ibid. (1870), 3:125.

39. Robert P. Harris, "Lessons from a study of the cesarean operation in the city and state of New York," *Am. J. Obst.* (1879), 12:82; Harris, "Special statistics of the cesarean operation in the United States," ibid. (1881), 14:349; Eastman (n.33), pp. 925–29.

40. Edoardo Porro, "Dell' amputazione utero-ovarica come complemento di taglio cesareo," *Ann. univ. di med. e chir.* (1876), 237:291–350.

41. The first successful cesarean section in the famous Dublin Rotunda took place on June 24, 1889, according to O'Donel T. D. Browne, *The Rotunda Hospital, 1745–1945* (Edinburgh: E. and S. Livingstone, 1947), p. 276. By 1923–24 Gibbon Fitzgibbon of the Rotunda reported nineteen cesarean sections with no maternal mortality but with loss of two infants, according to Spencer, *Caesarean section* (n.31), p. 12. Said the New York surgeon James W. Markoe in 1919, "The curse of cesarean section is that it is too easy and too dangerous." *JAMA*, 73:94.

42. James A. O'Leary and Charles M. Steer, "A 10 year review of cesarean hysterectomy," *Am. J. Obstet. Gynec.* (1964), 90(1):227–31.

43. Milton D. Klein, Raymond Robbins, and Leon Gabaeff, "Primary cesarean section in the multipara," *Am. J. Obstet. Gynec.* (1963), 87(1):251. In an analysis of 500 consecutive cesarean sections at the Chicago Lying-in Hospital in affiliation with the University of Chicago, Edwin F. Daily found a 1 percent mortality between May 1931 and September 1934. No black patients were at that period admitted to the University of Chicago hospitals. *Am. J. Obstet. Gynec.* (1935), 30:204.

44. Louis M. Hellman and Jack A. Pritchard, *Williams obstetrics*, 14th ed. (New York: Appleton-Century-Crofts, 1971), p. 1187.

Further Readings

Case, B. D.; Jeffcoate, Norman; and Randle, G. H. Caesarean section and its place in modern obstetric practice. *J. Obstet. Gynaec. Br. Commonw.* (1971), 78:203–14.

Fasbender, Heinrich. *Geschichte der Geburtshülfe.* Jena: Gustav Fischer, 1906. Reprint. Hildesheim: Georg Olm, 1964.

Foster, John W., Jr. Caesarean operation from the *Armamentarium Chirurgicum* by J. Scultetus, 1666. *J. Hist. Med.* (1972), 27:206–7.

Sänger, Max. *Der Kaiserschnitt bei Uterusfibromen nebst vergleichender Methodik der Sectio Caesarea und der Porro-Operation.* Leipzig, 1882.

Speert, Harold. Historical highlights. In *Textbook of obstetrics and gynecology*, ed. David N. Danforth, pp. 12–14. 3d ed. New York: Harper and Row, 1977.

Williams, J. Whitridge. Critical analysis of twenty-one years' experience with cesarean section. *Johns Hopkins Hosp. Bull.* (1921), 32:173–84.

Chapter 11. Ectopic Pregnancy

Notes

1. Albucasis, *On surgery and instruments*, trans. and ed. M. S. Spink and G. L. Lewis (Berkeley: Univ. California Press, 1973), pp. 480–82.

2. Abraham Cyprian, *Epistola historiam exhibens foetus humani post xxi menses ex uteri tuba, matre salva ac superstite, excisi* (Leyden, 1700), pp. 5–15. Cyprian (ca. 1655–1730) was professor of anatomy and surgery in the University of Franeker, Holland, when he attended this interesting patient. He later returned to his native city of Amsterdam and practiced lithotomy. The case is somewhat garbled in a retelling by J.-F. Simon, who even said the infant was removed alive. *Mém. Acad. roy. chir.*, Paris (1753), 2:328–29.

3. A famous case was that of Marguerite Mathieu, wife of a clothworker of Toulouse, who in 1652, after an apparent nine-month pregnancy, failed to deliver. For twenty-six years she continued to protest that she was carrying an unborn child and begged her surgeon to incise her belly and remove it. After her death in 1678 a partially macerated extrauterine fetus weighing 8 pounds was found in her abdomen. A report of the case from a Toulouse physician, François Bayle, and an engraving of the lithopedion were published in *J. des sçavans* (1678), 6:160–61. See also James Yonge's account in *Phil. Trans.* (1709), 26:424–31. There are many later versions. Felix Plater (1536–1614), a well-known surgeon and university professor in Basel, described several ectopic pregnancies in *Observationum in hominis affectibus* (Basel, 1614), pp. 211–16.

4. John G. Steig[h]ertahl, "An account of a foetus, that continued 46 years in the mother's body," *Phil. Trans.* (1721), 31:126–28. The author illustrates the postmortem specimen, preserved in the Cabinet of Rarities of the Duke of Württemberg, and says that Professor Camerarius of Tübingen conjectured it concerned an extrauterine pregnancy of the left fallopian tube. Steighertahl came to England from Hanover on the accession to the throne of George I, to whom he was "physician in ordinary," Munk's *Roll*, 2:38–39.

5. Robert Houstoun, "An account of an extra-uterine foetus, taken out of a woman after death, that had continued five years and a half in the body," *Phil. Trans.* (1723), 32:387–90. For a well-documented biography of Robert Houstoun (1678–1734), a little-known but remarkable Scottish surgeon, see C. John Mackinlay, *J. Obstet. Gynaec. Br. Commonw.* (1973), 80:193–200. Houstoun's account of the ovarian tumor appears in chapter 12, note 10.

6. Starkey Myddleton, "An account of a child being taken out of the abdomen, after . . . 16 years," *Phil. Trans.* (1747), 44:617–21.

7. John Bard's report of this case in a letter to John Fothergill, London, was read to the Society of Physicians in 1760 and published in their *Medical Observations* (1762), 2:369–72. An earlier account of the case, dated January 17, 1759, sent to a Philadelphia colleague, was published in *Eclectic Repertory* (1818), 8:540–42. Bard was a New York surgeon and the father of the distinguished Samuel Bard who studied under Fothergill. For another interesting American case, see B. F. Baer, "Report of a case of pregnancy in the right horn of a uterus bicornis treated successfully by a modified caesarean operation, twelve months after the death of the child at the full term of gestation," *Trans. Am. Gynec. Soc.* (1888), 13:455–70.

8. Ernst L. Heim, "Von einer Bauch-Schwangerschaft, bei welcher das Kind zu vollen Tagen ausgetragen, und durch den Bauchschnitt zur Welt gebracht wurde," *Mag. f. d. ges. Heilk.*, Berlin (1818), 3:1–19.

9. Johann H. G. Zwanck, *Beschreibung eines Bauchschnittes bei Graviditas extrauterina abdominalis mit glücklichem Ausgange für Mutter und Kind* (Hamburg, 1854). Zwanck was apologetic for the eighteen-year delay in reporting, occasioned by his large active practice.

10. André Levret, *Observations sur les causes et les accidens de plusieurs accouchemens laborieux*, 2d ed. (Paris, 1750), p. 243; ibid., 4th ed. (1770), pp. 248–49; John S. Parry, *Extra-uterine pregnancy* (Philadelphia, 1876), pp. 91, 119; John W. Taylor, *Extra-uterine pregnancy: A clinical and operative study* (London, 1899), p. 142. André Levret (1703–80), the accoucheur to the mother of Louis XVI, was also a surgeon and a member of the Royal Academy of Surgery. He invented a curved forceps (1747).

11. Willard M. Allen, May 13, 1975, personal communication. Allen has pursued the subject of extrauterine pregnancy, "this extraordinary natural phenomenon," first as a house officer in obstetrics at the University of Rochester, later as chairman of the Department of Obstetrics and Gynecology, Washington University, St. Louis, and more recently at the University of Maryland.

12. H. Hudnall Ware, Jr., "Observations on thirteen cases of late extrauterine pregnancy," *Am. J. Obstet. Gynec.* (1948), 55:577–78.

13. This indication was noted in 1723 by Houstoun (n.5), p. 387.

14. Maurice H. Friedman, "Mechanism of ovulation in the rabbit," *Am. J. Physiol.* (1929), 90:617–22; F. K. Beller, M. Maki, and M. D. Epstein, "Incoagulability of intraperitoneal blood," *Am. J. Obstet. Gynec.* (1968), 102:1121–27. In the Friedman test, 4 ml. of patient's urine is injected intravenously into unmated mature female rabbits twice daily for two days; hemorrhagic corpora lutea in the rabbits' ovaries denote a positive reaction.

15. Methods are reviewed in John Strahan, *The diagnosis and treatment of extra-uterine pregnancy* (Philadelphia, 1889), pp. 79–82; Parry, *Extra-uterine pregnancy* (n.10), pp. 199–209; J. Clarence Webster, *Ectopic pregnancy* (New York, 1895), pp. 207–11. Syphilization of the mother or loading her abdomen with bags of sand to crush the fetus were suggestions that probably remained untried. A near-starvation diet to lower the vital powers of the mother was also deemed likely to kill the fetus.

16. Paulin Cazeaux, *Traité théorique et pratique de l'art des accouchements*, 3d ed. (Paris, 1850), p. 274. Cazeaux is incorrectly cited as "Pierre" Cazeaux in many English indices.

17. Odoardo Bacchetti, "Nuova applicazione del'ago-elettro-puntura in un caso guidicato gravidanza extra-uterina tubaria," *Gazz. med. ital. feder. tosc.*, Florence (1853), 2s., 3:137–40, trans. Henry J. Garrigues in *Trans. Am. Gynec. Soc.* (1882), 7:191–92; Abram Brothers, "Treatment of extra-uterine pregnancy by electricity," *Am. J. Obst.* (1888), 21:474–84.

18. The account of Simpson's debacle appears in *Edinb. Med. J.* (1864), 9:865.

19. J. Désiré Joulin, *Des cas de dystocie appartenant au foetus* (Paris, 1863), p. 96; Joulin, *Traité complet d'accouchements* (Paris, 1867), p. 968; Nickolaus F. Friedreich, "Ueber einen Fall höchst wahrscheinlicher Extrauterinschwangerschaft mit günstigem Ausgang durch eine neue Behandlungsmethode," Virchow's *Arch. f. path. Anat. [etc.]* (1864), 29:312–20.

20. Strahan, *Extra-uterine pregnancy* (n.15), pp. 77–81; J. Matthews Duncan and J. Mason, "Cases of extra-uterine foetation," *St. Barth. Hosp. Rep.* (1883), 19:35–44, including notes by Steavenson on the electric treatments; and Lawson Tait, *Lectures on ectopic pregnancy and pelvic haematocele* (Birmingham, 1888), pp. 75–76.

21. O. Rennert, "Extrauterinschwangerschaft im fünften Monate: Tödtung des Fötus mittels Morphium-injection: Heilung," *Arch. Gynaek.* (1884), 24:266–80. Others included T. Gaillard Thomas, *Trans. Am. Gynec. Soc.* (1882), 7:219–42; ibid. (1884), 9:161–88; J. H. Aveling, *Br. M. J.* (1886), 2:1091–92; and A. H. Buckmaster, *Med. News,* Philadelphia (1888), 53:66–69. C. H. F. Routh, formerly a pupil of Semmelweis, was another who practiced electric shock therapy to kill the fetus, *Trans. Obstet. Soc. London* (1879), 21:93–115.

22. Tait, *Ectopic pregnancy* (n.20), pp. 76, 105. "After the fetus is dead a diseased mass is left behind," said J. M. Baldy of Philadelphia in a discussion of electrical therapy, *Trans. Am. Assoc. Obst. & Gynec.* (1888), 1:326.

23. G. Ernest Herman, "On delivery by the vagina in extra-uterine gestation," abstract, *Trans. Obstet. Soc.*, London (1887), 29:429–45.

24. Parry, *Extra-uterine pregnancy* (n.10), pp. 238–39. Parry's publication, appearing the year of his death (1876) at age thirty-three, was highly praised by Tait for its scholarly approach and influenced Tait's attack on the subject. He said, however, that Parry's "delusive use of statistics" had led Parry astray. Tait, *Ectopic pregnancy* (n.20), p. 4.

25. Tait, *Ectopic pregnancy* (n.20), pp. 7, 19–20, 24, 45, 70; Tait, "Five cases of extra-uterine pregnancy operated upon at the time of rupture," *Br. M. J.* (1884), 1:1250–51; Tait, discussion, *Br. M. J.* (1886), 2:1094; W. J. Stewart McKay, *Lawson Tait: His life and work* (London: Baillière, Tindall, and Cox, 1922), 207, 213–16, 318; I. Harvey Flack, *Lawson Tait, 1845–1899* (London: William Heinemann, 1949), pp. 27–29.

26. In 1889 Strahan, *Extra-uterine pregnancy* (n.15), p. 70, said that only one successful operation for tubal rupture had been performed before 1883. To whom was Strahan referring? Certainly not Tait, for in the fourth edition of his *Diseases of the ovaries* (New York, 1883) it is obvious that Tait, although experienced in the management of ovarian tumors, had then precious little to say concerning management of extrauterine pregnancy. Strahan may have been referring to T. R. Jessop. In discussing abdominal pregnancy, Tait (p. 79) said, "Only one such fortunate case is as yet, however, on record — that which recently has been published by Mr. Jessop, of Leeds." In two brief reports J. Knowsley Thornton alluded to a single personal success reported at sessions of the Obstetrical Society of London. *Br. M. J.* (1882), 1:426, 581.

27. A. Wiegand, "Statistisches über Extrauteringravidität," *Mschr. Geburtsh. Gynäk.* (1920), 52:316–25.

28. Ware (n.12), pp. 561–82.

29. Jørgen Lund, *Konservativ behandling af tidlig ectopisk graviditet* (Copenhagen: Arnold Busck, 1950), Univ. Copenhagen thesis.

30. Allen E. Winer, William D. Bergman, and Charles Fields, "Combined intra- and extra-uterine pregnancy," *Am. J. Obstet. Gynec.* (1957), 74(1):170–78.

31. J. T. Armstrong, Seward H. Wills, Jack Moore, and A. E. Lauden, "Ectopic pregnancy: A review of 481 cases," *Am. J. Obstet. Gynec.* (1959), 77:364–70. The hospitals concerned were the Jefferson Davis and the Hermann.

32. Herman D. Webster, Jr., David L. Barclay, and Charles K. Fischer, "Ectopic pregnancy, a seventeen-year review," *Am. J. Obstet. Gynec.* (1965), 92(1):23–34; Thomas W. McElin, "Ectopic pregnancy," in David N. Danforth, ed. *Obstetrics and Gynecology*, 3d ed. (New York: Harper and Row, 1977), p. 349.

33. Woodard D. Beacham, William C. Hernquist, Dan W. Beacham, and Herman D.

Webster, "Abdominal pregnancy at Charity Hospital in New Orleans," *Am. J. Obstet. Gynec.* (1962), 84(2):1257–70.

34. Jerold M. Rosenblum, Robert W. Dowling, and Allan C. Barnes, "Treatment of tubal pregnancy," *Am. J. Obstet. Gynec.* (1960), 80:274–77.

35. M. Leo Bobrow and Hugh G. Bell, "Ectopic pregnancy: A 16-year survey of 905 cases," *Obstet. Gynec.* (1962), 20:500–6.

Further Readings

Osiander, Friedrich Benjamin. *Handbuch der Entbindungskunst.* 4 vols. Tübingen, 1818–25.

Sandmire, H. F., and Randall, J. H. Ectopic pregnancy: A review of 182 cases. *Obstet. Gynec.* (1959), 14:227–33.

Tait, Lawson. *Lectures on ectopic pregnancy and pelvic haematocele.* Birmingham, 1888.

Vehaskari, Allan. The operation of choice for ectopic pregnancy with reference to subsequent fertility. *Acta obstet. gynec. scand.* (1960), vol. 39, suppl. 3.

Chapter 12. Ovariotomy (Excision of Ovarian Cyst)

Notes

1. Ephraim McDowell, "Three cases of extirpation of diseased ovaria," *Eclect. Repert.* (1817), 7:242–44. Samuel D. Gross appended a short biography of McDowell (1771–1830) to his report on Kentucky surgery in the 1851 *Transactions* of the Kentucky State Medical Society (1:122–45), reprinted in his *Lives of eminent American physicians and surgeons of the nineteenth century* (Philadelphia, 1861). In his account, substantiated by "extensive local research," Gross "created Ephraim McDowell's status in medical history," remarks the historian Genevieve Miller, *Bull. Hist. Med.* (1973), 47:594. Throughout this chapter we have relied extensively on Gross's authoritative report and on August Schachner's *Ephraim McDowell* (Philadelphia: J. B. Lippincott, 1921), a more detailed biography. McDowell's granddaughter, Mary Y. Ridenbaugh, gathered a number of pertinent articles in her *Biography of Ephraim McDowell* (New York, 1890). McDowell's house and adjoining apothecary shop have been faithfully restored and offer a wealth of information to visitors interested in the Danville surgeon and frontier medicine in America. McDowell's skill as a lithotomist was mentioned earlier (chapter 4).

2. Gross, *Lives* (n.1), pp. 209–10. Gross was unable to learn whether McDowell got a degree at Edinburgh; he was inclined to believe not.

3. James McDowell, a nephew, assisted Ephraim McDowell in the procedure, starting the external incision at his uncle's direction. Later, claims were made that the nephew had performed the ovariotomy, although James himself, who died young (1812), apparently made no such assertion. To counter these attacks on his veracity, Ephraim sent printed cards to various medical colleagues in 1826, stating that he had done the entire intra-abdominal segment of the operation; he included corroborating certificates from Mrs. Crawford, her nurse, and a witness. This material, quoted by Gross, has disappeared. A defamatory opinion was published by another nephew, Joseph N. McDowell, in *Trans. AMA* (1860), 13:427–66. He included the tale of an old Indian hunter, John King of Kentucky, who earned his livelihood spaying farm animals and, reputedly, in 1808 opened the abdomen of a woman with an ovarian tumor, ligated the pedicle, and removed the tumor, saving her life.

4. McDowell (n.1), p. 244.

5. Schachner, *McDowell* (n.1), p. 66.

6. Ephraim McDowell, "Observations on diseased ovaria," *Eclect. Repert.* (1819), 9:546–53. In this publication McDowell related that the second patient he described in 1817 had a recurrence; he had not been able to complete the excision of the tumor and had merely made an incision to extract its contents.

7. John Lizars, "Observations on extirpation of the ovaria, with cases," *Edinb. M. & S. J.* (1824), 22:247–56. Lizars's patient survived the unnecessary abdominal operation. Lizars's

Observations on extraction of diseased ovaria (Edinburgh, 1825) is listed among his "lesser writings" in his obituary in *Lancet*, June 9, 1860, p. 582.

8. These words have puzzled many. In his biography of McDowell (n.1) Schachner (pp. 68, 137) took pains to explain that McDowell may have been away on a case or at his country retreat for five days; Mrs. Crawford had said that the nephew did her dressings. A modern reader will not doubt the patient's ability to return home so soon. Making the bed was good early ambulatory therapy. Postoperative care in all major surgery is now recognized as an important determinant in success or failure, a development that slowly emerged with elective surgery in hospitals (ca. 1885). For Johnson's comments, see *Med.-Chir. Rev.* (1825), 2:215–17; (1826), 5:620.

9. Charles Clay, "Ovariotomy, another case of extirpation of diseased ovary by the major operation," *Med. Times* (1843–44), 9:4.

10. Washington L. Atlee, "A table of all the known operations of ovariotomy from 1701 to 1851, comprising 222 cases, and giving a synoptical history of each case," *Trans. AMA* (1851), 4:286–314. Why the date 1701? It may have been a misprint for 1781, the likely date of Laumonier's operation, or Atlee may have planned to include an operation performed in 1701 by Houstoun on a fifty-eight-year-old woman in Renfrew, Scotland, who had a tumor so large it filled her abdomen from umbilicus to pubis. She had been bedridden for three months. Houstoun made a 4-inch opening in her belly with a lancet, incising the cyst wall. He improvised an instrument from a fir splinter used in the countryside as a candle, wrapped one end in lint, thrust it into the wound, and extracted 2 yards of thick gelatinous substance about 10 inches wide, followed by 9 quarts of matter, usually found in steatomatous tumors. After he had squeezed out all possible gelatinous material, Houstoun closed the wound with three sutures and applied a balsam dressing dipped in French brandy. The patient was restored to health and survived until 1714. See *Phil. Trans.* (1726), 33:8–15. Houstoun obviously left the capsule of the cyst behind. The operation, therefore, was not a true ovariectomy, although it was so named by Tait and some others. See James Finlayson, "Dr. Robert Houston [sic], of Glasgow, the first ovariotomist," *Janus*, Amsterdam (1896), 1:216–18. Houstoun's account of an ectopic pregnancy is given in chapter 11.

11. L'Aumonier [Jean-Baptiste Laumonier], "Observation sur un dépôt de la trompe, et sur l'extirpation de l'ovaire," *Hist. Soc. roy. de méd., 1782–83* (1787), 5:296–300. Laumonier (1749–1818) was surgeon in chief at the Hôtel-Dieu, Rouen, and professor of anatomy and surgery, Rouen. Lizars (n.7) listed Laumonier's case as an ovariotomy. Achille Chereau (1847) said that ovariotomy had yet to be done in France and that Laumonier's case concerned an abscess (*Union méd.* 1:398). Gross agreed (n.1, 1851), pp. 128–29. Atlee later wrote of McDowell as the founder of ovariotomy.

12. Atlee's mortality rate (1870) was 30 percent in his first 200 ovariotomies; in the next 36, he lost 15 patients (41.6 percent), according to J. Ewing Mears, who reported Atlee's cases in *Am. J. Med. Sci.* (1870–72). See especially the entry for 1870, vol. 59, p. 99.

13. William Jeaffreson, "A case of ovarian tumour successfully removed," *Trans. Prov. M. & S. Assoc.* (1837), 5:239–45; John A. Shepherd, "William Jeaffreson (1790–1865): Surgical pioneer," *Br. M. J.* (1965), 2:1119–20. Jeaffreson mentions Nathan Smith's successful ovariotomy in New Haven, Connecticut, and Lizars's cases, but not McDowell's, yet Lizars's report had described McDowell's first operations. The large tumor is still on exhibit at St. Bartholomew's Hospital, London. Jeaffreson's case was soon followed by several fortunate attempts by colleagues in Suffolk.

14. Charles Clay, "Cases of peritoneal section," *Med. Times* (1842), 7:45, 59, 154; Clay, "Ovariotomy and its results," *Edinb. M. J.* (1856), 2:1096; Clay, "Ovariotomy and ovariotomists," *Lancet*, February 25, 1865, p. 200; John A. Shepherd, *Spencer Wells* (Edinburgh: E. and S. Livingstone, 1965), pp. 37, 42–53. Isaac Baker Brown (1812–73) helped Wells in some of his early cases. French visitors were impressed by Brown's technique, which was often mentioned in Paris discussions.

15. The account of the ancient Lydian practice is given in M.-L. Negroni, *Aperçu sur*

l'ovariotomie, Paris thesis, 1866, pp. 27–31. Negroni also noted that castrated women with masculine singing voices were entertainers in India in 1841.

16. T. Spencer Wells, "Some causes of excessive mortality after surgical operations," *Br. M. J.* (1864), 2:384–88.

17. "Ovariotomy," unsigned editorial, *Br. M. J.* (1880), 1:931–32; Shepherd, *Spencer Wells* (n.14), p. 97. Wells attributed his final achievement to use of improved surgical techniques rather than to adoption of antisepsis.

18. T. Spencer Wells, "Personal experience of aseptic and antiseptic surgery," *Br. M. J.* (1892), 1:1178.

19. J. Marion Sims, "Thomas Keith and ovariotomy," *Am. J. Obst.* (1880), 13:292–93.

20. Thomas Keith, "Results of ovariotomy before and after antiseptics," *Br. M. J.* (1878), 2:590–93. By 1879 Keith had performed 70 successive ovariotomies without a death. "A great deed in surgery," unsigned editorial, *Br. M. J.* (1879), 2:915.

21. J. Marion Sims wrote his wife from Aberdeen on his first trip abroad (August 10, 1861) that he had watched Keith "perform a half dozen surgical operations, as I have seldom ever seen equaled anywhere." Sims, *The story of my life* (New York, 1884; reprint, New York: Da Capo Press, 1968), p. 408.

22. Sims (n.19), pp. 290–303. Sims's report constitutes the best source of information on Keith's practices. See also Keith's obituary, *Br. M. J.* (1895), 2:1003–5.

23. "Sur les kystes ovariques," *Bull. Acad. imp. de méd.* (1856–57), 22:25, 181–82, 200. The discussions began at a séance in October 1856 and continued into February 1857, filling many pages of the *Bulletin*. As late as 1857, punctures of ovarian cysts, followed by injection of iodine to sclerose the sac, were considered in a lengthy editorial in *Bull. gén. de thérap.*, 52:22–32. The report concerns 132 patients from many sources; 25 died shortly after the puncture; within a year, 71 (53 percent) were dead — as high a mortality rate as was observed to attend ovariotomy a decade later. Jules Worms wrote in justification of ovariotomy in 1860, saying it had been tried only two or three times recently in France (*Gaz. hebd. méd.* 7:642–43).

24. Jean-Nicolas Demarquay, "L'ovariotomie à Londres," *Union méd.* (1862), 14:515–23. Nélaton, who was also attending operations in London, declared that they could be done in Paris. *Union méd.* (1861), 12:459.

25. Nélaton, eager to announce his success, presented the patient's multicellular cyst to the Academy, eight days postoperatively, declaring that the French would no longer have to envy their neighbors across the Channel. *Union méd.* (1862), 14:604.

26. Felix-J. Delstanche, "Visite a M. le docteur Nélaton," *J. de méd., chir., et pharmacol.*, Brussels (1869), 48:318–22. In this interview of October 10, 1868, Nélaton told Delstanche that McDowell first tried ovariotomy as an experiment on slaves at the behest of the owners who wanted to save their valuable property and that ovariotomy was therefore the result of avarice. Delstanche's report was undoubtedly the source of Nélaton's oft-repeated remarks about McDowell, which Schachner tried to locate (*McDowell* [n.1], pp. 132–33). Nélaton may have confused McDowell's operations with those of Sims for vesicovaginal fistula, or perhaps he was just misquoted. An even more garbled account appears in Louis Gallez, *Histoire des kystes de l'ovaire* (Brussels, 1873), pp. 426–27.

27. Eugène Koeberlé, *De l'ovariotomie* (Paris, 1865), pp. 31–34; Pierre Huard, "Eugène Koeberlé, pionnier de l'asepsie," *Episteme*, Milan (1968), 2:219–43. Koeberlé's first operation was done in June 1862; two years later he reported success in 9 of 12 cases (25 percent mortality). Koeberlé employed careful washing of instruments, utensils, and sponges in charcoal-filtered water. He also washed his hands often during the course of an operation.

28. Alfred Hegar, "Zur Ovariotomie," *Samml. klin. Vortr.* (1876), no. 109 (Gynäk. 36), pp. 811–30; Ernst Sonntag, "Alfred Hegar," *Arch. Gynaek.* (1914), 103:v–xi [final pages in the volume]; and Sonntag, "Alfred Hegar," *Dt. med. Wschr.* (1930), 56(1):57–62.

29. Chlorine is by no means completely innocuous. It is readily absorbed by visceral peritoneal and pleural surfaces. Halsted operated upon the famous Hopkins anatomist Franklin Paine Mall for gallstones in 1917. Mall's death a few days later was probably from

overuse of intraperitoneal injections of Dakin's solution. During World War I Halsted, not a military surgeon, had become enamored of Dakin's solution in wound management.

30. Hegar (n.28), p. 820.

31. Alfred Hegar, *Castration der Frauen* (Leipzig, 1878), pp. 82–83; Hegar and Rudolf Kaltenbach, *Operative Gynäkologie* (Erlangen, 1874), pp. 139–42. There is no mention of Semmelweis in either of these tracts. In his 1876 presentation (n.28) Hegar outlined for the first time his complete adherence to and reliance upon the Semmelweis technique in performing ovariotomy for ovarian cysts. Semmelweis is discussed fully in chapter 21.

32. Charles A. L. Reed, "The life and character of Lawson Tait," *Am. J. Obst.* (1899), 40:841; W. J. Stewart McKay, *Lawson Tait: His life and work* (London: Baillière, Tindall, and Cox, 1922), pp. 19, 157–68; I. Harvey Flack, *Lawson Tait, 1845–1899* (London: Heinemann, 1949), pp. 14–15.

33. Flack, *Tait* (n.32), p. 88; Lawson Tait, "One hundred and thirty-nine consecutive ovariotomies performed between January 1st, 1884, and December 31st, 1885, without a death," *Br. M. J.* (1886), 1:923.

34. In a letter in *Lancet* (1883), Tait prodded the sensitive wound of Wells. Tait had reported that Wells had a mortality rate of 25 percent with ovariotomy. Wells had written the editor of *Lancet*, suggesting that Tait was lying concerning Wells's statistics. Tait replied, "The facts are that between February, 1858, and February, 1878, Mr. Wells operated 892 times; and, according to his own tables of these cases, 220 died, giving a mortality of 24.66." *Lancet* (1883), 1:370, 520. John Homans II of Boston did 5 ovariotomies without benefit of antiseptics between 1872 and 1875; the patients all died. In 1877 he adopted Listerian antiseptic methods. Over the next ten years he removed ovarian cysts in an additional 277 patients, of whom 34 died, a mortality of 12.2 percent, a figure not rivaling the achievement of Hegar or Tait but exceeding that of Spencer Wells, whose writings Homans commended to readers of his small book, *Three hundred and eighty-four laparotomies for various diseases* (Boston, 1887).

35. Tait shunned use of the clamp which was employed by Wells and the French surgeons Koeberlé and Péan. The clamp would be left in situ for several days; the jaws of the clamp were then released with the clamp in place for some hours; if no bleeding occurred, the clamp was removed.

36. Lawson Tait, *General summary of conclusions from one thousand cases of abdominal section* (Birmingham, 1884), pp. 4–6.

37. An abridged report of Tait's address (1890) appears in McKay, *Tait* (n.32), pp. 403–16.

38. Another source of worry that compounded Tait's problems of failing health in his last years was the claim of a nurse at his hospital that he was the father of her daughter. Tait denied the accusation, saying "I will spend my last penny in defending myself. Nay, more, my wife is willing to sacrifice her wedding ring to help in paying the costs." Tait weathered the unfavorable publicity but at great cost to his reputation, professional stature, and practice. He was obliged to sell his New Forest house. Flack, *Tait* (n.32), pp. 114–17.

Further Readings

Cianfrani, Theodore. *A short history of obstetrics and gynecology*. Springfield, Ill.: Charles C Thomas, 1960.

Cutter, Irving S., and Viets, Henry R. *A short history of midwifery*. Philadelphia and London: W. B. Saunders, 1964.

Koeberlé, Eugène. De l'ovariotomie. *Mém. Acad. imp. méd.*, Paris (1863), 26:321–472.

Shepherd, John A. *Lawson Tait*. Kansas City, Kan.: Coronado Press, forthcoming.

Smellie, William. A collection of cases and observations in midwifery. In *A treatise on the theory and practice of midwifery*, vol. 2. New ed. London, 1779.

Storer, H. R. *Successful removal of the uterus and both ovaries by abdominal section*. Boston, 1866.

Tait, Lawson. *The pathology and treatment of diseases of the ovaries*. London, 1874.

Thoms, Herbert. *Classical contributions to obstetrics and gynecology*. Springfield, Ill.: Charles C Thomas, 1935.

Chapter 13. Vesicovaginal Fistula

Notes

1. Johann F. Dieffenbach, "Ueber die Heilung der Blasen-Scheiden-Fisteln und Zerreissungen der Blase und Scheide," *Med. Ztg.*, Berlin (1836), 5:117–24, 173–75, 177–80. Dieffenbach's curiosity concerning his handiwork prompted him to make daily examinations of the operative site, obviously not a wise procedure, especially when employing a nonsterile speculum. His use of the lithotomy position for surgical exposure was another obstacle to success. Dieffenbach was professor of surgery and ophthalmology at the University of Berlin, 1840–47.

2. J. Marion Sims, *The story of my life* (New York, 1884; reprint, New York: Da Capo Press, 1968); Seale Harris, *Woman's surgeon, the life story of J. Marion Sims* (New York: Macmillan, 1950). Sims's autobiography gives a full account of his early career and experiments with vesicovaginal fistula.

3. Sims's father wanted him to become a lawyer and, when the young man decided on medicine, he said to his son, "If I had known this I certainly should not have sent you to college," a reflection of the general public's appraisal of medicine as a profession in the early decades of the nineteenth century. Sims, *Life* (n.2), p. 116.

4. Sims named his oldest son for Pattison — Granville Sharp Sims. Pattison's contributions to urology are discussed in chapter 4.

5. Clarence Dennis, now of Stony Brook Medical School, Long Island, an ardent student of diarrhea in surgical cases, agrees that Sims did not have ulcerative colitis, that the most likely cause of his problem was contaminated drinking water. Dennis, May 31, 1974, personal communication.

6. Henry Graham (1841) described a large rubber bag which, when inflated and kept within the vagina, prevented escape of urine, with the patient in the dorsal recumbent position. He apparently used the method on one patient with success. *Edinb. M. & S. J.*, 56:378–79.

7. As late as 1877 Adolf Dirnhofer operated for vesicovaginal fistula without anesthesia, the patients having only slight pain. *Med.-chir. Centralbl.*, Vienna (1877), 12:148–49.

8. After years of failure, Sims relates in his autobiography (p. 242), his brother-in-law Dr. Rush Jones came to tell him to quit this foolishness and devote himself to his practice.

9. Sims, *Life* (n.2), pp. 244–46.

10. J. Marion Sims, "On the treatment of vesico-vaginal fistula," *Am. J. Med. Sci.* (1852), 23:59–82.

11. Sims, *Life* (n.2), pp. 309, 408.

12. As C. Lee Buxton pointed out in his foreword to the 1968 reprint of Sims's autobiography (p. x), it is not always possible to pinpoint Sims's foreign travels in these recollections of his life. Sometimes the dates conflict with those in the appended letters.

13. Edmond Souchon, "Reminiscences of Dr. J. Marion Sims in Paris," *Med. Record* (1894), 46:705–8. Slightly different versions appear in Sims, *Life* (n.2), pp. 319–25, and in Sims's letter to his wife, November 21, 1861, printed in the appendix, pp. 412–13. As a boy Nélaton had observed that mice overanesthetized with chloroform and apparently dead could be revived by swinging them by their tails in the inverted posture. L.-E. d'Heurle related that Nélaton used the head-down maneuver twice during an ovariotomy in 1862. The patient, who was receiving chloroform, had two attacks of syncope and her breathing stopped twice; the head-down maneuver was employed and the patient survived. Heurle, "Ovariotomie pratiquée avec succès par M. Nélaton," *Gaz. hôp.*, Paris (1862), 35:385.

14. Willy Meyer first described Trendelenburg's use of the posture in *Arch. klin. Chir.* (1885), 31:511–24. Meyer, later a well-known thoracic surgeon in New York, was then an assistant in the Trendelenburg Clinic in Bonn. Trendelenburg's own paper on the subject appeared in *Samml. klin. Vortr.* (1890), Chir. no. 109, pp. 3373–92. He emphasized its role in providing good surgical exposure for lower abdominal operations and in the resuscitation of patients in shock. Earlier uses of the position are mentioned in chapter 6.

15. An early report was that of Paul Bloc of Montpellier, *Étude clinique sur le traitement de la fistule vésico-vaginale* (Montpellier, 1862). Bloc followed what he called the American operation in all details, including posture of patient, speculum, and suture. His professor, A. Courty (1865), reported six successful cases operated upon by Sims's method, employing steel sutures. One patient had a subsequent pregnancy without difficulty. Another patient, illustrated in the publication, had complete loss of the vesicovaginal septum from urethra to cervix. Courty successfully repaired the defect (*Montpell. méd.*, 15:316–37).

16. J. Marion Sims, *The Woman's Hospital in 1874, a reply* (New York: [June 1] 1877). Sims could be difficult, but the self-serving statement (May 5, 1877) of three of his associates — Thomas A. Emmet, Edmond R. Peaslee, and T. Gaillard Thomas — does them no credit. Sims's mortality rate for ovariotomy was approximately 60 percent in 1874. Obviously, therefore, despite long experience, he had not yet capitulated to prophylactic surgical antisepsis. *Reply to Dr. J. Marion Sims' pamphlet . . . [of] June 1, 1877* (New York, 1877), p. 14. The fatal outcome in Sims's cholecystotomy (1878) was owing primarily to postoperative hemorrhage in a jaundiced patient. *Br. M. J.* (1878), 1:811–15.

17. Sims's election to the presidency of the AMA (1876–77) served to ease the hurt and injury to his dignity. Eleven years after his death in 1883 his statue, supported by subscriptions of $1 each from physicians throughout the land, was unveiled in Bryant Park, New York. It now stands on Fifth Avenue, opposite the New York Academy of Medicine. Woman's Hospital established an affiliation with St. Luke's a few blocks away in 1952, the latter having neither an obstetric service nor a gynecologic service of its own. In 1971 St. Luke's Hospital Center negotiated an amended affiliation agreement with the Columbia College of Physicians and Surgeons. Charles W. Davidson, July 30, 1974, personal communication.

18. J. Marion Sims, *Silver sutures in surgery, the anniversary discourse, before the New York Academy of Medicine* (New York, 1858), p. 8; D. L. Gravens, H. W. Margraf, H. R. Butcher, Jr., and Walter F. Ballinger, "Antibacterial effect of treating sutures with silver," *Surgery* (1973), 73:122–27. In 1897 Benno Credé of Dresden wrote of the sterilizing effect of silver sutures in the repair of vaginal defects (*Arch. klin. Chir.*, 55:861–71).

19. Montague Gosset, "Advantages of the gilt-wire suture," *Lancet* (1834), 1:345–46; *Dictionary of national biography*, s.v. "Gosset, Montague." John Russell described use of silver sutures in a leg amputation at Guy's Hospital in 1835 — the wires were painful and interfered with search for a postoperative bleeder. *Br. M. J.* (1858), p. 1043.

20. A London surgeon named Luke "of Charing Cross" is reported to have operated successfully for vesicovaginal fistula employing silver sutures prior to Sims's publication (1852). See Naguib Mahfouz, *J. Obstet. Gynaec. Br. Emp.* (1957), 64:24. We have found a report of James Luke operating "successfully" at London Hospital for a vesicovaginal fistula. His report, however, leaves the matter of permanent success somewhat in doubt. He operated first in early January 1830, repairing a medium-sized fistula with placement of interrupted sutures. Suppuration occurred around them with subsequent leakage of urine. Luke reoperated in March, placing one suture in the middle of the circular fistula. The patient was dismissed "cured" in six days. There is no mention of silver sutures. *London Med. Gaz.* (1831), 9:31–32.

21. Sims (n.10), p. 62; George Hayward, "Case of vesico-vaginal fistula, successfully treated by an operation," *Am. J. Med. Sci.* (1839), 24:283–88; Hayward, "Cases of vesico-vaginal fistula treated by operation," *Boston M. & S. J.* (1851), 33:209–24. Hayward (1791–1863), a Harvard Medical School professor, performed the first major operation under ether, amputating a thigh, on November 7, 1846.

22. John P. Mettauer, "Vesico-vaginal fistula," *Boston M. & S. J.* (1840), 22:154–55; Mettauer, "On vesico-vaginal fistula," *Am. J. Med. Sci.* (1847), 14:117–21. See also William Bickers, "John Peter Mettauer of Virginia," *JAMA* (1963), 184:870–71.

23. Dupuytren (1829) closed such a fistula in a thirty-year-old woman after two treatments with cautery at the Hôtel-Dieu (*Clinique*, Paris, 1:173). A number of cases are summarized by Paul Bontemps in a Strasbourg thesis of 1858, *De la fistule vésico-vaginale*, and in a Paris thesis

of 1860 by Pierre Boitelle, *Quelques réflexions sur les fistules vésico-utero-vaginales.* Dieffenbach found cauterization the least acceptable method. *Am. J. Med. Sci.* (1839), 23:229.

24. Auguste Bérard, "De l'oblitération du vagin appliquée au traitement de la fistule vésico-vaginale," *Bull. Acad. roy. de méd.* (1845), 10:407–10; J. Herrgott, "De l'oblitération du vagin comme moyen de guérison de l'incontinence d'urine dans les grandes pertes de substance de la vessie," *Arch. de tocol.*, Paris (1875), 2:336–50; Sims (n.10), p. 61.

25. Jules Rochard, *Histoire de la chirurgie française au XIXe siècle* (Paris, 1875), p. 288. A good description of Jobert's method is given in his "Mémoire sur les fistules vésico-vaginales, et sur leur traitement par une nouvelle méthode opératiore," *Gaz. méd. Paris* (1836), 4:225–27. Later revisions of the technique were called "autoplastie par glissement."

26. Gustav Simon, *Mittheilungen aus der chirurgischen Klinik des Rostocker Krankenhauses während der Jahre 1861–1865* (Prague, 1868), 2:128–30; Trendelenburg (n.14). Simon's first such repair was in 1861.

27. Leopold Dittel, "Abdominale Blasenscheidenfistel-Operation," *Wien. klin. Wschr.* (1893), 6:449–52; Maurice H. Collis, "Further remarks upon a new and successful mode of treatment for vesico-vaginal fistula," *Dubl. Quart. J. Med. Sci.* (1861), 31:302–16.

28. J. Chassar Moir, "Vesicovaginal fistulae, review of 100 consecutive cases," *Lancet* (1954), 1:61. Mahfouz (n.20) cited Sänger (1888) also as favoring the two-layer closure over the Sims method. However, the Sänger paper related solely to historic aspects of perineorraphy (*Zntbl. Gynäk.*, 12:765).

29. D. E. Derry, "Note on five pelves of women of the Eleventh Dynasty in Egypt," *J. Obstet. Gynaec. Br. Emp.* (1935), 42:490–95.

30. Henry van Roonhuyze [Roonhuisen], *Some observations and practices relating . . . to women in travel [labor]*, trans. from Dutch (London, 1676), pp. 132–35.

31. Howard A. Kelly, *Operative gynecology*, 2d ed. (New York: Appleton, 1912), 1:413. Kelly could find no clear reference to vesicovaginal fistula before the sixteenth century.

Further Readings

Flack, I. Harvey [Harvey Graham]. *Eternal Eve.* London: Heinemann, 1950.
Leonardo, Richard A. *History of gynecology.* New York: Froben Press, 1944.
Ricci, James V. *The development of gynaecological surgery and instruments . . . from the Hippocratic age to the antiseptic period.* Philadelphia: Blakiston, 1949.
———. *Genealogy of gynaecology; history of the development of gynaecology throughout the ages.* 2d ed. Philadelphia: Blakiston, 1950.
Speert, Harold. *Obstetric and gynecologic milestones.* New York: Macmillan, 1958.
———. *Iconographica gyniatrica; a pictorial history of gynecology and obstetrics.* Philadelphia: F. A. Davis, 1973.

Chapter 14. Phlebotomy

Notes

1. Joseph Bauer, *Geschichte der Aderlässe* (Munich, 1870; reprint, Munich: W. Fritsch, 1966), pp. 1–9; Fielding H. Garrison, "History of bloodletting," *N. York M. J.* (1913), 97:432–35; *Hippocrates*, with an English translation by W. H. S. Jones (Cambridge: Harvard Univ. Press, Loeb Classical Library, 1962), 1:271; Celsus, *De medicina*, with an English translation by W. G. Spencer (Cambridge: Harvard Univ. Press, Loeb Classical Library, 1971), 1:159–65; Albucasis, *On surgery and instruments*, trans. and ed. M. S. Spink and G. L. Lewis (Berkeley: Univ. California Press, 1973), p. 624. Celsus admitted that the patient's disease might sometimes demand bloodletting when his body seemed scarcely able to bear it, yet it was "better to try a doubled-edged remedy than none at all."

2. Townsend W. Thorndike, "History of bleeding and leeching," *Boston M. & S. J.* (1927), 197:473–75; John J. Abel, "Experimental and chemical studies of the blood," *Science* (1915), 42:135–41. Abel was the distinguished pharmacologist of the original Hopkins faculty. John Harington's English version of the *Regimen* is published with historical studies by Francis R. Packard and Fielding H. Garrison in *The School of Salernum* (London: Humphrey Milford, Oxford Univ. Press, 1922). A venesection calendar by Johannes Muncz for the year 1495 is

one of the treasures of the Municipal Ervin Szabó Library of Budapest. The Minnesota Biomedical Rare Book Collection is fortunate to have a facsimile, a gift of the Budapest library.

3. Leonardo Botallo, *De cvratione per sangvinis missionem liber* (Antwerp, 1583), p. 143 (1st ed., 1577).

4. Georges Cornu, *A l'hôpital il y a deux siècles; l'Hôtel-Dieu, les compagnons chirurgiens et externes*, Paris thesis, 1897, pp. 31–32, 42; Charles Coury, February 28, 1972, personal communication.

5. Alain René Le Sage, *Adventures of Gil Blas of Santillane*, trans. Tobias Smollett (New York: Bigelow, Brown [n.d.]), 1:94–96. The character of Sangrado is reputedly drawn after Dr. Philippe Hecquet (1661–1737), dean of the Faculty of Medicine of Paris. F. Hobill Cole, "Doctors in fiction," *Intercolon. M. J. Australasia* (1906), 11:638.

6. D'Arcy Power, *William Harvey* (New York, 1898), pp. 214–19; John Hunter, *Treatise on the blood, inflammation, and gun-shot wounds* (Philadelphia, 1796), 2:287–88; Astley Cooper, *Lectures on the principles and practice of surgery*, with additional notes and cases by Frederick Tyrrell, 3d Am. ed. (Boston, 1831), 1:50–52.

7. George Munro Smith, *History of the Bristol Royal Infirmary* (Bristol: Arrowsmith, 1917), pp. 54–55; J. G. Swayne, quoted in Augustin Prichard, "The early history of the Bristol Medical School," *Bristol M.-Chir. J.* (1892), 10:287; John A. Shepherd, *Simpson and Syme of Edinburgh* (Edinburgh: E. and S. Livingstone, 1969), pp. 23–24.

8. The first issue of *Lancet* carried no editorial comment upon the significance of the chosen name.

9. James Craik and Elisha C. Dick [account of the death of General Washington], *Med. Reposit.*, New York (1800), 3:311–12; J. H. Mason Knox, Jr., "The medical history of George Washington, his physicians, friends and advisers," *Bull. Inst. Hist. Med.* (1933), 1:174–91; Creighton Barker, "A case report," *Yale J. Biol. Med.* (1936), 9:185–87; George W. Corner, *The autobiography of Benjamin Rush* (Princeton: Princeton Univ. Press, for the American Philosophical Soc., 1948), pp. 248–49. A recent account of this national tragedy credits Rush with being present at Washington's death and doing the bleedings! See *JAMA* (1970), 214:901. Ironically, as Corner points out, the only physician (Dick) to object to the final bleedings was trained in Rush's University of Pennsylvania Medical School. See also chapter 8 on tracheostomy.

10. James G. Mumford, *A narrative of medicine in America* (Philadelphia: J. B. Lippincott, 1903), pp. 213–14.

11. John Brown to his brother William, October 1, 1838, in *Letters of Dr. John Brown*, ed. by his son and D. W. Forrest (London: Adam and Charles Black, 1907), pp. 39–40. See chapter 22 on the surgical amphitheatre.

12. Paul B. Beeson, "Infectious diseases (microbiology)," in John Z. Bowers and Elizabeth F. Purcell, eds., *Advances in American medicine: Essays at the Bicentennial* (New York: Josiah Macy, Jr. Foundation, 1976), 1:102. Chase was subsequently secretary of the treasury, chief justice of the Supreme Court, and an unsuccessful candidate for the presidency.

13. Fielding H. Garrison, *Introduction to the history of medicine*, 4th ed. (Philadelphia: W. B. Saunders, 1929), p. 410; Guillaume Dupuytren, *Leçons orales de clinique chirurgicale* (Paris, 1832), 2:297; John T. Morse, Jr., *Life and letters of Oliver Wendell Holmes* (Boston, 1896), 1:92. François J. V. Broussais (1772–1838), a pupil of Bichat, after an active career in the Napoleonic Wars became physician-in-chief at Val-de-Grâce, Paris, where he ardently applied his debilitating therapy. J. B. Bouillaud (1797–1881), called the last of the great bloodletters, was an able clinician, especially in cardiac diseases.

14. Johann H. Baas, *Grundriss der Geschichte der Medicin* (Stuttgart, 1876), p. 694; Elie Masson, *Elève des sangsues* (Paris, 1854), p. 23. Baas adds that in the same year (1833) 9 or 10 million leeches were being *exported* from France. Masson tabulated that in 1852 France was importing 10,415,000 leeches, chiefly from Turkey, England, Spain, and Germany. According to G. Rochette of Montpellier (*Essai médical sur les sangsues*, Paris thesis, 1803), Hippocrates did not mention leeches; Rochette said that the first report of using leeches to draw blood is in Themison and that Pliny applied leeches for gout and against all sorts of fevers (pp. 23–24). Themison of Laodicea lived in the first century B.C.

15. William Brockbank, *Portrait of a hospital (1752–1948) . . . Bi-centenary of the Royal Infirmary, Manchester* (London: Heinemann, 1952), pp. 73–75; George Horn, *An entire new treatise on leeches* (London, 1798). D'Arcy Power gives the figures for leeches at St. Bartholomew's in "Dr. Marshall Hall and the decay of bloodletting," *Practitioner* (1909), 82:320–31. Anna Dostoevsky, *Reminiscences,* trans. Beatrice Stillman (New York: Liveright, 1977), p. 10.

16. Joannes B. van Helmont, *Ortus medicinae, id est initia physicae inaudita,* 4th ed. (Lyons, 1655); Robert Rosenthal, "An early opponent of venesection [Johann G. Wolstein]," *Med. Life,* New York (1922), 29:585–90.

17. Nathaniel Rumsey, "Fever, sometimes the effect of depletion, by bleeding," *Edinb. M. & S. J.* (1819), 15:55–58; John Hutton Balfour, *Probationary essay on purulent deposits after wounds and operations* (Edinburgh, 1833), pp. 5–16. Balfour (1808–84) later won distinction as a botanist. For typical accounts of death after venesection, see Nathaniel Chapman, *Eclect. Repert.,* Philadelphia (1812), 2:360–67, and reports from St. George's and St. Bartholomew's hospitals, *London M. Gaz.* (1828), 2:155–57, 796–97.

18. Elaine Eyster and James Bernene, "Nosocomial anemia," *JAMA* (1973), 223(1):73–74.

19. Pierre C. A. Louis, "Recherches sur les effets de la saignée dans plusieurs maladies inflammatoires," *Arch. gén. de méd.* (1828), 18:321–36 (this article formed the first chapter of Louis's definitive publication in 1835 under the same title); Marshall Hall, *Researches principally relative to the morbid and curative effects of loss of blood* (London, 1830); Leon S. Bryan, Jr., "Bloodletting in American medicine, 1830–1892," *Bull. Hist. Med.* (1964), 38:516–29. D'Arcy Power (n.15) sketched Hall's versatile career, including his physiological research in reflex action.

20. Louis Stromeyer, *Gunshot fractures,* trans. S. F. Statham (Philadelphia, 1862), pp. 25–26. Stromeyer found leeches helpful in reducing the inflammatory swelling of fractures, preferring them to phlebotomy. "The curative effects of bloodletting" were the subject of discussion at a meeting of the New York Academy of Medicine in 1867. A number of prominent surgeons recalled cases in which they felt phlebotomy had been beneficial; several said they always carried a lancet, though they rarely used it. One member asserted that if indications for bloodletting "were palpable, he could restrain from it no more than he could from pulling a child back from a precipice." *Bull. N.Y. Acad. Med.* (1868), 3:266–72.

21. William Osler, *The principles and practice of medicine* (New York, 1892), p. 530. In the sixteenth edition (1947) Henry A. Christian qualified the endorsement somewhat (p. 69) by saying that bleeding at the onset of pneumonia in robust individuals "possibly still is a good practice." Harry H. LeVeen presented his thesis at the University of Minnesota Veterans Hospital Seminar, May 4, 1978.

22. O. H. Wangensteen, "Anti- or prophlogistic treatment of acute infections," *Surgery* (1938), 4:140–44.

23. Augustus Waller, "Microscopic examination of some of the principal tissues of the animal frame," *Phil. Mag.* (1846), 29:271–87. William Addison (1843) postulated migration of leucocytes through capillary blood vessels, but it was Waller who first observed with the microscope the actual penetration of and migration of leucocytes through the endothelial vessel walls. Strangely, neither Garrison nor *Garrison-Morton* cites Waller for this amazing and significant observation. Waller (1816–70), an English physician who gave up practice to pursue experimental research abroad, was primarily a neurophysiologist and made the observation quite accidentally, but obviously realized fully its significance. His primary discoveries concerned the nervous system. Lister (1858) demonstrated stasis in and dilatation of the blood vessels of the web of the frog's foot and in the wings of bats when mustard or other irritant was applied, but missed the migration of leucocytes through the endothelial capillary walls that Waller had demonstrated twelve years earlier (*Phil. Trans.,* 148:645–702).

24. Julius Cohnheim, "Ueber Entzündung und Eiterung," Virchow's *Arch. f. path. Anat.* [etc.] (1867), 40:1–79; Rudolf Virchow, *Die Cellularpathologie in ihrer Begründung auf physiologische und pathologische Gewebelehre* (Berlin, 1858); L. J. Rather, "Rudolf Virchow's views

on pathology, pathological anatomy, and cellular pathology," *Archs Path.* (1966), 82:197–204; Rather, "The place of Virchow's 'cellular pathology' in medical thought," pp. v–xxvii, in Rudolf Virchow, *Cellular pathology as based upon physiological and pathological histology*, trans. Frank Chance (New York: Dover Publications, 1971).

25. Elie Metchnikoff, "Beitrag zur Lehre über den Kampf der Phagocyten gegen Krankheitserreger," Virchow's *Arch. f. path. Anat.* [etc.] (1884), 96:177–95; Joseph Lister, "Address on the present position of antiseptic surgery," *Br. M. J.* (1890), 2:377; Ernst Ziegler, "Immunität des menschlischen Organismus gegen Infectionskrankheiten," *Beitr. path. Anat.*, Jena (1889), 5:419–38.

26. William Addison, *Experimental and practical researches on inflammation and on the origin and nature of tubercles of the lungs* (London, 1843).

27. Gert H. Brieger, Introduction, pp. ix–xxxi, in Elie Metchnikoff, *Immunity in infective diseases*, trans. F. G. Binnie, Sources of science, no. 61 (Cambridge Univ. Press, 1905; reprint, New York: Johnson Reprint Corp., 1968); Benjamin W. Zweifach, Lester Grant, and Robert T. McCluskey, eds., *The inflammatory process* (New York and London: Academic Press, 1965); J. V. Hurley, *Acute inflammation* (Edinburgh and London: Churchill Livingstone, 1972).

Further Readings

Eleven pages of references on bloodletting are cited in The Surgeon General's *Index-Catalogue* (Washington, D.C., 1881), pp. 175–85. There are nine additional pages in the second series (1897), 2:478–86. Many authors in the latter group deplored the practice.

Chapter 15. Vascular Surgery

Notes

1. Galen, *Opera omnia*, ed. C. G. Kühn (Leipzig, 1826), 11:313. Galen's "De aneurysmate et sydratione" has been edited and translated by John E. Erichsen in *Observations on aneurism* (London: Sydenham Soc., vol. 5, 1844), p. 3.

2. Celsus, *De medicina*, with an English translation by W. G. Spencer (Cambridge: Harvard Univ. Press, Loeb Classical Library, 1938), 3:405–7; Ambroise Paré, *The workes of that famous chirurgion Ambrose Parey*, trans. Thomas Johnson (London, 1634), pp. 459–63; Jacques Guillemeau, *The French chirurgerye*, trans. A. M. (Dordrecht [Dort], 1597), fol. 38 recto and verso; Jean-Louis Petit, "D'un nouvel instrument de chirurgie," *Mém. Acad. roy. d. sci.* (1718), pp. 252–55. See chapter 2 on amputation (n.31).

3. Rudolph Matas, "Traumatic aneurism of the left brachial artery," *Med. News*, Philadelphia (1888), 53:462–66. In *L'art de succer les plaies* (Amsterdam, 1707), Dominique Anel wrote of ligating the brachial artery for aneurysm (p. 20). The details of the operation apparently were described later (1710). The subtitle of this 1707 effort led the reader to believe that the author was about to reveal a secret of curing syphilis. Anel rambles on for 20 pages about this, but in the end keeps the secret to himself. See also chapter 9 on empyema (n.26).

4. Xavier Bichat, *Oeuvres chirurgicales, ou exposé de la doctrine et de la practique de P. J. Desault* (Paris, 1801), 2:553–62, 568–71; Alexis Boyer, *Traité des maladies chirurgicales*, 2d ed. (Paris, 1818), 2:143–45. See also George J. Guthrie, *On the diseases and injuries of arteries, with the operations required for their cure* (London, 1830), pp. 146–47.

5. *Biographisches Lexikon der hervorragenden Arzte* (1962), 1:680, indicates that Pierre B. Brasdor became an *agrégé* in surgery in Paris in 1752 and professor of surgery shortly thereafter. It credits him with the origination of proximal ligation for aneurysm which, in fact, was Anel's innovation in 1710; also with the suggestion of distal ligation. We have failed to locate a Brasdor publication on the matter. Fielding H. Garrison also credits Brasdor with having originated distal ligation for aneurysm. *Introduction to the history of medicine*, 3d ed. (Philadelphia: W. B. Saunders, 1922), pp. 349, 517.

6. Joseph-F. L. Deschamps (1740–1825) was chief of surgery at La Charité. His account of the operation is given in Bichat, *Oeuvres de Desault* (n.4), 2:572–80. Among those present were Boyer and Brasdor; no mention is made of Brasdor having performed or advocated distal ligation for aneurysm. Of the nine consultants, three advised incision of the tumor, six favored distal ligation. Boyer, who opposed the operation, also describes the occasion in *Maladies chirurgicales* (n.4), 2:145–64.

7. Guthrie, *Arteries* (n.4); James Wardrop, "Case of carotid aneurism, successfully treated by tying the artery above the aneurismal tumour," *Med.-Chir. Trans.* (1825), 13:217–26.

8. Everard Home, "An account of Mr. Hunter's method of performing the operation for the popliteal aneurism," *London M. J.* (1786), 7:391–406; Garrison, *History of medicine* (n.5), p. 355.

9. The second part of Giovanni Maria Lancisi's *De motu cordis et aneurysmatibus* (Rome, 1745) has been revised and translated by Wilmer Cave Wright and published under the auspices of the New York Academy of Medicine as *De aneurysmatibus, opus posthumum* (New York: Macmillan, 1952). When the unprinted anatomical plates of Bartolomeus Eustachius (1552) were discovered in the Library of the Vatican, Lancisi edited and published them. Eustachius, *Tabulae anatomicae* (Rome, 1714).

10. Lancisi (n.9), pp. 119–23, 143–75.

11. Astley Cooper, "A case of aneurism of the carotid artery," *Med.-Chir. Trans.* (1809), 1:1–12, and "Second case of carotid aneurism," ibid., pp. 224–35. The reports were read before the Medical and Chirurgical Society, January 29, 1806, and February 21, 1809, respectively. See also Cooper's "Account of the first successful operation, performed on the common carotid artery, for aneurism, in the year 1808: With the post-mortem examination in 1821," *Guy's Hosp. Rep.* (1836), 1:53–58.

12. John Abernethy, *Surgical observations* (London, 1809), pp. 234–92, the first published report of the 1796 operation. Cooper's appreciation of Abernethy's contribution is expressed in Charles Mingay Syder, ed., *Series of lectures . . . by Astley Cooper*, 1st Am. ed. (Boston, 1823), p. 180. The work was published originally by Charles William Jones, a former pupil of Cooper.

13. Emile Holman showed that the division of an artery and ligature or suture of both ends is less likely to be accompanied by leakage than is mere simple ligation. See his "War injuries to arteries and their treatment," *Surg. Gynec. Obstet.* (1942), 75:186, and "Further observations on surgery of the large arteries," ibid. (1944), 78:286.

14. Such rupture is more readily achieved if the arterial inflow at the site of ligature is temporarily arrested.

15. William Osler, "Sir Astley Cooper's case of ligature of the abdominal aorta," *Guy's Hosp. Gaz.* (1911), 25:277. Osler quotes a letter written by his Uncle Edward at the time.

16. George Tully Vaughn (1921) reported a successful distal ligature of the aorta for aneurysm in *Ann. Surg.*, 74:308–12.

17. Benjamin Travers, "On wounds and ligatures of veins," in Astley Cooper and Travers, *Surgical essays*, 1st Am. ed. (Philadelphia, 1821), pp. 167–214.

18. J.-L. Jaillot, *De la ligature dans les hémorrhagies artérielles consécutives, compliquant les blessures par armes à feu*, Paris thesis, 1857.

19. John G. Crosse kept a "Black Book of Surgery," in which he noted errors seen during his practice. One such entry described an aneurysm at the elbow, the result of an apothecary's opening the artery instead of the vein during bloodletting. V. Mary Crosse, *A surgeon of the early nineteenth century . . . John Green Crosse* (Edinburgh: E. & S. Livingstone, 1968), p. 143.

20. Robert Liston, *Practical surgery*, with notes by George W. Norris (Philadelphia, 1838), pp. 129–37.

21. Valentine Mott: "Reflections on securing in a ligature the arteria innominata," *Med. & Surg. Reg.*, New York (1818), 1:9–54; "Case of aneurism of the right subclavian artery, in which that vessel was tied within the scaleni muscles," *Am. J. Med. Sci.* (1833), 12:354–59;

"Aneurism of the arteria innominata involving the subclavian and the root of the carotid, successfully treated by tying the carotid artery," ibid. (1829), 5:297–300; and "Case of diffused femoral aneurism, for which the external iliac artery was tied," ibid. (1831), 8:393–97.

22. "Valentine Mott," *Lancet* (1865), 1:553.

23. George W. Norris: "Table showing the mortality following the operation of tying the iliac arteries," *Am. J. Med. Sci.* (1847), 13:13–26, and "Statistics of the mortality following the operation of tying the carotid arteries and arteria innominata," ibid., 14:13–40. In 30 cases of wounds of the carotid artery, 15 (50 percent) died. The first operation was performed by Fleming, a ship's surgeon, in 1803; the last, by F. Le Gros Clark, 1846, according to Norris. Of ligature of the carotid artery, during extirpation of tumors, Norris reported 6 deaths (44 percent mortality). The first operation was done by Mason F. Cogswell, 1803; the last reported, 1844, by Charles Bell Gibson, son of William Gibson. In both papers there were some instances in which pulsation in the aneurysm returned. When hemorrhage followed ligature of the carotid or external iliac arteries, the outcome was usually fatal.

24. Luigi Porta, *Delle alterazioni patologische delle arterie per la legatura e la torsione* (Milan, 1845).

25. Paul Broca, *Des anévrysmes et de leur traitement* (Paris, 1856), pp. 269–70, 300.

26. C. Pravaz [letter to the editor], *Gaz. méd. Paris* (1831), 2:20. See also R. Marjolin's biography of Charles-G. Pravaz (1791–1853) in *Mém. Soc. chir. Paris* (1857), 4:714–22. Pravaz was a surgeon who sought to apply the laws of chemistry and physics to surgical therapy. His work was continued by his son.

27. William Stewart Halsted, *Surgical papers*, ed. Walter C. Burket, 2 vols. (Baltimore: The Johns Hopkins Press, 1924), 1:311–586.

28. Halsted: "Ligation of the first portion of the left subclavian artery and excision of a subclavio-axillary aneurism," *Johns Hopkins Hosp. Bull.* (1892), 3:93–94 (*Surgical papers*, 1:311–13), and "Partial occlusion of blood-vessels, especially of the abdominal aorta," ibid. (1905), 16:346–47 (*Surgical papers*, 1:314–17).

29. Halsted, "Results of the complete and incomplete occlusion of the abdominal and thoracic aortas by metal bands," *JAMA* (1906), 47(2):2147–48 (*Surgical papers*, 1:318–20). The account of William W. Keen's operation for abdominal aneurysm and death of the patient from hemorrhage appears in *Am. J. Med. Sci.* (1900), 120:251–77.

30. Halsted: "Clinical and experimental contributions to the surgery of the thorax," *Trans. Am. Surg. Assoc.* (1909), 27:111–15 (*Surgical papers*, 1:321–24), and Discussion, ibid. (1910), 28:49–52 (*Surgical papers*, 1:325–28).

31. Halsted, "The effect of ligation of the common iliac artery on the circulation and function of the lower extremity," *Trans. Am. Surg. Assoc.* (1912), 30:196–286 (*Surgical papers*, 1:329–97). William Gibson (1788–1868) succeeded Physick as professor of surgery at the University of Pennsylvania in 1819.

32. Halsted: *Surgical papers*, 1:398–420, and "Der partielle Verschluss grosser Arterien," *Verh. dt. Ges. Chir.*, Berlin (1914), 43(2):349–67 (*Surgical papers*, 1:421–34). An attempt made by Halsted to ligate the aorta, proximal as well as distal to an aortic aneurysm, before a large and distinguished group of visiting German surgeons at The Hopkins was recounted by George Heuer, who was Halsted's senior surgical resident at the time. During the manipulation Halsted broke into the aneurysm with his aneurysm needle. Heuer stopped the bleeding manually by compression of the proximal aorta while Halsted mobilized the aorta proximal to the aneurysm and tied it. The German surgeons, says Heuer, "were vastly impressed." The patient survived for forty-eight hours; Heuer commented, "the proximal ligature around the aorta had occluded one and probably the other renal artery." Heuer, "Dr. Halsted," *Bull. Johns Hopkins Hosp.*, suppl. (1952), 90:50.

33. Halsted, "As to the cause of the dilatation of the subclavian artery observed in some cases of cervical rib," and "Experimental study of circumscribed dilation of an artery immediately distal to a partially occluding band," *Trans. Am. Surg. Assoc.* (1916), 34:273–88 (*Surgical papers*, 1:437–52). A supplemental article appears in *Surgical papers*, 1:453–56. Sev-

eral additional papers on arterial venous aneurysms and on lymphogenous cysts in the neck are reprinted in *Surgical papers*, 1:457–82.

34. Halsted, "Ligations of the left subclavian artery in its first portion," *Johns Hopkins Hosp. Rep.* (1921), 21:1–96 (*Surgical papers*, 1:483–572); Oribasius, *Oeuvres*, ed. U. C. Bussemaker and Charles Daremberg (Paris, 1862), 4:52–56. R. W. Livingstone was the author of *Meaning of the Greek genius* (1915). His translation appears in Osler's "Remarks on arteriovenous aneurysm," *Lancet* (1915), 1:950–51. Halsted referred to Gurlt's translation of Antyllus's method of treating aneurysms in *Geschichte der Chirurgie* (1898), 1:483.

35. The first ligation was done by J. Kearney Rodgers and published in *N. York J. M.* (1846), 7:102–3.

36. Jay McLean, "The thromboplastic action of cephalin," *Am. J. Physiol.* (1916), 41:250–57.

37. Halsted, *Surgical papers*, 1:487.

38. Alexander Jassinowsky, "Ein Beitrag zur Lehre von der Gefässnaht," *Arch. klin. Chir.* (1891), 42:816–41. The work was done at the Physiological Institute at Dorpat.

39. Julius Dörfler, "Ueber Arteriennaht," *Beitr. klin. Chir.* (1899), 25:781–825; F. Villar and Brachet, "Suture des veines: Étude expérimentale," *J. de méd. de Bordeaux* (1895), 25:585–88; Lothar Heidenhain, "Über Naht von Arterienwunden," *Centralbl. f. Chir.* (1895), 22:1113–15.

40. Alexis Carrel, "La technique opératoire des anastomoses vasculaires et la transplantation des viscères," *Lyon méd.* (1902), 98:859–64.

41. Alescis [Alexis] Carrel: "The surgery of blood vessels, etc.," *Johns Hopkins Hosp. Bull.* (1907), 18:18–28, and "Results of the transplantation of blood vessels, organs and limbs," *JAMA* (1908), 51:1662–67. If the award had been given just for Carrel's technique of blood vessel suture, the prior work of Jassinowsky and Dörfler should have been recognized by the Nobel committee. Carrel (1873–1944) had become identified in his research with Charles Claude Guthrie (1880–1963) at the University of Chicago before going to the Rockefeller Institute; they were joint authors of several published papers. Friends of Guthrie have expressed disappointment that he was not recognized in the Nobel Award with Carrel. As a young surgeon at Lyons, Carrel (1902) had already described his technique of arterial suture (*Lyon méd.*, 98:859–64). He was seven years older than Guthrie and their period of collaboration at the University of Chicago was less than two years; it is not unlikely that Carrel regarded Guthrie as his "assistant" rather than partner in the research. See also Serge J. Dos, "The Carrel-Guthrie controversy," *Surgery* (1975), 77:330–32.

42. Reynaldo dos Santos et al., "L'artériographie des membres de l'aorte et de ses branches abdominales," *Medna contemp.*, Lisbon (1929), 47:93–96; Werner T. O. Forssmann, "Die Sondierung des rechten Herzens," *Klin. Wschr.* (1929), 8:2085–87, 2287. A. J. Benatt wrote a brief historical review of cardiac catheterization in *Lancet* (1949), 1:746–47. A. F. Cournand, D. W. Richards, and Forssmann were awarded the Nobel Prize for their work on cardiac catheterization in 1956.

43. McLean (n.36). William H. Howell and Emmett Holt gave heparin its name. *Am. J. Physiol.* (1918), 47:328–41.

44. A. F. Charles and D. A. Scott, "Preparation of heparin," *J. Biol. Chem.* (1933), 102:425–29; D. A. Scott and A. F. Charles, "Purification of heparin," ibid., pp. 437–48; J. Erik Jorpes, "The chemistry of heparin," *Biochem. J.* (1935), 29:1817–30; D. W. Gordon Murray, L. B. Jaques, T. S. Perrett, and C. H. Best, "Heparin and the thrombosis of veins following injury," *Surgery* (1937), 2:163–87; J. Erik Jorpes, "On the dosage of the anticoagulants, heparin and dicumarol, in the treatment of thrombosis," *Acta chir. scand.* (1950), suppl. 149, p. 1.

45. Emile Holman, "Experimental studies in arteriovenous fistula," *Arch. Surg.* (1924), 9:822–55, 856–79; C. W. Lillehei, J. R. R. Bobb, and M. B. Visscher, "Occurrence of endocarditis with valvular deformities in dogs with arteriovenous fistulas," *Ann. Surg.* (1950), 132:577–90.

46. Nikolai V. Eck, [Ligature of the portal vein], *Voyenno-med. J.*, St. Petersburg (1877),

130(2):1–2, trans. C. Gardner Child III, *Surg. Gynec. Obstet.* (1953), 96:375–76; Allen O. Whipple, "Problem of portal hypertension in relation to hepatosplenopathies," *Ann. Surg.* (1945), 122:449–75; John F. Perry, Jr., Harlan D. Root, Fletcher A. Miller, and Richard L. Varco, "Total removal of the intrathoracic esophagus and antethoracic jejunal replacement for treatment of esophageal varices due to extrahepatic portal block," *Ann. Surg.* (1963), 158:126–28.

47. Max Schede, "Operative Behandlung der Unterschenkelvaricen," *Berl. klin. Wschr.* (1877), 14:85–89; Fr. Trendelenburg, "Unterbindung der Vena saphena magna bei Unterschenkelvaricen," *Beitr. klin. Chir.* (1890), 7:195–210; John Homans, "Operative treatment of varicose veins and ulcers, based upon a classification of these lesions," *Surg. Gynec. Obstet.* (1916), 22:143–58; Homans, "Etiology and treatment of varicose ulcer of the leg," ibid. (1917), 24:300–11; Homans, *N. Engl. J. Med.* (1934), 211:993–97; (1941), 224:179–86.

48. S. Jacobsson, U. Rothman, G. Arturson, K. Ganrot, K. Haeger, and I. Juhlin, "A new principle for the cleansing of infected wounds," *Scand. J. Plast. Reconstr. Surg.* (1976), 10:65–72.

49. L. Rehn, "Ueber Perikardiale Verwachsungen," *Medsche Klin.* (1920), 16:999–1003; Franz Volhard and Victor Schmieden, "Über Erkennung und Behandlung der Umklammerung des Herzens durch Schwielige Perikarditis," *Klin. Wschr.* (1923), 2:5–9; Schmieden and H. Fischer, "Die Herzbeutelentzündung und ihre Folgezustände," *Ergebn. Chir. Orthop.* (1926), 19:98–216; Edward D. Churchill, "Decortication of the heart (Delorme) for adhesive pericarditis," *Arch. Surg.* (1929), 19:1457–69; Edmond Delorme, "Sur un traitement de la symphyse cardo-péricardique," *Bull. mém. Soc. chir. Paris* (1898), 24:918–22. Delorme suggested but did not perform pericardiectomy, invoking his earlier suggestion of visceral pleurectomy to mobilize a collapsed lung following chronic empyema.

50. Robert E. Gross and John P. Hubbard, "Surgical ligation of a patent ductus arteriosus," *JAMA* (1939), 112(1):729–31; Gross, "Complete surgical division of the patent ductus arteriosus, a report of 14 successful cases," *Surg. Gynec. Obstet.* (1944), 78:36–43; Clarence Crafoord and G. Nylin, "Congenital coarctation of the aorta and its surgical treatment," *J. Thorac. Surg.* (1945), 14:347–61; Gross and Charles A. Hufnagel, "Coarctation of the aorta, experimental studies regarding its surgical correction," *New Engl. J. Med.* (1945), 233:287–93; Gross, "Surgical relief for tracheal obstruction from a vascular ring," ibid. (1945), 233:586–90; Gross, "Surgical treatment for dysphagia lusoria," *Ann. Surg.* (1946), 124:532–34.

51. Alfred Blalock and Helen B. Taussig, "The surgical treatment of malformations of the heart in which there is pulmonary stenosis or pulmonary atresia," *JAMA* (1945), 128:189–202.

52. Charles Dubost, Michel Allary, and Nicolas Oeconomos, "A propos du traitement des anévrysmes de l'aorte," *Mém. Acad. chir.* (1951), 77:381–83; Michael E. DeBakey and Denton A. Cooley, "Surgical treatment of aneurysm of abdominal aorta by resection and restoration of continuity with homograft," *Surg. Gynec. Obstet.* (1953), 97:257–66; Henry T. Bahnson, "Definitive treatment of saccular aneurysms of the aorta with excision of sac and aortic suture," *Surg. Gynec. Obstet.* (1953), 96:383–402; Erich Lexer, *Dt. Ges. Chir.* (1907), 36(2):215–33; ibid. (1912), 41(1):132–35; ibid. (1913), 42(1):113–16.

53. Clarence Crafoord, "Two cases of obstructive pulmonary embolism successfully operated upon," *Acta chir. scand.* (1928), 64:172–86; Martin Kirschner, "Ein durch die Trendelenburgsche Operation geheilter Fall von Embolie der Art. pulmonalis," *Arch. klin. Chir.* (1924), 133:312–59.

54. Thomas J. Fogarty, John J. Cranley, Raymond J. Krause, R. J. Strasser, Edward S. Strasser, and Charles D. Hafner, "Method for extraction of arterial emboli and thrombi," *Surg. Gynec. Obstet.* (1963), 116:241.

55. John H. Gibbon: "An oxygenator with a large surface-volume ratio," *J. Lab. Clin. Med.* (1939), 24:1192–98, and "Application of a mechnical heart and lung apparatus to cardiac surgery," *Minn. Med.* (1954), 37:171–80, 185.

56. Herbert E. Warden, Morley Cohen, Raymond C. Read, and C. Walton Lillehei, "Controlled cross circulation for open intracardiac surgery," *J. Thorac. Surg.* (1954), 28:331–43; Lillehei, "Controlled cross circulation for direct-vision intracardiac surgery," *Postgrad. Med.* (1955), 17:388–96; Warden, Richard A. DeWall, Read, Joseph B. Aust, Cohen, Richard L. Varco, and Lillehei, "Total cardiac by-pass utilizing continuous perfusion from reservoir of oxygenated blood," *Proc. Soc. Exp. Biol. Med.* (1955), 90:246–50; Warden, Read, DeWall, Aust, Cohen, Newell R. Ziegler, Varco, and Lillehei, "Direct vision intracardiac surgery by means of a reservoir of 'arterialized venous' blood," *J. Thorac. Surg.* (1955), 30:649–57; Lillehei, DeWall, Read, Warden, and Varco, "Direct vision intracardiac surgery in man using a simple disposable artificial oxygenator," *Dis. Chest* (1956), 29:1–8; Lillehei, DeWall, Vincent L. Gott, and Varco, "Direct vision correction of calcific aortic stenosis," *Dis. Chest* (1956), 30:123–32. In 1961 DeWall wrote the history of pump oxygenators and was surprised to learn that Waldemar Schröder had built a similar apparatus in 1882. *Surgery* (1961), 50:935.

57. F. John Lewis and Mansur Taufic, "Closure of atrial septal defects with the aid of hypothermia . . . report of one successful case," *Surgery* (1953), 33:52–59.

58. Clarence Dennis, Dwight S. Spreng, Jr., George E. Nelson, Karl E. Karlson, Russell M. Nelson, John V. Thomas, Walter P. Eder, and R. L. Varco, "Development of a pump-oxygenator to replace the heart and lungs; an apparatus applicable to human patients, and application to one case," *Ann. Surg.* (1951), 134(2):709–21. Dennis was probably the first to employ the pump oxygenator clinically; a girl of six years with a large interatrial septal defect, cyanosis, and pulmonary edema did not survive the operative procedure performed April 5, 1951.

59. An editorial in the December 16, 1967, issue of the *South African Medical Journal* 41(4):1181 announced that Christiaan N. Barnard and the Groote Schuur Hospital Transplant Team had performed a successful cardiac transplant December 3, 1967. In presenting Barnard to the University Chancellor for the degree of Doctor of Science Honoris Causa, it was said, "If the University of Cape Town was Barnard's alma mater, Minnesota was his fairy godmother." (Ibid., December 30, 1967, p. 1259.) Barnard's description of the operation appeared on pp. 1271–74. The patient, Louis Washkansky, died December 21, 1967.

60. Richard R. Lower and Norman E. Shumway, "Studies on orthotopic homotransplantation of the canine heart," *Surg. Forum* (1961), 11:18–19; Shumway, July 25, 1976, personal communication. In 1964 Shumway and his associates reported that of four orthotopic reimplantations of excised canine hearts, cardiac reinnervation was complete and myocardial function normal. Restoration of cardiac innervation fails to attend homograft cardiac transplants (*Surgery*, 56:270–74).

Further Readings

Ballance, Charles A., and Edmunds, Walter. *A treatise on the ligation of the great arteries in continuity with observation on the nature, progress, and treatment of aneurism.* London, 1891.

Biggs, Rosemary, and Macfarlane, Robert G. *Human blood coagulation and its disorders.* 3d ed. Philadelphia: F. A. Davis, 1962.

Birnstingl, Martin, ed. *Peripheral vascular surgery.* Philadelphia: J. B. Lippincott, 1973.

Brock, Russell. *The life and work of Astley Cooper.* Edinburgh and London: E. and S. Livingstone, 1952.

Butler, Richard L.; Byles, Peter; and Port, Lawrence. Intrathoracic pressure as a tourniquet to tamponade bleeding esophageal varices. *Am. J. Gastroent.* (1976), 66:441–47.

Colles, Abraham. On the operation of tying the subclavian artery. *Edinb. M. & S. J.* (1815), 11:1–25.

Cooley, Denton A.; Mahaffey, Daniel E.; and DeBakey, Michael E. Total excision of the aortic arch for aneurysm. *Surg. Gynec. Obstet.* (1955), 101:667–72.

Cotton, L. T., and Roberts, V. C. Prevention of deep vein thrombosis, with particular reference to mechanical methods of prevention. *Surgery* (1977), 81:228–35.

Dale, W. Andrew. *Autogenous vein grafts and related aspects of peripheral arterial disease.* Springfield, Ill.: Charles C Thomas, 1959.

Dennis, Clarence. Disaster following femoral vein ligation for thrombophlebitis, relief by fasciotomy. *Surgery* (1945), 17:264–69.

Dorsey, John Syng. Inguinal aneurism cured by tying the external iliac artery in the pelvis. *Eclect. Repert.* (1811), 2:111–15.

Edwards, W. Sterling. *Plastic arterial grafts.* Springfield, Ill.: Charles C Thomas, 1957.

Engelberg, Hyman. *Heparin: Metabolism, physiology, and clinical application.* Springfield, Ill.: Charles C Thomas, 1963.

Goor, Daniel A., and Lillehei, C. Walton. *Congenital malformations of the heart.* New York: Grune and Stratton, 1975.

Green, Richard M.; DeWeese, James A.; and Rob, Charles G. Arterial embolectomy before and after the Fogarty catheter. *Surgery* (1975), 77:24–33.

Gross, Robert E. *Surgical treatment for abnormalities of the heart and great vessels.* American lecture series, no. 3. Springfield, Ill.: Charles C Thomas, 1947.

Gross, Samuel D. *Memoir of Valentine Mott.* Philadelphia and New York, 1868.

Guthrie, George J. Case of a wound of the peroneal artery successfully treated by a ligature. *Med.-Chir. Trans.* (1816), 7:330–37.

Haimovici, Henry, ed. *Surgical management of vascular diseases.* Philadelphia: J. B. Lippincott, 1970.

Hodgson, Joseph. *Treatise on the diseases of arteries and veins, containing the pathology and treatment of aneurisms and wounded arteries.* London, 1815.

Holden, William D. *Acute peripheral arterial occlusion.* American lecture series, no. 141. Springfield, Ill.: Charles C Thomas, 1952.

Holman, Emile. *Arteriovenous aneurysm; abnormal communications between the arterial and venous circulations.* New York: Macmillan, 1937.

————. *New concepts in surgery of the vascular system.* American lecture series, no. 271. Springfield, Ill.: Charles C Thomas, 1955.

Johnson, Shirley A., and Seegers, Walter H., eds. *Physiology of hemostasis and thrombosis.* Springfield, Ill.: Charles C Thomas, 1967.

Jorpes, J. Erik. *Heparin; its chemistry, physiology, and application in medicine.* London: Oxford Univ. Press, 1939.

————. *Heparin in the treatment of thrombosis; an account of its chemistry, physiology, and application in medicine.* 2d ed. London: Oxford Univ. Press, 1946.

Kwaan, J. H. M.; Jones, R. N.; and Connolly, J. E. Simplified technique for management of refractory varicose ulcers. *Surgery* (1976), 80:743–47.

Lawrence, D.; Fish, S. J.; and Kakkar, V. V. Blood-flow in incompetent perforating veins. *Lancet* (1977), 1:117–18.

Linton, Robert R. John Homans' impact on diseases of the veins of the lower extremity, with special reference to deep thrombophlebitis and the post-thrombotic syndrome with ulceration. *Surgery* (1977), 81:1–11.

Lister, Joseph. Observations on ligature of arteries on the antiseptic system. *Lancet* (1869), 1:451–55.

Little, J. M. *Major amputations for vascular disease.* Edinburgh and New York: Churchill Livingstone, 1975.

Macilwain, George. *Memoirs of John Abernethy.* New York, 1853.

Maunoir, Jean-Pierre. *Mémoires physiologiques et pratiques sur l'anéurisme et la ligature des artères.* Geneva, 1802.

Mott, Valentine. Ligature of the arteria iliaca communis, at its origin. *Phila. J. M. & Phys. Sci.* (1827), 14:176.

Norman, John C., ed. *Cardiac surgery.* 2d ed. New York: Appleton-Century-Crofts, 1972.

Post, Wright. Successful ligation of the femoral artery; 1796. *Am. M. & Phil. Reg.* (1814), 4:452.

Ravitch, Mark M. Sir Astley Paston Cooper. *Bull. Am. Coll. Surg.* (1977), 62:17–20.
Shumacker, Harris B., Jr. A moment with Matas. *Surg. Gynec. Obstet.* (1977), 144:93–98.
Silver, Donald, and Sabiston, David C., Jr. Role of vena caval interruption in the management of pulmonary embolism. *Surgery* (1975), 77:1–10.
Swan, Kenneth G., ed. *Venous surgery in the lower extremities.* St. Louis: Warren H. Green, 1975.
Syme, James. Case of iliac aneurism. *Med.-Chir. Trans.* (1862), 45:381–87.
Thornton, John L. *John Abernethy; a biography.* London: Simpkin Marshall, 1953.
Warren, Richard, and Record, Eugene E. *Lower extremity amputations for arterial insufficiency.* Boston: Little, Brown, 1967.

Chapter 16. Anesthesia

NOTES

1. Sydney Smith, *Wit and wisdom of the Rev. Sydney Smith* (London, n.d.), p. 37; Ralph Waldo Emerson, "The American scholar," an oration delivered before the Phi Beta Kappa Society, Cambridge, 1837. Smith's provocative rebuke appeared in an editorial in the *Edinburgh Review* (1820), of which he was a founder. It was printed on the title page of the *Philadelphia Journal of the Medical and Physical Sciences* from its opening issue in 1820 until 1824.

2. No attempt has been made in this chapter to trace all facets in the intricate history of anesthesia; we have selected a few events which most directly affected the surgeon's practice and the progress of surgery. Among the numerous volumes devoted to the discovery and study of anesthetic agents and the conflicts over priority, a small selection will be found in the further readings.

3. Henry J. Bigelow, "Insensibility during surgical operations produced by inhalation," *Boston M. & S. J.* (1846), 35:309–17. Bigelow adds (p. 316) that the invention had been patented under the names of Charles T. Jackson and W. T. C. Morton, with the latter as proprietor. For John Collins Warren's account, see *Boston M. & S. J.* (1846), 35:375–79.

4. According to John F. Fulton and Madeline E. Stanton, *Centennial of surgical anesthesia* (New York: Schuman, 1946), p. 20, the earliest account of Cordus' discovery appears in his posthumous works, published by Conrad Gesner in 1561 at Strasbourg. An English translation was provided by Guy K. Tallmadge, "The third part of the *De extractione* of Valerius Cordus," *Isis* (1925), 7:394–411. In the same volume of *Isis* (pp. 14–24) Chauncey D. Leake gives an account of Cordus and his discovery of ether.

5. Crawford W. Long, "An account of the first use of sulphuric ether by inhalation as an anaesthetic in surgical operations," *South. M. & S. J.* (1849), 5:705–13. The article contained certified affidavits suggesting that Long intended to claim priority of discovery. See also Hugh H. Young, "Long, the discoverer of anaesthesia: A presentation of his original documents," *Johns Hopkins Hosp. Bull.* (1897), 8:174–84.

6. Morrill Wyman in a letter (February 15, 1877) to J. Collins Warren, grandson of the Warren who did the operation under ether. The letter appears in Warren's 1897 presidential address to the American Surgical Association, *Trans. Am. Surg. Assoc.* (1897), 15:11.

7. Humphry Davy, *Researches, chemical and philosophical, chiefly concerning nitrous oxide* (London, 1800), pp. 456, 556; F. F. Cartwright, *The English pioneers of anaesthesia: Beddoes, Davy, and Hickman* (Bristol: Wright, 1952). Davy (1778–1829), celebrated chemist and physicist, started as an assistant in Thomas Beddoes's Medical Pneumatic Institute in Bristol. Prominent literary and social leaders, including Samuel Taylor Coleridge, participated in some of Davy's experiments with the gas. An interesting analysis of the shifting attitudes revealed by the many biographers of Davy throughout the years has been made by J. Z. Fullmer, *Science* (1967), 155:285–91. The authors do not regard Henry H. Hickman's suspended animation (1824) as a form of anesthesia. Inhalation of carbon dioxide without air or oxygen is simple asphyxia, a serious threat to the viability of the vital centers. See Hickman's *Letter on suspended animation* (Ironbridge, 1824), listed in *Garrison-Morton*, #5647.

8. Horace Wells, *History of the discovery of the application of nitrous oxide gas, ether, and other vapors, to surgical operations* (Hartford, Conn., 1847); W. Harry Archer, "Chronological history of Horace Wells, discoverer of anesthesia," *Bull. Hist. Med.* (1939), 7:1140–69. Wells and Morton shared a partnership in dentistry during the winter of 1842–43, dissolved as unremunerative. Wells's first claim to priority in use of nitrous oxide for surgical anesthesia was his letter to the editor of the *Hartford Courant*, printed December 9, 1846.

9. Fulton and Stanton, *Centennial* (n.4), pp. 66–71. Jackson was a member of the Harvard faculty, and favorably known to the staff of the hospital; even so, he received no support from its staff in his desire to arrogate to himself sole credit for the achievement.

10. Fulton and Stanton, *Centennial* (n.4), pp. 32, 56.

11. Many of the conflicting views of priority in the Boston ether controversy are to be found in the reports of the Select Committee of Congress to whom the question of a memorial to the discoverer of anesthesia was referred. The claimants and their sponsors likewise printed numerous pamphlets stating their claims. On the occasion of the ether anesthesia centennial Fulton and Stanton (n.4) provided detailed bibliographical accounts of the sequence of events in the development of surgical anesthesia.

12. A. L. Cox, "Experiments with the Letheon in New York," *Boston M. & S. J.* (1846), 35:456–59.

13. James E. Eckenhoff, *Anesthesia from colonial times: A history of anesthesia at the University of Pennsylvania* (Philadelphia: Lippincott, 1966), pp. 26–28.

14. Barbara M. Duncum, *Development of inhalation anaesthesia* (London: Oxford Univ. Press for Wellcome Historical Medical Museum, 1947), pp. 120, 130–32; Francis Boott, letter to the editor, December 22, 1846, *Lancet* (1847), 1:8. Boott, an American-born general practitioner, had received his education at Harvard; he prepared the specifications for the inhaler used in the extraction. The first operation under ether in Ireland was performed eleven days after Liston's, January 1, 1847, by John MacDonnell at the Richmond Surgical Hospital, relates J. D. H. Widdess in *Ir. J. Med. Sci.* (1946), pp. 649–55.

15. Joseph Lister, then a medical student at University College Hospital, was in the audience. This has often been denied, but in 1896, during his presidency of the British Association for the Advancement of Science, Lister stated that he had witnessed the dramatic operation.

16. F. William Cock, "The first major operation under ether in England," *Am. J. Surg.* (1915), 29(anesthesia suppl.):98–106; William Squire, "The first operation under ether in Great Britain," *Br. M. J.* (1896), 2:142–43; W. R. Merrington, *University College Hospital and its medical school: A history* (London: Heinemann, 1976), pp. 31–35. Robert Liston died of an aneurysm of the arch of the aorta only a year after this operation (December 7, 1847). William Squire was a nephew of Peter Squire, the chemist who made Liston's ether inhaler. Cock (p. 104) also reported that in the pre-anesthetic era a patient granted Liston permission to operate upon him for vesical calculus. When the time came for the operation, the patient had locked himself in the toilet! Liston forced open the door, fastened the patient to the table, and proceeded with the perineal lithotomy. Liston was obviously a surgeon of determination.

17. Chloroform was the simultaneous finding of three different investigators in 1831: Samuel Guthrie in America, Eugène Souberian in France, and Justus Liebig in Germany. Thereafter its properties were explored by a number of other scientists. Simpson (1811–70), son of a Scottish farmer, entered Edinburgh University at age fourteen and was appointed to the chair of midwifery there at twenty-eight. He was the first to use chloroform in childbirth. His contributions in many other aspects of surgery and obstetrics as well as hospital salubrity are mentioned in other chapters.

18. James Y. Simpson, "Discovery of a new anaesthetic agent, more efficient than sulphuric ether," *London M. Gaz.* (1847), 5:934–37; Thomas E. Keys, *History of surgical anesthesia* (New York: Dover, 1963), p. 33.

19. See chapter 13 on vesicovaginal fistula.

20. Andreas Vesalius, *De humani corporis fabrica libri septem* (Basel, 1543), p. 658; Robert

Hooke, "An account of an experiment . . . preserving animals alive by blowing through their lungs with bellows," *Phil. Trans.* (1667), 2:539–40. Théodore Tuffier and Louis Hallion (1896) reported having maintained the lungs of dogs inflated during open pneumothorax, insufflating the lungs through a tracheostomy tube at 10 cm. water pressure (*Compt. rend. Soc. d. biol.*, 48:951–53). Trendelenburg's (1871) use of tracheostomy in inhalation anesthesia for jaw resections and other neck operations has been described in chapter 8 on tracheostomy.

21. George E. Fell, "Forced respiration," *JAMA* (1891), 16:325–30; Rudolph Matas, "Intralaryngeal insufflation for the relief of acute surgical pneumothorax," *JAMA* (1900), 34:1468–73; Samuel J. Meltzer and John Auer, "Continuous respiration without respiratory movements," *J. Exp. Med.* (1909), 11:622–25; Meltzer, "On subphrenic abscess," *N.Y. Med. J.* (1893), 57:692–96.

22. Ernst Ferdinand Sauerbruch, "Ueber die physiologischen und physikalischen Grundlagen bei intrathorakalen Eingriffen in meiner pneumatischen Operationskammer," *Verh. dt. Ges. Chir.* (1904), 33(2):105–15; Rudolf Nissen, *Erlebtes aus der Thorax-Chirurgie* (Stuttgart: Georg Thieme, 1955), pp. 24–27.

23. Stuart W. Harrington: "Intrathoracic new growths; results of treatment in twenty-four cases," *Surg. Gynec. Obstet.* (1930), 51:647–66, and "Surgical treatment of tumors of the lung and mediastinum," ibid. (1931), 52:417–27.

24. Albert Faulconer, Jr., and Thomas E. Keys, *Foundations of anesthesiology* (Springfield, Ill.: Charles C Thomas, 1965), 1:488–93. Johann F. Heyfelder (1798–1869) was professor of surgery and ophthalmology at the University of Erlangen at the time of his experiments with ethyl chloride. Camille Redard (1841–1910) of Geneva was pharmacist, physician, and dentist. The senior author used inhalation of ethyl chloride in the outpatient clinic over long years for brief surgical procedures such as opening abscesses, removal of foreign bodies, and reduction of dislocations of the elbow or shoulder.

25. Johann F. Dieffenbach, *Der Aether gegen den Schmerz* (Berlin, 1847).

26. Keys, *Anesthesia* (n.18), pp. 45, 71; Magendie's remarks appear in *Compt. rend. Acad. d. sc.* (1847), 24:134–38. He warned Pirogoff that rectal anesthesia might prove dangerous. J. J. Cole's advice to the military surgeon was: "Leave it [chloroform] with the medical store-keeper; place it on a high shelf in his warehouse, and if it be hot, remove the stopper from the bottle to keep it cool." See Cole, *Military surgery, or experience of field practice in India, 1848 and 1849* (London, 1852), p. 89.

27. Cushing was still at The Hopkins. He had visited Scipione Riva-Rocci's clinic in Pavia during his year abroad (1900–1). Riva-Rocci described his sphygmomanometer in 1896 (*Gazz. med. Torino*, 47:981–96, 1001–17). Cushing later wrote an amusing account of his experience in urging registration of blood pressure during operation in "Fashions in surgery," *Surg. Gynec. Obstet.* (1931), 52:266–68. The formal report of the committee appears in Division of Surgery of the Medical School of Harvard University, *Report of research work, 1903–1904* (Boston, March 1904), bull. 2, pp. 1–41. Cushing and Criles's innovation of blood pressure measurement during operation was the first monitoring device for the operating theatre.

28. Fletcher A. Miller, Allan Hemingway, A. O. Nier, Ralph T. Knight, E. B. Brown, Jr., and Richard L. Varco, "Development of, and certain clinical applications for a portable mass spectrometer," *J. Thorac. Surg.* (1950), 20:714–28; Joseph J. Buckley, Frederick H. Van Bergen, Miller, Hemingway, Howard L. Demorest, Knight, and Varco, "Portable mass spectrometer for continuous alveolar gas analysis," *Anesthesiology* (1952), 13:455–64. Use of the mass spectrograph in operation to assess concentration of anesthetic gases was a direct windfall from the Minnesota weekly surgical-physiologic conference. Visscher knew of Nier's important work on uranium 235 with the apparatus. An hour's conference of the three of us in Nier's laboratory left no doubt that the apparatus could be useful in augmenting the safety of simultaneous inhalation of several anesthetic gases.

29. John Snow (1813–58) was the first to practice anesthesia as a full-time profession. A member of the Royal College of Surgeons (1838), he also passed the examination for apothecaries and, in 1844, qualified as a doctor of medicine. Snow's finest publication ap-

peared posthumously, *On chloroform and other anesthetics, their action and administration* (London, 1858). Eckenhoff gives a good account of the establishment of the Department of Anesthesiology at the University of Pennsylvania in *Anesthesia from colonial times* (n.13), pp. 58–68.

30. Henry Oldenburg presented the account of Wren's experiment to the Royal Society in "An account of the rise and attempts, of a way to convey liquors immediately into the mass of blood," *Phil. Trans.* (1665), 1:128–30. Boyle told the story in "Some considerations touching the usefulness of experimental natural philosophy," available in his *Works*, ed. Thomas Birch, 3d ed. (Hildesheim: Georg Olms, 1966), 2:88.

31. Johann D. Major, *Chirurgia infusoria* (Kiel, 1667); Pierre-C. Oré, "De l'anesthesie produite chez l'homme par les injections de chloral dans les veines," *Compt. rend. Acad. d. sc.* (1874), 78:515–17, 651–54.

32. Ludwig Bogendörfer, "Ueber lösliche Schlafmittel der Barbitursäurereihe (Dial löslich)," *Schweiz. med. Wschr.* (1924), 54:437–38; Leon G. Zerfas, J. T. C. McCallum, H. A. Shonle, Edward E. Swanson, J. P. Scott, and George H. A. Clowes, "Induction of anesthesia in man by intravenous injection of sodium isoamyl-ethyl barbiturate," *Proc. Soc. Exp. Biol. Med.* (1929), 26:399–403; Martin Kirschner, "Eine pycheschonende und steuerbare Form der Allgemeinbetäubung," *Chirurg.*, Berlin (1929), 1:673–82.

33. Marc Dupuy, "Note sur les effets de l'injection de l'éther dans le rectum," *Compt. rend. Acad. d. sc.* (1847), 24:605–7; Nicolai I. Pirogoff, "Nouveau procédé pour produire, au moyen de la vapeur d'éther, l'insensibilité chez les individus soumis à des operations chirurgicales," *Compt. rend. Acad. d. sc.* (1847), 24:789; ibid., p. 1110. Frank Lahey and John Cunningham invoked the same method more than fifty years later. See *Boston M. & S. J.* (1905), 152:450–57.

34. John Syng Dorsey, *Elements of surgery* (Philadelphia, 1813), 1:197–99. In quoting Colin M'Kenzie's letter Dorsey said he believed "no other surgeon of this or former ages can boast" of success in a case of longer duration, adding that Desault's most chronic case was of three months' duration.

35. Monro added that the practice "has an appearance of cruelty, but it saves a vast deal of pain to the patient and makes the Chance of success at least much more greater." The quotations are from "Lecture 22" in "Monro's Surgery, Edinburgh 1779," a volume of unsigned handwritten lecture notes in the Moody Medical Library, Galveston. Almost identical wording appears in other manuscript notebooks which were undoubtedly written or at least used by students attending Monro's popular lectures. Two such copies in the library of the Liverpool Medical Institution are tentatively dated 1774. Both assign the material to "Lecture 114." A copy dated 1775 is in the possession of Edinburgh University (MS. Gen. 573, p. 150); another in the library of the Royal College of Physicians, Edinburgh, is probably later than 1783 (MS. 1(7), p. 1975). The Edinburgh copies are both verbatim from shorthand and corrected in Monro II's hand, according to D. W. Taylor, Chairman of Physiology, Otago Medical School, Dunedin, New Zealand, where the library of the Monro Collection, from the library of the three Monros, is housed. Monro III stated that his father, Monro II, for fifteen years did not use notes, but lectured from topic headings. In 1775 Monro II purchased a copy of his own lectures from John Thorburn, one of his pupils. Thorburn had full notes of Cullen and other lectures, which he sold for 5 guineas a copy. This may explain the similarity of the Monro notebooks. Alexander Monro III, *Essays and heads of lectures on anatomy, physiology, pathology, and surgery by the late Alexander Monro Secundus . . . with a memoir of his life* (Edinburgh, 1840), p. viii.

36. Astley Cooper, *Treatise on dislocations and on fractures of the joints*, 2d ed. (London, 1823), pp. 28–29; Alexander Monro III, *Elements of the anatomy of the human body* (Edinburgh, 1825), 1:248.

37. William P. Dewees, *An essay on the means of lessening pain, and facilitating certain cases of difficult parturition* (Philadelphia, 1806), pp. 63–95.

38. George W. Crile and William E. Lower, *Anoci-association* (Philadelphia: W. B. Saunders, 1915), pp. 108–21.

39. Alexander Forbes, R. McIntosh, and W. Sefton, "The effect of ether anaesthesia on the electrical activity of nerve," *Am. J. Physiol.* (1916), 40:503–13.

40. The quotations are from a translation of Dioscorides' *Herbal*, prepared in 1652–55 by John Goodyer, an English botanist of note. It remained in manuscript form at Magdalen College, unused by generations of classical tutors who preferred "the sterile joys of reading dead languages in the original," wrote Robert T. Gunther in his 1934 edition of the work (Oxford: Oxford Univ. Press, 1934), pp. 458, 473–74. Dioscorides, a military surgeon, collected many of his botanical specimens in the course of his army peregrinations.

41. Pliny, *Natural history*, trans. W. H. S. Jones (Cambridge: Harvard Univ. Press, Loeb Classical Library, 1966), 7:241 (bk. 25, cap. 94).

42. G. K. Tallmadge, "Some anesthetics of antiquity," *J. Hist. Med.* (1946), 1:518; Celsus, *De medicina*, with an English translation by W. G. Spencer (Cambridge: Harvard Univ. Press, Loeb Classical Library, 1935, 1938), 1:211, 297; 2:61.

43. Prudentius' poem, "Before sleep," is translated in Helen Waddell, *Mediaeval Latin lyrics* (Baltimore: Penguin, 1968), p. 53. We are indebted to Henrietta H. Warwick, author of *Vergil concordance* (Minneapolis: Univ. Minnesota Press, 1975), for pointing out this passage, as well as several in Vergil. In Homer's *Odyssey*, Helen poured "nepenthe" into the wine to cause Telemachus and other sorrowful guests to forget their grief and fall asleep. The ingredients of the drug, said to be of Egyptian origin, are unknown. See A. T. Murray's translation (Cambridge: Harvard Univ. Press, Loeb Classical Library, 1945), 1:122–23.

44. *The surgery of Theodoric, ca. A.D. 1267*, trans. Eldridge Campbell and James Colton (New York: Appleton-Century-Crofts, 1960), 2:212–13; Guy de Chauliac, *La grande chirurgie de Guy de Chauliac, composée en l'an 1363*, ed. Édouard Nicaise (Paris, 1890), p. 436. Recipes for soporific sponges have been found in ninth century documents. See Keys, *History of anesthesia* (n.18), pp. 7–8.

45. Oswald Heer, "Die Pflanzen der Pfahlbauten," An die zürcherische Jugend auf das Jahr 1866, *Naturforschenden Gesellschaft* (1866), 68:32.

46. Guido Majno, *The healing hand* (Cambridge: Harvard Univ. Press, 1975), pp. 109–11; *A treatise on the canon of medicine of Avicenna*, incorporating a translation of the first book by O. Cameron Gruner (London: Luzac, 1930), p. 527. Avicenna named as less powerful stupefacients mandrake, hemlock, hyoscyamus, deadly nightshade, lettuce-seed, snow-, and ice-water.

47. Arthur Dickson Wright, "The history of opium," *Trans. Stud., Coll. Physns Phila.* (1961), 29:22–27.

48. James Paget, "Case of colotomy," *Lancet* (1870), 1:835; Vincenz Kern, *Ueber die Handlungsweise bey Absetzung der Glieder*, 2d ed. (Vienna, 1826), pp. 30–35. See also chapter 6 on intestinal obstruction.

49. From John Collins Warren's "Biographical notes," quoted in Edward Warren, *Life of John Collins Warren* (Boston, 1860), 1:384. For an account of mesmerism, which John Collins Warren had found ineffectual for producing somnolence and insensitivity to pain during surgery, see Keys, *History of anesthesia* (n.18), pp. 12–14, and James Esdaile, *Mesmerism in India, and its practical application in surgery and medicine* (London, 1846).

50. Approximately 10 percent morphine or 0.08 to 1 grain of morphine.

51. Stephen Smith, "Reminiscences of two epochs — anaesthesia and asepsis," *Johns Hopkins Hosp. Bull.* (1919), 30:278.

52. Joh. N. Nussbaum, "Über Injection von Morphium in die Venen an sich selbst gemacht," *Dt. Ges. f. Chir.* (1872), 1:50–53. Read by President Langenbeck.

53. Carl Koller, "Vorläufige Mittheilung über locale Anästhesirung am Auge," *Klin. Mbl. Augenheilk.* (1884), 22:60–63. Koller (1857–1944) was working at the time in Freud's clinic. Koller's letter to M. G. Seelig appears in *JAMA* (1941), 117:1284. Seelig sent the letter to the editor, saying it was "not only of human interest but also of historical significance."

54. William S. Halsted, "Practical comments on the use and abuse of cocaine; suggested by its invariably successful employment in more than a thousand minor surgical oeprations,"

N. York M. J. (1885), 42:294–95. This article was not reprinted in Halsted's collected papers. The editor, Walter C. Burket, stated that it was "written while Dr. Halsted was ill" and would require "such reediting as is not deemed expedient." Halsted's priority for innovation of nerve conduction block with cocaine was confirmed in letter exchanges in 1920–21, a year before his death. Halsted, *Surgical papers* (Baltimore: The Johns Hopkins Press), 1:167–77.

55. Karl L. Schleich, "Infiltrations anästhesie (locale Anästhesie) und ihr Verhältniss zur allgmeinen Narcose (Inhalationsanästhesie)," *Verh. dt. Ges. Chir.*, 21 Congress, Berlin, June 8–11, 1892 (Berlin, 1892), pp. 121–28; Heinrich G. Brugsch, "Karl Ludwig Schleich," *New Engl. J. Med.* (1960), 263:696–97; Friedrich Trendelenburg, *Die ersten 25 Jahre der Deutschen Gesellschaft für Chirurgie* (Berlin: J. Springer, 1923), pp. 110–14. In Schleich's paper (1892) there is a brief addendum (pp. 127–28) printed with Bardeleben's approval in which Schleich explained that his presentation expressed only a personal opinion concerning the hazards of inhalation anesthesia, particularly chloroform, an attitude he would continue to defend. There are probably very few public announcements on record of important observations that have met with such ridicule by an experienced presiding officer. History has vindicated Schleich. Despite his emotional appeal, he deserved well at the hands of his audience. Schleich had a discontinuous and interrupted type of surgical training, first with Heinrich Helferich at Greifswald, then in pathology with Virchow in Berlin, followed by a continuance of surgical training under Bergmann in Berlin. Great innovator that he was, Schleich was unwilling to wait patiently in the academic arena for a university appointment. His mature professional life was spent in a private surgical clinic in Berlin.

56. Heinrich Braun, "Über einige neue örtliche Anaesthetica (Stovain, Alypin, Novocain)," *Dt. med. Wschr.* (1905), 31(2):1667–71. Novocaine was renamed procaine in World War I to obviate payment of German patent rights to the former title.

57. Heinrich I. Quincke, "Über Hydrocephalus," *Verh. d. Cong. f. innere Med.* (1891), 10:321–39; August Bier, "Versuche über Cocainisirung des Rückenmarkes," *Dt. Ztschr. Chir.* (1899), 51:361–69. When this surgeon spent a week at Bier's clinic at the Ziegelstrasse Clinic in Berlin in May 1928, Bier was not enthusiastic over spinal anesthesia and related his personal experience and trials with the method at the turn of the century.

58. J. Leonard Corning, "Spinal anaesthesia and local medication of the cord," *N.Y. Med. J.* (1885), 42:483–85. Faulconer and Keys believe that Corning achieved epidural rather than intradural spinal anesthesia. See *Foundations of anesthesiology* (n.24), 2:914–20. "Intraspinal cocainization" by Rudolph Matas, Felix A. Larue, Hermann B. Gessner, and Carroll Allen appears as "Medical News" in *JAMA* (1899), 33:1659.

59. Gaston Labat, "Elimination of dangers of spinal anesthesia," *Am. J. Surg.* (1928), 5:625–32. See discussion of the Trendelenburg position in chapter 13 on vesicovaginal fistula.

60. George P. Pitkin, "Controllable spinal anesthesia," *Am. J. Surg.* (1928), 5:537–53; Arthur E. Barker, "Clinical experiences with spinal analgesia in 100 cases," *Br. M. J.* (1907), 1:665–74.

61. A. Sicard, "Les injections médicamenteuses extra-durales par voie sacrococcygienne," *Compt. rend. Soc. d. biol.* (1901), 53:396–98.

62. Fernand Cathelin, "Une nouvelle voie d'injection rachidienne. Methode des injections épidurales par le procédé du canal sacré. Applications à l'homme," *Compt. rend. Soc. d. biol.* (1901), 53:452–53; Waldo B. Edwards and Robert A. Hingson, "Continuous caudal anesthesia in obstetrics," *Am. J. Surg.* (1942), 57:459–64.

63. James H. Cassedy, "Early uses of acupuncture in the United States, with an addendum (1826) by Franklin Bache, M.D.," *Bull. N.Y. Acad. Med.* (1974), 50:892–906; John Z. Bowers, "Acupuncture," *Proc. Am. Phil. Soc.* (1973), 117:143–51; Shanghai Acupuncture Anaesthesia Co-ordinating Group, *Acupuncture anaesthesia: An anaesthetic method by combination of traditional Chinese and Western medicine* (People's Republic of China, August 1973).

64. Frederick H. Van Bergen, April 15, 1975, personal communication. In a letter of March 22, 1976, Richard A. Theye, head of anesthesiology in the Mayo Clinic, stated that during 1975 nitrous oxide complemented with other inhalation anesthetic agents was used by

the Anesthesia Department in about 90 percent of approximately 50,000 anesthetics. Ether was administered in less than 100 cases. Richard J. Kitz, chief anesthetist at Harvard's Massachusetts General Hospital, in a letter of July 2, 1976, stated that 80 percent of operations there are done under inhalation anesthesia, approximately 20 percent under regional. Ether or cyclopropane is employed in 0.15 percent of cases. "Virtually all of the cases of general anesthesia involve the use of nitrous oxide, half of those are supplemented by an additional anesthetic agent, the other half by intravenous medication."

Further Readings

Cole, Frank. *Milestones in anesthesia; readings in the development of surgical anesthesia, 1665–1940.* Lincoln: Univ. Nebraska Press, 1965.

Davison, M. H. Armstrong. *The evolution of anaesthesia.* Baltimore: Williams and Wilkins, 1965.

Duffy, John. Anglo-American reaction to obstetrical anesthesia. *Bull. Hist. Med.* (1964), 38:32–44.

Ellis, Edgar S. *Ancient anodynes; primitive anaesthesia and allied conditions.* London: William Heinemann, 1946.

Heaton, Claude Edwin. History of anesthesia and analgesia in obstetrics. *J. Hist. Med.* (1946), 1:567–72.

Howard-Jones, Norman. A critical study of the origins and early development of hypodermic medication. *J. Hist. Med.* (1947), 2:201–49.

Jennings, William Oscar. *The morphia habit and its voluntary renunciation.* London: Baillière, Tindall, and Cox, 1909.

Lafargue, G. V. Recherches thérapeutiques sur les effets de quelques médicamens introduits sous l'épiderme. *Bull. gén. de thérap.* (1836), 11:329–35.

———. Des avantages thérapeutiques le l'inoculation de la morphine et de celle de quelques autres médicaments énergiques. *Bull. gén. de thérap.* (1847), 33:19–26; 182–91; 349–57.

Olmsted, James Montrose D. *François Magendie, pioneer in experimental physiology and scientific medicine in XIX century France.* New York: Schuman, 1945.

Rynd, Francis. Description of an instrument for the subcutaneous introduction of fluids in affections of the nerves. *Dubl. Quart. J. Med. Sci.* (1861), 32:12–13.

Warren, John C. *Etherization; with surgical remarks.* Boston, 1848.

Chapter 17. Antiseptics

Notes

1. Henry Dunbar, "The medicine and surgery of Homer," *Br. M. J.* (1880), 1:48–51; Ernst Gurlt, *Geschichte der Chirurgie* (Berlin, 1898), 1:89.

2. We are indebted to Dr. Matthew B. Smorstok of the University of Minnesota Health Service for pointing out this early reference which he noticed in Eugeniusz Sieńkowski, "Rozwój antyseptyki i aseptyki w polsce," *Studia i materialy z dziejow nauki polskiej*, Seria B, Z. 15, 1969, p. 4, undertaken on the 120th anniversary of the introduction of prophylactic antisepsis by Semmelweis (1847) and the 100th of Lister's use of carbolic acid for compound fracture. Place's use of the word antiseptic was also recalled by H. S. Wellcome in an address at the St. Louis 1910 AMA meeting: *The evolution of antiseptic surgery* (London: Burroughs Wellcome, 1910), pp. 48–50. We have been unable to find any information about Place himself.

3. John Pringle, "Some experiments on substances resisting putrefaction," *Phil. Trans.* (1750), 46:487, and *Observations on the diseases of the army, in camp and garrison,* 2d ed. (London, 1753), pp. 309–403. What a tragedy that these observations did not concern John Hunter as much as did Pringle's on gastromalacia, to the elucidation of which Hunter's interest and curiosity contributed so much. Pringle (1707–82), a Scot, received his medical degree at Leyden and became joint professor of pneumatics and moral philosophy at Edinburgh. After

his army career Pringle practiced in London and was well known in scientific circles there and in Europe. He was president of the Royal Society (1772–78). His most important work, in military medicine and sanitation, will be discussed later.

4. D. M. Macbride, *Experimental essays on medical and philosophical subjects* (London, 1764); William Alexander, *Experimental essays . . . I. On the external application of antiseptics in putrid diseases* (London, 1768), pp. 1–77; Thomas Henry, *Experiments and observations* (London, 1773).

5. This is probably not the first nor the last time that the best paper has received second prize. The traditionalism of the judges is always a factor. Third prize went to Guillaume L. Godart. The three presentations were published in a monograph, *Dissertations sur les antiseptiques, qui ont concouru pour le prix* (Dijon, 1769).

6. Pliny, *Natural history*, with an English translation by W. H. S. Jones (Cambridge: Harvard Univ. Press, Loeb Classical Library, 1966), 7:29, 31 (bk. 24). Terebinth resin came from *Pistacia terebinthus*, the terebinth tree, mentioned in the Old Testament and by Dioscorides (first century). See *The Greek herbal of Dioscorides*, ed. Robert T. Gunther (Oxford: Oxford Univ. Press, 1934), p. 49. In northern localities the source of turpentine was usually one of the pine family. The popular "Venice turpentine" came from the European larch, according to the pharmacologist Edme A. Bourgoin, "Térébenthine, chimie," *Dict. encycl. d. sc. méd.*, Paris (1886), 95:413–17. The remains of conifers which may have been gathered for medicinal purposes have been identified by Oswald Heer in the prehistoric Lake Dwellings of Switzerland (3000 to 2000 B.C.). "Die Pflanzen der Pfahlbauten," And die zürcherische Jugend auf das Jahr 1866, *Naturforschenden Gesellschaft* (1866), 68:32, 38–39.

7. *Hippocrates*, with an English translation by E. T. Withington (Cambridge: Harvard Univ. Press, Loeb Classical Library, 1948), 3:151, 163, 353, 431, 447; J.-F. Malgaigne, *De l'irrigation dans les maladies chirurgicales, concours* thesis, Paris, 1842, pp. 5–13.

8. Guy de Chauliac, *Ars chirurgica* (Venice, 1546), fol. 31 recto; Hieronymus Brunschwig, *Das Buch der Cirurgia* (Strasbourg, 1497; facsimile, with a study on Brunschwig by Henry E. Sigerist, Milan: Lier, 1923), fol. 30 verso; Felix Würtz, *An experimental treatise of surgerie*, trans. Abraham L. Fox (London, 1656), p. 300; Würtz, *Practica der Wundartzney* (Basel, 1596), p. 553.

9. John Woodall, *The surgeons mate or military & domestique surgery* (London, 1639), pp. 46, 388; John Arderne, *Treatises of fistula in ano, hemorrhoids, and clysters*, ed. D'Arcy Power (London: Frowde, 1910), pp. 31–32; Peter Lowe, *The whole course of chirurgerie* (London, 1597), treatise 6, chaps. 3 and 5; Richard Wiseman, *Severall chirurgicall treatises* (London, 1676), pp. 426, 446; James Yonge, *Currus triumphalis, è terebinthô* (London, 1679), pp. 51–86; Matthäus G. Purmann, *Chirurgica curiosa*, trans. (London, 1706), pp. 213–15. Turpentine and tar were common ingredients of applications for wounds and abscesses in London in the mid-eighteenth century. See *The modern practice of the London hospitals, viz. St. Bartholomew's, St. Thomas's, St. George's, and Guy's*, 2d ed. (London, 1766), pp. 32, 71, 84, 132. An ointment used at St. Bartholomew's (p. 32) calling for beeswax, mutton suet, linseed oil, and Venice turpentine is attributed to "P.P.," undoubtedly Percivall Pott.

10. Robert Esler, "Oakum as an antiseptic dressing," *Dublin J. M. Sc.* (1877), 64:324–30; Joseph Lister, "Case illustrating the present aspect of the antiseptic system of treatment in surgery," *Br. M. J.* (1871), 1:31. Oakum prepared from ships' riggings was still being used for dressings in hospitals in Port Arthur in the Russo-Japanese War of 1904–5. See Great Britain War Office, *The Russo-Japanese War: Medical and sanitary reports* (London: His Majesty's Stationery Office, 1908), p. 268.

11. The authors are indebted to Capt. Herbert B. Hechtman (1967) in the Office of the Surgeon General of the Army for uncovering Hachenberg's communication. For reports see *Br. M. J.* (1864), 2:11–12; *Bull. gén. de thérap.*, Paris (1864), 67:42–43; Frank H. Hamilton, *Treatise on military surgery and hygiene* (New York, 1865), pp. 579–80.

12. Waid Rogers, 1966, personal communication.

13. Solomon Solis-Cohen and Thomas S. Githens, *Pharmacotherapeutics, materia medica, and drug action* (New York: Appleton, 1928), p. 857.

14. Celsus, *De medicina*, with an English translation by W. G. Spencer (Cambridge: Harvard Univ. Press, Loeb Classical Library, 1961), 2:5; Antoine-F. Fourcroy, *Élémens d'histoire naturelle et de chimie* (Paris, 1786), 4:95.

15. Pliny, *Natural history* (n.6), p. 23; Guillaume Mauquest de la Motte, *Traité complet de chirurgie* (Paris, 1732), 3:338–44; Dominique-J. Larrey, *Mémoires de chirurgie militaire et campagnes* (Paris, 1812), 1:347; 2:343; William Adams, "The treatment of wounds upon the antiseptic and subcutaneous principles," *Med. Times & Gaz.* (1868), 1:257.

16. Amatus Lusitanus, *In Dioscoridis Anazarbei de medica materia libros quinque* (Venice, 1553), p. 34; Nicolo Monardes, *Dos libros. El uno trata de todas las cosas que traen de neustras Indias occidentales* (Seville, 1565), sig. C, fols. iii recto–[vii] verso, and *Joyfull newes out of the new founde worlde*, Englished by John Frampton, 1577 (London: Constable and Knopf, 1925), 1:22–27, 156–59; Michael Döring, [Diatribā] *de opobalsamo Syriaco, Judaico, Aegyptio, Peruviano, Tolutano et Europaeo* (Jena, 1620), p. 41. Balsam of Peru was obtained from *Myroxylon pereirai*, a tree in San Salvador. It was usually shipped to Europe via Peru and, confusingly, named for the country of final export. The Indian process of making the balsam is described by Charles Dorat in a letter to Carson, *Am. J. Pharm.* (1860), 32:302–6, and by Daniel Hanbury, *Pharm. J. & Trans.*, London (1863), 5:241–48, 315–17.

17. Eduard Wiss, "Therapeutische Mittheilungen," *Berl. klin. Wscher.* (1876), 13:696; Eduard Beck, *Beruht die gute Wundwirkung des Perubalsams auf einem Gehalt an Vitamin A?*, Berlin thesis, 1937.

18. Thomas Kirkland, *Thoughts on amputation* (London, 1780), p. 2.

19. *Hippocrates* (n.7), 3:151, 163; Frederick B. Lund, "Allusions to medicine in classical literature," *Bull. N.Y. Acad. Med.* (1929), 5:855; Gurlt, *Geschichte der Chirurgie* (n.1), 3:580.

20. Conrad Brunner, *Handbuch der Wundbehandlung* (Stuttgart: Enke, 1916), p. 40.

21. Johann L. Schmucker, "Untersuchung uber die Abnehmung der Glieder," in his *Vermischte chirurgische Schriften* (Berlin, 1776), 1:3–73; John Hunter, *Treatise on the blood, inflammation, and gun-shot wounds* (London, 1794), pp. 557–63.

22. Ambroise Paré, *The workes of that famous chirurgion Ambrose Parey*, trans. Thomas Johnson (London, 1634), pp. 52, 463, 582–86; John Hennen, *Principles of military surgery*, 1st Am. ed. (Philadelphia, 1838), pp. 104–5.

23. The account of Percivall Pott's fracture is told by James Earle in his edition of Pott's *Chirurgical works* (London, 1790), 1:14–16. Pott's "Remarks on the necessity . . . of amputation" (1762) appears in this edition (1:373–407). Edward Nourse (1701–72) lectured in anatomy and surgery at St. Bartholomew's.

24. Johannes U. Bilguer, *De membrorum amputatione rarissime administranda, aut quasi abroganda*, inaugural dissertation, Halle, 1761; Karl Vogeler, "Johann Ulrich Bilguer und der Streit um die Amputation im 18. Jahrhundert," *München. med. Wschr.* (1929), 76(1):754.

25. Silvester O'Halloran, *Complete treatise on gangrene and sphacelus with a new method of amputation* (London, 1765), pp. vii–ix. J. D. H. Widdess wrote the authors (April 17, 1978) that with other searchers he had recently located the grave of Silvester O'Halloran (1728–1807), heavily overgrown with vegetation, in an old Limerick cemetery. A limestone slab has been placed to commemorate O'Halloran.

26. Alexis Boyer, *Lectures upon diseases of the bones*, arranged by A. Richerand, trans. Farrell (Philadelphia, 1805), pp. 34–35; Gerard van Swieten, *Commentaries upon the aphorisms of Herman Boerhaave* (Edinburgh, 1776), 4:89–90; Foucard, "Observation de quatre fractures . . . du même sujet," *Rev. méd.-chir. de Paris* (1850), 7:143–49. See also D.-M. Rollande, "Des fractures comminutives très-graves peuvent être traitées et guéries sans l'amputation," *Bull. gén. de thérap.*, Paris (1833), 5:129–32. D. M. Carré expressed a similar opinion in the same journal (1834), 6:221–23. L.-J.-G. Seutin, a Belgian surgeon, said, "The art of making amputations unnecessary should precede the art of doing them well" and that Léon Legouest's "results were five times better in extremity injuries without amputation." *De l'abus des amputations et de l'utilité de la chirurgie conservatrice* (Bruxelles, 1860), pp. 1, 43.

27. J.-F. Malgaigne: "Études statistiques sur les fractures et les luxations," *Ann. d'hyg.*, Paris (1839), 22:241–69, and *Treatise on fractures*, trans. John H. Packard (Philadelphia, 1859), p. 597. Malgaigne's (1842) amputation study is discussed in chapter 2.

28. John E. Erichsen, *The science and art of surgery*, Am. ed. from 2d London ed., (Philadelphia, 1867), pp. 42–47.

29. Alexis Alquié, *Chirurgie conservatrice, et moyens de restreindre l'utilité des opérations* (Montpellier, 1850). J. M. C. Fourquet (1865) cited the experience of Pichorel's clinic in Le Havre, where primary amputation for compound fracture was accompanied by a mortality of 60 percent, almost twice that of conservative therapy (34.8 percent). *Quelques mots sur les pansements rares dans les fractures compliquées de plaie*, Montpellier thesis, 1865, p. 29.

30. John Crowther, "A successful mode of preventing gangrene in compound fractures," *Med. & Phys. J.*, London (1802), 7:307–10. Perusal of the pages of the *Medical and Physical Journal* for eighteen years following Crowther's publication failed to turn up any suggestion of trial with, or interest in, his technique by the profession.

31. Dominique-J. Larrey, *Relation médicale de campagnes et voyages, de 1815, à 1840* (Paris, 1841), pp. 16–17; Paul Triaire, *Napoléon et Larrey* (Tours: Mame, 1902), pp. 495, 521.

32. Dominique-J. Larrey, "Mémoire sur une nouvelle manière de réduire ou de traiter les fractures des membres compliquées de plaies," *J. compl. du dict. d. sc. méd.*, Paris (1824), 20:193–200. Reports of the séance appear in *Rev. méd. franç. et étrang.*, Paris (1824), 16:465, and *Arch. gén. de méd.*, Paris (1824), 6:460.

33. For reviews see *Rev. méd. franç. et étrang.*, Paris (1825), 18:454–55, and *Gior. di chir. prat.*, Trient (1826), 2:44–46.

34. Ludovic Biencourt, *Considérations sur le traitement des fractures compliquées de plaie*, Paris thesis, 1873, p. 14.

35. William Adams, *Sketch of the principles and practice of subcutaneous surgery* (London, 1857), pp. 15–18; Sampson Gamgee, *On the treatment of wounds and fractures* (London, 1883), p. 125.

36. *Oswestry Advertizer*, April 28, 1869.

37. Believing that a surgeon's son, even in the late 1700s, would probably have attended a boy's school, we addressed an inquiry to a hypothetical "Headmaster of the Oswestry School." Fortunately such a school did exist, although its old records had been destroyed. The headmaster's wife, Mrs. Audrey Gern, put a notice of our search in the local newspaper, where it was noted by Miss Whitfield. From her we learned that besides his medical career Bennion took interest in the Welsh Bards and was a judge at some of their singing contests. Moreover, a book on Welsh folklore credits him with a local reputation of possessing the "black art," the power to raise devils. Bennion gave his secret as follows: "Publish it abroad that you can raise the Devil, and the country will believe you, and will credit you with many miracles. All you have to do afterwards is be silent, and you will then be as good a raiser of Devils as I am." Apparently the doctor possessed a touch of the psychologist as well as unusual surgical skill. Rev. Elias Owen, *Welsh folk-lore . . . the prize essay of the National Eisteddfod, 1887* (Oswestry, n.d.), p. 216.

38. Thomas Bryant: "Contributions to the subject of compound fracture," *Med.-Chir. Trans.* (1861), 44:19–28, and "Cases of compound fracture in which the wounds were closed with compresses soaked in compound tincture of benzoin," *Lancet* (1876), 2:747–48, 781–82, 821–22.

39. Edmund O. Lippmann has reviewed the bibliography of alcohol and brandy for wound therapy extending back to the fourteenth and fifteenth centuries in *Chemiker-Zeitung* (1913), 37:1313, 1346, 1358, 1419, 1428.

40. Galen, *Medicorum graecorum opera quae exstant*, ed. C. G. Kühn (Leipzig, 1830), 18(2):366–67, 567; Theodoric, "Chirurgia" in *Ars chirurgica Guidonis Cauliaci* (Venice, 1546), fols. 135 verso, 136 recto, 140; Lanfranc, "Chirurgia parva," in ibid., fol. 201 recto; William of Saliceto, "Chirurgia" in ibid., fol. 325 verso; Henri de Mondeville, *Chirurgie composée de 1306 à 1320*, ed. Édouard Nicaise (Paris, 1893), pp. 214, 373–74.

41. Distillation had undoubtedly been known to the Arabs earlier. In several books of the Old Testament including Numbers, Deuteronomy, Proverbs, and Ezekiel, there are references to "wine and strong drink."

42. E. Nicaise, "Propos général des plaies et solutions de continuité par Guy de Chauliac," *Rev. de chir.*, Paris (1891), 11:69; Paré (n.22), pp. 408–9, 1143.

43. Giuseppe Lanzoni, "De vulnere aqua vitae curato," *Miscellanea curiosa* (1692), 2 s., 10:225; Lanzoni, "De viribus acquae vitae," *Ephemerides naturae curiosorum* (1715), 3 s., pp. 43–44; Lorenz Heister, *A general system of surgery*, trans., 4th ed. (London, 1750), 1:37, 45, 53; Johannes Juncker, *Conspectus therapiae generalis cum notis in materiam medicam* (Halle, 1725), p. 477; Theodor Kappenhagen, *De insigni usu spiritus vini in sanandis vulneribris* (Altdorf, Switzerland, 1745); Félix Hutin, *Fragmens historiques et médicaux sur l'Hôtel national des Invalides* (Paris, 1851), p. 42.

44. Walter F. Atlee, *Clinical lectures on surgery by M. Nélaton* (Philadelphia, 1855), p. 111. Atlee wrote his monograph on surgical practices of the Nélaton Clinic from notes made during his three-year visit. He stated that he had observed alcohol dressings applied to wounds there in 1852 and that in 1855 it was Nélaton's practice to treat furuncles with alcohol.

45. J. F. Bataihé and Ad. Guillet, *De l'alcool et des composés alcooliques en chirurgie* (Paris, 1859), p. 12; Jules Le Coeur, *Des pansement a l'aide de l'alcool et des teintures alcooliques* (Caen, 1864), p. 78. Batailhé and Guillet published extensively on the use of alcohol for wounds in France. Their 1859 monograph was announced in *Br. M. J.*, September 10, 1859, p. 747. It appeared in English in 1860 as *Alcohol and alcoholic preparations in surgery* (Paris, 1860).

46. S. A. Chédevergne, "Du traitement des plaies chirurgicales et traumatiques par les pansements à l'alcool," *Bull. gén. de thérap.*, Paris (1864), 67:249–62, 302–8, 346–57; Jean de Gaulejac, *Du pansement des plaies par l'alcool*, Paris thesis, 1864. Jules Le Coeur, *Des pansements de l'alcool* (n.45), pp. 36–44, gives a detailed account of the alcohols then available. He lists two types of camphorated alcohol, one at 34° Cartier corresponding to 86 percent alcohol by volume, the other at 21° Cartier, or 56 percent alcohol, probably the one which Nélaton used largely. John Green (1863), former assistant surgeon of the U.S. Army, alluded to the use of strong alcohol in France in wound management (36° Cartier) which he interpreted as 89.2 percent alcohol by volume (*Boston M. & S. J.*, 68:459). Frederick E. Shideman, professor of pharmacology at the University of Minnesota, has confirmed the accuracy of these conversions (July 7, 1967; personal communication).

47. De Gaulejac, *Pansement* (n.46), pp. 43–53; Chédevergne (n.46), pp. 349–55.

48. By 1867, Nélaton was able to report that in 97 operations, 2 purulent infections ("with some question in one of those") and 5 mild cases of erysipelas had been observed, without mention of hospital death. Le Coeur's monograph (n.46), pp. 19–22, contains a letter to Batailhé, dated September 10, 1859, setting forth Le Coeur's ideas of preventing infection in wounds by application of alcohol dressings. [A. Nélaton], "Exposé des progrès accomplis dans le traitement des blessés et des opérés," in C. P. Denonvilliers, A. Nélaton, A. Velpeau, Félix Guyon, and Léon Labbé, *Rapport sur les progrès de la chirurgie* (Paris, 1867), p. 729. Lestocquoy of Arras was using alcohol dressings on wounds as early as 1848, according to J. Rochard, *Histoire de la chirurgie française au XIXe siècle* (Paris, 1875), p. 649. P. V. Marvy enthusiastically endorsed alcohol in management of wounds and surgical infections in a Strasbourg thesis, *Du pansement des plaies par l'alcool*, 1864.

49. W. W. Cheyne, *Antiseptic surgery* (London, 1882), p. 406.

50. Unsigned editorial, *Bull. gén. de thérap.* (1865), 68:181; Léon Labbé, "Rapport sur un travail intitulé: De l'imbibition et de son rôle en pathologie . . . par M. Marc Sée," *Bull. Soc. imp. de chir., Paris* (1867), 7:504–7; discussion, pp. 507–8. Nélaton's efforts to avoid contamination of the wound are mentioned in chapter 6 on intestinal obstructions. But see also chapter 23.

51. Alf. Velpeau, *Lessons upon the diagnosis and treatment of surgical diseases, 1865*, ed. A. Regnard, trans. W. C. B. Fifield (Boston, 1866), pp. 102–3; Larrey, *Mémoires de chirurgie militaire* (n.15), 2:343. It is not without interest that O'Halloran, a vigorous opponent of

primary amputation for compound fracture, also admonished against use of alcohol in such wounds because it retarded suppuration. See his *Gangrene and sphacelus* (n.25), pp. 168, 174–75.

52. Félix Guyon, "Eloge d'Auguste Nélaton," *Bull. et mém. Soc. de chir. Paris* (1876), 2:76–95; J. Béclard, *Notice historique sur M. Nélaton* (Paris, 1878), p. 33. In 1910 Francis Dowling wrote: "He [Nélaton] is said to have received the largest fees of any surgeon in France; the Sultan of Turkey once paid him fifty thousand dollars for operating upon him in Constantinople." When Nélaton died "his estate was valued at twelve million francs," — a rather tidy sum for a surgeon raised in an impoverished family and whose mother, widowed by war, took in sewing to meet her children's needs. Poverty in a modest man like Nélaton obviously can foster a spirit of avarice when one might more reasonably have looked for traces of benevolent generosity (*Lancet-Clin.*, Cincinnati, 104:611).

53. Chédevergne (n.46), pp. 306–8. The papers of Nélaton, Batailhé and Guillet, and Le Coeur were reviewed in England and the United States. See Augustin Prichard, "The alcoholic treatment of wounds," *Br. M. J.*, November 3, 1860, pp. 860–61; W. Lockwood Bradley, *Proc. Connect. M. Soc.* (1867), 2:253–57. A brief note on Nélaton's use of alcohol in *Pacific M. & S. J.* (1867) was reprinted in *M. & S. Reporter*, Philadelphia (1867), 16:53.

54. Prichard (n.53).

55. Antonio M. Barbosa, "Note statistique des grandes opérations faites à l'hôpital national et royal de Saint-Joseph pendant les douze dernières années," pp. 234–69 in *Congrès médical international de Paris, 1867* (Paris, 1868).

56. Alexander G. Gibson, *History of the Radcliffe Infirmary* (1926), p. 211; David Blair, "On whisky as an antiseptic dressing in surgery," *Glasg. Med. J.* (1870), 2:204–9. J. L. Suesserott of Pennsylvania said that whisky was used "with wonderful effects" by his grandmothers and "other more ancient dames" for wound dressings. *Phila. M. Times* (1874), 4:775.

57. Ed. Willm, "Glycérine (chimie)," *Dict. encycl. d. sc. méd.* (Paris, 1883), 9:318. Michel E. Chevreul (1786–1889) was an active French chemist for eighty years.

58. Jean-Nicolas Demarquay, *Mémoire sur la glycérine et ses applications* (Paris, 1859), pp. 6–25; A.-J. Desormeaux, "Nouveau mode de pansement," [review], *Bull. Soc. de chir. Paris* (1862), 2:369.

59. Manuel E. Lichtenstein, "Suppurative wounds, the use of glycerine as a topical application," *Illinois Med. J.* (1929), 56:425–26. The studies quoted are those of C. E. A. Winslow and Dorothy Holland, *Proc. Soc. Ex. Biol. Med.* (1918), 16:91.

60. John Stomfay-Stitz, "Honey: An ancient yet modern medicine," *Sci. Couns.*, Dec. 1960, p. 110; Celsus, *De medicina* (n.14), 2:5, 35.

61. John Partington, *History of chemistry* (London: Macmillan, 1961), 2:13, 99, 705.

62. Joseph Lister, "Corrosive sublimate as a surgical dressing," *Br. M. J.* (1884), 2:803–7; Emil Behring, "Über Desinfection, Desinfectionsmittel, und Desinfectionsmethoden," *Ztschr. f. Hyg.* (1890), 9:404, 417–19.

63. William S. Halsted, "The treatment of wounds," *Johns Hopkins Hosp. Rep.* (1891), 2:309; A. C. Abbott, "Corrosive sublimate as a disinfectant against the Staphylococcus pyogenes aureus," *Johns Hopkins Hosp. Bull.* (1891), 2:50–60.

64. John Higginbottom, *An essay on the application of the lunar caustic in the cure of certain wounds and ulcers* (London, 1826), and *A practical essay on the use of the nitrate of silver, in the treatment of inflammation, wounds and ulcers*, 3d ed. (London, 1865), pp. 5–6. Higginbottom (1788–1876) asks his question in the preface of the 1826 edition. Throughout his long and active career as a general practitioner in Nottingham, Higginbottom continued his research on silver nitrate. He was a fellow of the Royal College of Surgeons of England and of the Royal Society; the latter honor came in recognition of his studies on the physiology of tritons and tadpoles. *Br. M. J.* (1876), 1:553.

65. John Ferguson, *Bibliotheca chemica* (London, 1954), 1:81. Basil Valentine's "Quomodo Sal Lunae conficiendum est" appears in his *Haliographia* (Bologna, 1644), pp. 6–8.

66. Alexander Read, *The chirurgicall lectures of tumors and ulcers* (London, 1635), p. 148;

Léon Briele, ed., *Collection de documents pour servir à l'histoire des hôpitaux de Paris* (Paris, 1881), 1:149. Read, a Scot, received his M.D. at Oxford in 1620.

67. Antoine Maître-Jan, *Traité des maladies de l'oeil* (Troyes, 1707), pp. 499–500; Charles de Saint-Yves, *Nouveau traité des maladies des yeux* (Paris, 1722), pp. 220–21; Carl Sigmund Franz Credé, *Die Verhütung der Augenentzündung der Neugeborenen* (Berlin, 1884). Maître-Jan has been called the father of scientific ophthalmology in France. Saint-Yves (1667–1733), a French surgeon who specialized in cataract operations, is said to have removed 571 cataracts in one year (1708). *Dict. encyl. d. sc. méd.* (1878), 85:190.

68. François Quesnay, *Traité de la suppuration* (Paris, 1764), p. 336; Joseph Lieutaud, *Précis de la matière médicale* (Paris, 1776), 2:167; Busmann, "Von der Wirkung des Höllensteins zur Hebung einiger äusserer veralteter Schäden," *Mag. f. d. Wundarzneiw.* (1798–99), 2:180; Everard Home, *Practical observations on the treatment of ulcers on the legs* (London, 1797), pp. 59, 63–64, 110–11; Charles William Jones, *A series of lectures on . . . surgery, principally derived from the lectures delivered by Astley Cooper*, ed. Charles Mingay Syder, 1st Am. ed. (Boston, 1823), pp. 56, 79.

69. Albucasis, *On surgery and instruments*, trans. and ed. M. S. Spink and G. L. Lewis (Berkeley: Univ. California Press, 1973), p. 530; Brunschwig, *Cirurgia* (n.8), fol. 30 verso; Hans Gersdorff, *Feldtbůch der Wundartzney* (Strasbourg, 1526), fols. 80–81; Mauquest de la Motte, *Traité de chirurgie* (n.15); Barthélemi Vigarous, *Oeuvres de chirurgie-pratique* ([posthumous] Montpellier, 1812). Vigarous died in 1790. His son, Joseph-M.-J. Vigarous, edited his works, including an undated "Aperçu-pratique sur les bons effets de l'eau de chaux dans le traitement des plaies et des ulcères" (pp. 342–56).

70. M.-J.-Gaston Blache, "Effets du chlore et des chlorures alcalins sur l'organisme," *Dict. de méd.*, 2d ed. (Paris, 1834), 7:410–36; P.-F. M. Dupouy, *De l'emploi des chlorures de chaux et de soude, sous le point de vue thérapeutique*, Paris thesis, 1833. François Chaussier (1746–1828), of Dijon, worked with Fourcroy (1794) in reorganizing the Écoles de Santé, later held professorial positions in the Faculty of Paris.

71. Antoine-Germain Labarraque, *De l'emploi des chlorures d'oxide de sodium et de chaux* (Paris, 1825); Ernest Geoffrey, "Clinique chirurgicale . . . de M. Lisfranc. Observations sur l'emploi de chlorure de chaux dans les brûlures," *Rev. méd. franç. et étrang.*, Paris (1826), 22:373–80; Thomas Alcock, *Essay on the use of chlorurets of oxide of sodium and of lime, as powerful disinfecting agents, and of the chloruret of oxide of sodium . . . in the treatment of hospital gangrene . . . and various other diseases* (London, 1827); *Lancet* (1827), 2:643–47. Labarraque (1822) originally introduced hypochlorite for curing catgut for violin strings, thus saving an important French industry.

72. See chapter 24.

73. Francis C. Kelly, "Iodine in medicine and pharmacy," *Proc. R. Soc. Med.*, London (1961), 54:831–36.

74. John Davies, *Practical remarks on the use of iodine* (London, 1839), pp. 15–16, 28–31, 57–62.

75. Alph.-Alex. Boinet, "Mémoire et observations sur l'efficacité des injections iodées," *J. conn. méd.-chir.*, Paris (1846), 14(1):49, 97; Boinet, *Iodothérapie* (Paris, 1855), pp. 622–26; Amédée Bonnet, "De l'absorption et des effets généraux de l'iode," *Gaz. méd. Paris* (1852), 7:310–13; C. J. Marchal (de Calvi), "Note sur l'emploi de l'iode désinfectant et anti-septique," *Union méd.* (1859), 3:276–80.

76. Nicholas Senn, "Iodine in surgery," *Surg. Gynec. Obstet.* (1905), 1:7; Antonio Grossich, "Eine neue Sterilisierungsmethode der Haut bei Operationen," *Zentbl. Chir.* (1908), 35:1289–92.

77. Antoine J. Balard, "Sur une substance particulière contenue dans l'eau de la mer," *Ann. de chim.*, Paris (1826), 32:337–81; Pourché, "Observations sur l'emploi du brôme et de l'hydrobromate de potasse dans les scrofules et le goître," *Ephém. méd. Montpel.* (1828), 8:45–53; Middleton Goldsmith, *Report on hospital gangrene, erysipelas and pyaemia* (Louisville, 1863), p. [95]. The *American Medical Times* during 1863 ran a number of reports by Goldsmith and

others on the success of bromine in treating hospital gangrene. See also M. O. Terry, "The value of bromine in military surgery," *Internat. J. Surg.*, New York (1895), 8:233–35.

78. Karl Reichenbach, "De la créosote et de ses propriétés thérapeutiques," *Bull. gén. de thérap.*, Paris (1832), 5:205–11.

79. *Bull. gén. de thérap.* (1833), 5:205–6, 219–22, 311–15, 338–43, 555–56; *London M. Gaz.* (1834), 13:869.

80. Friedlieb F. Runge, "Ueber einige Produkte der Steinkohlendestillation," *Ann. d. Phys. u. Chem.* (1834), 31:65–78; 32:308–33.

81. *Br. M. J.* (1859), p. 818. Pertinent material appears in *Compte rendu des séances de l'Académie des sciences*, Paris, for 1859–60 (vols. 49–50). See Demeaux and Edm. Corne (49:127–28), Velpeau, Chevreul, et al. (49:145–61), and other reporters (50:279–302). As Velpeau had suggested in 1859 (p. 147), the powder was tried on the wounded in the military hospitals in Italy, evoking an enthusiastic memoir from Jacquemont in Milan in 1860 (*Compt. rend.*, 50:676–77), but a later publication of J.-C. Chenu, including various army surgeons' assessments, was less encouraging. *Statistique médico-chirurgicale de la campagne d'Italie en 1850 et 1860* (Paris, 1869), 2:363–95.

82. Jules Lemaire, *Du coaltar saponiné, désinfectant énergique, arrêtant les fermentations* (Paris, 1860), and *De l'acide phénique . . . et de ses applications*, 2d ed. (Paris, 1865); Gilbert Déclat, *Nouvelles applications de l'acide phénique* (Paris, 1865); Enrico Bottini, "Dell'acido fenico nella chirurgia pratica," *Ann. univ. di med.*, Milan (1866), 198:385. In his 1865 publication Déclat said he made a successful public demonstration of the use of phenol dressing in management of a gangrenous wound in December 1861 (pp. 21–24). Déclat summarized his claims to priority in use of phenol in wound therapy in a monograph published in 1874.

83. F. Crace Calvert, "Note sur l'emploi du coal-tar en médecine," *Compt. rend. Acad. d. sc.*, Paris (1859), 49:262–64. During 1860–64 Calvert wrote seven publications in English medical journals on carbolic acid and its therapeutic uses. *Lancet* (1862), 1:86, stated that carbolic acid had been used by J. A. Ransome at Manchester Royal Infirmary for treating ulcers. Edward Lund, another surgeon at the Infirmary, described healing in a case of lupus with undiluted carbolic acid after several years of other unsuccessful treatment. He too found dilute carbolic acid beneficial for sloughing wounds, reported in *Br. M. J.* (1862), 1:344. Benjamin Godfrey (1862) found carbolic acid had many surgical uses, with action "speedy and marvelous," saying it deodorized and hastened healing of fetid wounds (*Med. Circ.*, London, 21:435).

84. F. Crace Calvert, "On the therapeutic properties of carbolic acid," *Lancet* (1863), 2:362–63. See ensuing letters, pp. 422, 464, 523.

85. James Watson, "Observations on some new remedies," *Edinb. M. J.* (1864), 9:625–27; J. R. Wolfe, "On the use of phenic acid for the cure of phthisis," *Med. Times & Gaz.* (1865), 31:572–73.

86. A.-M.-B. Burin du Buisson, *Traité de l'action thérapeutique du perchlorure de fer* (Paris, 1860), pp. 11–12, 49–53, 132. A negative opinion was voiced by some Paris authorities, notably Malgaigne. Burin du Buisson includes a history of the antiseptic, describing its use in a secret formula in Russian and French court circles in the eighteenth century.

87. Salleron, "Mémoire sur l'emploi du perchlorure de fer contre la pourriture d'hôpital," *Rec. de mém. de méd. . . . mil.*, Paris (1859), 2:280–82, 357, 415; Marie-P.-A. Bourot, *Considérations sur la pourriture d'hôpital observée en Orient et sur son traitement par le perchlorure de fer*, Strasbourg thesis, 1858, pp. 21–25. The wound was washed with a weak solution of ferric chloride, then covered with a dressing soaked in a solution of 34.65 percent of the iron salt and 65.35 percent water, kept in place twenty-four to forty-eight hours. On removal the wound was coagulated. Salleron also used the cautery, but found it demoralized the patient. The editor subtended a note at the end of Salleron's paper stating that the cautery had such remarkable success with hospital gangrene it must not be discarded.

88. A. Terreil, "Emploi du perchlorure de fer dans le traitement des plaies dites purulentes," *Compt. rend. Acad. d. sc.*, Paris (1859), 49:265–66; Duleau, "Remarques à l'occasion d'un mémoire de M. Jacquemont," *Compt. rend. Acad. d. sc.*, Paris (1860), 50:771; Bourgade,

"Des accidents généraux qui entrainent la mort après les opérations chirurgicalés," pp. 224–33, 302, in *Congrès médical international de Paris, 1867* (Paris, 1868). Bourgade adds that Fleury, professor of clinical surgery in the Medical School at Clermont, also had used this method with great success.

89. Dziewonski and Fix, "Antisepsie primitive sur le champ de bataille," *Rev. mil. de méd. et de chir.* (1881), 1:192.

90. Alfred North, "Report on sixty cases of hospital gangrene," *Am. M. Times,* New York (1863), 6:255–58; William Detmold, "Lectures on military surgery," *Am. M. Times* (1863), 6:98; J. Julian Chisolm, *Manual of military surgery,* 3d ed. (Columbia, S.C., 1864), p. 243. See also chapter 24.

91. Campbell de Morgan, "On the use of the chloride of zinc in surgical operations and injuries," *Br. & For. M.-Chir. Rev.* (1866), 37:201–14; Joseph Lister, "The antiseptic system of treatment in surgery," *Br. M. J.* (1868), 2:53–58. In 1848 in a marine hospital in Quebec, Thomas Stratton found the death rate from infectious fevers and dysentery was less in wards disinfected with Burnett's fluid than in others. *Edinb. M. & S. J.* (1848), 70:287–97.

92. Alexander Fleming, "The action of chemical and physiological antiseptics in a septic wound," *Br. J. Surg.* (1919), 7:99–129.

Further Readings

Brewer, George E. Some observations upon modern surgical technics, from an analysis of four hundred and twenty-one operative cases at the City Hospital. *Med. Record* (1898), 53:433–36.

Colebrook, Leonard. *Almroth Wright, provocative doctor and thinker.* London: William Heinemann, 1954.

Déclat, Gilbert. *Traitement des plaies au moyen de l'acide phénique, et des résultats . . . pendant le siége de Paris.* Paris, 1873.

Lister, Joseph. On a new method of treating compound fracture. *Lancet* (1867), 1:326–29, 357–59, 387–89, 507–9; 2:95–96.

Nussbaum, Johann. Lister's grosse Erfindung. *Aerztl. Int.-Bl.* (1875), 22:41–44.

———. Einfluss der Antiseptik auf die gerichtliche Medicin. *Aerztl. Int.-Bl.* (1880), 27:203–7, 215–19.

Wangensteen, O. H.; Wangensteen, S. D.; and Klinger, Charles F. Some pre-listerian and post-listerian antiseptic wound practices and the emergence of asepsis. *Surg. Gynec. Obstet.* (1973), 137:677–702.

Chapter 18. Early Hospital Practices

Notes

1. Charles Singer, *Short history of medicine* (New York: Oxford Univ. Press, 1928), pp. 48–50. Singer refers to a Roman military hospital (ca. 100 A.D.) that has been excavated at Düsseldorf.

2. John D. Thompson and Grace Goldin, *The hospital: A social and architectural history* (New Haven and London: Yale Univ. Press, 1975), pp. 4–6.

3. Theodor Meyer-Steineg and Karl Sudhoff, *Geschichte der Medizin im Überblick mit Abbildungen,* 2d ed. (Jena: Gustav Fischer, 1922).

4. Samuel Martyn, *A discourse on hospitals past and present* (London, 1862), pp. 13–17; Fielding H. Garrison, *Introduction to the history of medicine,* 4th ed. (Philadelphia: W. B. Saunders, 1929), pp. 176–79.

5. Garrison, *History of medicine* (n.4), p. 304; D. Slater Lewis, *Royal Victoria Hospital, 1887–1947* (Montreal: McGill Univ. Press, 1969), pp. 3–4; Arturo Castiglioni, *History of medicine,* trans. E. B. Krumbhaar (New York: Alfred A. Knopf, 1947), p. 393.

6. Hôtel-Dieu in Lyons is France's oldest hospital, founded in 542, according to Ernst Gurlt, *Geschichte der Chirurgie* (Berlin, 1898), 2:17.

7. Charles Coury, *L'Hôtel-Dieu de Paris: Treize siècles de soins, d'enseignement et de recherche* ([Paris]: L'Expansion Éditeur, 1969), pp. 7–11, 56–63, 72, 87. The interesting history of the Hôtel-Dieu (Paris) has been depicted in many monographs including those of Rondonneau de la Motte (1787), Jacques Tenon (1788), Armand Husson (1862), Ernest L. Coyecque (1889–91), Casimir Tollet (1892), and Coury (1969). La Charité was built primarily because of the black death (bubonic plague), caused by *Pasteurella pestis*, an infection transmitted to man by fleas from infected rats. The etiology was independently discovered by Shibasaburo Kitasato and Alexandre Yersin in 1894.

8. Armand Husson, *Étude sur les hôpitaux* (Paris, 1862), pp. 501–2. The great fire (1772) burned for eleven days and destroyed all the hospital between rue du Petit-Pont and St. Denis Square. Husson includes several excellent illustrations of the Hôtel-Dieu, including one facing the Petit-Pont "before the fire" (p. 482). More illustrations of the Hôtel-Dieu appear in Casimir Tollet, *Les édifices hospitaliers*, 2d ed. (Paris, 1892). Tollet supplies probable dates for many of the scenes.

9. Ernest L. Coyecque, *L'Hôtel-Dieu de Paris au moyen âge* (Paris, 1891), 1:81–93; Dorothy-Louise Mackay, *Les hôpitaux et la charité a Paris au XIIIe siècle* (Paris: Champion, 1923), pp. 63–67; Ellen N. La Motte, "The Hôtel-Dieu of Paris — an historical sketch," *Med. Libr. Hist. J.*, Brooklyn (1906), 4:230–32. The three pints of wine (1,500 ml.) at the usual 12 percent alcohol content is the equivalent of 180 ml. of alcohol, or approximately 12 ounces of whisky, certainly enough to provoke somnolence and a state of intoxication; calculated at a 10 percent alcoholic content, the whisky equivalence would be 10 ounces.

10. Mackay, *Hôpitaux* (n.9); Phyllis Allen Richmond, "The Hôtel-Dieu of Paris on the eve of the Revolution," *J. Hist. Med.* (1961), 16:338; Charles Graves, *The story of St. Thomas's, 1106–1947* (London: Faber and Faber, 1947), p. 13. According to Graves, "Beds did not become common until the end of the thirteenth century, when they were occupied by two to even three patients who, in those days wore no night clothes at all."

11. Coyecque, *L'Hôtel-Dieu au moyen âge* (n.9), 1:104, 116–17; Rondonneau de la Motte, *Essai historique sur l'Hôtel-Dieu de Paris* (Paris, 1787), pp. 239–43.

12. Marcel Fosseyeux, *Hôtel-Dieu de Paris au XVIIe et au XVIIIe siècles* (Paris: Berger-Levrault, 1912), p. 286.

13. Jacques Tenon, *Mémoires sur les hôpitaux de Paris* (Paris, 1788), pp. 287, 290–95; Henriette Carrier, *Origines de la maternité de Paris* (Paris, 1888), pp. 53–54. Tenon's report and its repercussions will be discussed in the following chapter, as will John Howard's observations on the Hôtel-Dieu.

14. Coury, *Hôtel-Dieu* (n.7), p. 36; Rondonneau de La Motte, *Essai historique* (n.11), pp. 235–43; d'Alembert, "Hôtel-Dieu," in Denis Diderot, ed., *Encyclopédie* (Neufchatel, 1765), 8:319–20. The situation worsened in 1781 when wooden double beds with dividing partitions were introduced over the protests of the staff physicians and surgeons, who favored single beds. The new accommodations were most uncomfortable, particularly since more than two patients were sometimes placed in them. See A. Corlieu, "Les lits de L'Hôtel-Dieu avant la Révolution," *Gaz. méd. de Strasbourg* (1890), 49:110–11.

15. John Collins Warren, *Surgical pathology and therapeutics* (Philadelphia, 1895), p. 784.

16. Bernard Poyet, *Mémoire sur la nécessité de transférer et reconstruire l'Hôtel-Dieu de Paris* (Paris, 1785), pp. 3–4, 31; Tenon, *Hôpitaux* (n.13), p. 228.

17. Regnier, *Dénonciation des principaux abus de l'Hôtel-Dieu de Paris, à l'assemblée générale des citoyens* (Paris, 1789), pp. 7, 9, 19. Regnier's 1776 Paris publication, *Project d'une hôpital de malades ou Hôtel-Dieu*, favored single beds for all patients. The *Catalogue* of the Bibliothèque nationale lists Regnier as a "correspondent de plusieurs administrations provinciales." We have been unable to obtain any further information about him.

18. Johann N. Hunczovsky, *Medicinisch-chirurgische Beobachtungen auf seinen Reisen durch England und Frankreich, besonders über die Spitäler* (Vienna, 1783), pp. 79, 85, 112. Hunczovsky

reported that hospitalized soldiers in the military hospitals of Gros Caillou and Les Invalides fared considerably better, with an allowance of a pound of meat a day. The food portions for officers were greater, but the wine allotment was the same (pp. 126, 131–32).

19. Hunczovsky, *Beobachtungen auf Reisen* (n.18), pp. 112, 167–68. A ligature was passed by probe through the external fistulous opening into the internal opening and tied. This converted the tract into an open channel, permitting the fistula to heal.

20. Hunczovsky, *Beobachtungen auf Reisen* (n.18), pp. 84–85; Coyecque, *Hôtel-Dieu au moyen âge* (n.9), 1:25. See also Malgaigne's introduction to his edition of *Oeuvres complètes d'Ambroise Paré* (Paris, 1840), 1:cxxxii.

21. Coury, *Hôtel-Dieu* (n.7), pp. 87, 153–73.

22. Lanfranc, being married, also was denied the privilege of teaching in the Paris faculty.

23. Represented by Desault (1738–95), P. J. Pelletan (1747–1829), Dupuytren (1778–1835), J. N. Marjolin (1780–1850), Sanson (1790–1841), Roux (1780–1854), Velpeau (1795–1867), Jobert (1799–1867), Lembert (1802–51), Malgaigne (1806–65), Nélaton (1807–73), Maisonneuve (1809–97), Alphonse Guérin (1816–95), Just Lucas-Championnière (1843–1913), Tuffier (1857–1929), Henri Hartman (1860–1952), and a number of surgeons of the twentieth century who have continued to lend lustre to French surgery.

24. "Die Phlegmone nosocomialis cutanea, nach ihrem Vorkommen im Hôtel-Dieu zu Paris," *N. Jahrb. d. dt. Med. u. Chir.* (1824), 8:137–40.

25. Ulysse Trélat, "Mémoire historique et critique sur les hôpitaux," *J. de progr. d. sc. méd.*, Paris (1828), 11:207; F. Campbell Stewart, *Hospitals and surgeons of Paris* (New York, 1843), p. 32.

26. Georg Cless, "De la médecine en France et en Angleterre," *Arch. gén. de méd.* (1840), 7(1):379–80; Fosseyeux (n.12), pp. 318–19; Karl Hueter, "Die chirurgische Behandlung der Wundfieber bei Schusswunden," *Samml. klin. Vortr.* (1871), Chir. no. 7, p. 109.

27. Jules Rochard, *Histoire de la chirurgie française au XIXe siècle* (Paris, 1875), pp. 674–78; Léon Le Fort, "Résection de l'articulation coxo-fémorale dans les cas de coxalgie et de plaies par armes à feu," *Bull. Acad. imp. de méd.* (1860), 26:126–34. Ensuant discussions are scattered throughout the Academy's *Bulletin*, vol. 27, from October 15, 1861, through April 22, 1862. See especially pp. 194–202, 737. Malgaigne was suffering from arteriosclerosis. He had a stroke (January 1865) while presiding as president of the Academy of Medicine and died in October. See *Ann. méd. Nancy* (1965), 4:548–49.

28. *Bull. Acad. imp. de méd.* (1861–62), 27:260–61, 388–89.

29. Trélat's address appears in *Bull. Soc. de chir.* (1865), 5:493–500. The discussions follow. See especially pp. 525–26. Trélat believed 400 beds per hospital were enough, 800 were too many.

30. Louis X. Ollier, "Sur les complications nosocomiales des maladies chirurgicales," *Gaz. méd., Lyon* (1868), 20:455–58; Émile Vidal, "Rapport sur . . . l'isolement des malades," *Bull. mém. Soc. méd. hôp. Paris* (1864), 1:173–93.

31. Stewart, *Hospitals of Paris* (n.25), pp. 214–15.

32. A.-G. Maurice Raynaud, *Les médecins au temps de Molière*, 2d ed. (Paris, 1863), p. 22.

33. Émile Bégin, "Bibliographie analytique des écrits sur l'hygiène depuis 1792 jusqu'à nos jours," *J. d'hyg.*, Paris (1879), 4:157. Similarly in England, W. H. Corfield, professor of hygiene at University College, lamented the separation of practical medicine and surgery from hygiene. See *Br. M. J.* (1870), 1:617–19, 645–46.

34. Jean-François Rameaux, *Appréciation des progrès des l'hygiène publique, depuis le commencement du dix-neuvième siècle*, Strasbourg thesis, 1839; Johann Peter Frank (1745–1821), one of the founders of preventative medicine, stimulated considerable interest in public hygiene; his writings, published in 4 to 9 volumes, were widely read. *System einer vollständigen medicinischen Polizey*, 9 vols. (Mannheim, 1777–88; Vienna, 1779–1827); William Falconer, *Remarks on the influence of climate, situation, nature of country . . . on the disposition and temper . . . laws and custom, form of government . . . of mankind* (London, 1781).

35. Aimé Martin, *Essai sur les rapports de l'hygiène et de la prophilactique, avec la magistrature de police de salubrité*, Paris thesis, 1803.

36. Charles H. Talbot, *Medicine in medieval England* (London: Oldbourne, 1967), pp. 170–76; Rotha Mary Clay, *The mediaeval hospitals of England* (London: Methuen, 1909), pp. 1–4, 71, 252, 297–98; E. M. McInnes, *St. Thomas' Hospital* (London: George Allen, 1963); F. G. Parsons, *The history of St. Thomas's Hospital* (London: Methuen, 1932), 1:1. According to Clay, England at one time had sixteen St. Bartholomew hospitals, chiefly in the south. Parsons states at the opening of his three-volume monograph on St. Thomas's: "the harder we try to find out when and how it began, the farther does its origin fade away into the long past days when legend and tradition take the place of reliable records."

37. Herbert Bloye, *Story of Bart's, the mother hospital of the Empire* (London: East and Blades, 1923); D'Arcy Power, *A short history of St. Bartholomew's Hospital, 1123–1923* (London, 1923), pp. 5–8, 29.

38. Walter Besant, Introduction in A. Egmont Hake, *Suffering London* (1892), pp. xxxviii–xl; Norman Moore, *St. Bartholomew's Hospital in peace and war* (Cambridge Univ. Press, 1915), p. 13. The priory of St. Bartholomew was surrendered October 5, 1539, states T. Winyard, *The Priory Church of St. Bartholomew the Great* (1974), p. 6. St. Thomas's Hospital was surrendered to the king in 1540 and remained closed for ten years. Although it was again to be known as "St. Thomas's Hospital," its patron became St. Thomas the Apostle, not St. Thomas the Martyr (à Becket), explains McInnes, *St. Thomas'* (n.36), pp. 22–24.

39. James Knowles, "Architecture," in Victor Cornelius Medvei and John L. Thornton, eds., *The Royal Hospital of Saint Bartholomew, 1123–1973* (London: St. Bartholomew's Hospital, 1974), pp. 278–83. Several excellent pictures of the old and new buildings are included.

40. D'Arcy Power, *St. Bartholomew's* (n.37), pp. 20, 32–35.

41. John Langdon-Davies, *Westminster Hospital, two centuries of voluntary service, 1719–1948* (London: John Murray, 1952); Peter Eade, *The Norfolk & Norwich Hospital, 1770 to 1900* (London: Jarrold, 1900). Langdon-Davies (pp. 42–43) said the word "filth" characterized the lives of nine out of every ten people living in rotting mansions, in the hovels of the poor, and on the wharves in the seventeenth century. Continued Davies, a martyr would find little pleasure in sitting "through a meal beside the Virgin Queen," a reference to the prevalence of general insalubrity of households and personal hygiene in the Elizabethan period. Eade (p. 61) related that in compliance with the exhortation of King George IV, the Norfolk and Norwich Hospital economized in the use of bread in 1800. "Potatoes were substituted for bread at dinner in the wards and household department of the hospital," and rice was used instead of bread in the patients' broth at supper once or twice a week.

42. D'Arcy Power, *St. Bartholomew's* (n.37), pp. 29–43. John Howard mentioned the burial fee that was exacted at admission, except in "case of sudden accidents" at St. Bartholomew's and gave details of other fees there. See his *Account of the principal lazarettos in Europe . . . foreign prisons and hospitals* (Warrington, 1789), p. 132. His crusade for prison and hospital reform is reviewed in chapter 19.

43. *The modern practice of the London hospitals, viz. St. Bartholomew's, St. Thomas's, St. George's, and Guy's*, 2d ed. (London, 1766).

44. D'Arcy Power, *St. Bartholomew's* (n.36), pp. 51–52.

45. Frank B. Berry, Introduction in John of Mirfield, *Surgery*, trans. James B. Colton (New York: Hafner, auspices of Library of the New York Academy of Medicine, 1969); Talbot, *Medieval England* (n.36), pp. 200–1.

46. William Clowes, *A short and profitable treatise touching the cure of the disease called (Morbus Gallicus) by unctions* (London, 1579), sig. B, fol. ii, verso. For Clowes's thigh amputation (1588) and Woodall's work, see chapter 2 on amputation.

47. Percivall Pott, *Chirurgical observations relative to the cataract . . . the cancer of the scrotum* (London, 1775); William Lawrence, *Treatise on the diseases of the eye* (London, 1833); James Paget, "On disease of the mammary areola preceding cancer of the mammary gland," *St. Barth. Hosp. Rep.* (1874), 10:87–89; Paget, "On a form of chronic inflammation of bones

(osteitis deformans)," *Med.-Chir. Trans.* (1877), 60:37–64; (1882), 65:225–36. Abernethy's vascular surgery is discussed in chapter 15.

48. D'Arcy Power, *St. Bartholomew's* (n.37), pp. 49–50.

49. George W. Callender, "Two years of hospital practice," *St. Barth. Hosp. Rep.* (1873), 9:1–46; Callender, "Seven years of hospital practice," ibid. (1878), 14:183–95; Holmes Coote, "On the treatment of wounds," ibid. (1870), 6:113–17. Callender, one of the senior surgeons at St. Bartholomew's during this period, was an early convert to Listerian practices; his results with amputation, given in the hospital's reports, were very satisfactory.

50. From a speech by Berkeley Moynihan, "The most gentle profession," Leeds, January 21, 1921, reprinted in his *Selected writings: A centenary volume* (London: Pitman, for the Osler Club of London, 1967), p. 126.

51. Frederick Treves, letter to Viscount Knutsford, May 15, 1919, printed in *Lond. Hosp. Gaz.* (1919), 22:223–25. Howard, *Lazarettos* (n.41), p. 181, said that at Haslar Naval Hospital any nurse who got drunk was discharged. The regulations for nurses there forbade them to wash in water closets.

52. "Lancet Sanitary Commission for investigating the state of the infirmaries of workhouses," *Lancet* (1865), 2:14–16. "Report of the Lancet Sanitary Commission on the surgical wards of St. Bartholomew's Hospital," ibid. (1874), 1:246–47.

53. The editors were still continuing their attack in 1864. See *Br. M. J.* (1864), 2:581–83.

54. John Erichsen: "On the nature and causes of the mortality after surgical operations," *Med. Circ.* (1859), 14:241, and "Hospitalism and the causes of death after operations," *Br. M. J.* (1874), 1:65–67, 97–100, 131–34, 193–96.

55. William Farr, "Mortality in hospitals," letter to the editor, *Lancet* (1864), 1:420–22.

56. Meyer-Steineg and Sudhoff, *Geschichte der Medizin* (n.3), p. 220.

57. Rudolf Virchow, *Ueber Hospitäler und Lazarette* (Berlin, 1869), pp. 3, 28.

58. Ignaz Neudörfer, "Ueber Hospitalismus," *Wien. med. Presse* (1869), 10:1069–71.

59. Andreas M. Adam, "Notes on the hospitals of Munich," *Edinb. M. J.* (1860), 6:25–35.

60. Friedrich Oppert: *Die Einrichtung von Krankenhäusern* (Berlin, 1859), and "The progress of sanitary improvement in existing hospitals," *Med. Press & Circ.* (1868), 6:21–25. This surgeon spent some months in Bern (1927–28) at Bois Fleury, a four-story pension heated solely by a single large *kachelofen* on the ground floor. The warmest temperature of the upper floors during January and February was usually around 55° F.

61. Christoph Ludwig Hoffmann, *Bestättigung der Nothwendigkeit, einem jeden Kranken in einem Hospitale sein eigenes Zimmer zu geben* (Mainz, 1788).

62. W. H. W., "The hospitals of Berlin," *Clinic*, Cincinnati (1877), 13:130–32.

63. Theodor Billroth, *Chirurgische Briefe aus den Kriegs-Lazarethen in Weissenburg und Mannheim, 1870* (Berlin, 1872), pp. 60–61; Alexander Primrose, "Notes on a recent visit to surgical clinics in Germany and Switzerland," *Canad. Practnr Rev.* (1909), 34:214.

64. Gustav Neuber, *Die aseptische Wundbehandlung in meinen chirurgischen Privat-Hospitälern* (Kiel, 1886); Ernst Bergmann, "Die antiseptische Wundbehandlung in der Kgl. chirurgischen Universitäts Klinik zu Berlin," *Klin. Jahrb.* (1889), 1:147–66; Curt Schimmelbusch, *Anleitung zur aseptischen Wundbehandlung* (Berlin, 1892), pp. 11–12. See also chapter 20.

65. Stephen Smith, "Reminiscences of two epochs — anaesthesia and asepsis," *Johns Hopkins Hosp. Bull.* (1919), 30:273–78. Smith was ninety-five years of age when he made his presentation at The Hopkins. Some of the narrative, therefore, may not be completely factual.

66. Stephen Smith, "The comparative results of operations in Bellevue Hospital," *Med. News* (1885), 47:469–71.

67. Robert F. Weir, "Personal reminiscences of the New York Hospital from 1856 to 1900," in Society of the New York Hospital, *General Bull.* (1917), 1:3, 23–26. Weir was attending surgeon (1876–1900) and later a consulting surgeon. A junior walker at the New York Hospital was a medical graduate doing his first eight months of hospital service; during the next eight months he was a senior walker. See D. B. St. John Roosa, *The Old Hospital and other papers* (New York, 1889), pp. 13–14.

68. Edwin R. Maxson, "Hospitals: British, French, and American," *Med. & Surg. Reporter*, Philadelphia (1868), 18:258.

69. Arthur A. Bliss, *Blockley days: Memories and impressions of a resident physician, 1883–1884* (Springfield, Mass., 1916), pp. 21–22, 48. Bliss related he watched over a postoperative patient in an empty ward one night and heard rats in the walls; a cat came to sit with him.

70. Leroy Brown, "Our operating-rooms and methods of preparing patients," *Med. Record* (1891), 40:97.

71. Allan E. Dumont, "Halsted at Bellevue, 1883–1887," *Ann. Surg.* (1970), 172:934.

72. William M. Polk, chairman, "Report of the Committee of the Medical Board of Bellevue Hospital, appointed January 2, 1901, to investigate and report upon questions relating to the general administration of the Hospital," *Med. News* (1901), 78:489–90.

73. Hunter Robb, "The air of the operating room as a possible factor in the infection of wounds," *Trans. Am. Gynec. Assoc.* (1909), 34:550–64. Robb was a trainee in gynecology of Howard A. Kelly at The Hopkins. His endorsement of rubber gloves for all members of the operative team is discussed in chapter 23.

74. Edward W. Sheldon, "Historical address," in Society of the New York Hospital, 1771-1921, *Commemoration . . . 1921* (1922), pp. 24–25.

75. William E. Quine, "Early history of the Cook County Hospital to 1870," *Plexus*, Chicago (1910), 16:582–97; John A. Hornsby, "Chicago as a medical and surgical center. III. The hospitals of Chicago," *Surg. Gynec. Obstet.* (1913), vol. 17 (insert, "Clinical Congress of Surgeons of North America, fourth annual session . . . 1913 [program]," pp. 2–12). Robert E. Scully (1976) reported that the trustees of prestigious Massachusetts General Hospital provided a microscope costing $50 for the use of the admitting physician in 1847; the hospital did not have a full-time pathologist until many years later. *New Engl. J. Med.*, 295:1428.

76. Edmund Andrews, "The sum and substance of antiseptic surgery," *Chicago M. Exam.* (1869), 10:732–39.

77. Lester R. Dragstedt, "Christian Fenger and the Midwestern School of Surgery," *Guthrie Clin. Bull.* (1963), 33:13–24; Henry T. Ricketts, "Forty years of full-time medicine at University of Chicago," *JAMA* (1969), 208:2069–73.

78. James L. Cabell, "On sanitary conditions in relation to the treatment of surgical operations and injuries [and discussion]," *Trans. Am. Surg. Assoc.* (1882), 1:23–82; B. A. Watson, "Lister's system of aseptic wound treatment versus its modifications [and discussion]," ibid. (1883), 1:205–23.

79. John Shaw Billings, Introduction, pp. v–xxxiii, in *Circular No. 4, a report on barracks and hospitals; with descriptions of military posts* (Washington, D.C., 1870); Billings et al., *Hospital plans, for the use only of the Trustees of The Johns Hopkins Hospital 1875* (Baltimore, 1875); Billings, "Plans and purposes of The Johns Hopkins Hospital," *Med. News* (1889), 54:505–10. In Circular no. 4, Woodward said, "Never before in the History of the World has the mortality in military barracks been so low and the barracks so ample for the care of the sick, who remain free of diseases within their walls." Billings commented that the mortality rate should have been low, because the soldiers were a screened group of healthy persons (p. xxxii).

80. Zachary Cope, "John Shaw Billings, Florence Nightingale and The Johns Hopkins Hospital," *Med. Hist.*, London (1957), 1:367–68.

81. Jean-Baptiste Le Roy, *Précis d'un ouvrage sur les hôpitaux, dans lequel on expose les principes résultant des observations de physique et de médecine qu'on doit avoir en vue dans la construction de ces édifices* ([1777]); Charles Rauge, *Étude sur les hôpitaux à pavillons isolés et sans étages*, Paris thesis, 1879; Michel Lévy, *Bull. Acad. imp. de méd.*, Paris (1862), 27:593–620; Gustave Chantreuil, "Étude sur quelques points d'hygiène hospitalière," *Arch. gén. de méd.*, Paris (1868), 2:385–407, 548–69.

82. Douglas Galton, *An address on the general principles which should be observed in the construction of hospitals, delivered to the British Medical Association at Leeds, July 29, 1869, with the discussion which took place thereon* (London, 1869); Lewis A. Stimson, "Bacteria and their influence upon

the origin and development of septic complications of wounds," *N. York M. J.* (1875), 22:144–45.

83. Friedrich Sander, *Ueber Geschichte, Statistik, Bau und Einrichtung der Krankenhäuser. Nebst einem Bericht über das Krankenhaus der Stadt Barmen* (Köln, 1875).

84. Félix Rochard: *Projet de création d'une ambulance sur la Seine* (Paris, 1871), and "Rapport sur la construction des hôpitaux," *Ann. d'hyg.*, Paris (1883), 9:423–45; 10:73, 179.

85. Oppert (n.60).

86. Y. W. Jastreboff, "Communication sur les antiseptiques et l'installation d'un hôpital, au point de vue antiseptique," *Ann. d'hyg.*, Paris (1885), 13:80–82.

87. Alphonse Laveran, "De la contagion dans les salles d'hôpital, quelques desiderata de l'hygiène hospitalière," *Méd. mod.* (1889–90), 1:221–25.

88. I. P. Semmelweis, *Die Aetiologie . . .* (1861), p. 270.

Further Readings

Ackerknecht, Erwin H. *Medicine at the Paris hospital, 1794–1848.* Baltimore: Johns Hopkins Press, 1967.

Beck, R. Theodore. *The cutting edge: Early history of the surgeons of London.* London: Humphries, 1974.

Bonner, Thomas. *American doctors and German universities.* Lincoln, Neb.: Univ. Nebraska Press, 1963.

Brieger, Gert H., ed. *Theory and practice in American medicine.* New York: Science History Publications, 1976.

Brock, Russell. The operating theatre of old Guy's Hospital. *Guy's Hosp. Rep.* (1964), 113:131–35.

Browne, O'Donel T. D. *The Rotunda Hospital, 1745–1945.* Edinburgh: E. and S. Livingstone, 1947.

Churchill, Edward D., ed. *To work in the vineyard of surgery; the reminiscences of J. Collins Warren (1842–1927).* Cambridge: Harvard Univ. Press, 1958.

Clendening, Logan. *Source book of medical history.* New York: Paul B. Hoeber, 1942.

Collection of essays on American medicine in revolutionary times. *JAMA*, Bicentennial issue (1976), 236:26–88.

Corlieu, Auguste. *Centenaire de la Faculté de médecine de Paris (1794–1894).* Paris, 1896.

Corner, George W. *Two centuries of medicine; a history of the School of Medicine, University of Pennsylvania.* Philadelphia and Montreal: J. B. Lippincott, 1965.

Dainton, Courtney. *The story of England's hospitals.* London: Museum Press, 1961.

Denny, Lionel. The Royal Hospitals of the City of London. *Ann. R. Coll. Surg.*, England (1973), 52:86–101.

Earle, Arthur S. *Surgery in America: from the colonial era to the twentieth century.* Philadelphia and London: W. B. Saunders, 1965.

Fifield, James C. *American and Canadian hospitals.* Minneapolis: Midwest Publishers, 1933.

Flack, I. Harvey [Harvey Graham]. *Surgeons all.* London: Rich and Cowan, 1939.

Franklin, Benjamin. *Some account of the Pennsylvania Hospital.* Philadelphia, 1754. Facsimile. Baltimore: Johns Hopkins Press, 1954.

Gelfand, Toby. *The training of surgeons in eighteenth-century Paris.* Ann Arbor, Mich.: Xerox University Microfilms, 1974.

Girard, A. C. Report on materials used in Lister's system of wound treatment. Circular Orders No. 3. Surgeon General's Office, Washington, D.C., August 20, 1877.

Goldhahn, Richard. *Spital und Arzt von Einst bis Jetzt.* Stuttgart: Ferdinand Enke, 1947.

Grois, Bernhard. *Das Allgemeine Krankenhaus in Wien und seine Geschichte.* Vienna: W. Maudrich, 1965.

Innes Smith, Robert W. *English-speaking students of medicine at the University of Leyden.* Edinburgh and London: Oliver and Boyd, 1932.

Killian, Hans, and Krämer, G. *Meister der Chirurgie und die Chirurgenschulen im Deutschen Raum.* Stuttgart: G. Thieme, 1951.

Leistikow, Dankwart. *Ten centuries of European hospital architecture; a contribution to the history of hospital architecture.* Ingelheim am Rhein: C. H. Boehringer, 1967.

Lindpainter, Julius. Ergebnisse der Lister'schen Wundbehandlung. *Dt. Z. Chir.* (1876), 7:187–273.

Marty, Alan T. The pagan roots of Western hospitals. *Surg. Gynec. Obstet.* (1971), 133(2):1019–22.

Moore, Norman. *History of the study of medicine in the British Isles.* Oxford: Clarendon Press, 1908.

Morton, Thomas G. *History of the Pennsylvania Hospital, 1751–1895.* Philadelphia, 1895.

Mumford, James G. *A narrative of medicine in America.* Philadelphia and London: J. B. Lippincott, 1903.

Neuburger, Max. *British medicine and the Vienna School: Contacts and parallels.* London: William Heinemann, 1943.

Ober, William B. *Great men of Guy's.* Metuchen, N.J.: Scarecrow Reprint, 1973.

Osler, William. *The principles and practice of medicine.* New York, 1892.

Packard, Francis R. *History of medicine in the United States.* 2 vols. 2d ed. New York: Paul B. Hoeber, 1931. Reprint. New York: Hafner, 1963.

Shryock, Richard H. *Medicine in America; historical essays.* Baltimore: Johns Hopkins Press, 1966.

Smith, Stephen. The evolution of American surgery. In *American practice of surgery,* ed. Joseph D. Bryant and Albert H. Buck, vol. 1, pp. 3–67. New York: William Wood, 1906.

Van der Star, P. History of thermometry in medicine. *Biblthca radiol.* (1969), no. 5, pp. 1–7.

Williams, William H. *America's first hospital: The Pennsylvania Hospital, 1751–1841.* Wayne, Pa.: Haverford House, 1976.

Woollcott, Joan, ed. *Classics in medical literature from the University of Pennsylvania, 1765–1965.* Philadelphia: Univ. Pennsylvania, Medical Affairs, 1965.

Chapter 19. Hospital Reformers, Sanitarians, and Surgical Accountability

Notes

1. John Aikin, *A view of the character and public services of the late John Howard* (London, 1792). Aikin, a physician, was a friend and consultant of Howard. John Howard came into possession of a considerable inheritance at age twenty-five, a bequest from his father, a successful Smithfield businessman. Howard was twice married, first at age twenty-six, to a fifty-three-year-old widow who died within three years. His second marriage (1758) gave him his "only years of true enjoyment," but his wife died when their only child, a son, was born in 1765. During her lifetime Howard spent much of his time and income in building new houses for the tenants on his property near Bedford. Thereafter his fortune was dedicated to the cause of prison and hospital reforms and his necessary travel. Howard was created a Fellow of the Royal Society in 1756. His biographer, Aikin, explains (p. 21) that the honor was not given for any extraordinary proficiency in science, but in "conformity to the laudable practice of that society, of attaching gentlemen of fortune and leisure to the interests of knowledge, by incorporating them into their body." See also *Dictionary of national biography*, s.v. "Howard, John."

2. John Howard, *The state of the prisons in England and Wales, with . . . an account of some foreign prisons* (Warrington, 1777). Additional material on prisons as well as descriptions of some foreign hospitals was published as an *Appendix* in 1780. We have used the fourth edition of Howard's *Prisons* (1792), which includes accounts of his hospital visits.

3. John Howard, *An account of the principal lazarettos in Europe with . . . observations on some foreign prisons and hospitals* (Warrington, 1789).

4. Howard, *Prisons* (1792), pp. 6–8, 26, 61, 138, 211, and *Lazarettos* (1789), p. 206.

5. Howard, *Prisons* (1792), pp. 1–5, and *Lazarettos* (1789), pp. 24–25, 231–32. Howard found debtors among the "most pitiable objects in our gaols." In 1787 Howard gave an inquiring physician his health regimen: He rose early, took a cold water sponge, head to toe, always breakfasting before hospital visits. A total abstainer, he ate two meals a day, took no animal food other than milk, which together with tea and a twopenny loaf of bread constituted his sustenance, and said Howard, he was capable of great exertion. Alexander G. Gibson, *The Radcliffe Infirmary* (London: Oxford Univ. Press, 1926), p. 102.

6. Howard, *Lazarettos*, pp. 10–12, 22, 27, 32. Howard stressed the economic advantages for England in getting cotton directly from Turkey. The methods of fumigation were sometimes rather bizarre. At Malta a letter from Turkey was received with "iron tongs, dipped in vinegar, and then put into a case, and laid for about a quarter of an hour on wire grates, under which straw and perfumes had been burnt," before it was delivered (p. 8).

7. Howard, *Prisons*, pp. 176, 179, 342; Howard, *Lazarettos*, pp. 138, 192; Nathaniel W. Faxon, "A history of hospitals," *Bull. Am. Hosp. Assoc.* (1929), 3:30.

8. Aikin, *Howard* (n.1), pp. 189–98, 227. Burke is quoted in William A. Guy, *Public health; a popular introduction to sanitary science* (London, 1870), p. 192. Sevastopol, the site of sieges in the Crimean War (1854–56) and World War I, was reduced to rubble in World War II, but rebuilt as a great military naval base. It is no longer accessible to visitors, as the authors learned when at nearby Yalta in September 1973.

9. Georges Cuvier, "Éloge historique de Jacques Tenon," in *Recueil des éloges historiques* (Strasbourg, 1819), 2:269–304. Cuvier says (p. 294) that Tenon went "toise à la main" into the hospitals, and adds that he never saw Tenon attending the funeral of a confrere without his measuring the grave to see if it conformed to regulations. *Toise*, meaning a "fathom measure," has been freely translated by the authors as "yardstick."

10. Two fine articles on Tenon and his hospital studies have been prepared by Louis S. Greenbaum: "*The commercial treaty of humanity.* La tournée des hôpitaux anglais par Jacques Tenon en 1787," *Rev. d'hist. sci. applic.* (1971), 24:317–50, and "'Measure of civilization,' the hospital thought of Jacques Tenon on the eve of the French Revolution," *Bull. Hist. Med.* (1975), 49:43–56.

11. The Hôtel-Dieu also had small beds, for one or sometimes two occupants, but there were many more of the large type.

12. Jacques Tenon, *Mémoires sur les hôpitaux de Paris* (Paris, 1788), pp. 135, 220–37.

13. Tenon's mortality table showed that 1 in every 4.5 patients died at the Hôtel-Dieu. He believed that the rate was actually higher (pp. 278–79). It should be considered, however, that dying patients dismissed from other hospitals often found their way to the Hôtel-Dieu. By a decree of 1803 each French hospital was obliged to have a separate room for operations. Pierre Huard and Mirko Drazen Grmek, *La chirurgie moderne* (Paris: Dacosta, 1968), p. 35.

14. Louis S. Greenbaum, "The humanitarianism of Antoine Laurent Lavoisier," *Studies on Voltaire and the eighteenth century* (1972), 88:651–75. See chapter 20 on germ theory.

15. From a quotation by Sir John Simon, colleague and successor in public health work, in Samuel E. Finer, *Life and times of Sir Edwin Chadwick* (New York: Barnes and Noble, 1952), the definitive biography of Chadwick (p. 515).

16. Edwin Chadwick, "An essay on the means of insurance against the casualties of sickness, decrepitude, and mortality," *Westminster Rev.* (1828), 9:417.

17. *Report . . . from the Poor Law Commissioners on an inquiry into the sanitary condition of the labouring population of Great Britain* (London, 1842), pp. 1, 47, 154–61, 212, 369–70. A new edition of the *Report*, with an introduction by M. W. Flinn, was published in 1965 by the Edinburgh University Press. Chadwick was not a great statistician and inevitably came into conflict in such matters with his assistant, William Farr. Richard Lewis, *Edwin Chadwick and the public health movement, 1832–1854* (London: Longmans, Green, 1952), p. 32.

18. Edwin Chadwick, "Progress of sanitation, civil and military," *J. Soc. Arts* (1888), 36(2):1030–34.

19. "The pestilential state of the Thames," *Br. M. J.* (1858), 2:535; Carleton B. Chapman, "The year of the great stink," *Pharos* (1972), 35:90–105. See also: *Lancet* (1858), 1:632; 2:41, 43, 67, 77; *Br. M. J.* (1858), pp. 545, 547. We are indebted to Charles Talbot of the Wellcome Institute of the History of Medicine for information on the 1858 Thames controversy.

20. Chadwick's belief that untreated sewage could be profitably and safely used as field manure is explained in Flinn's introduction to the 1965 edition of *Report into the sanitary condition*, p. 59. See also Finer's *Life and times of Chadwick* (1952).

21. Chadwick, "Progress of sanitation" (1888), p. 1031.

22. Edwin Chadwick, *The general history of principles of sanitation* (London, 1889), pp. 6–11.

23. Edwin Chadwick's reply, read by Lord Fortescue, appears in the *Sanitarian* (1889), 22:387–95.

24. Royston Lambert, *Sir John Simon, 1816–1904, and English social administration* (London: MacGibbon and Kee, 1963); H. Willoughby Lyle, *King's and some King's men* (Oxford: Oxford Univ. Press, 1935), pp. 61–63. John Simon at age seventeen became one of Joseph H. Green's dressers at King's College and St. Thomas's Hospital, for which privilege his family paid Green the handsome fee of 500 guineas. Originally identified with both institutions, Simon left King's to become assistant surgeon at St. Thomas's in 1853; he was promoted surgeon in 1863. Simon was president of the Royal College of Surgeons in 1878. Liverpool was the first English town to appoint a medical officer of health; London was the second.

25. See chapter 5 on prostatic obstruction.

26. Simon's superb English "made sanitary reform a branch of English literature." His *English sanitary institutions* (1890) deserved to be read side by side with Buckle's *History of civilisation*, wrote Victor G. Plarr, librarian of the Royal College of Surgeons, in *Lancet* (August 13, 1904, pp. 488–89), citing especially a passage on St. Francis in Simon's introduction.

27. As a youth Simon had studied in Europe and acquired an interest in literature, art, and music. In later travels he met many leading European scientists of the day. Sir John and Lady Simon were fond of entertaining and their salons were attended by literary celebrities and artists — Thackeray, Tennyson, and Rossetti among others. *Lancet*, July 30, 1904, pp. 320–25.

28. John Simon, *Reports relating to the sanitary condition of the City of London* (London, 1854), pp. xxvi–xxvii, xxxii, xl.

29. *Sixth report of the Medical Officer of the Privy Council, 1863* (London, 1864), pp. 38–39. The early hospital records of the Royal Bristol Infirmary that originated in 1735 were used as old paper. Fortunately some were rescued for the benefit of a hospital historian. J. Paul Bush, *Bristol M.-Chir. J.* (1908), 26:193–206.

30. Simon, *Sixth report, 1863* (n.29), pp. 39–40, 52, 57. Pierre Chalvet died at the age of forty (1871). A physician of great scientific curiosity but little means, he had turned his living room into a laboratory.

31. C. H. F. Routh, "On the causes of the endemic puerperal fever of Vienna," *Med.-Chir. Trans.* (1849), 32:27–40. Simon had also referred briefly to Routh's article in *Papers relating to the sanitary state of the people of England* (London, 1858), p. 305. See also chapter 23 on preparations for operation.

32. See especially Simon, *Sixth report, 1863* (n.29), pp. 52, 59, 65–74.

33. William Robinson, *Story of the Royal Infirmary, Sunderland* (Sunderland, 1934), p. 16.

34. *Br. M. J.* (1904), 2:267.

35. *Report of the Commissioners appointed to inquire into the regulations affecting the sanitary condition of the Army, the organization of military hospitals, and the treatment of the sick and wounded*, Blue book (London, 1858), p. 361. See Edward Cook, *Life of Florence Nightingale*, 2 vols. (London: Macmillan, 1913), 1:416–19. Cook's is the most complete biography of this distinguished woman and is the source of much of the information in this section.

36. Pastor Theodor and Friederike Fliedner in 1833 turned the gardenhouse of his pastorate into an asylum for discharged female prisoners, and in 1836 founded the first school for deaconesses. It became the model for similar institutions in Germany. Elizabeth Fry visited

Fliedner's hospital in 1840 during her tour for prison reform in Europe. Her niece described the young nurses (deaconesses) as a "capital set of women." *Elizabeth Fry's journeys on the Continent 1840–1841, from a diary kept by her niece Elizabeth Gurney*, ed. R. Brimley Johnson (London: John Lane the Bodley Head, 1931), p. 100.

37. Cook, *Nightingale* (n.35), 1:147, 149.

38. Scutari and Constantinople are now Üskürdar and Istanbul, respectively.

39. John Howard had approved of women nurses in the military Haslar Hospital. "All the nurses here, and in the hospital at Plymouth, are women, which is very proper, as they are more cleanly and tender; and they more easily pacify the patients, who are seafaring men." *Lazarettos* (n.2), p. 180.

40. Quoted in Cook, *Nightingale* (n.35), 1:183–84.

41. *Report of the Commissioners* (n.35), p. 365; Florence Nightingale, *Notes on nursing* (London, 1860), pp. 29–30.

42. Cook, *Nightingale* (n.35), 1:186, 236. Miss Nightingale's letters and notes occupy 150 volumes at the British Museum, according to Zachary Cope, *Florence Nightingale and the doctors* (London: Museum Press, 1958), p. 151.

43. *Letters of Florence Nightingale in the History of Nursing Archive, . . . Boston University Libraries*, ed. Lois A. Monteiro (Boston: Boston University, Mugar Memorial Library, 1974), letter 66, p. 35. Sir Andrew Clark (1826–93) was knighted in 1883. For twenty years he was one of the senior physicians at the London Hospital and had one of the most lucrative practices in London. He left £200,000. His services were widely sought; hypochondriacs called him "their dearest friend"; his funeral was almost a public event, a portion of which was held at Westminster Abbey. A. E. Clark-Kennedy, *The London, a study in the voluntary hospital system* (London: Pitman, 1962), 2:133; *Dictionary of national biography*, s.v. "Clark, Sir Andrew, M.D."

44. Florence Nightingale, *Notes on hospitals*, 3d ed. (London, 1863), pp. 56, 101–2. Miss Nightingale wrote Dr. Pattison Walker, April 1866, "See what harm the German pathologists have done us. There are no specific diseases, there are specific disease conditions. . . . It is a great thing for weak minds — the doctrine of contagion." Quoted in Cope, *Nightingale and the doctors* (n.42), p. 16.

45. Smith was active in the New York Academy of Medicine during the last (ninety-ninth) year of his life.

46. Stephen Smith, *The city that was* (New York: Allaben, 1911; reprint under auspices of the New York Academy of Medicine: Scarecrow, 1973), pp. 34–39. Smith also tells the story in "The history of Public Health, 1871–1921," in P. Ravenel Mazyck, ed., *A half century of public health* (New York: Am. Public Health Assoc., 1921), p. 1.

47. Gert H. Brieger, "Sanitary reform in New York City: Stephen Smith and the passage of the Metropolitan Health Bill," *Bull. Hist. Med.* (1966), 40:407–29. Brieger explains that in 1860 New York's city inspector and his forty-four health wardens were in charge of the city's sanitation. The position was bought and sold; several of the wardens admitted they did not personally inspect cases of disease (p. 416). This was the era of Tammany.

48. Most of the inspectors were young physicians from charitable dispensaries who knew the areas and many of the inhabitants well through their practice. They received a token $40 a month for the task which they undertook with enthusiasm "as a purely scientific study." Smith, *City that was* (n.46), pp. 52–57; Brieger (n.47), p. 421.

49. Citizen's Association of New York, *Report of the Council of Hygiene and Public Health of the Citizen's Association of New York upon the sanitary condition of the city* (New York, 1865); Smith, *City that was* (n.47), pp. 59–73.

50. Stephen Smith, "On the limitations and modifying conditions of human longevity, the basis of sanitary work," in Am. Public Health Assoc., *Reports and papers . . . 1873* (New York, 1875), 1:13–16.

51. Edward H. Sieveking, "Harvey, and the unity of the profession," *Lancet* (1862), 1:117; Alexander Monro I, "Remarks on the amputations of the larger extremities," *Med.*

Essays & Obs., Edinburgh (1737), 4:342; (1752), 4:276; Joseph-François Malgaigne, "Études statistiques sur les résultats des grandes opérations dans les hôpitaux de Paris," *Arch. gén. de méd.* (1842), 13:389–418; 14:50–81.

52. James Paget, "Address in surgery," *Br. M. J.* (1862), 2:157. John C. Warren also heard the account from Cooper, who told him the Paris surgeon was Larrey. See Howard Payson Arnold, *Memoir of Jonathan Mason Warren, M.D.* (Boston, 1886), p. 85.

53. Lawson Tait, "Address in surgery," *Br. M. J.* (1890), 2:272.

54. A discussion of some of the current problems on "medical audit and recertification" appeared in *Br. M. J.*, February 16, 1974, pp. 255–57, 271–82.

Further Readings

Astruc, Pierre. Florence Nightingale. *Progrès méd.*, Paris (1954), 82:112–13.

Baly, Monica E. Florence Nightingale's influence on nursing today. *Nurs. Times* (1969), 65:1–4.

Belt, Elmer. Florence Nightingale's role in history. In the Elmer Belt Florence Nightingale Collection, University of California Biomedical Library Catalogue. Los Angeles, 1958.

Bishop, William J., and Goldie, Sue. *A bio-bibliography of Florence Nightingale.* London: Dawsons of Pall Mall for International Council of Nurses, 1962.

Brown, James B. *Memoirs of the public and private life of John Howard, the philanthropist.* 2d ed. London, 1823.

Cartwright, F. F. Miss Nightingale's dearest friend. *Proc. R. Soc. Med.*, London (1976), 69:169–75.

Dudley, Hugh. Necessity for surgical audit. *Br. M. J.* (1974), 1:275–77.

Field, John. *Life of John Howard with comments on his character and philanthropic labours.* London, 1850.

Hawley, Katharine J. The contributions of Florence Nightingale to hygiene and sanitation. M.P.H. thesis. Yale, 1938.

Marston, Maurice. *Sir Edwin Chadwick.* London: Leonard Parsons, 1925.

Payne, Joseph F. Sir John Pringle (1707–1782). In *Dictionary of national biography*, vol. 16, pp. 386–88. London: Oxford Univ. Press, 1896.

Pickering, George. Florence Nightingale's illness. Letter to the editors. *Br. M. J.* (1974), 4:656.

Pringle, John. *Observations on the diseases of the Army in camp and garrison.* 2d ed. London, 1753.

Richardson, Benjamin W. *The health of nations. A review of the works of Edwin Chadwick, with a biographical dissertation.* 2 vols. London, 1887.

Sanazaro, P. J. Medical audit, experience in the U.S.A. *Br. M. J.* (1974), 1:271–74.

Seaton, Edward. The achievements of public preventive medicine in the Victorian era. *Practitioner* (1897), 58:703–9.

Simon, John. *Filth-diseases and their prevention.* 1st Am. ed. Boston, 1876. Towards medical audit. Editorial. *Br. M. J.* (1974), 1:255–57.

Volkmann, Richard. Ueber den antiseptischen Occlusivverband und seinen Einfluss auf den Heilungsprocess der Wunden. *Samml. klin. Vortr.* (1874), Chir. no. 30, pp. 759–812.

Woodham-Smith, Cecil. *Florence Nightingale: 1820–1910.* New York: McGraw-Hill, 1951.

Chapter 20. Germ Theory of Infection and Disease

Notes

1. Girolamo Fracastoro, *De contagione et contagiosis morbis et eorum curatione* [Contagion, contagious diseases and their treatment], trans. with notes by Wilmer C. Wright (New York: Putnam, 1930), pp. vii–xxi; Fielding H. Garrison, letter to the editor, *Science* (1910), 31:500. Wright gives Fracastoro's birth as probably 1478; he died in 1553. His family had been

prominent citizens of Verona for generations. Fracastoro first studied mathematics, then medicine at the University of Padua, and became one of Verona's leading physicians. *De contagione* was published in 1546, after his retirement. Osler called Fracastoro's *Syphilis* the "most successful medical poem ever written." *Proc. Charaka Club* (1906), 2:5.

2. Fracastoro, *Contagione* (n.1), pp. 7, 187, 193. Wright (p. 302) translated "germs" as the closest English equivalent of "seminaria."

3. Francesco Redi, *Esperienze intorno alla generazione degl'insetti* (Florence, 1668). Antonj van Leeuwenhoek (1632–1723) lived practically all his long and creative life in Delft. He was a self-taught microscopist, without any formal scientific education. Many of his remarkable discoveries were communicated by letters in Dutch to the Royal Society of London, of which he was made a Fellow in 1680, and were published in translation in the Society's *Philosophical Transactions*. See especially his "Observations . . . concerning little animals . . . observed in rain- well- sea- and snow-water," *Phil. Trans.* (1677), 12:821–31. An excellent biography is Clifford Dobell's *Antony van Leeuwenhoek and his "little animals"* (London: Harcourt, Brace, 1932).

4. [John] Tubervill[e] Needham, "Summary of some late observations upon the generation, composition, and decomposition of animal and vegetable substances," *Phil. Trans.* (1748), 45:615–66; Lazaro Spallanzani, *Saggio di osservazioni microscopiche relative al sistema della generazione* (Modena, 1767); Spallanzani, *Opusculi di fisica animale e vegetabile*, 2 vols. (Modena, 1776). René J. Dubos has stated that Spallanzani's failure to inoculate his media occasioned him to overlook the great potential of his work, that otherwise he might have been the founder of experimental microbiology. Dubos, "Evolution of medical microbiology," in Dubos and James G. Hirsch, eds., 4th ed., *Bacterial and mycotic infections of man* (Philadelphia: Lippincott, 1965), p. 2.

5. Franz Schulze, "Vorläufige Mittheilung der Resultate einer experimentellen Beobachtung über Generatio aequivoca," *Ann. d. Phys. u. Chem.* (1836), 39:487–89. Theodor Schwann, "Vorläufige Mittheilung, betreffend Versuche über die Weingährung und Fäulniss," *Ann. d. Phys. u. Chem.* (1837), 41:184–93. Marcel Florkin reports that an entry in Schwann's unpublished journal of experiments in January 1836 reads: "Alcoholic fermentation is the work of a living organism and this living organism must be of vegetable origin since tincture of nux vomica does not influence it." *Bull. Acad. roy. méd. Belg.* (1952), 17:166.

6. Charles Cagniard-Latour, "Mémoire sur la fermentation vineuse," *Compt. rend. Acad. d. sc.* (1837), 4:905–6; Schwann (n.5); Friedrich T. Kützing, "Microscopische Untersuchungen über die Hefe und Essigmutter," *J. f. prakt. Chem.* (1837), 11:385–409; Johann J. Berzelius, "Weingährung," *Jahresb. ü. d. Fortschr. d. phys. Wissensch.* (1839), 18:400–3; Justus Liebig, "Über die Erscheinungen der Gährung, Fäulniss und Verwesung und ihre Ursachen," *Ann. d. Phys. u. Chem.* (1839), 18:106–50; [Liebig and F. Wöhler], "Das enträthselte Geheimniss der geistigen Gährung" [Riddle of vinous fermentation], *Ann. d. Pharm.* (1839), 29:100–4. The story is well told by William Bulloch, *History of bacteriology* (London: Oxford Univ. Press, 1938; reprint 1960), pp. 46–57. Cagniard-Latour's findings were first presented at several meetings of the Société philomathique (1836–37).

7. Hermann Helmholtz, "Ueber das Wesen der Fäulniss und Gährung," *Arch. f. Anat. Physiol. u. wissensch. Med.* (1843), pp. 453–62.

8. Heinrich Schröder and Theodor Dusch, "Ueber Filtration der Luft in Beziehungen auf Fäulniss und Gährung," *Ann. d. Chem. u. Pharm.* (1854), 89:232–43; Louis Pasteur, "Suite à une precédente communication relative aux générations dites spontanées," *Compt. rend. Acad. d. sc.* (1860), 51:675–78.

9. John Tyndall's papers (1876–77) initially appearing in *Philosophical Transactions* of the Royal Society and other journals were published in a monograph, *Essays on the floating-matter of the air, in relation to putrefaction and infection* (London, 1881).

10. Leeuwenhoek bequeathed 26 microscopes to the Royal Society, which have since disappeared, and left behind at least 247 finished microscopes, as well as 172 mounted lenses, according to Dobell, *Leeuwenhoek* (n.3), pp. 320–21.

11. Rudolf Virchow, "Rokitansky, Handbuch der allgemeinen pathologischen Anatomie," *Preuss. Med.-Ztg.* (1846), no. 49, pp. 237–38, no. 50, pp. 243–44; Virchow, "Die neue Auflage von Rokitansky's allgemeiner pathologischer Anatomie," *Wien. med. Wschr.* (1855), 5:401–5, 417–21; L. J. Rather, "Virchow's review of Rokitansky's *Handbuch* in the *Preussiche Medizinal-Zeitung*, Dec. 1846," *Clio Med.* (1969), 4:127–40.

12. Athanasius Kircher, *Scrutinium physico-medicum contagiosae luis, quae pestis dicitur* (Rome, 1658); Friedrich Löffler, *Vorlesungen über die geschichtliche Entwickelung der Lehre von den Bacterien* (Leipzig, 1887), p. vi; Dobell, *Leeuwenhoek* (n.3), pp. 243–49.

13. Louis Joblot, *Observations d'histoire naturelle, faites avec le microscope* (Paris, 1754), 1(2):40. The first edition appeared in 1718.

14. Marcello Malpighi, *De pulmonibus observationes anatomicae* (Bologna, 1661); Robert Hooke, *Microphagia, or some physiological descriptions of minute bodies made by magnifying glasses* (London, 1665); Nehemiah Grew, *Musaeum Regalis Societatis, or a catalogue and description of the . . . rarities belonging to the Royal Society . . . whereunto is subjoyned the comparative anatomy of stomachs and guts* (London, 1681).

15. Ivan Pavlov, *The work of the digestive glands* (London, 1902), pp. 177–78.

16. Christian G. Ehrenberg, *Die Infusionsthierchen als vollkommene Organismen; ein Blick in das tiefere organische Leben der Natur* (Leipzig, 1838).

17. Julius Vogel, *Über Eiter, Eiterung und die damit verwandten Vorgänge* (Erlangen, 1838); Emanuel Kreipl, *Ueber Eiter und Eiterung* (Vienna, 1839); Hubert Luschka, *Entwickelungsgeschichte der Formbestandtheile des Eiters und der Granulationen* (Freiburg im Breisgau, 1845).

18. Jacob Henle, "Miasmen und Contagien," pp. 1–82 in his *Pathologische Untersuchungen* (Berlin, 1840); George Rosen, "Social aspects of Jacob Henle's medical thought," *Bull. Hist. Med.* (1937), 5:509–37; Elie Metchnikoff, *The founders of modern medicine* (New York: Walden, 1939), p. 26.

19. Simon Flexner and James Thomas Flexner, *William Henry Welch and the heroic age of American medicine* (New York: Viking Press, 1941), p. 94.

20. Arnold Hiller, "Ein experimenteller Beitrag zur Lehre von der organisirten Natur der Contagien und von der Fäulniss," *Arch. klin. Chir.* (1875), 18:697. In 1876 Hiller concluded that pus might contain injurious putrefactive ferments or substances, but he was not willing to admit the pathogenic character of bacteria. *Centralb. f. Chir.* (1876), 3:227–30.

21. Lawson Tait, "One hundred and thirty-nine consecutive ovariotomies performed between January 1st, 1884, and December 31st, 1885, without a death," *Br. M. J.* (1886), 1:921–24.

22. Joseph Gerlach, "Ueber die Einwirkung von Farbstoff auf lebende Gewebe," *Wissensch. Mitth. d. phys.-med. Soc. zu Erlang.* (1858), 1(1):5–12; Carl Weigert, "Über eine Mykose bei einem neugeborenen Kinde," *Jahresb. d. schles. Gesellsch. f. väterl. Kult., 1875* (1876), 53:229–30.

23. Hermann Klencke, *Untersuchungen und Erfahrungen im Gebiete der Anatomie, Physiologie, Mikrologie und wissenschaftlichen Medicin* (Leipzig, 1843), pp. 108–11; H. R. Ranke, "Die Bacterien-Vegetation unter dem Lister'schen Verbande," *Centralbl. f. Chir.* (1874), 1:193–94, amplified in *Dt. Z. Chir.* (1877), 7:63–68; Friedrich Fehleisen, "Ueber Erysipel," *Dt. Z. Chir.* (1882), 16:391–97.

24. P.-F.-O. Rayer, "Inoculation du sang de rate," *Compt. rend. Soc. de biol.* (1850), 2:141–44. Casimir J. Davaine (1812–82) was associated with Rayer (1793–1867) in the research and later said that he had composed the report. See *Bull. Acad. de méd.* (1875), 4:581–83.

25. Casimir J. Davaine, "Bactérie, bactéridie," *Dict. encycl. d. sc. méd.* (1868), 8:19, 23; Bulloch, *History of bacteriology* (n.6), p. 144.

26. Edwin Klebs, "Die Ursache der infectiösen Wundkrankheiten," *Cor.-Bl. f. schweiz. Aerzte* (1871), 1:241–46; Klebs, *Beiträge zur pathologischen Anatomie der Schusswunden* (Leipzig, 1872), pp. 97–113; Rudolf Virchow, *Die Fortschritte der Kriegsheilkunde, besonders im Gebiete Infectionskrankheiten* (Berlin, 1874); Virchow [discussion], *Programm der XXXVI Versammlung*

deutscher Naturforscher und Aerzte in Speyer 1861. Section Gynäkologie, pp. 56–58; Franz Bruck, "Semmelweis und Virchow," *Sudhoff's Arch. Gesch. Med.* (1930), 23:387–88.

27. Léon Coze and Victor Feltz, "Récherches expérimentales sur la présence des infusoires et l'état du sang dans les maladies inféctieuses," *Gaz. méd. Strasbourg* (1866), 26:61–64, 115–25, 208–9, 225–29; (1867), 27:217–20; (1869), 29:1–3, 27–30, 38–42.

28. Ferdinand Cohn, *Ueber Bacterien, die kleinsten lebenden Wesen* (Berlin, 1872). Otto F. Müller's *Animalcula infusoria fluviatilia et marina* (Copenhagen, 1786) was published two years after the death of the great naturalist.

29. Agnostino Bassi, *Del mal del segno calcinaccio o moscardino malattia che affligge i bachi da seta e sul modo di liberarne le bigattaje anche le più infestate*, 2 vols. (Lodi, 1835–36); Félix Dujardin, *Histoire naturelle des zoophytes* (Paris, 1841); Ferdinand Cohn, *Bacteria, the smallest of living organisms*, trans. Charles S. Dolley, 1881 (Baltimore: The Johns Hopkins Press, 1939), p. 18. Bassi was one of the first to recognize bacteria to be of plant rather than animal origin.

30. Cohn, *Bacteria* (n.29), pp. 19, 33.

31. Charles E. Sédillot, "De l'influence des découvertes de M. Pasteur sur les progrès de la chirurgie," *Compt. rend. Acad. d. sc.* (1878), 86:634. Correspondence between Sédillot and Littré concerning the term "microbe" is quoted in René Vallery-Radot, *Life of Pasteur* (Garden City, N.Y.: Doubleday, Doran, 1928), pp. 266–67.

32. Bernard Gaspard, "Mémoire physiologique sur les maladies purulentes et putrides," *J. de physiol. expér.*, Paris (1822), 2:1–45; Gaspard, "Second mémoire physiologique et médical sur les maladies putrides," ibid. (1824), 4:24; François Magendie, "Remarques sur la notice précédente, avec quelques expériences sur les effets des substances en putréfaction," *J. de physiol. expér.*, Paris (1823), 3:81–88. Pringle's experiments are discussed in chapter 17 on antiseptics.

33. Peter Ludvig Panum, "Bidrag til Laeren om den saakaldte putride eller septiske Infection," *Biblioth. f. Læger* (1856), 8:253–85; Panum, "Studier over Gäring och Farrådnelse," *Nord. med. Ark.* (1876), 8(25):11–35; (1878), 10:1–53; Edouard P. M. Chassaignac, *Traité pratique de la suppuration et du drainage chirurgical* (Paris, 1859), 1:2, 9. Panum's initial studies were made in Kiel.

34. Bergeret, "Études sur le pus," *Gaz. hôp.*, Paris (1854), 27:386.

35. "Existence de micrococcus et de bactéries sur les murs des salles d'hôpitaux," *Union méd.*, Paris (1877), 23:610–11; [abstract], *Med. Times & Gaz.* (1877), 1:435.

36. Pasteur, "Communication [on Bergeron's work]," *Bull. Acad. de méd.* (1875), 4:192–97.

37. W. Watson Cheyne, "On the relation of organisms to antiseptic dressings," *Trans. Path. Soc. London* (1879), 30:558; Alexander Ogston, "Micro-organisms in surgical diseases," *Br. M. J.* (1881), 1:373. Ogston referred to Cheyne's conclusion that ordinary forms of micrococcus were harmless.

38. Claude Pouteau, *Oeuvres posthumes* (Paris, 1783), 3:264–66. For Delpech's work, see the section on cautery as antiputrefactive device in chapter 2. S.-N. Vautier, a former army surgeon, presented a number of pertinent observations on transference of infection in *Sur la pourriture d'hôpital*, a Paris thesis of 1812.

39. Alexandre-François Ollivier, *Traité expérimental du typhus traumatique, gangrène ou pourriture des hôpitaux* (Paris, 1822), pp. xxxii–liv, 51, 197–204, 236–47. This book of 473 pages, a rarity in American medical libraries, merits recognition as an astute early analysis of the spread of infection. It is also the tragic account of a young scientist's disillusionment: "In a word, as a reward for my services I was copied [plagiarized], insulted, annulled, denounced, dismissed, and finally scoffed at" (p. xviii).

40. Sixteen pages on wigs in a medical dictionary does seem a bit overdone, or, as Ollivier remarked, "Quelle hygiène!" But Percy's humor enlivened the accounts of his most mundane case history and he does not fail us here. Thumbing through Panckoucke's many tomes one welcomes something not exactly scientific yet somehow related to medicine. Percy tells us that

the most magnificent wigs were those worn by the surgeons Martinière, Hévin, and Louis and that Brasdor nearly expired with discomfort under a new wig at his wedding banquet. The article is signed by Percy and his nephew Charles-N. Laurent, but, as Ollivier stated, the style is unmistakably Percy's. *Dictionaire des sciences médicales*, 60 vols. (Paris: C. L. F. Panckoucke, 1812–22).

41. John Thomson, *Lectures on inflammation* (London, 1813), pp. 484–85.

42. John Rollo: *An account of two cases of the diabetes mellitus* (London, 1797), 2:267, 275–80, and *Short account of the Royal Artillery Hospital at Woolwich* (London, 1801), pp. 73, 117.

43. Alexander C. Hutchison, *Practical observations in surgery*, 2d ed. (London, 1826), pp. 202–3, 219. Blackadder's experiments (1818) on preventing spread of hospital gangrene have been noted in chapter 2.

44. Karl Garré, "On the etiology of acute purulent inflammations (osteomyelitis, furuncle, and whitlow)," in W. Watson Cheyne, ed., *Recent essays by various authors on bacteria in relation to disease* (London: New Sydenham Soc., vol. 115, 1886), pp. 439–44; Cheyne, "Lectures on suppuration and septic diseases," *Br. M. J.* (1888), 1:407.

45. The passage appears in a stanza of Rudyard Kipling's "Our Fathers of Old."

> They took their lives in their lancet-hand
> And, oh, what a wonderful war they waged!
> Yes, when the crosses were chalked on the door —
> (Yes, when the terrible dead-cart rolled!)
> Excellent courage our fathers bore —

46. Velpeau, quoted in Vallery-Radot, *Pasteur* (n.31), p. 234; John Syng Dorsey, *Elements of surgery*, 3d ed. (Philadelphia, 1823), 2:489; Louis C. Chouvet, *De la piqûre anatomique* (Paris, 1865); John Shaw, "On the treatment of wounds received during dissection," *London M. & Phys. J.* (1825), 53:369–79. Nitre is potassium nitrate, or saltpeter, which is used in the manufacture of gunpowder. After a dissection wound, Shaw suggested the following: Wash it well with soap and water, suck it, then bathe it in spirits of alcohol or turpentine. If the patient should become symptomatic, give calomel and pledgets dipped in laudanum and Goulard's solution of lead acetate. Valentine Mott's putting his finger in his mouth after such a wound was recalled by a student (see chapter 2).

47. Jakob Kolletschka's death is recorded in *Vrtljschr. f. d. prakt. Heilk.*, Prague 5 Jg. (1848), 2:132–33.

48. John D. Muter, *On dissection-wounds*, Glasgow thesis, 1839. The death of Marc Girard of Bordeaux, a surgeon of great promise, who died at age thirty-five following a slight scratch of a finger sustained while disarticulating a patient's shoulder for suppuration, was reported in *N. York M. J.* (1873), 18:112. The famous Paris surgeon Jobert (de Lamballe) in 1864, while operating upon a woman with syphilis, cut a finger and contracted syphilis, from which he died a few years later. Robert Le Sage, *Un grand chirurgien Breton, Jobert (de Lamballe) 1799–1867*, Paris thesis, 1938, p. 37.

49. Rex E. Wright-St. Clair, *Doctors Monro, a medical saga* (London: Wellcome Historical Medical Library, 1964), p. 29; James Paget, "Notes for a clinical lecture on dissection poisons," *Lancet* (1871), 1:735–36, 774–76. Sir William Lawrence, remarked Paget, said he had not known of a patient recovering after having been seen by more than seven consultants. Paget commented he had nine and expressed the belief there is safety in a multitude of counselors.

50. Joseph Lister, "On a case illustrating the present aspect of the antiseptic system of treatment in surgery," *Br. M. J.* (1871), 1:31. In this paper Lister also spoke of using "cheap muslin gauze" dipped in oakum as a dressing. In his next paper (1871) Lister spoke of using rags, linen rags, carbolated cotton wool, and gauze (ibid., 2:226–27).

51. Pouteau, *Oeuvres posthumes* (n.38), 3:231–35; Alexander G. Gibson, *The Radcliffe Infirmary* (London: Oxford Univ. Press, 1926), p. 199.

52. S. J. Brugmans and J. Delpech, *Ueber den Hospitalbrand* (Jena, 1816), pp. 24–25; Alexis Boyer, *Treatise on surgical diseases*, trans. Alexander H. Stevens (New York, 1815), 1:162;

William Henry, "Further experiments on the disinfecting powers of increased temperatures," *Phil. Mag.* (1832), 11:25–26; Isabelle M. Z. Elliott and James R. Elliott, *A short history of surgical dressings* (London: Pharmaceutical Press, 1964), p. 81.

53. *Br. M. J.* (1878), 1:686; (1885), 1:907.

54. W. P. Ruysch, "Rapport sur les chiffons infectés, un danger national et international," *Congress internat. d'hyg. et de démog. 1884* (The Hague, 1885), 2:73–90.

55. William M. Smith, "Contagious diseases propagated by rags, and the necessity of disinfection," *Sanitarian*, N.Y. (1885), 15:481–87. A. J. Martin (1887) noted that some bales of rags to be sterilized weighed up to twenty tons (*Rev. d'hyg.*, Paris, 9:806–13).

56. "Report of the Committee on Disinfection of Rags," in American Public Health Association, *Papers and reports . . . 14th annual meeting . . . 5–8 Oct. 1886* (Concord, N.H., 1887), 12:170–92.

57. George M. Sternberg's letter to J. H. Raymond, December 22, 1886, follows the above report (pp. 192–96).

58. C. F. Withington, *Inquiry into the transmission of infectious diseases through the medium of rags* (Boston, 1887); Ax. Ulrik, "Kvantitativ Undersøgelse af Luftens Kim i Kludesorteringslokaler," *Biblioth. f. Læger* (1890), 82:123–30.

59. Wurtz, "Sur la suppression du chiffonage à Paris," *Bull. Acad. de méd.* (1916), 75:429–34. This report was the outgrowth of a letter from a commissioner of the Paris Museum of Hygiene (1915) to the president of the French Academy of Medicine, calling attention to the need for stricter regulations in the gathering and disposing of rags.

60. *Lancet* (1877), 2:240–42; (1898), 2:502–3; E. Beaugrand, "Blanchisseurs, blanchisseuses, hygiène professional," *Dict. encycl. d. sc. méd.* (1868), 9:567–71. Beaugrand said that Fourcroy had warned of the hazard of pinpricks in soiled linen.

61. G. W. Blanch, an Edinburgh surgeon, wrote a letter to the *Medical Times*, London (1849), 20:207, concerning the hazards of the "modern usage" of families in large cities sending out laundry.

62. M. C. Schroeder and S. G. Southerland, *Laundries and the public health*, Public Health Report no. 385 (Washington, D.C., 1917).

63. Friedrich Riegler, *Das Neue oder das Zweckmässige im Baue . . . der Spitäler* (Vienna, 1851), pp. 105–18.

64. *Lancet* (1861), 2:434–35.

65. Friedrich Oppert, "The progress of sanitary improvement in existing hospitals," *Med. Press & Circ.*, London (1868), 6:21–25.

66. Susanna Meredith, "Washing for the sick," letter to the editor, *Lancet* (1877), 2:300.

67. André Vincent, *Traitement des plaies infectées et des foyers de suppuration par le savon*, Paris thesis, 1937.

68. Richard Reithoffer, "Ueber die Seifen als Desinfectionsmittel," *Arch. f. Hyg.* (1896), 27:350–64. See also *Am. J. Med. Sci.* (1897), 114:247–49.

69. P. G. Unna, "Ueber medicinische Seifen," *Samml. klin. Vortr.* (ca. 1886), Innere Med., no. 87, pp. 2292–94.

Further Readings

Alexander, J. W. Nosocomial infections. *Curr. Probl. Surg.* (August 1973).

Alibert, Jean-Louis. Éloge historique de Lazare Spallanzani. In *Éloges historiques composés pour la Société médicale de Paris.* Pp. 1–186. Paris, 1806.

Behring, Emil Adolf. Ueber ein neues Diphtherieschutzmittel. *Dt. med. Wschr.* (1913), 39:873–76; (1914), 40:1139.

Behring, Emil Adolf, and Kitasato, Shibasaburo. Ueber das Zustandekommen der Diphtherie-Immunität und der Tetanus-Immunität bei Thieren. *Dt. med. Wschr.* (1890), 16:1113–14, 1145–48.

Bennett, John Hughes. *On the atmospheric germ theory and origin of infusoria.* Edinburgh, 1868.

Brock, Thomas D., ed. *Milestones in microbiology*. Englewood Cliffs, N.J.: Prentice-Hall, 1961.

Clay, Reginald Stanley, and Court, Thomas H. *The history of the microscope*. London: Griffin, 1932.

Cole, Rufus. Francesco Redi (1626–1697), physician, naturalist, poet. *Ann. Med. Hist.* (1926), 8:347–59.

Conant, James Bryant. *Pasteur's and Tyndall's study of spontaneous generation*. Cambridge: Harvard Univ. Press, 1953.

Conn, Harold Joel. *History of staining*. 2d ed. Geneva, N.Y.: Biotech Publications, 1948.

Crookshank, Edgar March. *An introduction to practical bacteriology based upon the methods of Koch*. London, 1886.

Ehrlich, Paul. Beiträge zur Kenntniss der Anilinfärbungen und ihrer Verwendung in der mikroskopischen Technik. *Arch. f. mikr. Anat.* (1877), 13:263–77.

Forbes, R. J. *Short history of the art of distillation, from the beginnings up to the death of Cellier Blumenthal*. Leyden: E. J. Brill, 1948.

Freund, Hugo, and Berg, Alexander, eds. *Geschichte der Mikroskopie*. 3 vols. Frankfurt am Main: Umschau, 1963–66.

Gram, Hans Christian J. Ueber die isolirte Färbung der Schizomyceten in Schnitt- und Trockenpräparaten. *Fortschr. d. Med.* (1884), 2:185–89.

Great Britain. Medical Research Council. *A system of bacteriology*. 9 vols. London: H. M. Stationery Office, 1929–31.

Hektoen, Ludvig. The influence of the x-ray on the production of antibodies. *J. Infect. Dis.* (1915), 17:415–22.

Henle, Jacob. Theodor Schwann. *Arch. f. mikr. Anat.* (1882), 21:i–xlix.

Herelle, Felix Hubert d'. *Le bactériophage*. Paris: Masson, 1921.

His, Wilhelm, Sr. Beschreibung eines Mikrotoms. *Arch. f. mikr. Anat.* (1870), 6:229–32.

Joklik, Wolfgang K., and Smith, David T., eds. *Zinsser-microbiology*. 15th ed. New York: Appleton-Century-Crofts, 1972.

Lankester, Edwin Ray. Elias Mecznikow. *Proc. Roy. Soc. London* (1917), 89:li–lix.

Lechevalier, Hubert A., and Solotorovsky, Morris. *Three centuries of microbiology*. New York: McGraw-Hill, 1965.

Lister, Joseph Jackson. On some properties in achromatic object-glasses applicable to the improvement of the microscope. *Phil. Trans.* (1830), 120:187–200.

Metchnikoff, Elie. Zur Geschichte der Phagocytenlehre. In *Handbuch der Immunotätsforschung und experimentellen Therapie*, ed. Rudolf Kraus and C. Levadite, Lieferung 1:124–9. 2d ed. Jena: G. Fischer, 1914.

Poynter, F. N. L., ed. *Medicine and science in the 1860s: Proceedings of the sixth British Congress on the History of Medicine . . . 1967*. London: Wellcome Institute of the History of Medicine, 1968.

Puschmann, Theodor. *Die Geschichte der Lehre von der Ansteckung*. Vienna, 1895.

Roux, P. P. Émile, and Martin, André L. F. J. Contribution à l'étude de la diphthérie (sérumthérapie). *Ann. de l'Inst. Pasteur* (1894), 8:609–39.

Roux, P. P. Émile, and Yersin, A. E. J. Contribution à l'étude de la diphthérie. *Ann. de l'Inst. Pasteur* (1888), 2:629–61; (1889), 3:273–88; (1890), 4:385–426.

Salmon, Daniel Elmer, and Smith, Theobald. On a new method of producing immunity from contagious diseases. *Proc. Biol. Soc. Wash.* (1886), 3:29–33.

Schick, Bela. Kutanreaktion bei Impfung mit Diphtherietoxin. *München. med. Wschr.* (1908), 55:504–6.

Shwartzman, Gregory. Studies on Bacillus typhosus toxic substances. I. Phenomenon of local skin reactivity to B. typhosus culture filtrate. *J. Exp. Med.* (1928), 48:247–68.

Twort, Frederick William. An investigation on the nature of ultra-microscopic viruses. *Lancet* (1915), 2:1241–43.

Welch, William H. Morbid conditions caused by Bacillus aërogenes capsulatus. *Johns Hopkins Hosp. Bull.* (1900), 11:185–204.

Wells, Harry Gideon. *The chemical aspects of immunity.* New York: Chem. Catalog., 1925.
Wilson, Graham S., and Miles, A. A., eds. *Topley and Wilson's principles of bacteriology and immunity.* 2 vols. 5th ed. Baltimore: Williams and Wilkins, 1964.

Chapter 21. Nineteenth-Century Discoverers and Discoveries

NOTES

1. *Hippocrates,* trans. W. H. S. Jones (Cambridge: Harvard Univ. Press, Loeb Classical Library, 1962), 1:193–95 (Epidemics 1, case 4); J.-A.-F. Ozanam, *Histoire médicale . . . des maladies épidémiques,* 2d ed. (Paris, 1835), 2:14; James H. Burtenshaw, "The fever of the puerperium (puerperal infection); a chronological review," *N. York M. J.* (1904), 79:1137–38; C. H. Peckham, "Brief history of puerperal infection," *Bull. Hist. Med.* (1935), 3:187–91.

2. William Harvey, *Exercitationes de generatione animalium* (Amsterdam, 1651), p. 354. See also Arnold W. Lea, *Puerperal infection* (London: Oxford Univ. Press, 1910), p. 41; Erwin Kehrer, "Anatomie und Physiologie der Schwangerschaft," in Ludwig Seitz and Alfred I. Amreich, eds., *Biologie und Pathologie des Weibes, ein Handbuch der Frauenheilkunde und der Geburtshilfe,* 2d ed. (Berlin: Urban and Schwarzenburg, 1952), 7(1):354–55. According to Lea, the parturient uterus at delivery is a wound approximately 900 sq. cm. in area; Kehrer is in general agreement: the placental attachment, the segment of greatest denudation, constitutes about one-third the area.

3. Claude Pouteau, *Mélanges de chirurgie* (Lyons, 1860), p. 182. Pouteau made the observations in 1850 during an outbreak of puerperal fever in Lyons.

4. Charles White, *Treatise on the management of pregnant and lying-in women* (London, 1773), pp. 4–10, 112, 130. White (1728–1813) founded a small hospital which became the famous Manchester Royal Infirmary. He believed in early ambulation — the parturient should be out of bed, the sooner the better, by the second or third day (p. 131). White's treatise was popular and is said to have had a wide influence. Thomas Kirkland (1722–98) of Leicestershire, in a work intended as a postscript to White's treatise, also stressed the importance of cleanliness in lying-in hospitals, the comparison of the uterus immediately after delivery to a large wound, and the similarity between puerperal and hospital fever. Kirkland, *Treatise on child-bed fevers* (London, 1774), pp. 45–46, 73–75.

5. Alexander Gordon, *A treatise on the epidemic puerperal fever of Aberdeen* (London, 1795), pp. 3, 62–64, 80–85; Ian A. Porter, *Alexander Gordon, M.D., of Aberdeen, 1752–1799* (Edinburgh: Oliver and Boyd for Univ. Aberdeen, 1958). Gordon was a well-trained obstetrician, who, besides his medical education in Aberdeen and Edinburgh, had studied in London and seen puerperal fever there. He pointed out the analogy between dissection wounds and puerperal fever, stating that in either case the introduction of putrid material gave rise to suppuration, in the uterus to puerperal fever. To prevent the spread of infection, he recommended burning or thoroughly purifying an affected patient's clothing and bedding, and that attendants wash carefully and fumigate their clothing. Gordon believed that if he could see the patient within the first twelve hours, there was an excellent chance of cure — the remedy was bleeding of 20 to 24 ounces and purgation! Gordon's frankness in listing cases and attendants to prove the validity of his thesis won enmity among his peers. He returned to active duty with the navy and died of pulmonary tuberculosis at the age of forty-seven. Herbert Thoms, *Our obstetric heritage, the story of safe childbirth* (Hamden, Conn.: Shoe String Press, 1960), pp. 105–7.

6. Joseph Clarke, "Observations on the puerperal fever," *Med. Comment.,* Edinburgh (1790), 5:299–324; Robert Collins, *Practical treatise on midwifery* (Philadelphia, 1838), pp. 188–93; O'Donel T. D. Browne, *The Rotunda Hospital, 1745–1945* (Edinburgh: E. and S. Livingstone, 1947, pp. 32–34, 109–10. Clarke attributed the rotation system to a suggestion of John Howard. Semmelweis had planned to work at the Rotunda and was studying English during the winter of 1846–47, a project he never realized, according to Alan F. Guttmacher, in

his introduction to the 1966 reprint of Semmelweis's *Die Aetiologie, der Begriff und die Prophylaxis des Kindbettfiebers* (New York: Johnson Reprint Corp., 1966), pp. xxvii, xxx.

7. Pehr G. Cederschjöld, "Berättelse om förhållandet å Allmänna Barnbördschuset från och med år 1826 till och med år 1830," *Svensk. Läk.-Sällsk. Handl.* (1833), 12:105; Ernst Nachmanson, *Bidrag till kännedomen om Pehr Gustaf Cederschjölds liv och verksamhet* (Stockholm: Isaac Marcus, 1927); Oliver Wendell Holmes, "The contagiousness of puerperal fever," *New Engl. Quart. J. M. & S.* (1843), 1:503–30. Two unsigned letters to Humphreys Storer are quoted (pp. 516–20).

8. Kr. Brandt, "Lucas Johann Boër," *Norsk mag. Laegevidensk.* (1906), 67:1165; Erna Lesky, *Die Wiener medizinische Schule im 19. Jahrhundert* (Grätz: Böhlaus, 1965), pp. 71–77. Boër (1751–1835) was conservative in his methods and followed the expectant plan of noninterference during descent of the unborn infant upon the mother's pelvic floor, as opposed to instrumental delivery. He is often referred to as the founder of modern obstetrics. The story of obstetrics and obstetricians in Vienna from the founding of the University (1365) and the establishment of the first chair in obstetrics (1754) is well told by Isidor Fischer in *Geschichte der Geburtshilfe in Wien* (Leipzig: Deuticke, 1909).

9. Erna Lesky, "Ignaz Philipp Semmelweis, Legende und Historie," *Dt. med. Wschr.* (1972), 97:627–32; Guttmacher (n.6); Ignaz Philipp Semmelweis, *Die Aetiologie, der Begriff und die Prophylaxis des Kindbettfiebers* (Pest, Vienna, and Leipzig, 1861), pp. 52, 103, 269.

10. Karl Haller, "An die geehrten Leser," *Ztschr. d. k.-k. Gesellsch. d. Aerzte zu Wien* (1847), 4(1):xxxb; Haller, "Aerztlicher Bericht über das k. k. allgemeine Krankenhaus in Wien," ibid. (1849), 5(2):538; Lesky, *Wiener medizinische Schule* (n.8), p. 215.

11. Semmelweis, *Aetiologie des Kindbettfiebers* (n.9), pp. 76–81, 108. Josef Skoda gave a full report of the rabbit experiments in the Vienna *Sitzungsb. d. k. Akad. d. Wissensch. Math.-naturw. Cl.* (1849), 3(2):168–82, and *Ztschr. d. k.-k. Gesellsch. d. Aerzte zu Wien* (1850), 6:107–17.

12. In a very perceptive analysis Erna Lesky, professor of the history of medicine at the University of Vienna, has dissected the events leading up to Semmelweis's dismissal, showing it was not simply a matter of difference between Semmelweis and his superior, Klein, but a power struggle in the faculty between the old and the new. The crafty maneuverer Rosas and Klein represented the old; Rokitansky, dean of the faculty, Skoda, F. Hebra, Haller, and others, the new. The fact that two undistinguished members of a great faculty could offset the judgment and recommendations of Dean Rokitansky and a brilliant staff defies understanding. Lesky, *Ignaz Philipp Semmelweis und die Wiener medizinische Schule* (Vienna: Böhlaus, 1964, Österreichischen Akademie der Wissenschaften, Philosophisch-historische Klasse, vol. 245, no. 3).

13. Semmelweis, *Aetiologie des Kindbettfiebers* (n.9), pp. 103, 269. The title sheet carries the dateline 1861, but the book actually appeared simultaneously in late 1860 in Pest, Vienna, and Leipzig. Buda and Pest became a united city in 1872.

14. William J. Sinclair, *Semmelweis, his life and his doctrine* (Manchester: Manchester Univ. Press, 1909), p. 265.

15. Lesky, *Semmelweis und die Wiener Schule* (n.12), pp. 83–93.

16. Walter Radcliffe in his *Milestones in midwifery* (Bristol: Wright, 1967) relates that Semmelweis's monograph of 1861 was disappointing and that Semmelweis considered puerperal fever as a form of pyemia, produced by decomposed "animal-organic matter" and repeatedly stated that it was not a contagious disease (p. 79). Obviously, Radcliffe missed Semmelweis's 1861 observations that all materials coming in contact with the parturient canal and especially the accoucheur's hands, unless cleansed by the Semmelweis technique, were potential agents of puerperal fever and that living microorganisms constituted the animal organic matter.

17. Friedrich Wieger, "Des moyens prophylactiques mis en usage au grand hôpital de Vienne contre l'apparition de la fièvre puérperale," *Gaz. méd. Strasbourg* (1849), vol. 9, cols. 96–105; *De la fièvre puérperale: De sa nature et de son traitement: Communications a l'Académie impériale de médecine* (Paris, 1858).

18. Ignatio Phil. Semmelweis, *Tractatus de vita plantarum*, Vienna, 1844; also in *Semmelweis' gesammelte Werke*, ed. Tiberius Győry (Jena: Gustav Fischer, 1905), pp. 1–18. Semmelweis's doctorate is a very rare item. The authors know of only two copies, one in the Semmelweis Library in Budapest, the other in the Historical Section of the University of Minnesota's Biomedical Library. Minnesota came by its copy in an unusual manner. At the end of World War II the senior author learned that Budapest's well-known surgeon, Eugen Pólya, had been dispatched by the Nazis in November 1944 and that his widow was clerking in a store in Sydney, Australia. He persuaded nineteen American gastric surgeons to join him in a purse of $2,000 to Frau Pólya. Her touching response was overwhelming, and thus it was that the beautiful copy of the Semmelweis Vienna thesis came to reside on the library shelves of the University of Minnesota. See Charles F. Klinger, "A review of Ignác Philipp Semmelweis' *Tractatus de vita plantarum* (1844)," *Bio-Med. Libr. Bull.* [Minnesota], no. 42, September 1975, pp. 5–14.

19. Louis Pasteur's writings were edited and reprinted by his grandson, Pasteur Vallery-Radot, in *Oeuvres de Pasteur*, 7 vols. (Paris: Masson, 1922–39). In citing Pasteur's publications we have, when possible, given the original source as well as that in the *Oeuvres*.

20. A number of excellent biographies of Pasteur are listed in further readings. For details of his early life, the authors found the accounts by his son-in-law, René Vallery-Radot (1928), and by René J. Dubos (1950) particularly useful.

21. Louis Pasteur, "Mémoire sur la fermentation appelée lactique," *Ann. de chim. et phys.* (1858), 52:404–18 (*Oeuvres*, 2:3–13). The paper was presented at a meeting in Lille, August 3, 1857.

22. Pasteur: "Mémoire sur les corpuscules organisés qui existent dans l'atmosphère. Examen de la doctrine des générations spontanées," *Ann. d. sc. nat., zool.* (1861), 16:5–98 (*Oeuvres*, 2:210–94), and "Nouvel exemple de fermentation déterminée par des animalcules infusories pouvant vivre sans gaz oxygène libre, et en dehors de tout contact avec l'air de l'atmosphère," *Compt. rend. Acad. d. sc.* (1863), 56:416–21 (*Oeuvres*, 2:159–64).

23. Pasteur's "Lettre au Colonel Favé" was published for the first time in *Oeuvres* (1939), 7:8–9.

24. Pasteur, "Recherches sur la putréfaction," *Compt. rend. Acad. d. sc.* (1863), 56:1189–94 (*Oeuvres*, 2:175–81). See also Pasteur's "Animalcules infusoires vivant sans gaz oxygène libre et determinant des fermentations," *Compt. rend. Acad. d. sc.* (1861), 52:344–47 (*Oeuvres*, 2:136–38).

25. Pasteur, "Conférence faite aux 'Soirées scientifiques de la Sorbonne,' le 7 avril 1864," *Rev. d. cours scient.* (1863–64), 1:257–65 (*Oeuvres*, 2:328–46).

26. Pasteur: *Études sur le vin* (Paris, 1866), *Oeuvres*, 3:111–381; *Études sur le vinaigre* (Paris, 1868), *Oeuvres*, 2:78–106; *Études sur la bière* (Paris, 1876), *Oeuvres*, 5:1–307.

27. "Visite de l'Empereur au laboratoire de chimie de l'École Normale supérieure et à la Sorbonne," *Moniteur universel*, January 28, 1868, p. 128 (*Oeuvres*, 7:196–98).

28. The argument between Jules R. Guérin and Pasteur terminated in a bitter exchange (October 5, 1880) in which Guérin was restrained by H. Larrey from throwing himself upon Pasteur; the meeting ended in tumult. Pasteur resolved the controversy in a letter to the chairman of the Academy in which he said he had no intention of injuring a colleague in such discussions, being only interested in defending the exactitude of his own work. The "Discussions sur la variole et la vaccine" at the weekly meetings of the Academy of Medicine from May 18 to July 29 and September 28 to October 5, 1880, are reprinted in *Oeuvres*, 6:471–89. The physician Jules R. Guérin (1801–86) is often confused with the surgeon Alphonse F. M. Guérin.

29. Discussion, *Bull. Acad. de méd.* (1878), 7:139–67 (*Oeuvres*, 6:108–10). See also Léon Le Fort, "Le germe ferment et le germe contage," *Bull. gén. de thérap.* (1882), 102:449–73, 497–504, 103:6–22, an address at the Hôtel-Dieu clinics in which Le Fort summed up his stand on the germ theory. He gave a good review of wound treatment practices from the beginning of the century, recalling his presentation on hip resection (1860) that provoked the celebrated

discussion on hospital hygiene at the Academy of Medicine. See chapter 18 on hospital practices.

30. Pasteur, with the collaboration of Jules F. Joubert and Charles E. Chamberland, "La théorie des germes et ses applications à la médecine et à la chirurgie," *Compt. rend. Acad. d. sc.* (1878), 86:1037–43 (*Oeuvres*, 6:112–30). In an earlier presentation (1874) Pasteur had stated, "If I had the honor of being a surgeon, I would never introduce into a human body an instrument that had not been passed through boiling water, and better yet a flame, just before operation, and rapidly cooled." Pasteur, "A l'occasion de la note de MM. Gosselin et A. Robin," *Compt. rend. Acad. d. sc.* (1874), 78:46 (*Oeuvres*, 6:71).

31. F. H. Arneth, "Note sur le moyen proposé et employé par M. Semmeliveis [sic] pour empécher le développement des épidémies puerpérales dans l'hospice de la maternité de Vienne," *Ann. d'hyg.* (1851), 45:281–90.

32. *Berl. klin. Wschr.* (1905), 42:673–75.

33. Rickman J. Godlee, *Lord Lister* (London: Macmillan, 1917); G. T. Wrench, *Lord Lister, his life and work* (London: Unwin, 1913). Godlee (1849–1925), himself a distinguished surgeon, was Lister's nephew. He drew on family records and letters, many of which were later destroyed or have disappeared, to write this definitive and sensitive account, "the outstanding biography of a medical man in modern times" (*Dictionary of national biography,* s.v. "Godlee, Rickman J."). Wrench wrote the first biography of Lister; it contains some material not found in later accounts. Numerous works dealing with reminiscences of Lister by former students and colleagues are also of great help to the student of the Lister story.

34. The Listers' honeymoon included over three months' travel abroad, with visits to most of the principal medical centers on the Continent. They were in Vienna for two weeks, where Rokitansky, a guest in Lister's home many years before, returned the Lister hospitality generously. It was at this time that Semmelweis, then in Budapest, was being considered for the Chair of Obstetrics, as successor to Klein, who had just died.

35. Hector Clare Cameron, *Reminiscences of Lister and of his work in the wards of the Glasgow Royal Infirmary 1860–1869* (Glasgow: Jackson, Wylie, 1927), pp. 8–9.

36. T. Spencer Wells, "Some causes of excessive mortality after surgical operations," *Br. M. J.* (1864), 2:384–88.

37. *Testimonials in favour of Joseph Lister, Esq. . . . Candidate for the Professorship of Surgery in University College, London* [1866], p. 21; New Sydenham Society, *Biennial retrospect of medicine, surgery, and their allied sciences for 1865–6* (London, 1867), 32:219. The notice was dated Glasgow, July 1866.

38. Joseph Lister, "On a new method of treating compound fracture, abscess, etc.," *Lancet* (1867), 1:326–29, 357–59, 387–89, 507–9, 2:95–96; reprinted in *Collected papers of Joseph, Baron Lister* (Oxford: Clarendon Press, 1909), 2:1–36; Lister, "Address in surgery," *Br. M. J.* (1871), 2:225–33 (*Collected papers*, 2:172–98); Abraham Wallace, *Reminiscences of Lister* (Manchester: Two Worlds, 1928), pp. 9–10. For the reader's convenience, in listing Lister's publications we have cited, when possible, the original source and the *Collected papers.* Some slight editorial changes may occasionally be observed in the latter. The origin of Lister's spray is summarized in Richard B. Fisher, *Joseph Lister, 1827–1912* (London: Macdonald and Jane's, 1977), pp. 164, 184–85. It was an adaptation of earlier instruments — Richardson's spray, a sort of large scent bottle, and a spray used by Thomas Nunn of the Middlesex Hospital.

39. Joseph Lister: "The present position of antiseptic surgery," *Br. M. J.* (1890), 2:377–79 (*Collected papers*, 2:336–37), "Antiseptic management of wounds," *Br. M. J.* (1893), 1:161–62, 277–78, 337–39 (*Collected papers*, 2:349–64), and [presidential address] "On the interdependence of science and the healing art" (*Collected papers*, 2:489–514). The evolution of Lister's capitulation to prophylactic antisepsis is analyzed by the present authors and C. F. Klinger in *Surg. Gynec. Obstet.* (1973), 137:694–96.

40. Victor Bruns, "Fort mit dem Spray!" *Berl. klin. Wschr.* (1880), 17:609; Johann Mikulicz, "Erfahrungen über den Dauerverband und die Wundheilung ohne Drainage," *Klin.*

Jahrb. (1889), 1:169–70; Theodor Kocher, *Operative surgery* (New York, 1894), p. 20. In 1887 John Homans of Boston wrote that he was still using the carbolic acid spray "though I think it unnecessary, yet I hate to give it up." *Three hundred and eighty-four laparotomies for various diseases* (Boston, 1887), p. 4. See chapter 24 on the surgery of war.

41. Rickman J. Godlee, "Lord Lister and antiseptic surgery," in *Surg. Clin. John B. Murphy, Mercy Hospital, Chicago* (1914), 3:94; F. F. Cartwright, "Lister — the man," *Br. J. Surg.* (1967), 54(1):405–10. On the occasion of the Lister Centenary (1967) a number of tributes signaled Lister's first publication on surgical antisepsis, including this account of Lister's progression through three professoriates presented by Cartwright, anesthesiologist at King's College Hospital, Lister's London workshop.

42. Jules Lemaire, *Du coaltar saponiné désinfectant énergique, arrêtant les fermentations* (Paris, 1860); Gilbert Déclat, *Nouvelles applications de l'acide phénique* (Paris, 1865). See also chapter 17 on antiseptics.

43. Lister had offered himself as a candidate in 1864 for the Chair of Systematic Surgery at Edinburgh without success. Lister's father died on October 24, 1869, and James Syme on June 26, 1870, occurrences of grave concern to Lister.

44. Joseph Lister, "On the effects of the antiseptic system of treatment upon the salubrity of a surgical hospital," *Lancet* (1870), 1:4–6, 40–42. Secretary Henry Lamond, reporting for the directors, complained that Lister had disparaged the Glasgow Royal Infirmary, January 29, *Lancet* (1870), 1:175. Lister replied, February 5, ibid., pp. 210–11.

45. Richard Volkmann, "Ueber den antiseptischen Occlusivverband und seinen Einfluss auf den Heilungsprocess der Wunden," *Samml. klin. Vortr.* (1874), Chir. 30, pp. 759–812; Johann Nussbaum, "Lister's grosse Erfindung," *Aertzl. Int.-Bl.* (1875), 22:41–44; Godlee, *Lister* (n.33), pp. 367–68.

46. "Letter from Philadelphia," *Boston Med. & Surg. J.* (1876), 95:366. The discussions and Lister's presentation appear in *Transactions of the International Medical Congress of Philadelphia, 1876* (Philadelphia, 1877), pp. 517–44. See also Godlee, *Lister* (n. 33), pp. 390–91. F. H. Gerrish, Portland, Maine, privately published his results (1880) in operations over a four-month period with "the Lister method"; wounds healed promptly without suppuration; in 7 breast operations in the same hospital by other surgeons without antisepsis, all wounds suppurated.

47. "International Congress of Medical Science, Amsterdam," *Br. M. J.* (1879), 2:453; Congrès périodique international des sciences médicales, 6th session, Amsterdam, September 1879, *Compte-rendu*, 1:411.

48. John J. Packard, "The great advances in surgery, and how they have been made," *Phila. M. Times* (1885), 15:297–304. Wrench told of Lister's visit to Bergmann's Ziegelstrasse Clinic during the 10th Congress (1890) held in Berlin. Bergmann, eager to reveal the triumphal results of his therapy, presented some cases of mastectomy to indicate how nicely wounds healed without instillation of antiseptics. "Von Bergmann rolled back the dressing from the first case, from the second, from each one in turn, and each case revealed, not a sweet, clean wound, but the old picture of suppuration and decomposition. By some chance each case had become infected, and there was no antiseptic to kill the infection at its birth." Wrench, *Lister* (n.33), p. 331.

49. "The vacant chair at King's College," unsigned editorial, *Br. M. J.* (1877), 1:212–13. For the controversial story of the events preceding Lister's coming to King's see especially Godlee, *Lister* (n.33), pp. 395–421, and Fisher, *Lister* (n.38), pp. 224–33. Fisher's account adds valuable information from the Minutes of the Hospital Board.

50. Godlee (n.41), pp. 92–94. According to Lyle, "The only personal preparations made by Lister [for operations] were to button up his coat — a frock-coat of broadcloth — turn up the collar and sleeves, and purify his hands. He never wore an overall, mask, or gloves. Professor Lister was a slow operator and, when faced with any temporary difficulty during operation, sweated profusely. The theatre sister had to stand by with a towel and wipe his forehead." H. Willoughby Lyle, *King's and some King's men* (London: Oxford Univ. Press, 1935), p. 191.

51. St. Clair Thomson, "Lister: A house-surgeon's memories," *Br. M. J.* (1927), 1:661.

52. Stephen Smith, "Reminiscences of two epochs — anaesthesia and asepsis," *Johns Hopkins Hosp. Bull.* (1919), 30:277. See chapter 23 on preparations for operation.

53. John Rudd Leeson, *Lister as I knew him* (London: Baillière, Tindall, and Cox, 1927), p. 51; Godlee, *Lister* (n.33), p. 607; Cartwright (n.41), p. 409.

54. Agnes Lister recounted her husband's preparation for a lecture on spontaneous gangrene delivered at a meeting of the Edinburgh Medico-Chirurgical Society on March 18, 1858. "When we went to dinner the paper was in a most incomplete state . . . about 7 we resumed our labours . . . Joseph . . . keeping me writing as fast as I possibly could, and the sentences flowing out so smoothly . . . at 10 minutes past 8, a cab was sent for . . . and off went Joseph and the manuscript." Lister arrived just as his predecessor on the program sat down. Godlee, *Lister* (n.33), pp. 72–73.

55. Lister left £10,000 to each of the following: the Royal Society, King Edward's Hospital Fund, King's College Hospital, and North London and University College Hospital, and £20,000 to the Lister Institute of Preventive Medicine. The Edinburgh memorabilia are on display in a case at the entry to the University Library. Lister's will may be seen at Somerset House, London.

56. There is a photograph of Park House, Walmer, in A. Logan Turner, ed., *Joseph Baron Lister, Centenary volume, 1827–1927* (Edinburgh: Oliver and Boyd, 1927), p. 20. The iron fence fronting the street in the illustration has been removed; the stone wall remains. The entry to the kitchen has a beautiful curved door made of thick mahogany, now painted over, which the owner believes was the door to the library before the house was split. According to Felix Hull, Kent Archivist, Maidstone, the house was built sometime between 1826 and 1842; it was listed as Park House, one of four houses on a road known as The Beach, in 1842. He found no record of Lister's owning the house.

57. Godlee, *Lord Lister* (n.33), pp. 139–41; William Bulloch, *History of bacteriology* (London: Oxford Univ. Press, 1938), p. 142.

58. Semmelweis's "Open letters" have been reprinted in Györy, *Semmelweis' Werke* (n.18), pp. 431–511.

59. E. C. J. Siebold, *Geburtshülfliche Briefe* (Braunschweig, 1862), p. 79; Joseph Späth, "Historische Ueberblicke der Vorkommnisse im Wiener Gebärhause seit 1784 bis 1863, mit besonderer Berücksichtigung der Puerperal-Erkrankungen," *Wien. med. Wschr.* (1864), 14:164–67; Friedrich W. Scanzoni, *Lehrbuch der Geburtshilfe*, 4th ed. (Vienna, 1867), 3:436. Translations of Späth's report appeared abroad. See *Br. M. J.* (1864), 1:476–77 and *Am. J. Med. Sci.* (1865), 49:533–34. Späth had noted the low mortality among *Gassengeburten* ("alley births"), patients who delivered before reaching the hospital.

60. Ignaz P. Semmelweis, "On the origin and prevention of puerperal fever," *Med. Times & Gaz.*, vol. 1 for 1862, pp. 601–2, reprinted in W. Braithwaite's *Retrospect of practical medicine and surgery* (New York, 1863), 46:150–53; Charles H. F. Routh, "On the causes of the endemic puerperal fever of Vienna," *Lancet* (1848), 2:642–43; reviews in *Am. J. Med. Sci.* (1849), 17:509–10, and *Edinb. M. & S. J.* (1851), 75:244–51; Arneth (n.31); Arneth, "Evidence of puerperal fever depending upon the contagious inoculation of morbid matter," *Month. J. M. Sc.*, Edinburgh (1851), 12:505–11; "Hofrat Dr. Franz Hektor Ritter v. Arneth," *Rote Kreuz*, Vienna (1906), 22:49–50. Edward W. Murphy, professor of midwifery, University College, London, described Semmelweis's findings in the *Dublin Quart. J. Med. Sci.* (1857), 24:1–30. See also a translation from Josef Skoda in *Lond. J. Med.* (1850), [2]:700–3, and *Am. J. Med. Sci.* (1850), 20:529–32. Routh's review was quoted by John Simon, sanitarian. When one of Michaelis's patients succumbed to puerperal fever, he suffered a severe depression and committed suicide. Semmelweis, learning of this tragedy, said a monument should be erected to Michaelis's conscientiousness. See Rudolf Dohrn, *Geschichte der Geburts hülfe der Neuzeit* (Tübingen, 1903), p. 59; Sinclair, *Semmelweis* (n.14), pp. 76–77.

61. Lesky, *Semmelweis und die Wiener Schule* (n.12), p. 41.

62. Lister (n.38), 1:327 (*Collected papers*, 2:3). Cheyne summarized Lister's antiseptic practices in a well-known monograph of 616 pages entitled *Antiseptic surgery, its principles,*

practice, history and results, published in 1882. Cheyne, unlike Lister, demonstrated himself to be a good historian of earlier ideas and practices in wound treatment. Despite the thoroughness of his review, Cheyne completely overlooked Semmelweis; in fact, he did not mention him.

63. See chapter 17 on antiseptics.

64. While serving as his house surgeon, Lister made it a practice to report some of Syme's lectures in *Lancet*. Adams took exception to Lister's interpretation of Syme's tenotomy of the tibialis posticus muscle for young patients with clubfoot. It has been said that Lister did not engage in polemics or sophistry. His debate with Adams concerned Syme, not himself. Possibly from this experience, and the knowledge that Syme was a noted and often unsuccessful controversialist, and probably too through exhortations from his father, Lister learned the folly of such dialectics and only rarely deigned thereafter to reply to critics when his own innovations became a matter of heated debate. See especially William Adams, letter to the editor, *Med. Times & Gaz.* (1855), 10:419–20, and Joseph Lister, letters to the editor, *Lancet* (1855), 2:204–5, 447–50.

65. William Adams, *Sketch of the principles and practice of subcutaneous surgery* (London, 1857), pp. 15–18, and "Treatment of wounds upon the antiseptic and subcutaneous principles," *Med. Times & Gaz.* (1868), 1:257. Adams delivered his 1857 oration before the Medical Society of London. See chapter 17 on antiseptics.

66. *Pest. med.-chir. Presse* (1883), vol. 19, cols. 895–96; *Prager med. Wschr.* (1883), 8:407; Wrench, *Lister* (n.33), p. 341. Plans for the Budapest statue of Semmelweis, unveiled on September 30, 1906, are discussed in *Lancet* (1892), 2:267, 897, 1012–13. See also *Br. M. J.* (1893), 1:26; 2:160, 434.

67. This matter is discussed at length by the authors in "Lister, his books, and evolvement of his antiseptic wound practices," *Bull. Hist. Med.* (1974), 48:100–28.

68. An obituary of Charles Henry Routh (1822–1909), consulting physician to the London Samaritan Free Hospital, appears in *J. Obstet. Gynaec. Br. Emp.* (1909), 15:251–56. Semmelweis's letter is included.

69. Alfred Hegar, "Zur Ovariotomie," *Samml. klin. Vortr.* (1876), no. 109 (Gynäk. 36), p. 820; Lawson Tait, "One Hundred and thirty-nine consecutive ovariotomies performed . . . without a death," *Br. M. J.* (1886), 1:922–23; John Shepherd, "Lister and the development of abdominal surgery," in F. N. L. Poynter, ed., *Medicine and science in the 1860s: Proceedings of the Sixth British Congress on the History of Medicine, 1967* (London: Wellcome Institute of the History of Medicine, 1968), p. 113. The first biography of Semmelweis was Hegar's *Ignaz Philipp Semmelweis, sein Leben und seine Lehre* (Freiburg, 1882). See also chapter 12 on ovariotomy.

70. O. H. Wangensteen, S. D. Wangensteen, John J. Alpar, and Charles F. Klinger, "New light on the Semmelweis-Lister controversy," *Acta Congressus Internationalis XXIV Historiae Artis Medicinae . . . 1974* (1976), 1:453–60. See also *Bull. N.Y. Acad. Med.* (1970), 46:581.

71. István Benedek, *Semmelweis és kora* (Budapest: Gondolat, 1967), p. 427, translated for the authors by Paul Rupprecht, director of the Boynton Student Health Service, University of Minnesota.

72. Almroth E. Wright, "Address on wound infections; and on some new methods for the study of the various factors which come into consideration in their treatment," *Proc. R. Soc. Med.*, London (1915), 8:41–86; Alexander Fleming, "The action of chemical and physiological antiseptics in a septic wound," *Br. J. Surg.* (1919), 7:99–129. See chapter 24 on war surgery.

73. Sinclair, *Semmelweis* (n.14), p. 367.

74. Godlee, *Lister* (n.33), pp. 55, 139; Adolf Kussmaul, *Jugenderinnerungen eines alten Arztes*, 18th ed. (Stuttgart: Bonz, 1931), p. 383. Kussmaul knew and greatly admired Semmelweis (pp. 385–90).

75. *Orvosi hetilap* (1861), vol. 5, cols. 184–86, 225–28, 267–70. Dr. John Alpar of Amarillo, Texas, in early 1974 kindly translated the review for the authors.

76. Godlee, *Lister* (n.33), pp. 660–63.

77. Ferdinand Hebra, "Höchst wichtige Erfahrungen über die Ätiologie der in

Gebäranstalten epidemischen Puerperalfieber," *Ztschr. d. k. k. Gesellsch. d. Aerzte zu Wien* (1847), 4(2):242–44, and *Geschichtliche Darstellung der grösseren chirurgischen Operationen mit besonderer Rücksicht auf Edlen von Wattmann's Operations-Methoden* (Vienna, 1842).

78. There are a number of competent biographies of Robert Koch (1843–1910). The ones most useful to the authors in this brief sketch are listed in further readings. Koch's publications have been reprinted in *Gesammelte Werke von Robert Koch*, ed. Georg Gaffky and E. Pfuhl, 2 vols. in 3 (Leipzig: George Thieme, 1912). For the reader's convenience, both the original article and the reprinted article are cited when possible.

79. William W. Ford, "The life and work of Robert Koch," *Johns Hopkins Hosp. Bull.* (1911), 22:419; Lawrason Brown, "Robert Koch (1843–1910), an American tribute," *Ann. Med. Hist.* (1935), 7:103; Donald Fleming, *William H. Welch and the rise of modern medicine* (Boston: Little, Brown, 1954), pp. 33–34; Simon Flexner and James Thomas Flexner, *William Henry Welch and the heroic age of American medicine* (New York: Viking Press, 1941), pp. 94–96. Ford implies that Welch witnessed Koch's original 1876 presentation; actually Welch was not in Breslau until April 1877. Welch, in an address at the New York Academy of Medicine, on the occasion of his 80th birthday celebration, said: "That was a remarkable group that I was associated with for eight months in Breslau. . . . It was the dawn of Koch's work on anthrax. He came to Breslau and showed us his work. I shall never forget his coming, with Ferdinand Cohn, through the room with Cohnheim. I often reminded Koch of it." This remark appears in the stenographic report of Welch's address in Victor O. Freeburg, ed., *William Henry Welch at eighty, a memorial record of celebrations around the world in his honor* (New York: Milbank Memorial Fund for the Committee on the Celebration, 1930), p. 68.

80. Robert Koch, "Die Ätiologie der Milzbrand-Krankheit, begründet auf die Entwicklungsgeschichte des Bacillus anthracis," *Beitr. Biol. Pfl.* (1876), 2:277–310 (*Gesammelte Werke*, 1:5–25).

81. Robert Koch, "Verfahren zur Untersuchung, zum Konservieren und Photographieren der Bacterien," *Beitr. Biol. Pfl.* (1877), 2:399–434 (*Gesammelte Werke*, 1:27–50).

82. Robert Koch, *Untersuchungen über die Ätiologie der Wundinfektionskrankheiten* (Leipzig, 1878) (*Gesammelte Werke*, 1:61–108).

83. Robert Koch, "Zur Untersuchung von pathogenen Organismen," *Mitt. k. Gesundh-Amte* (1881), 1:1–48 (*Gesammelte Werke*, 1:112–45).

84. Koch's appearance is not officially included in the *Transactions* of the Seventh International Medical Congress; however, Lister in a discussion referred to Koch's kindness in making the two presentations (vol. 1, pp. 311–12). *Lancet* (1881) mentioned his exhibit of the potato medium at King's College (vol. 2, pp. 291, 299). Garrison and others refer to Pasteur's remark, which must also have occurred at King's. *Introduction to the history of medicine*, 4th ed. (Philadelphia: W. B. Saunders, 1929), p. 579.

85. Robert Koch, "Die Ätiologie der Tuberkulose," *Berl. klin. Wschr.* (1882), 19:221–30 (*Gesammelte Werke*, 1:428–45). A more detailed account appeared in 1884 in *Mitt. k. Gesundh-Amte* 2:1–88 (*Gesammelte Werke*, 1:467–565).

86. Robert Koch, "Über Desinfektion," *Mitt. k. GesundhAmte* (1881), 1:234–82 (*Gesammelte Werke*, 1:301–32). W. Watson Cheyne selected and edited for a New Sydenham Society publication several essays on *Bacteria in relation to disease* (London, 1886). In this he included three papers by Koch and associates on disinfection, abstracted by Dr. Whitelegge from Koch's official reports to the Berlin Institutes of Health (*Mitt. k. GesundhAmte*). The abstract of Koch's disinfection paper appears in Cheyne, pp. 493–518.

87. Emil Behring, "Über Desinfection, Desinfectionsmittel und Desinfectionsmethoden," *Ztschr. f. Hyg.*, Leipzig (1890), 9:404, 417–19. See also chapter 17 on antiseptics.

88. Robert Koch and Gustav Wolffhügel, "Untersuchungen über die Desinfektion mit heisser Luft," *Mitt. k. GesundhAmte* (1881), 1:301–21, and Koch, Georg Gaffky, and Friedrich Löffler, "Versuche über die Verwerthbarkeit heisser Wasserdämpfe zu Desinfektionszwecken," ibid., pp. 322–40 (*Gesammelte Werke*, 1:339–59, 360–79). Abstracts appear in Cheyne (n.86), pp. 519–33.

89. Nicolas Appert: *L'art de conserver, pendant plusieurs années, toutes les substances animales et végétales* (Paris, 1810), and *The art of preserving all kinds of animal and vegetable substances for several years*, trans. (London, 1811). Leonard G. Wilson, chairman of the Department of the History of Medicine, University of Minnesota, in a series of lectures on Pasteur in 1969, referred to the importance of Appert's work. See also Bulloch, *Bacteriology* (n.57), pp. 44–45. Appert (1750–1841), despite his remarkable innovation, died in poverty.

90. "The International Medical Congress in Berlin," *Lancet* (1890), 2:355–56. Koch's presentation, "Ueber bakteriologische Forschung," is given in *Verhandl. X internat. med. Congress, 1890* (Berlin, 1892), 1:35–47, and in *Wien. med. Bl.* (1890), 13:531–35 (*Gesammelte Werke*, 1:650–60).

91. Robert Koch, "Weitere Mittheilungen über ein Heilmittel gegen Tuberculose," *Dt. med. Wschr.* (1890), 16:1029–32; (1891), 17:101–2, 1189–92 (*Gesammelte Werke*, 1:661–82).

92. Gotthold Pannwitz, "Koch's Standpunkt in der Frage nach den Beziehungen Zwischen Menschen- und Rindertuberculose" [Washington 1908 Tuberculosis Conference, including discussion by Koch], *Berl. klin. Wschr.* (1908), 45:2001–6 (*Gesammelte Werke*, 1:624–35); J. Arthur Myers and James H. Steele, *Bovine tuberculosis control in man and animals* (St. Louis: W. H. Green [1969]).

93. N. Howard-Jones, "Gelsenkirchen typhoid epidemic of 1901, Robert Koch, and the dead hand of Max von Pettenkofer," *Br. M. J.* (1973), 1:103–5.

94. Robert Muir, "Paul Ehrlich (1854–1915)," *J. Path & Bacteriol.* (1915–16), 20:350–60; Ehrlich, "Ueber das Methylenblau und seine klinisch-bakterioskopische Verwerthung" [intravital staining], *Zt. klin. Med.* (1881), 2:710–13; Ehrlich, "Methodologische Beiträge . . . der verschiedenen Formen der Leukocyten" [differential leucocyte blood counts], ibid. (1879–80), 1:553–60; Ehrlich, "Die Wertbemessung des Diphtherieheilserums" [side-chain theory], *Klin. Jahrb.* (1897), 6:299–326; Ehrlich and Sakachiro Hata, *Die experimentelle Chemotherapie der Spirillosen* [salvarsan, 606, for syphilis and yaws] (Berlin: Springer, 1910); Ehrlich, *Gesammelte Arbeiten zur Immunitätsforschung* (Berlin: Hirschwald, 1904).

Further Readings

SEMMELWEIS:

Adami, John George. *Charles White of Manchester (1728–1813), and arrest of puerperal fever.* New York: Paul B. Hoeber, 1923.

Berger, Alfred. *Semmelweis: Eine österreichische Geschichte.* Schriften zur aufklärung und Weiterbildung der Gemeinde- und Staatsarbeiter, no. 2. Berlin: Gemeinde and Staatsarbeiter, 1922.

Gortvay, György, and Zoltán, Imre. *Semmelweis, his life and work.* Budapest: Akadémiai Kiadó, 1968.

Lesky, Erna. Die Wiener geburtshilflich-gynäkologische Schule: Geist und Leistung. [Vienna, 1961.] Read at the Third World Congress of the International Federation of Gynaecology and Obstetrics.

Schürer von Waldheim, Fritz. *Ignaz Philipp Semmelweis, sein Leben und Wirken.* Vienna and Leipzig: A. Hartleben, 1905.

Slaughter, Frank G. *Immortal Magyar: Semmelweis, conqueror of childbed fever.* New York: Schuman, 1950.

Zweifel, Paul. *I. P. Semmelweis. Ätiologie, Begriff, und Prophylaxis des Kindbettfiebers (1861).* Leipzig: J. A. Barth, 1912.

PASTEUR:

Compton, Piers. *The genius of Louis Pasteur.* New York: Macmillan, 1932.

Cuny, Hilaire. *Louis Pasteur, the man and his theories.* Trans. Patrick Evans. Profiles in science. London: Souvenir Press, 1965.

Descour, L. *Pasteur and his work.* Trans. A. F. and B. H. Wedd. London: T. Fisher Unwin, 1922.

Dubos, Rene J. *Louis Pasteur, free lance of science.* Boston: Little, Brown, 1950.

Duclaux, Émile. *Pasteur, the history of a mind.* Trans. Erwin F. Smith and Florence Hedges. Philadelphia and London: W. B. Saunders, 1920.

Institut Pasteur. *1822–1922, Pasteur: Centième anniversaire de la naissance de Pasteur, 27 decembre 1922.* Paris: Hachette, 1922.

Paget, Stephen. *Pasteur and after Pasteur.* London: Adam and Charles Black, 1914.

Vallery-Radot, René. *The life of Pasteur.* Trans. R. L. Devonshire. Garden City, N.Y.: Doubleday, Doran, 1928.

LISTER:

Cameron, Hector C. *Joseph Lister, friend of man.* London: Heinemann, 1948.

Cheyne, W. Watson. *Lister and his achievement.* London: Longmans, Green, 1925.

Chiene, John. *Looking back.* 2d ed. Edinburgh: Darien, 1908.

Dukes, Cuthbert. *Lord Lister (1827–1912).* London: Leonard Parsons, 1924.

Guthrie, Douglas. *Lord Lister, his life and doctrine.* Edinburgh: E. and S. Livingstone, 1949.

Henley, William E. *Poems.* 7th ed. Poems 15 and 16. New York: Charles Scribner, 1904.

KOCH:

Bochalli, Richard. *Robert Koch, der Schöpfer der modernen Bakteriologie.* Stuttgart: Wissenschaftliche Verlagsgesellschaft, 1954.

Heymann, Bruno. *Robert Koch.* Leipzig: Akademische Verlagsgesellschaft, 1932.

Knopf, S. Adolphus. Robert Koch (1843–1910), father of the modern science of tuberculosis. *Johns Hopkins Hosp. Bull.* (1911), 22:425–28.

Schaaf, Paul. *Robert Koch und Emil v. Behring. Ursprung und Geist einer Forschung.* Leipzig and Berlin: Lühe-Verlag, 1944.

HENLE:

Bardeleben, Karl. Jacob Henle. *Dt. med. Wschr.* (1885), 11:463–64, 483–84.

Gozzi, Guido. Jakob Henles Zürcher Jahre (1840–44). *Zürch. Med.-gesch. Abh.* (1974), no. 103.

Robinson, Victor. *The life of Jacob Henle.* New York: New York Medical Life, 1921.

COHNHEIM:

Klebs, Erwin. Julius Cohnheim nekrolog. *Arch. f. exper. Path. u. Pharmakol.*, Leipzig (1884), 18:i–x.

Kühne, Willy. Zur Erinnerung an Julius Cohnheim. In Julius Cohnheim, *Gesammelte Abhandlungen*, ed. E. Wagner, pp. ix–li. Berlin, 1885.

Salomonsen, Carl J. Lebenserinnerungen aus dem Breslauer Sommersemester 1877. *Berl. klin. Wschr.* (1914), 51:485–90.

Sanderson, J. Burdon. A life devoted to medical science. *Lancet* (1885), 2:747–50.

Weigert, C. Nekrolog Julius Cohnheim. *Berl. klin. Wschr.* (1884), 21:564–66.

BEHRING:

Behring, Emil Adolf. *Gesammelte Abhandlungen zur ätiologischen Therapie von ansteckenden Krankheiten.* Leipzig, 1893.

Behring zum Gedächtnis, Philipps-Universität Marburg an der Lahn [Festschrift by multiple authors]. Berlin-Grunewald: B. Schultz, 1942.

Browning, C. H. Emil von Behring and Paul Ehrlich; their contributions to science. *Nature* (1955), 175:616–19.

Satter, Heinrich. *Emil von Behring.* Bad Godesberg: Inter Nationes, 1967.

Schadewaldt, H. Emil v. Behring (1854–1917). In *Dictionary of scientific biography*, vol. 1, pp. 574–78. New York: Charles Scribner, 1970.

Zeiss, Heinz, and Bieling, Richard. *Behring, Gestalt und Werk.* Berlin-Grunewald: B. Schultz, 1940.

EHRLICH:

Dolman, Claude E. Paul Ehrlich (1854–1915). In *Dictionary of scientific biography*, vol. 4, pp. 295–305. New York: Charles Scribner, 1971.

Ehrlich, Paul. *Beiträge zur experimentellen Pathologie und Chemotherapie*. Leipzig: Akademische Verlagsgessellschaft, 1909.

Lazarus, Adolf, et al. Internationale Beiträge zur Ehrung. Paul Ehrlich und Emil v. Behring. *Berl. klin. Wschr.* (1914), 51(1):481–91.

Loewe, Hans. *Paul Ehrlich, Schöpfer der Chemotherapie*. Stuttgart: Wissenschaftlich Verlagsgesellschaft, 1950.

Marquardt, Martha. *Paul Ehrlich als Mensch und Arbeiter*. Stuttgart: Deutsche Verlags-Anstalt, 1924.

Paul Ehrlich. Eine Darstellung, seines wissenschaftlichen Wirkens [Festschrift for Ehrlich's sixtieth birthday]. Jena: G. Fischer, 1914.

Roux, E., and Metchnikoff, Élie. L'oeuvre de Paul Ehrlich. *Berl. klin. Wschr.* (1914), 51:529–31.

Wassermann, August. Paul Ehrlich. *Dt. med. Wschr.* (1915), 41:1103–6, 1135–36.

METCHNIKOFF:

Brieger, Gert H. Élie Metchnikoff. In *Dictionary of scientific biography*, vol. 9, pp. 331–35. New York: Charles Scribner, 1974.

Metchnikoff, Élie. Über eine Sprosspilzkrankheit der Caphnien. Beitrag zur Lehre über den Kampf der Phagocyten gegen Krankheitserreger. *Virchow Arch. path. Anat. Physiol.* (1884), 96:177–95.

———. *L'immunité dans les maladies infectieuses*. Paris: Masson, 1901.

Metchnikoff, Olga. *Vie d'Élie Metchnikoff*. Paris: Hachette, 1920.

ROUX:

Bulloch, W. Émile Roux (1853–1933). *J. Path. & Bacteriol.* (1934), 38:99–105.

Dujarric de la Rivière, R. Émile Roux (1853–1933). In *Les biographies médicales*, ed. Maurice Genty, vol. 6, pp. 369–84. Paris: J.-B. Baillière, 1939.

Émile Roux, nécrologe. *Ann. de l'Inst. Pasteur* (1933), 51:545–52.

SMITH, THEOBALD:

Dolman, Claude E. Theobald Smith (1859–1934). In *Dictionary of scientific biography*, vol. 12, pp. 480–86. New York: Charles Scribner, 1975.

Salmon, Daniel Elmer, and Smith, Theobald. On a new method of producing immunity from contagious diseases. *Proc. Biol. Soc. Wash.* (1886), 3:29–33.

Smith, Theobald. A comparative study of bovine tubercle bacilli and of human bacilli from sputum. *J. Exp. Med.* (1898), 3:451–511.

Smith, Theobald, and Kilbourne, F. L. *Nature, causation, and prevention of Texas fever or southern cattle fever*. Washington, D.C., 1893.

WELCH:

Welch, William Henry. *Papers and addresses*. Ed. Walter C. Burket. 3 vols. Baltimore: Johns Hopkins Press, 1920.

Chapter 22. The Surgical Amphitheatre

Notes

1. Jacques Tenon, *Mémoires sur les hôpitaux de Paris* (Paris, 1788), pp. 221–30; John [G.] Cross[e], *Sketches of the medical schools of Paris* (London, 1815), pp. 69, 145; V. Mary Crosse, *A surgeon in the early nineteenth century, the life and times of John Green Crosse* (Edinburgh: E. and S. Livingstone, 1968), p. 79.

2. Gottfried Richter, "Das anatomische Theater," no. 16 in *Abh. Gesch. Med. Naturw.*, ed. Paul Diepgen (Berlin: Emil Ebering, 1936), pp. 21–43; Arturo Castiglioni, "The origin and development of the anatomical theater to the end of the Renaissance," *Ciba Symposia* (1941), 3:826–44; John A. Shepherd, July 17, 1974, personal communication.

3. H. Willoughby Lyle, *King's and some King's men* (London: Oxford Univ. Press, 1935), p. 119. For a further account of speed in amputation, see chapter 2.

4. A number of well-known surgeons of the twentieth century, including Cushing and Moynihan, left eloquent accounts of their admiration of Kocher's technique of careful operating. See A. C. Klebs, "Theodor Kocher, 1841–1917," *U.S. Naval Med. Bull.* (1918), 12:59–63.

5. See chapter 4 on lithotomy.

6. "Rab and his friends" is included in John Brown's *Horae subsecivae*, 2d ed. (Edinburgh, 1859), pp. 295–319. Alexander Peddie (1890) was able to locate the case of "Ailie" (a fictitious name) in the records of the Minto House Hospital for December 1830. See *Edinb. M. J.*, 35(2):1057. See also W. J. S. McKay, *Lawson Tait: His life and work* (London: Baillière, Tindall, and Cox, 1922), p. 538. Ruth J. Mann gives a brief account of Ailie's mastectomy and Syme's use of Minto House in "The hospital and the surgeon's reputation," *Mayo Clin. Proc.* (1976), 51:740.

7. J. Scultetus, *Arcenal de chirurgie* (Lyons, 1675), pp. 172–74. Joyce Hemlow et al., eds., *Journals and letters of Fanny Burney (Madame d'Arblay)* (Oxford: Clarendon Press, 1975), 6:596–616; Alan D. Steinfeld, "Historical report of a mastectomy for carcinoma of the breast," *Surg. Gynec. Obstet.* (1975), 141(2):616–17. Larrey, recognizing his great responsibility, called in Antoine Dubois, first obstetrician of Paris and a leading surgeon of that day. Mme. d'Arblay had previously consulted Dubois; he had told her husband that an operation would be necessary but was unable to take the case, being then in constant attendance on Marie Louise, Napoleon's empress. (Dubois safely delivered the empress on March 20, 1811.) Mme. d'Arblay relates that Larrey's face was ashen gray as the operation got under way. In neither the Larrey nor the Boylston breast amputation was a histologic examination performed, a refinement that awaited the development of tissue staining. See also a review of Fanny Burney's *Journals*, vol. VI, by O. H. Wangensteen, *Bull. Hist. Med.* (1977), 51:632–41.

8. See chapter 1.

9. Jacques Gondoin, *Description des écoles de chirurgie* (Paris, 1780).

10. Cross[e], *Medical schools of Paris* (n.1), pp. 24–25; Karl Otto's account is quoted in Mireille Wiriot, *L'enseignement clinique dans les hôpitaux de Paris entre 1794 et 1848* (Paris, 1970), pp. 93–94. Wiriot includes a number of other interesting reports of Dupuytren's famous clinic.

11. Louis Dulieu, *Essai historique sur l'hôpital Saint-Éloi de Montpellier, 1183–1950* (Montpellier: Déhan, 1953), p. 201.

12. Quoted from the hospital minute books, in Peter Eade, *The Norfolk & Norwich Hospital, 1770 to 1900* (London: Jarrold, 1900), pp. 69, 77.

13. Russell Brock, "The operating theatre of old Guy's Hospital," *Guy's Hosp. Rep.* (1964), 113:131; "Surgical amphitheater under reconstruction," *Pennsylvania Hospital Quill* (1976, fall), pp. 2–3; Benjamin H. Coates, "Brief account of the history and present state of the Pennsylvania Hospital," *Phila. J. M. & Phys. Sci.* (1824), 9:35–37; Seymour I. Schwartz, editorial, *Contemp. Surg.* (1974), 5:9.

14. Stephen Smith: "Shall not the operating theatres of hospitals be abolished?" *Sanitarian*, New York (1878), 6:35–37, and "Reminiscences of two epochs — anaesthesia and asepsis," *Johns Hopkins Hosp. Bull.* (1919), 30:275. The catlin was a double-edged sharp pointed knife used by early nineteenth-century amputationists striving for speed.

15. Lawson Tait, "Development of surgery and the germ theory," *Br. M. J.* (1887), 2:116.

16. Page Cooper, *The Bellevue story* (New York: Crowell, 1948), p. 113.

17. Ambroise Paré, "Epistle dedicatorie, 1579," in *The workes of that famous chirurgion Ambrose Parey*, trans. Thomas Johnson (London, 1634); Alexis Boyer, *Traité des maladies chirur-*

gicales, 2d ed. (Paris, 1818), 1:v; Berkeley Moynihan, "Before and after operation," *Lancet* (1926), 2:790.

18. "Middlesex Hospital: New operation theatre," unsigned editorial, *Lancet* (1895), 2:224; "New operating theatre at St. George's Hospital," unsigned editorial, ibid. (1897), 1:267.

19. Thomas L. Rhoads, "The technique of Professor Keen's Surgical Clinic in the Jefferson Medical College Hospital," *Therap. Gaz.* (1897), 21:156–64, 236–43.

20. David W. Cheever, "Opening of the new surgical amphitheatre at the Boston City Hospital," *Boston M. & S. J.* (1899), 140:173.

21. Theodor Billroth, *Aphorismen zum "Lehren und Lernen der medicinischen Wissenschaften"* (Vienna, 1886), pp. 50–69; R. U. Krönlein, "Die aseptischen Operationsräume der Züricher chirurgischen Klinik und ihre Bedeutung für den chirurgischklinischen Unterrichte," *Beitr. klin. Chir.* (1903), 37:661–63; John Duncan, "Modern operating theatres," *Br. M. J.* (1898), 2:299.

22. Alexander Primrose, "Notes on a recent visit to surgical clinics in Germany and Switzerland," *Canad. Practnr Rev.* (1909), 34:199–217; Max Saegesser, August 11, 1974, and Rudolf Nissen, June 27, 1974, personal communications.

23. J. Balandin, "Ein neuer Operationssaal, insbesondere für Laparotomien bestimmt," *Verhandl. d. X Internatl. Med. Cong. 1890* (1891), 3(8):96–100; "A model operating theatre," unsigned editorial, *Br. M. J.* (1893), 1:427; Belouet, "Le nouvel amphithéatre d'opérations de l'Hôpital Necker," *Rev. d'hyg.*, Paris (1894), 16:27–40; "New operating theatres at the Royal Free Hospital," unsigned editorial, *Lancet* (1908), 1:181.

24. Billroth, *Aphorismen* (n.21), pp. 50–69.

25. George T. Beatson, "On the construction of operating theatres," *Lancet* (1899), 2:713; Rickman J. Godlee, *Lord Lister* (London: Macmillan, 1917), p. 459.

26. In a large photograph of the scene contributed to the University of Minnesota Bio-Medical Library by Mrs. James A. Johnson, Rickman J. Godlee can be identified sitting in the operating arena with a few other visiting celebrities. Murphy's Clinic was also a host at the first session of the Clinical Congress (an antecedent of the American College of Surgeons), according to a somewhat similar photograph (November, 1910) in John A. Hornsby, "Chicago as a medical and surgical center. III. The hospitals of Chicago," *Surg. Gynec. Obstet.* (1913), vol. 17 (insert, "Clinical Congress of Surgeons of North America, fourth annual session . . . 1913 [program]," p. 4).

27. Jonathan E. Rhoads, February 2, 1972, Leland S. McKittrick, April 7, 1972, Alton Ochsner, June 14, 1974, Loyal Davis, June 27, 1974, B. Marden Black, January 11 and 19, 1973, and William Beck, June 18, 1974, personal communications.

28. Harvey Cushing: "Introduction," in C. M. Faris et al., "Comparative surgery, with illustrative cases," *Johns Hopkins Hosp. Bull.* (1905), 16:179–80, and "Instruction in operative medicine, with the description of a course in the Hunterian Laboratory of Experimental Medicine," ibid. (1906), 17:123–34.

29. Loyal Davis, June 27, 1974, personal communication.

Further Readings

Billroth, Theodor. *Antwort auf die Adresse des Leservereines der deutschen Studenten Wien's.* Vienna, 1875.

———. Wie sollen Uterrichtsräume einer chirurgischen Klinik in Wien beschaffen sein. *Wien. klin. Wschr.* (1889), 2:2–7, 24–27, 43–47.

Eckenhoff, James E. The anesthetists in Thomas Eakins' "Clinics." *Ann. Hist.* (1965), 26:663–66.

Fergusson, William. *Lectures on the progress of anatomy and surgery.* P. 286. London, 1867.

Fox, E. Margaret. *The nurse's duties before and during operations.* London: Scientific Press, 1913.

Halsted, William Stewart. The training of the surgeon. *Johns Hopkins Hosp. Bull.* (1904), 15:267–75.

Imbault-Huart, Marie-José. *L'École Pratique de Dissection de Paris de 1750 à 1822.* Paris thesis, 1973.

Wangensteen, O. H., and Wangensteen, S. D. The surgical amphitheatre, history of its origins, functions, and fate. *Surgery* (1975), 77:403–18.

Wangensteen, O. H.; Wangensteen, S. D.; and Klinger, C. F. Surgical cleanliness, hospital salubrity, and surgical statistics, historically considered. *Surgery* (1972), 71:477–93.

Chapter 23. Preparations for Operation

Notes

1. Ambroise Paré, *The workes of that famous chirurgion Ambrose Parey*, trans. Thomas Johnson (London, 1634), p. 463; Claude Pouteau, "Sur les moyens d'obvier dans les hôpitaux aux dangers d'inoculer par les pansemens, toutes sortes de virus," in his *Oeuvres posthumes* (Paris, 1783), 3:227–38. Britain's first great surgeon, John of Arderne (fourteenth century) spoke of the importance of clean hands and well-shaped nails for the aspiring surgeon, but his wording suggests he was thinking chiefly of social acceptability. See William Anderson, "John Arderne and his time," *Lancet* (1897), 2:1065. The earliest reference Edmond Delorme could find to clean hands in surgery was in *Le manuel du chirurgien d'armée* (Paris, 1643); the unidentified author, L. L. M. C., criticized army surgeons who did not clean and clip their nails and keep their hands clean. Delorme, *Traité de chirurgie de guerre* (Paris, 1888), 1:59.

2. James Syme, called the "safest surgeon of his time," was meticulous about hand washing, according to Tait. See W. J. Stewart McKay, *Lawson Tait: His life and work* (London: Baillière, Tindall, and Cox, 1922), pp. 14, 168, 364, 392. Valentine Mott "was scrupulously careful about washing his hands immediately prior to performing any surgical operation, and every instrument was thoroughly washed just before use," noted Frederic S. Dennis in *Med. Record* (1892), 42:638–39.

3. C. H. F. Routh, "On the causes of the endemic puerperal fever of Vienna," *Med.-Chir. Trans.* (1849), 32:35; F. H. Arneth, "Evidence of puerperal fever depending upon the contagious inoculation of morbid matter," *Month. J. M. Sc.*, Edinburgh (1851), 12:508; Friedrich Wieger, "Des moyens prophylactiques mis en usage au grand hôpital de Vienne contre l'apparition de la fièvre puérperale," *Gaz. méd. Strasbourg* (1849), vol. 9, col. 101; Alphonse Guérard, in *De la fièvre puèrperale . . . Communications à l'Académie impériale de médecine* (Paris, 1858), p. 11; Anton Fløystrup, *Den prophylaktiske og kurative Antiseptik under Fødsel og Barselseng* (Copenhagen, 1880), p. 39.

4. Thomas Watson, "Lectures on the principles and practice of physic," *London M. Gaz.* (1842), 29:806. Watson's *Lectures* were published in 1843 in London and became a popular text, reprinted many times in England and America.

5. John Shaw, "On the treatment of wounds received during dissection," *London M. & Phys. J.* (1825), 53:379; James Robert Liston, "A midwifery glove," letter to the editor, *Lancet* (1871), 1:673. Justine Randers-Pehrson in *The surgeon's glove* (Springfield, Ill.: Charles C Thomas, 1960) includes a number of glovelike devices used chiefly in obstetrical manipulations in early days. Her book has much pertinent material.

6. William S. Halsted, "The treatment of wounds: The management of dead spaces," *Johns Hopkins Hosp. Rep.* (1890–91), 2:308–10 (*Surgical papers*, 1:108–9). According to J. M. T. Finney, William H. Welch used in postmortems a pair of heavy rubber gloves he had brought from Germany, and Halsted got the idea of rubber gloves from these. J. M. T. Finney, *A surgeon's life* (New York: G. P. Putnam, 1940), p. 90.

7. W. W. Keen quoted Halsted's letter at a meeting of the Section on General Surgery of the College of Physicians of Philadelphia, November 12, 1897. He presented a sample of white cotton gloves which he believed superior to rubber, saying the latter diminished the sense of touch and were hard to fit, clumsy, and expensive ($2 a pair). *Ann. Surg.* (1898), 27:225.

8. Joseph C. Bloodgood, "Operations on 459 cases of hernia in The Johns Hopkins Hospital from June, 1889, to January, 1899," *Johns Hopkins Hosp. Rep.* (1899), 7:225, 304–5. Bloodgood was Halsted's surgical resident in the mid-1890s, subsequently an eminent cancer surgeon at The Hopkins.

9. Hunter Robb: "The use of rubber gloves and gauntlets as a means of preventing infection in surgery," *Cleveland M. Gaz.* (1900), 15:551–52, and *Aseptic surgical technique* (Philadelphia, 1894), pp. 54–57, 125–26; 2d ed. (1902) and 4th ed. (1906), same pages.

10. Richard W. TeLinde, March 1976, personal communication.

11. James F. Mitchell, "The introduction of rubber gloves for use in surgical operations," *Ann. Surg.* (1945), 122 (2):902–4; A. McGehee Harvey, *Adventures in medical research, a century of discovery at Johns Hopkins* (Baltimore: Johns Hopkins Univ. Press, 1976), p. 77; James Bordley and Harvey, *Two centuries of American medicine, 1776–1976* (Philadelphia: W. B. Saunders, 1976), p. 302.

12. William S. Halsted, "The results of operations for the cure of cancer of the breast performed at The Johns Hopkins Hospital from June, 1889, to January, 1894," *Johns Hopkins Hosp. Rep.* (1894), vol. 4, plate 12 (*Surgical papers*, 2: plate 51). Halsted refers to his picture, saying it was taken late in 1893 and "shows that gloves were not being regularly worn by us at that time," *JAMA* (1913), 60:1124.

13. George Blumer, "Reminiscences of an old-time doctor," *Yale J. Biol. Med.* (1955), 28:9–13; William S. Halsted, "Employment of fine silk in preference to catgut . . . also an account of the introduction of gloves, gutta-percha tissue and silver foil," *JAMA* (1913), 60:1119–26 (*Surgical papers*, 1:39).

14. Charles Talbot of the Wellcome Institute of the History of Medicine procured a copy of Forster's patent rights (No. 1532) for the authors. The patent was granted on October 1, 1878. Richard F. Cooke's letter, in the possession of the New York Academy of Medicine Rare Book Room, is quoted by Curt Proskauer, "Development and use of the rubber glove in surgery and gynecology," *J. Hist. Med.* (1958), 13:373–81. Samuel Guthrie, Sackets Harbor, New York, was a chemist, inventor, and physician. His findings on chloroform are mentioned in chapter 17 on anesthesia.

15. William Acton, "On the advantages of solutions of caoutchouc and gutta percha in protecting the skin against the contagion of animal poisons," *Lancet* (1848), 2:589.

16. "M. Blatin montre des gants," *Gaz. hôp.*, Paris (1846), 8:415, also in *London M. Gaz.* (1846), 3:634; Thomas Cattell, "Precautionary measures which may be employed in dissections and postmortem examinations," *Lancet* (1847), 1:645. Blatin of the Hôtel-Dieu must have been an inventor or gadgeteer; various other items, including a douche, were exhibited by him before the same society over the years.

17. J. Lynn Thomas, "On the value of gloves in operative work, with a note on the cleansing of the hands," *Br. M. J.* (1899), 1:140–42; Théodore Tuffier, [discussion], *Bull. et mém. Soc. de chir., Paris* (1900), 26:810. Said Thomas, "The use of gloves is of high antiquity for it is recorded that Cyrus, King of the Persians, about 2,500 years ago, went without his gloves."

18. J. Lynn Thomas, "Modern fashions in surgery," *Br. M. J.* (1905), 2:1628–30; Russell S. Fowler, *The operating room and the patient* (Philadelphia: W. B. Saunders, 1906).

19. Johann Mikulicz, "Das Operieren in sterilisierten Zwirnhandschuhen und mit Mundbinde," *Centralbl. f. Chir.* (1897), 24:713–17. Werner Zoege-Manteuffel (1898) used linen gloves. See [discussion], *Dt. Gesellsch. f. Chir.* (1898), 27:15. During a few months' stay at the University Surgical Clinic in Bern in 1927–28, the senior author wore cotton gloves when assisting at operations. Only the surgeon and his first assistant wore rubber gloves. This custom obviously was in part traditional and also an exercise in economy. By running water over the external surface of rubber gloves, their safe removal without tearing is ensured.

20. Herbert Fox and Edward A. Schumann, "Permeability to bacteria of surgeons' rubber gloves," *Am. J. Med. Sci.* (1905), 130:656–58. Alexander Primrose, "Notes on a recent visit to surgical clinics in Germany and Switzerland," *Canad. Practnr Rev.* (1909), 34:216; Berkeley Moynihan, "The ritual of a surgical operation," *Br. J. Surg.* (1920), 8:30.

21. Carl E. Black, "Some experiments with rubber gloves," *Surg. Gynec. Obstet.* (1916), 22:701–5. It took an average of twenty-two seconds longer to read one hundred words in Braille, wearing gloves, than with bare fingers.

22. J. W. Kennedy, "Has the rubber glove solved the question of hand infection?" *Am. J. Surg.* (1921), 35:61–63; Robert T. Morris, "Gloves for aseptic surgery," letter to the editor, *Med. Record* (1898), 53:608; Morris, "Where the rubber glove is behind the times," *Am. J. Obstet. Gynec.* (1921), 1:334–37. Kennedy advised that assistants wear rubber gloves because they failed to scrub adequately. He used six scrub brushes in as many basins to prepare his hands; certainly everywhere today surgeons scrub their hands in running water. In 1924, when the senior author was an exchange surgical fellow at the Mayo Clinic, the senior surgeons of the staff, including Drs. W. J. and C. H. Mayo, regularly performed vaginal examinations with an ungloved but well-soaped hand. Rectal examinations were conducted with a finger cot on the index finger. Since disposable gloves have become readily available, these austere practices have vanished.

23. E. Stanmore Bishop, "Are gloves and masks advisable in modern surgery?" *Surg. Gynec. Obstet.* (1908), 7:250–52.

24. John B. Murphy, "A method of dispensing with rubber gloves and the adhesive rubber dam," *JAMA* (1904), 42:765–66.

25. Charles McBurney, "The use of rubber gloves in operative surgery," *Ann. Surg.* (1898), 28:113–14. In a footnote McBurney related that Halsted in a recent personal communication had indicated "that since 1891 all assistants at his operations have been expected to wear gloves," a statement not quite in accord with published accounts.

26. George E. Brewer: "Some observations upon modern surgical technics, from an analysis of four hundred and twenty-one operative cases at the City Hospital," *Med. Record* (1898), 53:433–36, "Operative surgery at the City Hospital," *N. York M. J.* (1896), 65:573, and "Studies in aseptic technic with a report of some recent observations at the Roosevelt Hospital," *JAMA* (1915), 64:1372.

27. Horace Packard, "The use of rubber gloves in surgery," *New Engl. M. Gaz.* (1899), 34:202–13; John M. Howard, chairman, "Postoperative wound infections . . . Report of an *ad hoc* committee," *Ann. Surg.* (1964), 160: no. 2 (August), suppl. The 1964 report is discussed in chapter 3 on debridement.

28. G. W. Theobald and J. W. Bigger, "In which it is contended that gloves may be sterilized without resorting to heat," *J. Obstet. Gynaec. Br. Emp.* (1924), 31:62–65. Theobald concludes this remarkable sequence (p. 59) by saying "*After lunch* [our italics] I motored to Trinity College, removed the gloves which had been on for five and a half hours, when 90 organisms were grown from my right hand and 120 from my left." How reminiscent of that enigmatic quip of Halsted's in a letter to Garrison (December 1, 1920): "I am putting on my aseptic rubber gloves in the car to save time at the hospital." Halsted implies that the quotation is from a novel by Willa Cather, but a thorough search by Professor Susan Turner of Vassar College failed to discover such a remark in Cather's published works.

29. Primrose (n.20), p. 216.

30. Edgar R. McGuire, "Are antiseptics of any value in hand disinfection?" *Am. Med.* (1903), 5:331–35; Gerhard Leopold, "Zur Verhütung des Kindbettfiebers," *Dt. med. Wschr.* (1887), 13:541–42; ibid. (1888), 14:389–91. Leopold insisted that all personnel in obstetrical deliveries scrub fingers, hands, and forearms with a brush for a full five minutes in soap and warm water, followed by a scrub of three minutes in warm 1:2,000 sublimate and immersion of the hands in 1:1,000 sublimate for thirty seconds; observance of his plan enabled him to report a series of more than 1,000 deliveries without mortality.

31. Robert Koch, "Über Desinfektion," *Mitt. k. GesundhAmte* (1881), 1:234–82 (*Gesammelte Werke*, 1:287–338); Emil Behring, "Über Desinfection, Desinfectionsmittel und Desinfectionsmethoden," *Ztschr. f. Hyg.* (1890), 9:404, 417–19.

32. Carl W. Walter and Ruth B. Kundsin, "Bacteriologic study of surgical gloves from 250 operations," *Surg. Gynec. Obstet.* (1969), 129:952. The senior author recalls a surgical

intern of four decades ago, whose hands, upon completion of conventional scrubbing, uniformly had surprisingly high bacterial counts.

33. Gabriel Fallopius, "De preservatione a carie gallica," *Opera . . . omnia* (Frankfurt, 1584), p. 833. The identity of the condom remains in doubt. Hans Ferdy, a German writer (1905), related that Condom was an English physician at the court of Charles II. Yet the English claim no knowledge of him. Ferdy, "Zur Geschichte des Coecal-Condoms," *Ztschr. f. Bekämpf. d. Geschlechtskrankh.* (1905), 3:144–47.

34. W. W. Keen, "Military surgery in 1861 and in 1918," *Ann. Am. Acad. Polit. Sc.* (1918), 80:11. When Richard Hebb was appointed pathologist to Westminster Hospital (1888), one of the surgeons sent him his old operating coat, "to do duty as a post-mortem garment. Hebb called a porter, picked the awful object off the floor with a pair of tongs and told him to take it away and burn it." J. G. Humble and Peter Hansell, *Westminster Hospital, 1716–1966* (London: Pitman, 1966), p. 86.

35. David L. Edsall, "The transformation in medicine," *South. M. J.* (1931), 24:1104–5. These leaders whose surgical practices failed to match their professional zeal for antisepsis were identified by Joseph C. Aub forty years later (1970), respectively, as John Ashhurst, Jr., and J. William White. Aub and Ruth K. Hapgood, *Pioneer in modern medicine, David Linn Edsall of Harvard* (Cambridge: Harvard Medical Alumni Assoc., 1970), p. 15.

36. Berkeley Moynihan's letter appears in *Lancet* (September 18, 1915), 2:674, and is reprinted in his *Selected writings: A centenary volume* (London: Pitman, for the Osler Club of London, 1967), p. 151. When the senior author visited St. George's Krankenhaus in Leipzig in 1928, Ernst Heller employed greenish blue; Cushing during the same period used gowns and wound drapes of gray.

37. Henri-François Le Dran, *Operations in surgery*, trans. Thomas Gataker, 2d ed. (London, 1752), p. 234; "Heroes of medicine, Robert Liston," *Practitioner*, London (1899), 10:548; William S. Halsted, [discussion], *N. York M. J.* (1884), 40:497. Saul Jarcho, New York physician-historian, enumerated some of these early mouth-to-hand practices of surgeons in *Bull. N.Y. Acad. Med.* (1970), 46:643–45.

38. W. W. Keen, "The contrast between the surgery of the Civil War and that of the present war," *N. York M. J.* (1915), 101:820.

39. Carl Flügge, "Ueber Luftinfection," *Ztschr. f. Hyg.* (1897), 25:179–224; Wilhelm Hübener, "Ueber die Möglichkeit der Wundinfection vom Munde aus und ihre Verhütung durch Operationsmasken," *Ztschr. f. Hyg.* (1898), 28:360–65.

40. P. Laschtschenko, "Ueber Luftinfection durch beim Husten, Niesen und Sprechen verspritzte Tröpfchen," *Ztschr. f. Hyg.* (1899), 30:128–31; Mendes de Leon, "Ueber die Gefahren der Wundinfection durch das Sprechen bei Operationen," *Arch. f. klin. Chir.* (1904), 72:920–23; Josef Riese, "Stummes Operieren," *Zentbl. Chir.* (1936), 63:1874–90, 1922–39.

41. Brewster C. Doust and Arthur B. Lyon, "Face masks in infections of the respiratory tract," *JAMA* (1918), 71:1216–19; David A. Haller and Raymond C. Colwell, "The protective qualities of the gauze face mask," *JAMA* (1918), 71:1213–15; Lloyd Arnold, "A new surgical mask, a bacteriologic air filter," *Arch. Surg.* (1938), 37:1008–16; M. W. Jennison and H. E. Edgerton, "Droplet infection of air: High-speed photography of droplet production by sneezing," *Proc. Soc. Exp. Biol. Med.* (1940), 43:455–58; John W. Hirshfeld and Paul J. Laube, "Surgical masks, an experimental study," *Surgery* (1941), 9:720–30.

42. For each operative setup after World War II, the senior author included a sterile pencil and writing tablet upon which the first scrub nurse or the first surgical assistant, both of whom understood the needs during every phase of the operation, could indicate to a circulating nurse what was desired. Angelo M. May (1974), a San Francisco surgeon, was working with an auditory amplifier to augment and elevate soft-spoken words during operations to diminish droplet wound infections.

43. Felix Würtz, *An experimental treatise of surgerie*, trans. A. L. Fox (London, 1656), p. 59; William Fergusson, *Lectures on the progress of anatomy and surgery* (London, 1867), p. 286; Carl Walter et al., "The infector on the surgical team," *Clin. Neurosurg.* (1967), 14:376. Wrote

Würtz: "A surgeon ought . . . to turn away his mouth from the Wound, or ought to put a cloth before his mouth, if need, for such breathing may cause that a water [droplet] may stick to the Wound, and incline it to a rottenness." In 1908 Bishop (n.23) wrote that "absolute silence during operative work" was "almost universally the rule in all well-regulated theaters" (p. 252). In the 1905–6 period at The Hopkins, Cushing emphasized the use of the experimental laboratory for teaching surgery to undergraduate students, *Johns Hopkins Hosp. Bull.* (1905), 16:179–80; (1906), 17:123. After he became Harvard's professor of surgery at the Peter Bent Brigham Hospital, Cushing did operate before spectators, but over long years he mandated total silence from the operating team. Loyal Davis, June 27, November 5, 1974, and Wesley W. Spink, February 26, 1975, personal communications.

44. John Pringle, *Observations on the diseases of the army, in camp and garrison* (London, 1753), p. viii. J. Y. Simpson (1859), in discussing whether it was advisable for a patient requiring a surgical operation for a chronic condition to become "acclimated to the hospital by a residence in it of a few days' duration," concluded that it was better for the patient to be operated upon immediately rather than "live for a time in the vitiated air of an hospital" (*Med. Times & Gaz.*, 39:489). Jastreboff's hospital plans are mentioned in chapter 18, n.86.

45. *Ordonnance du Roi, portant règlement général concernant les hôpitaux militaires, du 2 mai 1781* (Paris, 1781), p. 75.

46. On Pasteur, see chapter 21, n.30.

47. Louis Pasteur and Léon Colin, "Études publiques de desinfection," (1878–80) (*Oeuvres*, 7:115–19); Charles E. Chamberland, "Recherches sur l'origine et le développement des organismes microscopiques," *Annales scientifiques de l'École Normale supérieure* (Paris, 1878), 7 (suppl.):3–94; Chamberland, "Résistance des germes de certains organismes à la température de 100 degrés; conditions de leur développement," *Compt. rend. Acad. d. sc.* (1879), 88:659–61; Paul Redard, "Appareil pour la désinfection des instruments chirurgicaux et des objets de pansements," *Gaz. méd. de Paris* (1886), 25:292–93; Redard, "De la désinfection des instruments chirurgicaux et des objets de pansement," *Rev. chir.* (1888), 8:360–71, 494–509; Hugo Davidsohn, "Wie soll der Arzt seine Instrumente desinficieren?" *Berl. klin. Wschr.* (1888), 25:697–703; F. Jayle, "Les appareils de stérilisation chirurgicale," *Presse méd.* (1934), 2:1219–20, 1709. See also chapter 21, n.88. Redard is sometimes erroneously spelled Bedard.

48. Arthur Newsholme, *Fifty years in public health* (London: Allen and Unwin, 1935), 1:56; John R. Leeson, *Lister as I knew him* (London: Baillière, Tindall, and Cox, 1927), pp. 5–6. Simon retired from active surgery at St. Thomas's in 1876.

49. Information provided by Marilyn Lande, director of University of Minnesota's Hospital Operating Suite.

50. See chapter 20 on the germ theory of infection and disease.

51. Walter (n.43), pp. 361–79.

52. R. Blowers, "Source and routes of surgical infections," *Bull. Soc. int. chir.* (1971), 30:90–107; R. A. Shooter (London), "Infection arising in the operating room," ibid., pp. 108–117; R. E. O. Williams (London), "The role of the hospital ward in the etiology of surgical infections," ibid., 30:129–143.

53. John Charnley, "A clean-air operating theatre enclosure," *Br. J. Surg.* (1964), 51:202–5; Charnley, "Operating-theatre ventilation," *Lancet* (1970), 1(2):1053–54; Charnley and N. Eftekhar, "Penetration of gown material by organisms from the surgeon's body," *Lancet* (1969), 1:172–73. In orthopedic operations involving expenditure of energy, penetration of operating room gowns by bacteria is readily demonstrable — Charnley and Eftekhar advise wearing extra nonpenetrable gowns over the usual gowns or a closely woven textile to minimize penetration from the surgeon's body to the wound. See also chapter 25 on surgical specialization, orthopedic section.

54. Joseph A. Moylan, Edward Balish, and John Chan, "Intraoperative bacterial transmission," *Surg. Gynec. Obstet.* (1975), 141:731–33.

Further Readings

Altemeier, William A., et al., Committee on Control of Surgical Infections, American College of Surgeons. *Control of infections in surgical patients*. Philadelphia and Toronto: J. B. Lippincott, 1976.

Cheyne, W. Watson. On the relation of organisms to antiseptic dressings. *Trans. Path. Soc. London* (1879), 30:557–82.

Colebrook, Leonard, and Kenny, Méave. Treatment of human puerperal infections, and of experimental infections in mice, with prontosil. *Lancet* (1936), 1:1279–86.

Dakin, Henry Drysdale, and Dunham, Edward Kellogg. *Handbook on antiseptics*. New York: Macmillan, 1917.

Domagk, Gerhard. Ein Beitrag zur Chemotherapie der bakteriellen Infektionen. *Dt. med. Wschr.* (1935), 61:250–53.

Fleming, Alexander. The action of chemical and physiological antiseptics in a septic wound. *Br. J. Surg.* (1919), 7:99–129.

———. On the antibacterial action of cultures of a penicillium, with special reference to their use in the isolation of *B. influenzae*. *Br. J. Exp. Path.* (1929), 10:226–36.

Flügge, Carl. *Micro-organisms with special reference to the etiology of the infective diseases*. Trans. W. Watson Cheyne. 2d ed. London: New Sydenham Soc., 1890.

Gordon-Taylor, Gordon. The Fergusson tradition. *Br. M. J.* (1957), 2:817–18.

Klebs, Arnold C. Theodor Kocher, 1841–1917. *U.S. Naval Med. Bull.* (1918), 12:59–63.

Kocher, Theodor. On some conditions of healing by first intention, with special reference to disinfection of hands. *Trans. Am. Surg. Assoc.* (1899), 17:116–42; discussion, 143–51.

Masks or silence. Editorial. *Br. M. J.* (1960), 1:1339–40.

Mikulicz, Johann. Ueber die neusten Bestrebungen, die aseptische Wundbehandlung zu vervollkommen. *Arch. klin. Chir.* (1898), 57:243–79.

Pasteur, Louis. Sépticémie puerpérale. *Bull. Acad. de méd.*, Paris (1879), 8:505–8.

Saffron, Morris H. The Tilton affair. *JAMA*, Bicentennial issue (1976), 236:67–72.

Schweitzer, Robert T. Mask wiggling as a potential cause of wound contamination. *Lancet* (1976), 2:1129–30.

Shooter, R. A.; Smith, M. A.; and Hunter, C. J. W. A study of surgical masks. *Br. J. Surg.* (1959), 47:246–49.

Thal, Alan P.; Brown, E. B.; Hermreck, Arlo S.; and Bell, Hugh H. *Shock; a physiologic basis for treatment*. Chicago: Year Book Medical Publishers, 1971.

Tréfouël, J.; Tréfouël, Mme. J.; Nitti, F.; and Bovet, D. Activité du p-amino-phénylsulfamide sur les infections streptococciques expérimentales de la souris et du lapin. *Compt. rend. Soc. de Biol.* (1935), 120:756–58.

Watson-Jones, Reginald. Masks or silence. Letter to the editor. *Br. M. J.* (1960), 1:1501.

Chapter 24. Surgery of War

Notes

1. Theodor Billroth, *Historical studies on the nature and treatment of gunshot wounds from the fifteenth century to the present time . . . Berlin, 1859*, trans. C. P. Rhoads (New Haven, Conn.: Nathan Smith Medical Club, 1933), pp. 2–3. The "wound man" is discussed by the authors and Charles Klinger in "Wound management of Ambroise Paré and Dominique Larrey," *Bull. Hist. Med.* (1972), 46:218. See also Elizabeth M. Lewis, ed., *Military medicine and the wound man* (West Point, N.Y.: U.S. Military Academy, Library bull. no. 15, 1976). Lewis depicts a number of early "wound men," beginning with one from a Latin manuscript, ca. 1400. She believes that the first "wound man" with a gunshot wound (shown by a bump on his head) appears in Johannes de Ketham, *Fasciculus medicinae* (Venice, 1491).

2. George R. Callender, "Wound ballistics," *War Med.* (1943), 3:337–50; Pierre A. Finck, "Ballistic and forensic pathologic aspects of missile wounds," *Milit. Med.* (1965), 130:545–69; Ralph W. French and Callender, "Ballistic characteristics of wounding agents," and E. N. Harvey, J. H. McMillen, E. G. Butler, and W. O. Puckett, "Mechanism of wounding," in Medical Department, U.S. Army, *Wound ballistics* (Washington, D.C.: Govt. Printing Office, 1962), pp. 91–141, 143–235; Louis B. Wilson, *Firearms and projectiles; their bearing on wound production* (Washington, D.C.: Govt. Printing Office, 1927). Kocher's cans had been preserved and could be seen on shelves of the surgical clinic in Bern in October 1927.

3. A. J. Forsyth (1769–1843), Scottish inventor of the percussion cap that ignited gunpowder, was offered £20,000 by Napoleon for the secret; Forsyth refused. *Columbia encyclopedia*, 3d ed., s.v. "Forsyth, Alexander John."

4. Charles-N. Laurent, "Notice historique sur M. Percy," *Rev. méd. franç. et étrang.* (1825), 18:171; Bonnette, "Le Baron Percy, chirurgien en chef des armées impériales (1754–1825)," *Aesculape* (1912), 2:274–79.

5. Dominique-Jean Larrey, *Mémoires de chirurgie militaire, et campagnes* (Paris, 1812), 1:65–66, 150–58, 278; "Jean Dominique Larrey, 1766–1842," *U.S. Naval Med. Bull.* (1919), 13:267–69; Wangensteen et al. (n.1), pp. 220–30. Larrey's ambulance was drawn by one or two horses and was light enough to travel rapidly over difficult terrain. It superseded Percy's *Wurz*, which required up to six horses and carried materials for 1,200 dressings, as well as eight assistant surgeons and as many servants (some rode the horses); it followed the artillery into the midst of battle. Operating under cannon fire was possible since the volleys marked a parabolic curve over the surgeons' heads, not to be risked in front of direct musket fire. Percy's vehicles brought quick aid but had no provision for immediate transport of the wounded to the rear.

6. Both Percy and Larrey were at Friedland. Percy said that it was impossible to number the wounded: one hundred surgeons worked all evening and night, and more than one hundred sixty amputations were performed. Émile Longin, *Journal des campagnes du Baron Percy . . . publié d'après les manuscrits inédits*, 2d ed. (Paris: Plon, 1904), pp. 291–92.

7. Larrey, *Mémoires de chirurgie militaire* (n.5), 4:1–283; Joseph Romain Louis de Kirckhoff [Kerckhove], *Observations médicales, faites pendant les campagnes de Russie en 1812 et d'Allemagne en 1813*, 2d ed. (Utrecht, 1822). Other medical accounts include: Heinrich U. L. Roos, *Mit Napoleon in Russland* (Stuttgart, [1911]), of which there are several editions including a French translation of 1913 (an early account appeared in 1832); Carpon, "Un chapitre inédit de la retraite en Russie. Les morts de Wilna," (letter to Larrey), *France méd.* (1902), 49:357–63; Bonnette, "Les sépulcres de la Grande Armée, 1812–1813," *Aesculape* (1914), 4:12–15. Even in the days of Napoleon's victories, the medical arrangements were often very inadequate. Percy found the surgeon general at Marienbourg (1807) amputating with an ordinary knife and workman's saw. Added Percy, "O Shame, O Calamity: Detestable administration." Longin, *Percy* (n.6), p. 327.

8. Seminar by O. H. Wangensteen in Leonard G. Wilson's History of Medicine Lecture Series, titled "Dominique Larrey and the Napoleonic campaigns," May 1, 1972, unpublished. The research of Claude Ollivier is discussed in chapter 20 on the germ theory of disease; for Jacques Delpech see chapter 2 on amputation.

9. J. F. B. Maurice Treille, *Propositions médico-chirurgicales pratiques*, Paris thesis, 1816, pp. 12–15. Treille said he frequently called the attention of his superiors, including Broussais, to the condition of these patients in the Toulouse hospital.

10. Salleron, "Mémoire sur l'emploi du perchlorure de fer contre la pourriture d'hôpital," *Rec. de mém., de méd. . . . mil.*, Paris (1859), 2:278–414; Marie-P.-A. Bourot, *Considérations sur la pourriture d'hôpital observée en Orient et sur son traitement par le perchlorure de fer*, Strasbourg thesis, 1858.

11. George H. B. Macleod, *Notes on the surgery of the war in the Crimea* (Philadelphia, 1862), pp. 328–33.

12. John Shepherd, "The surgeons in the Crimea, 1854–1856," *J. R. Coll. Surg.*, Edin-

burgh (1972), 17:280–81; Edward T. Cook, *Life of Florence Nightingale* (London: Macmillan, 1913), 1:158–59, 185.

13. T. Spencer Wells, "Introductory lecture . . . Smyrna Hospital," *Med. Times & Gaz.* (1855), 10:430–33. John Howard visited the Haslar Hospital on July 8, 1788, and wrote that women were in attendance there and also at the Plymouth Hospital to nurse the sick. John Howard, *Account of the principle lazarettos in Europe* (Warrington, 1789), p. 180.

14. John Shaw Billings, "Medical reminiscences of the Civil War" and W. W. Keen, "Surgical reminiscences of the Civil War," *Trans. Coll. Physns Phila.* (1905), 27:115–21 and 95–114 respectively. The modern clinical thermometer was introduced by Allbutt in 1870. Clinical thermometry dates back to Sanctorius (1625).

15. Jean Henri Dunant, *Un souvenir de Solferino* (Geneva, 1862); John Pringle, *Observations on the diseases of the army* (London, 1753), p. viii. Percy had proposed a pledge by belligerents that the wounded of both sides be treated equally and that hospitals be inviolate and sacred to both. See Étienne Pariset, "Éloge de M. le Baron Percy," *Mém. Acad. roy. de méd.* (1833), 2:18.

16. United States War Dept. Surgeon General's Office, *Medical and surgical history of the War of the Rebellion, 1861–65*, 3 vols. in 6 (Washington, 1870–88). *Surgical history* is pt. 1, vol. 2 (1875), pt. 2, vol. 2 (1876), and pt. 3, vol. 2 (1883), prepared under the direction of Joseph K. Barnes, Surgeon General, U.S. Army, by George A. Otis (pt. 1, vol. 2 and pt. 2, vol. 2), and by Otis and D. L. Huntington (pt. 3, vol. 2).

17. See chapter 17 on antiseptics. On p. 105 of his "reminiscences" (n.14), Keen referred to Goldsmith's success but did not mention bromine.

18. Alfred North, "Report of sixty cases of hospital gangrene," *Am. M. Times*, N.Y. (1863), 6:255–58; William Detmold, "Lectures on military surgery," ibid., p. 98; J. J. Woodward, "Hospital gangrene," letter to Professor Detmold, ibid., p. 179.

19. Keen (n.14), p. 100.

20. Otis and Huntington, *Surgical history of War of the Rebellion* (n.16), p. 877.

21. See note 79 of chapter 2 on amputation.

22. Edmund Andrews, "Hospital gangrene," *Chicago M. Exam.* (1861), 2:515–16.

23. Otis and Huntington, *Surgical history of War of the Rebellion* (n.16), pt. 3, vol. 2, p. 887.

24. Percy M. Ashburn, *History of the medical department of the United States Army* (Boston: Houghton Mifflin, 1929), pp. 83–84; D. L. Griffiths, "Medicine and surgery in the American Civil War," *Proc. R. Soc. Med.* (1966), 59:204–8.

25. Rudolf Virchow, *Die Fortschritte der Kriegsheilkunde* (Berlin, 1874), p. 7; Hippolyte Larrey, [discussion], *Compt. rend. Acad. d. sci.*, Paris (1874), 78:84–85.

26. Léon Legouest, *Le service de santé des armées americaines pendant la guerre des États-Unis, 1861 à 1866* (Paris, 1866), p. 29; *World almanac* (1948), p. 568.

27. J. Julian Chisolm, *Manual of military surgery, for the use of surgeons in the Confederate States Army*, 3d ed. (Columbia, S.C., 1864), pp. 264–414.

28. An account of Napoleon III's illness and death is given in chapter 4 on lithotomy.

29. Joseph Lister, "A method of antiseptic treatment applicable to wounded soldiers in the present war," *Br. M. J.* (1870), 2:243–44 (*Collected papers*, 2:161); Richard Geissel, "Kriegschirurgie Reminiscenzen von 1870 bis 1871," *Dt. Ztschr. Chir.* (1875), 5:25–61; Medizinal-Abtheilung des königlich preussischen Kriegsministeriums, *Die Verwundungen durch Kriegswaffen bei den deutschen Heeren im Kriege gegen Frankreich 1870/71* (Berlin, 1890), 3(2):203.

30. Orieulx de la Porte, *Alphonse Guérin, sa vie, ses oeuvres* (Laval, 1897), pp. 5–7; William MacCormac, "Operation rooms, past and present," *Bristol M.-Chir. J.* (1898), 16:304; O. H. Wangensteen and S. D. Wangensteen, "Military surgeons and surgery, old and new," *Surgery* (1967), 62:1118–19.

31. Carl Reyher's contribution is discussed in chapter 3 on debridement.

32. Alfred Blalock, "Experimental shock; the cause of the low blood pressure produced by muscle injury," *Arch. Surg.* (1930), 20:959–96.

33. [Reports of Inter-Allied Surgical Conference], *Br. M. J.* (1917), 2:666, 838; Berkeley Moynihan, *American addresses* (Philadelphia: W. B. Saunders, 1917), pp. 44–48, 76.

34. Henry D. Dakin, "On the use of certain antiseptic substances in the treatment of infected wounds," *Br. M. J.* (1915), 2:318–20; Alexis Carrel and G. Dehelly, *Le traitement des plaies infectées* (Paris: Masson, 1917). Dakin, English-born, retained his British citizenship, although he spent most of his professional life in New York. He became a distinguished biochemist. Herter died in 1910; in 1916 Dakin married Herter's widow and continued to live in New York.

35. William S. Halsted, "Carrel-Dakin method of the treatment of infected wounds," letter to William W. Keen, December 14, 1917, in Halsted's *Surgical papers* (Baltimore: Johns Hopkins Press, 1924), 1:64–67; W. W. Keen, *Treatment of war wounds*, 2d ed. (Philadelphia: W. B. Saunders, 1918), pp. 86–110, 252–59. Keen wrote a little book of forty-three pages, *A sketch of the early history of practical anatomy* (Philadelphia, 1874), which enjoyed warm praise in high sources. Keen's account makes fascinating reading. Keen related (p. 36) how William Hunter embalmed the body of Mrs. Martin Van Butchell at her husband's request, restoring color to her cheeks by placement of vermilion in the oil of turpentine injected into her arteries to perserve the body from decay. She was placed in a glass case and the widowed husband placed her in his dining room to assuage his loneliness. On a visit to the Museum of the Royal College of Surgeons during the first International London Cancer Conference in August 1928, Sir Arthur Keith, curator of the museum, showed a few members of the American contingent Hunter's beautiful handiwork, relating that Mr. Van Butchell ultimately found more comfort in a vibrant second wife than in the remains of his first.

36. Alexander Fleming, "The action of chemical and physiological antiseptics in a septic wound," *Br. J. Surg.* (1919), 7:99–129.

37. Alexander Fleming, "On lysozyme, a bacteriologic ferment found normally in tissues and secretions," *Lancet* (1929), 1:217–20, and "On the antibacterial action of cultures of a penicillium, with special reference to their use in the isolation of *B. influenzae*," *Br. J. Exp. Path.* (1929), 10:226–36. After the death of his devoted wife Sarah (1949), Fleming suffered great loneliness until he married (1953) a talented Greek microbiologist, Dr. Amalia Voureka, who was doing productive research in his laboratory; this was also a very felicitous marriage, but Fleming, who had been an inveterate cigarette smoker throughout his adult life, succumbed to a coronary thrombosis on March 11, 1955. He was mourned by an appreciative nation and admirers throughout the world. See André Maurois, *The life of Sir Alexander Fleming, discoverer of penicillin*, trans. Gerard Hopkins (London: Jonathan Cape, 1959).

38. U.S. Library of Congress. Congressional Research Service. Roger Swanson and Robert Goldrich, "U.S. military personnel and casualties in principal U.S. wars: By branch of service from the Revolutionary War to the Vietnam War; by preservice home state from World War I to the Vietnam War," revised August 2, 1973, 19 pp.

39. Ernst B. Chain, Howard W. Florey, et al., "Penicillin as a chemotherapeutic agent," *Lancet* (1940), 2:226–28.

40. Norman T. Kirk, "Development of amputation," *Bull. Med. Libr. Assoc.* (1944), 32:162. See also chapter 3 on debridement.

41. Harris B. Shumacker, Jr., "Arterial aneurysms and arteriovenous fistulas: Sympathectomy as an adjunct measure in operative treatment," pp. 318–60 in Daniel C. Elkin and Michael E. DeBakey, eds., *Vascular surgery in World War II* (Washington, D.C.: Office of the Surgeon General — *Surgery in World War II*, vol. 2, 1955).

42. Leonard D. Heaton et al., "Military surgical practices of the United States Army in Viet Nam," *Curr. Probl. Surg.*, November 1966, pp. 19, 58.

43. Elisheva Simchen and Theodor Sacks, "Infection in war wounds: Experience during the 1973 October War in Israel," *Ann. Surg.* (1975), 182:754–61.

44. W. T. Sherman and Robert E. Lee are quoted by H. L. Mencken, *New dictionary of quotations* (New York: Alfred A. Knopf, 1946), p. 1266.

45. Gaston Bodart, "Losses of life in modern wars: Austria-Hungary, 1618–1913," pp. 3–156, in Carnegie Endowment for International Peace, Harald Westergaard, ed., *Losses of life in modern wars* (Oxford: Clarendon Press, 1916).

46. General Frederick Weyand quoted in *World almanac* (1974), p. 991.

47. Pasteur quoted in René Vallery-Radot, *Life of Pasteur* (Garden City, N.Y.: Doubleday, Doran, 1928), p. 451.

Further Readings

Adams, George Worthington. *Doctors in blue, medical history of the Union Army in the Civil War.* New York: Schuman, 1952.

Bayne-Jones, Stanhope. *Evolution of preventive medicine in the United States Army, 1607–1939.* Washington, D.C.: Office of the Surgeon General, 1968.

Blanco, Richard L. *Wellington's surgeon general: Sir James McGregor.* Durham, N.C.: Duke Univ. Press, 1974.

Borchard, August, and Schmieden, Victor. *Die deutsche Chirurgie im Weltkrieg, 1914–1918.* 2d ed. Leipzig: J. A. Barth, 1920.

Cabanès, Augustin. *Chirurgiens et blessés à travers l'histoire, des origines à la Croix-rouge.* Paris: Albin Michel, 1918.

Cash, Phillip. Medical men at the siege of Boston, April 1775–April 1776. Philadelphia: American Philosophical Soc., 1973.

Cunningham, Horace. *Field medical services at the battles of Manassas.* Athens, Georgia: Univ. Georgia Press, 1968.

Diffenbaugh, Willis G. Military surgery in the Civil War. *Milit. Med.* (1965), 130:490–96.

Duncan, Louis C. *Medical men in the American Revolution (1775–1783).* Carlisle Barracks, Pa.: Medical Field Service School, 1931. Reprint. New York: Augustus M. Kelley, 1970.

Edmonds, S. Emma E. *Nurse and spy in the Union Army: Comprising the adventures and experiences of a woman in hospitals, camps, and battlefields.* Hartford, Conn.: W. S. Williams, 1865.

Fischer, Hermann E. Handbuch der Kriegschirurgie. *Dt. Chir.* Stuttgart (1882), vol. 17 (2 vols. in 1).

Franz, Carl. *Lehrbuch der Kriegschirurgie.* 2d ed. Berlin: Julius Springer, 1936.

Gibson, James E. *Dr. Bodo Otto and the medical background of the American Revolution.* Springfield, Ill.: Charles C Thomas, 1937.

Gribel, Friedrich. Die Entwicklung der Wundbehandlung von der Mitte des 18. bis zur Mitte des 19. Jahrhunderts. *Abh. Gesch. Med. Naturur.* (1936), vol. 15.

Grosland, Maurice. Science and the Franco-Prussian War. *Social studies of science* (1976), 6:185–214.

Guthrie, George J. *A treatise on gun-shot wounds.* 2d ed. London, 1820.

Hampton, Oscar P., Jr. *Orthopedic surgery in the Mediterranean Theater of Operations.* Surgery in World War II. Washington, D.C.: Office of the Surgeon General, 1957.

Kiel, Frank W. Hazards of military parachuting. *Milit. Med.* (1965), 130:512–21.

King, Clyde L., ed. Rehabilitation of the wounded. *Ann. Am. Acad. Polit. and Soc. Sci.* (1918), vol. 80.

Medical notes from the Far East (from a special correspondent). *Lancet* (1904), 2:982–84; (1905), 1:256–58.

Pincoffs, Peter. *Experiences of a civilian in eastern military hospitals with observations on the English, French, and other medical departments and the organization of military medical schools and hospitals.* London and Edinburgh, 1857.

Rose, Achilles. *Napoleon's campaigns in Russia, anno 1812; medico-historical.* New York: A. Rose, 1913.

Ryerson, G. Sterling. Some experiences in the war in South Africa. *Canad. Practnr Rev.* (1900), 25:525–30.

Schaefer, Friedrich. Die Lanze, eine geschichtliche und kriegschirurgische Studie. *Arch. klin. Chir.* (1900), 62:599–658.

Seaman, Louis Livingston. *The real triumph of Japan.* New York: D. Appleton, 1908.

Sédillot, Charles E. *Du traitement des fractures des membres par armes à feu.* Strasbourg, 1871.

Stevenson, William F. *Wounds in war, mechanism of their production and treatment.* New York, 1898.
Thomson, John. *Report of observations made in the British military hospitals in Belgium after the Battle of Waterloo.* Edinburgh, 1816.
Trueta, José. *Principles and practice of war surgery.* St. Louis: C. V. Mosby, 1943.
U.S. Army Medical Service. *Wound ballistics.* Prepared and published under the direction of Leonard D. Heaton. Ed. James Boyd Coates, Jr., and James C. Beyer. Washington, D.C.: Office of the Surgeon General, 1962.
Woodward, Joseph J. *Outlines of chief camp diseases of the United States armies.* Philadelphia, 1863. Reprint. New York: Hafner, 1964.

Chapter 25. Surgical Specialization

Notes

1. Burton Chance, *Ophthalmology* (New York: Paul B. Hoeber, 1939), p. 35.

2. Wilhelm Stricker, "Studien zur Geschichte der Augenheilkunde," *Arch. f. path. Anat.* (1869), 47:519; Guy de Chauliac, *La grande chirurgie de Guy de Chauliac, composée en l'an 1363*, ed. Édouard Nicaise (Paris, 1890), pp. ciii, 485; Louis Dulieu, *La chirurgie à Montpellier de ses origines au début de XIXe siècle* (Avignon: Presses universelles, 1975), p. 40. The blind King John was killed at the Battle of Crécy when he rode his steed into the thick of the fight.

3. Georg Bartisch, *Augendienst* (Dresden, 1583); Richard Banister, *Treatise of one hundred and thirteene diseases of the eyes and eye-liddes*, 2d ed. (London, 1622); Michel Brisseau, *Traité de la cataracte et du glaucoma* (Paris, 1709); Antoine Maître-Jan, *Traité des maladies de l'oeil* (Troyes, 1707); Jacques Daviel, "Sur une nouvelle méthode de guérir la cataracte par l'extraction du cristalin," *Mém. Acad. roy. chir.* (1753), 2:337–54.

4. Jacques Guillemeau, *Traité des maladies de l'oeil* (Paris, 1585); William Cheselden, "An account of some observations made by a young gentleman who was born blind, or . . . had no remembrance of ever having seen, and was couch'd between 13 and 14 years of age," *Phil. Trans.* (1728), 35:447–52; Samuel Sharp, "Description of a new method of opening the cornea, in order to extract the crystalline humour," *Phil. Trans.* [for 1753] (1754), 48(1):161–63; 322–31; Antonio Scarpa, *Saggio di osservazioni e d'esperienze sulle principali malattie degli occhi* (Pavia, 1801); Dominique Jean Larrey, *Mémoire sur l'ophthalmie régnante en Égypte* (Cairo, [1802]); Benjamin Travers, *Synopsis of the diseases of the eye* (London, 1820); George J. Guthrie, *Lectures on the operative surgery of the eye* (London, 1823); William Lawrence, *Treatise on the diseases of the eye* (London, 1833); Johann Dieffenbach, *Ueber das Schielen und die Heilung desselben durch die Operation* (Berlin, 1842).

5. Edward Delafield's (1795–1875) contribution is described in Alvin A. Hubbell, *Development of ophthalmology in America, 1800 to 1870* (Chicago: W. T. Keener, 1908).

6. Hermann Helmholtz, *Beschreibung eines Augen-Spiegels zur Untersuchung der Netzhaut im lebenden Auge* (Berlin, 1851).

7. Hans Killian and G. Krämer, *Meister der Chirurgie und die Chirurgenschulen im deutschen Raum* (Stuttgart: G. Thieme, 1951), p. 178.

8. Eduard Michaelis, *Albrecht v. Graefe; sein Leben und Werken* (Berlin, 1877); Fielding H. Garrison, *Introduction to the history of medicine*, 3d ed. (Philadelphia: W. B. Saunders, 1922), p. 656.

9. Albrecht Graefe: "Vorläufige Notiz über das Wesen des Glaucoms," *Arch. f. Ophth.* (1854), 1(1):371–82; "Ueber die Iridectomie bei Glaucom und über den glaucomatösen Process," ibid. (1857), 3(2):456–555; (1858), 4(2):127–61; (1862), 8(2):242–313; "Ueber Complication von Sehnervenentzündung mit Gehirnkrankheiten," ibid. (1860). 7(2):58–71; "Ueber modificirte Linearextraction," ibid. (1865), 11(2):1–106; (1866), 12(1):150–223; (1868), 14(2):106–48; *Symptomenlehre der Augenmuskellähmungen* (Berlin, 1867). Michaelis,

Graefe's biographer, related that Graefe died at 3:00 A.M., July 20, 1870. He was struggling for air; his physician, Traube, was called and arrived as he was breathing his last. Michaelis said that Graefe had taken care of many thousands of patients from all over the world, eye surgeons from everywhere in large numbers had visited his clinic. So passed quickly one of the great ophthalmologists of all time.

10. Chevalier Jackson, *Tracheo-bronchoscopy, esophagoscopy and gastroscopy* (St. Louis: Laryngoscope Co., 1907).

11. R. Scott Stevenson and Douglas Guthrie, *History of oto-laryngology* (Edinburgh: E. and S. Livingstone, 1949), p. 123.

12. Anton Troeltsch, "Die Untersuchung des Gehörgangs und Trommelfells. Ihre Bedeutung. Kritik der bisherigen Untersuchungsmethoden und Angabe einer neuen," *Dt. Klinik* (1860), 12:113–15, 121–23, 131–35, 143–46, 151–55. William Wilde, father of the playwright Oscar Wilde, had shown that mastoiditis was a complication of middle ear disease. Wilde, *Practical observations on aural surgery* (London, 1853).

13. Julius Lempert, "Improvements of hearing in cases of otosclerosis: A new, one-stage surgical technic," *Archs Otolar.* (1938), 28:42–97; Samuel Rosen, "Mobilization of the stapes to restore hearing in otosclerosis," *N.Y. St. J. Med.* (1953), 53:2650–53; John R. Lindsay, "Otosclerosis," pp. 205–30, in Michael M. Paparella and Donald A. Shumrich, eds., *Otolaryngology*, vol. 2, *The Ear* (Philadelphia: W. B. Saunders, 1973).

14. Prosper Menière, "Mémoire sur des lésions de l'oreille interne donnant lieu à des symptomes de congestion cérébrale apoplectiforme," *Gaz. méd. Paris* (1861), 16:88–89, 239–40, 379–80, 597–601.

15. Gaspare Tagliacozzi, *De curtorum chirurgia per insitionem* (Venice, 1597); Martha T. Gnudi and Jerome P. Webster, *Life and times of Gaspare Tagliacozzi* (New York: Herbert Reichner, 1950); Eduard Zeis, *Die Literatur und Geschichte der plastischen Chirurgie* (Leipzig, 1863; reprint, Bologna: A. Forni, 1963), pp. 188, 201–8.

16. René-J.-C. Garengeot, *Traité des operations de chirurgie*, 2d ed. (Paris, 1731), 3:55–56; J. F. Dieffenbach, *Surgical observations on the restoration of the nose* [with] *notes and additional cases by John Stevenson Bushnan* (London, 1833), p. 13. William Balfour reported the case in 1814.

17. J. Braid, "Case of reunion of a separated portion of the finger," *Edinb. M. & S. J.* (1816), 12:428–29; [note on Carlizze], *Lancet* (1834), 1:437; John Mackenzie, communication, *Edinb. M. & S. J.* (1837), 47:335. *Lancet* took the Carlizze account from a Sicilian medical journal.

18. John Denny, "Re-union of fingers after their total separation by incision," *Lancet* (1849), 2:295–96; Zeis, *Plastischen Chirurgie* (n.15), pp. 201–8.

19. Jacques Reverdin, "Greffe épidermique. Expérience faite dans le service de . . . Guyon à l'hôpital Necker," *Bull. Soc. imp. de chir. Paris, 1869* (1870), 10:511–15; ibid. (1871), 12:28; Louis Xavier Ollier, "Greffes cutanées ou autoplastiques," *Bull. Acad. de méd.*, Paris (1872), 1:243–50.

20. Carl Thiersch, "Über die feineren anatomischen Veränderungen bei Aufheilung von Haut auf Granulationen," *Verh. dt. Ges. Chir.* (1874), 3(2):69–75.

21. John R. Wolfe, "A new method of performing plastic operations," *Br. M. J.* (1875), 2:360–61; Wolfe, "The transplantation of tissues," *Chicago Clin. Rev.* (1893), 3:83–88. The latter reference concerns a demonstration of Wolfe's at the Pan-American Medical Congress in Washington, D.C., September 1893. A biographic sketch and portrait of Wolfe appear in the same journal (pp. 83, 114–16). He was then professor of ophthalmology at Glasgow's Royal Infirmary. Wolfe had earlier worked in Aberdeen where he apparently conducted the study of carbolic acid and wounds (1865) mentioned in chapter 17 on antiseptics.

22. J. F. Esser, "Studies in plastic surgery of the face," *Ann. Surg.* (1917), 65:297–315; Harold D. Gillies, *Plastic surgery of the face* (London: H. Frowde, 1920); V. P. Blair and James Barrett Brown, "The use and uses of large split skin grafts of intermediate thickness," *Surg. Gynec. Obstet.* (1929), 49:82–97; Earl C. Padgett, "Calibrated intermediate skin grafts," *Surg. Gynec. Obstet.* (1939), 69:779–93.

23. Ronald A. Malt and Charles F. McKhann, "Replantation of severed arms," *JAMA* (1964), 189:716–22; Malt, J. P. Remensnyder, and William H. Harris, "Long-term utility of replanted arms," *Ann. Surg.* (1972), 176:334–42; Malt, February 21, 1976, personal communication; Report of American Replantation Mission to China, Harry J. Buncke, Jr., chairman, "Replantation surgery in China," *Plastic & Reconstr. Surg.* (1973), 52:476–89.

24. Erich Lexer, "Ueber freie Transplantationen," *Arch. klin. Chir.* (1911), 95:827–51; Zeis, *Plastischen Chirurgie* (n.15); Peter B. Medawar, "The behaviour and fate of skin autografts and skin homografts in rabbits," *J. Anat.*, London (1944), 78:176–99. See also chapter 15 on vascular surgery.

25. Earl Padgett, "Is iso-skin grafting practicable?" *South. Med. J.* (1932), 25:895–900; Archibald McIndoe and A. Franceschetti, "Reciprocal skin homografts in a medico-legal case of familial identification of exchanged identical twins," *Br. J. Plast. Surg.* (1950), 2:283–89.

26. G. Elliot Smith, "The most ancient splints," *Br. M. J.* (1908), 1:732–34; Smith, "Alleged discovery of syphilis in prehistoric Egyptians," *Lancet* (1908), 2:521–24; Frederic Wood Jones, "Postmortem staining of bone produced by the antemortem shedding of blood," *Br. M. J.* (1908), 1:734; Jones, "Examination of the bodies of 100 men executed in Nubia in Roman times," ibid. (1908), 1:736 and plate; Smith and Warren R. Dawson, *Egyptian mummies* (London: G. Allen and Unwin, 1924), p. 161.

27. Lorenz Böhler, *Technik der Knochenbruchbehandlung* (Vienna: W. Maudrich, 1929); Professors Lorenz and Jörg Böhler, supplemental volume on *Treatment of fractures*, trans. Alfred Wallner (New York and London: Grune and Stratton, 1966).

28. William Eton, *Survey of the Turkish Empire*, 3d ed. (London, 1801), p. 212.

29. Antonius Mathijsen, *Nieuwe wijze van aanwending van het gips-verband bij beenbreuken. Eene bijdrage tot de militaire chirurgie* (Haarlem, 1852). A facsimile of this and the French edition (Liége, 1854) has been published in one volume with an introduction by G. J. Bremer (Nieuwkoop: de Graaf, 1962); see p. 11. Bruno Valentin of Rio de Janeiro (1956) cited a number of persons who had used plaster in some form before Mathijsen, including Dieffenbach (1834). See Valentin, *Geschichte des Gipsverbandes*, suppl. to *Ztschr. f. Orthop.* (1956), vol. 87.

30. William Cheselden, *Anatomy of the human body*, 6th ed. (London, 1741), p. 38.

31. Dominique-J. Larrey, "Mémoire sur une nouvelle manière, de réduire ou de traiter les fractures des membres compliquées de plaies," *J. compl. du dict. d. sc. méd.*, Paris (1824), 20:193–200; Johann F. Dieffenbach, *Mag. f. d. ges. Heilk.* (1834), 41:278–95.

32. William R. Beaumont, *Observations and experiments on a new mode of treating fractures of the leg and fore-arm, especially compound fractures* (London, 1831), reviewed in *Med.-Chir. Rev.* (1832), 16:247–51.

33. Vittorio Putti, "The utilization of the muscles of the stump to actuate artificial limbs: Cinematic amputations," *Br. M. J.* (1918), 1:635–38; Hugh Owen Thomas, *Diseases of the hip, knee and ankle joints, with their deformities, treated by a new and efficient method* (Liverpool, 1875). Robert Jones is quoted in Edgar Milton Bick, *Source book of orthopaedics*, 2d ed. (Baltimore: Williams and Wilkins, 1948), p. 464.

34. Henri Comte, *Résultats éloignés des résections du coude selon la méthode d'Ollier* (Lyons: Bosc and Riou, 1926), p. 19.

35. Arbuthnot Lane, "On the operative treatment of fractures," *Clin. J. Lond.* (1903), 22:161–67, 181–87, 196–201, 218–24; E. W. Hey Groves, "An experimental study of the operative treatment of fractures," *Br. J. Surg.* (1913), 1:438–501; Arthur A. Zierold, "Reaction of bone to various metals," *Arch. Surg.* (1924), 9:365–412. Lane provided elaborate illustrations of his treatment in the two editions (1905, 1914) of his monograph, *The operative treatment of fractures.*

36. Gerhard Küntscher, *Practice of intramedullary nailing*, trans. H. H. Rinne (Springfield, Ill.: Charles C Thomas, 1967); Leonard F. Peltier, E. Y. Bickel, R. Lillo, and M. S. Thein, "The use of plaster of Paris to fill defects in bone," *Ann. Surg.* (1957), 146:61–69.

37. Marius N. Smith-Petersen, "Arthroplasty of the hip, a new method," *J. Bone Jt. Surg.*

(1939), 21:269–88; John Charnley, *Acrylic cement in orthopaedic surgery* (Baltimore: Williams and Wilkins, 1970).

38. Robert B. Osgood and Nathaniel Allison, *Fundamentals of orthopaedic surgery in general medicine and surgery (Harvard lectures)* (New York: Macmillan, 1931), p. 3.

39. Alexander H. Bennett and Rickman J. Godlee, "Case of cerebral tumour," *Med.-Chir. Trans.* (1885), 68:243–75, first reported in *Lancet* (1884), 2:1090–91; William Macewen, "Intra-cranial lesions," *Lancet* (1881), 2:581–82; William R. Gowers and Victor A. Horsley, "A case of tumour of the spinal cord, removal, recovery," *Med.-Chir. Trans.* (1888), 71:377–430; Gilbert Horrax, *Neurosurgery, an historical sketch* (Springfield, Ill.: Charles C Thomas, 1952), p. 60. The tumor in Godlee's patient was an intracerebral glioma. Macewen's patient had a dural meningioma which he was able to excise completely.

40. Harvey Cushing: "Neurological surgeons: With the report of one case," *Archs Neurol. Psychiat.*, Chicago (1923), 10:385–86; "The special field of neurological surgery," *Bull. Johns Hopkins Hosp.* (1905), 16:77–87; and "The control of bleeding in operations for brain tumors. With the description of silver 'clips,'" *Ann. Surg.* (1911), 54:1–19. The Cushing-Bovie electrocautery is discussed in chapter 2 on amputation.

41. Walter E. Dandy, "Ventriculography following the injection of air into the cerebral ventricles," *Ann. Surg.* (1918), 68:5–11.

42. George E. Moore, William T. Peyton, Lyle A. French, and Walter W. Walker, "Clinical use of fluorescein in neurosurgery: Localization of brain tumors," *J. Neurosurg.* (1948), 5:392–98.

43. James L. Birley, "Traumatic aneurysm of the intracranial portion of the internal carotid artery, with a note by Wilfred Trotter," *Brain* (1928), 51:184–208; Norman M. Dott, "Intracranial aneurysms: Cerebral arterioradiography: Surgical treatment," *Trans. Med.-Chir. Soc. Edinb.* (1932–33), 47:219–34.

44. William G. Spiller and Charles H. Frazier, "The division of the sensory root of the trigeminus for the relief of tic douloureux," *Univ. Pa Med. Bull.* (1901), 14:342–52; Harvey W. Cushing, "A method of total extirpation of the Gasserian ganglion for trigeminal neuralgia . . . through the temporal fossa and beneath the middle meningeal artery," *JAMA* (1900), 34:1035–41; Achille M. Dogliotti, "Traitement des syndromes douloureux de la périphérie par l'alcoolisation sub-arachnoïdienne des racines postérieures a leur émergence de la moelle épinière," *Presse méd.* (August 1931), pp. 1249–52; Malt and McKhann (n.23). William Rose of King's College Hospital, London, removed the Gasserian ganglion for trigeminal neuralgia in 1890. *Lancet* (1890), 2:914–15.

45. Oscar Hirsch: "Operative Behandlung der Hypophysen-Tumoren," *17th International Medical Congress, London, 1913*, section 15, Rhinoplasty and Laryngology, pt. 1, pp. 189–96, and "Life-long cures and improvements after transsphenoidal operation of pituitary tumors (thirty-three patients, followed-up for 20–37 years)," *Acta Ophthal.* (1959), suppl. 56.

46. Walter E. Dandy, "Loose cartilage from intervertebral disk simulating tumor of spinal cord," *Arch. Surg.* (1929), 19:660–72.

47. Max Nitze, "Eine neue Beobachtungs- und Untersuchungsmethode für Harnröhre Harnblase und Rectum," *Wien. med. Wschr.* (1879), 29:649–52, 713–15, 779–82, 806–10.

48. Hugh Cabot, "Is urology entitled to be regarded as a specialty?" (and discussion), *Trans. Am. Urol. Assoc.* (1911), 5:1–20.

49. See chapter 5.

50. *Columbia encyclopedia*, 9th ed., s.v. "Edison, Thomas Alva (1847–1931)." Thomas Edison, without the advantage of a formal education, was self-trained. While a telegraph operator in the Boston area, he acquired a second-hand copy of Michael Faraday's two-volume work *Experimental researches in electricity*. Edison credits Faraday's important 1831 demonstration of induced electricity as having been the stimulus for his own interest and significant work in creating electric illumination. See also chapters 4, on lithotomy, and 5, on prostatic obstruction.

51. Quoted by Fielding H. Garrison, *Introduction to the history of medicine*, 3d ed. (Philadelphia: W. B. Saunders, 1922), p. 652.

52. Arnold Walker, "Midwife services (England and Wales)," in J. M. M. Kerr, R. W. Johnstone, and M. H. Phillips, eds., *Historical review of British obstetrics and gynaecology* (Edinburgh: E. and S. Livingstone, 1954), pp. 332–35.

53. A. M. Cooke, *History of the Royal College of Physicians of London* (London: Clarendon Press, 1972), 3:1044.

54. Berkeley G. A. Moynihan, *Abdominal operations*, 4th ed., 2 vols. (Philadelphia: W. B. Saunders, 1926).

55. O. H. Wangensteen, "Hemorrhoidectomy, frequently an unnecessary operation," *Am. J. Gastroenterol.* (1955), 24:521–22.

56. Henry Smith, "On the use of the clamp in the treatment of hemorrhoids and prolapsus," *Lancet* (1863), 2:506–7.

57. H. Willoughby Lyle, *King's and some King's men* (London: Oxford Univ. Press, 1935), p. 212.

58. O. H. Wangensteen, "We cannot escape history,'" *Ann. Surg.* (1969), 170:309–16.

Further Readings

Altemeier, William A. Crisis and apathy. *Trans. Am. Surg. Assoc.* (1970), 88:49–58.

Braasch, William F. *Early days in the Mayo Clinic.* Springfield, Ill.: Charles C Thomas, 1969.

Buck, Gurdon. *Contributions to reparative surgery.* New York, 1876.

Conway, Herbert, and Stark, Richard B. *Plastic surgery at the New York Hospital one hundred years ago.* New York: Paul B. Hoeber, 1953.

Daland, Judson. Depressed fracture and trephining of the skull by the Incas of Peru. *Ann. Med. Hist.* (1935), 7:550–58.

Davis, Loyal. *Fellowship of surgeons: A history of the American College of Surgeons.* Springfield, Ill.: Charles C Thomas, 1960.

Dissertationes in honorem Jens Christian Christoffersen . . . 1973 [historical essays on urology in Denmark by a number of authors]. *Acta chir. scand.* (1973), suppl. 433, pp. 62–168.

Fergusson, William. *Lectures on the progress of anatomy and surgery during the present century.* London, 1867.

Fox, J. DeWitt. Walter Dandy — super-surgeon. *Henry Ford Hosp. M. J.* (1977), 25:149–70.

Goodhill, Victor. *Stapes surgery for otosclerosis.* New York: Paul B. Hoeber, 1961.

Grabb, William C., and Smith, James W., eds. *Plastic surgery: A concise guide to clinical practice.* Boston: Little, Brown, 1968.

Gurdjian, Elisha S. *Head injury from antiquity to the present with special reference to penetrating head wounds.* Springfield, Ill.: Charles C Thomas, 1973.

Gussen, Ruth. The labyrinthine capsule: Normal structure and pathogenesis of otosclerosis. *Acta oto-lar.* (1968), suppl. 235.

Hall, Jens G. Otosclerosis in Norway. A geographical and genetical study. *Acta oto-lar.* (1974), suppl. 324.

Kelemen, George, and Linthicum, Fred H., Jr. Labyrinthine otosclerosis. *Acta oto-lar.* (1969), suppl. 253.

Koelbing, Huldrych M. *Renaissance der Augenheilkunde, 1540–1630.* Bern and Stuttgart: Hans Huber, 1967.

Macewen, William. *Growth of bone, observations on osteogenesis.* Glasgow: James Maclehose, 1912.

Maltz, Maxwell. *Evolution of plastic surgery.* New York: Froben Press, 1946.

Moore, Francis D. Freedom and organization. *Trans. Am. Surg. Assoc.* (1972), 90:39–48.

———. Manpower goals in American surgery. *Ann. Surg.* (1976), 184:125–44.

———. Surgery. In *Advances in American medicine: Essays at the Bicentennial*, ed. John Z. Bowers and Elizabeth F. Purcell, vol. 2, pp. 614–84. New York: Joseph Macy, Jr. Foundation, 1976.

Najarian, John S., and Simmons, Richard L., eds. *Transplantation*. Philadelphia: Lea and Febiger, 1972.

Nissen, Rudolf. *Erlebtes aus der Thorax chirurgie*. Stuttgart: Georg Thieme, 1955.

————. *Helle Blätter — dunkle Blätter, Erinnerungen eines Chirurgen*. Stuttgart: Deutsche Verlags-Anstalt, 1969.

Ollier, Leopold. *Traité expérimentale et clinique de la régénération des os et de la production artificielle du tissu osseux*. 2 vols. Paris, 1867.

Padgett, Earl C. *Skin grafting*. Springfield, Ill.: Charles C Thomas, 1942.

Politzer, Adam. Ein neues Heilverfahren gegen Schwerhörigkeit in Folge von Unwegsamkeit der Eustachischen Ohrtrompete. *Wien. med. Wschr.* (1863), 13:84–87, 102–4, 117–19, 148–52.

Rosen, George. *The specialization of medicine, with particular reference to ophthalmology*. New York: Froben Press, 1944.

Sabiston, David C., Jr. Major contributions to surgery from the South. *Ann. Surg.* (1975), 181:487–507.

Sachs, Ernest. *The history and development of neurological surgery*. New York: Paul B. Hoeber, 1952.

Shastid, Thomas Hall. *An outline history of ophthalmology*. Southbridge, Mass.: American Optical, 1927.

Soifer, N., et al. Otosclerosis, a review. *Acta oto-lar.* (1970), suppl. 269.

Sorsby, Arnold. *A short history of ophthalmology*. 2d ed. London and New York: Staples Press, 1948.

Toynbee, Joseph. *Diseases of the ear; their nature, diagnosis, and treatment*. London: J. Churchill, 1860.

Varco, Richard L. Fragmentation in medicine: Continuing proliferation in varieties of certificates of special competence. *Human Pathology* (January 1976), 7:1–2.

Wangensteen, O. H. Historical aspects of some surgical training programs: A plea to retain the surgical generalist in the academic arena. *Surgery* (1972), 72:692–98.

Zeis, Eduard. *History and annotated index of plastic surgery*. Trans. T. J. S. Patterson and ed. Frank McDowell. Baltimore: Williams and Wilkins, 1977.

Chapter 26. Retrospect and Prospect

Notes

1. In a memorial tribute to John Shaw Billings, William H. Welch (1913) called the Surgeon General's Library, its Index Catalogue, and the *Index Medicus* "America's greatest contribution to medicine," and, said he, "We owe it to this extraordinary man [Billings]," *Bull. N.Y. Public Library* (1913), 17:511; reprinted in Welch's *Papers and addresses* (Baltimore: Johns Hopkins Press, 1920), 3:400.

2. Claude Bernard and Charles Huette: *Précis iconographique de médecine opératoire* (Paris, 1848), and *Illustrated manual of operative surgery*, ed. W. H. Van Buren and C. E. Isaacs (New York, 1855). That Bernard's book on operative surgery was recognized as a guide for practical surgeons tells much about the quality of the book, at the same time pointing up the rarity of such texts during that period. Bernard's introduction to his class is quoted in J. M. D. Olmsted and E. Harris Olmsted, *Claude Bernard & the experimental method in medicine* (New York: Henry Schuman, 1952), p. 59.

3. James Lind, *A treatise of the scurvy* (Edinburgh, 1753); Balduinus Ronsseus, *De magnis Hippocratis lienibus, Pliniique stomacace, ac sceletyrbe, seu vulgo dicto scorbuto, libellus* (Antwerp, 1564). In the 1655 London edition of John Woodall's *Surgeons mate*, the beneficial effects of citrus fruits in preventing scurvy are discussed on pp. 39, 164–65.

4. Edward Jenner, *An inquiry into the causes and effects of the variolae vaccinae* (London,

1798). Jenner first sent his paper to the Royal Society; Sir Joseph Banks, its president, returned it with the explanation that he was protecting Jenner's reputation. Henry O. Marcy tells the anecdote about Napoleon and Jenner in a letter to the editor, *Boston M. & S. J.* (1920), 182:310.

5. Smallpox had been known since the tenth century. Lady Mary Wortley Montague had her three-year-old son inoculated while they were in Turkey (1718) and brought the idea to England. In America Cotton Mather and Zabdiel Boylston inaugurated inoculation against smallpox. Jenner's method of vaccination was introduced by Benjamin Waterhouse. See Mather, *An account of the method and success of inoculating the small pox in Boston in New England* (London, 1722); Boylston, *An historical account of the small-pox inoculated in New England* (London, 1726); Waterhouse, *A prospect of exterminating the small-pox*, 2 pts. (Boston, 1800–2).

6. Frederick G. Banting, J. J. Macleod, and C. H. Best, "The internal secretion of the pancreas," *Am. J. Physiol.* (1922), 59:479; Adolph M. Hanson, "An elementary chemical study of the parathyroid glands of cattle," *Milit. Surg.* (1923), 52:280–84. Hanson could be seen in the pharmacologic laboratory of Professor A. D. Hirschfelder once a week during the school year in the 1919–20 period.

7. Frieda S. Robscheit-Robbins and George H. Whipple, "Blood regeneration in severe anaemia. II. Favourable influence of liver, heart and skeletal muscle in diet," *Am. J. Physiol.* (1925), 72:408–18; George R. Minot and William P. Murphy, "Treatment of pernicious anemia by a special diet," *JAMA* (1926), 87:470–76; Edward L. Rickes, N. G. Brink, F. R. Koniuszy, T. R. Wood, and Karl Folkers, "Crystalline vitamin B_{12}," *Science* (1948), 107:396–97; Ernest Lester Smith, "Presence of cobalt in the anti-pernicious anaemia factor," *Nature*, London (1948), 162:144–45; William B. Castle, "Observations on the etiologic relationship of achylia gastrica to pernicious anemia," *Am. J. Med. Sci.* (1929), 178:748–64.

8. Carl Dam, "Isolierung des Vitamins K in hochgereinigter Form," *Helv. chim. acta* (1939), 22:310–13; Stephen B. Binkley, D. W. MacCorquodale, S. A. Thayer, and Edward A. Doisy, "The isolation of vitamin K," *J. Biol. Chem.* (1939), 130:219–34; Albert Szent-Györgyi, "Observations on the function of perioxidase systems and the chemistry of the adrenal cortex. Description of a new carbohydrate derivative," *Biochem. J.* (1928), 22:1387–1409; Philip S. Hench, Edward C. Kendall, Charles H. Slocumb, and Howard F. Polley, "The effect of a hormone of the adrenal cortex (. . . compound E) and of pituitary adrenocorticotropic hormone on rheumatoid arthritis," *Proc. Staff Meet. Mayo Clinic* (1949), 24:181–97; Tadeus Reichstein, "Über Bestandteile der Nebennieren-Rinde. VI. Trennungsmethoden sowie Isolierung der Substanzen Fa, H, und J.," *Helv. chim. acta* (1936), 19:1107–26.

9. In 1921 the senior author held a junior internship at St. Paul Gillette Orthopedic Hospital for Crippled Children. Approximately one-third of the one hundred patients were hospitalized for tuberculous cervical or mesenteric lymph nodes or for tuberculosis of bones and joints; two decades later both disorders had disappeared entirely owing to the complete elimination of bovine tuberculosis by pasteurization of marketed milk and slaughter of tuberculous cattle — a bold and innovative program of the U.S. Livestock Sanitary Board and Public Health authorities. J. A. Myers and J. H. Steele, *Bovine tuberculosis in man and animals* (St. Louis: W. H. Green, 1969).

10. Death benefits paid out in 1963 for poliomyelitis by the Metropolitan Life Insurance Company to American policyholders totaled $7,000, about 1 percent of the 1953 outlay ($648,000).

11. John Franklin Enders, Thomas H. Weller, and Fredrick C. Robbins, "Cultivation of the Lansing strain of poliomyelitis virus in cultures of various human embryonic tissues," *Science* (1949), 109:85–87; Albert Sabin, "Characteristics and genetic potentialities of experimentally produced and naturally occurring variants of poliomyelitis virus," *Ann. N.Y. Acad. Sci.* (1955), 61:924–38; Jonas Salk, "Principles of immunization as applied to poliomyelitis and influenza," *Am. J. Publ. Hlth* (1953), 43:1384–98. Several investigators mentioned in the above discussion were recipients of the Nobel Prize for their discoveries: Banting and Macleod in 1923; Whipple, Minot, and Murphy in 1934; Szent-Györygi in 1937; Doisy and Dam in 1943;

Hench, Kendall, and Reichstein in 1950; Enders, Weller, and Robbins for growing the poliomyelitis virus, which led the way to the preparation of an effective vaccine in the hands of Sabin and Salk (1954).

12. David Marine, "Simple goiter and its prevention," *JAMA* (1926), 87:1463–64; Marine, "Pathogenesis and prevention of simple or endemic goiter," ibid. (1935), 104:2334–41.

13. See chapter 23.

14. Howard Lilienthal, "The two-stage principle in operative surgery," *Ann. Surg.* (1910), 51:30–39.

15. Charles McBurney, "Experience with early operative interference in cases of disease of the vermiform appendix," *N. York M. J.* (1889), 50:676–84.

16. William S. Halsted, "Results of operations for the cure of cancer of the breast," *Johns Hopkins Hosp. Rep.* (1894), 4:297–350.

17. George T. Beatson: "Treatment of inoperable cases of carcinoma of the mamma," *Lancet* (1896), 2:104–7, 162–65, and "Treatment of cancer of the breast by oöphorectomy and thyroid extract," *Br. M. J.* (1901), 2:1145–48.

18. Michael J. Brennan, "Breast cancer," in James F. Holland and Emil Frei III, eds., *Cancer medicine* (Philadelphia: Lea and Febiger, 1973), pp. 1769–88.

19. Roy Hertz, Delbert M. Bergenstal, Mortimer B. Lipsett, Edward B. Price, and Theodore F. Hilbish, "Chemotherapy of choriocarcinoma and related trophoblastic tumors in women," *JAMA* (1958), 168:845–54; Hertz, John Lewis, Jr., and Lipsett, "Five years' experience with the chemotherapy of metastatic choriocarcinoma and related trophoblastic tumors in women," *Am. J. Obstet. Gynec.* (1961), 82:631–40.

20. Robert E. Gross, *Surgery of infancy and childhood* (Philadelphia: W. B. Saunders, 1953), p. 602; Gross and Edward B. D. Neuhauser, "Treatment of mixed tumors of the kidney in childhood," *Pediatrics* (1950), 6:843–52; W. W. Sutow et al., "Comparison of survival curves, 1956 versus 1962, in children with Wilms' tumor and neuroblastoma," *Pediatrics* (1970), 45:800–11.

21. Henry S. Kaplan, "On the natural history, treatment, and prognosis of Hodgkin's disease," *The Harvey lectures . . . 1968–1969*, series 64 (New York: Academic Press, 1970), pp. 215–59; W. W. Sutow and R. G. Martin, "Bone and cartilaginous tumors," Holland and Frei, eds., *Cancer medicine* (n.18), pp. 1863–79.

22. D. C. Dahlin and Mark B. Coventry, "Osteogenic sarcoma, a study of 600 cases," *J. Bone & Jt. Surg.* (1967), 49A:101–10; H. J. Mankin et al., "Massive resection and allograft transplantation in the treatment of malignant bone tumours," *New Engl. J. Med.* (1976), 294:1247–55; Erich Lexer, *Arch. klin. Chir.* (1908), 86:939–54; Lexer, *Surg. Gynec. Obstet.* (1925), 40:782–809.

23. Lars Andrén, Sture Frieberg, and Sölve Welin, "Roentgen diagnosis of small polyps in colon and rectum," *Acta radiol.* (1955), 43:201–8.

24. Victor Gilbertsen, Saturday Surgical Seminar, University of Minnesota, January 21, 1978.

25. Komei Nakayama, *Cancer* (1967), 12:778–88; Dan Gavriliu, "Aspects of esophageal cancer," *Curr. Probl. Surg.* (1975), vol. 12, no. 10.

26. O. H. Wangensteen, "Cancer of the colon and rectum with special reference to: 1) earlier recognition of alimentary tract malignancy; 2) secondary delayed re-entry of the abdomen in patients exhibiting lymph-node involvement; 3) subtotal primary excision of the colon; 4) operation in obstruction," *Wisc. Med. J.* (1949), 48:591–97.

27. King George V's "Reply" appears in *Report of the 1st International Conference on Cancer*, London, July 17–20, 1928 (New York: Wm. Wood, 1928), p. v.

28. A. R. Dochez, "President's address," *Trans. Am. Clin. Climat. Assoc.* (1939), 54:xviii–xxvi.

29. Thomas E. Starzl et al., "Orthopic liver transplantation in ninety-three patients," *Surg. Gynec. Obstet.* (1976), 142:487–504. There were no long-term survivors in the alcoholic cirrhosis group; the achievement in infants with congenital biliary atresia also was poor.

30. Alice Hamilton was the first woman appointed to the faculty of Harvard's Medical School in 1919. The strictures imposed upon Alice Hamilton's appointment by President Lowell, by current-day standards, appear ludicrous: she was not eligible for admission to the Harvard Club, she could not march in academic processions, and she was ineligible to receive a quota of tickets for Harvard football games. See Jean A. Curran, *Founders of the Harvard School of Public Health* (New York: Josiah Macy, Jr. Foundation, 1970), p. 18.

31. Samuel D. Gross, "Surgery," pp. 128, 146, 157, 189, in Edward H. Clarke et al., *A century of American medicine, 1776–1876* (Philadelphia, 1876). In a well-documented presentation, Francis D. Moore has skillfully sketched the progress of American surgery over two centuries in John Z. Bowers and Elizabeth F. Purcell, eds., *Advances in American medicine: Essays at the Bicentennial* (New York: Josiah Macy, Jr. Foundation, 1976), 2:614–84.

32. O. H. Wangensteen, "Some post-renaissance systems and schools of surgical training," *Proc. XXIII Congr. Hist. Med.* (London: Wellcome Institute, 1974), pp. 1017–23. Leyden, nurse and mother to Edinburgh's school of surgery, had a strong school of physicians dating from Hermann Boerhaave (1668–1738), but a parallel great school of surgery failed to develop. Petrus Camper (1722–89) of a later generation was one of Holland's first innovative surgeons.

Further Readings

Blake, John B., ed. *Education in the history of medicine*. New York: Hafner, 1968.

Clarke, Edward H.; Bigelow, Henry J.; Gross, Samuel D.; Thomas, T. Gaillard; Billings, John Shaw. *A century of American medicine (1776–1876)*. Philadelphia, 1876.

Flexner, Abraham. *I remember; the autobiography of Abraham Flexner*. New York: Simon and Schuster, 1940.

Gross, Samuel D. A century of American surgery. *Am. J. Med. Sci.* (1876), 71:431–84.

Hardy, James. American surgery, 1976. *Ann. Surg.* (1976), 184:245–52.

Huxley, Thomas H. *Science and education*. Chap. 2, p. 46. New York: Collier, 1902.

Moore, Francis D. Lessons we have learned from the transplant experience. *Surgery* (1977), 81:63–67.

Muller, William H. United we stand. *Trans. Am. Surg. Assoc.* (1975), 93:52–60.

Rhoads, Jonathan E. The quality of surgical scholarship. *Trans. Am. Surg. Assoc.* (1973), 91:24–30.

Rohrer, C. W. G. Julius Friedrich Cohnheim (1834–84), a trail-blazer in cancer research. *Researches in Cancer* (1934), 1:49–126.

Sarton, George. *A history of science*. Vol. 2, *Helenistic science and culture in the last three centuries B.C.* Cambridge: Harvard Univ. Press, 1959.

Scott, H. W., Jr. Professional freedom and governmental control. *Trans. Am. Surg. Assoc.* (1974), 92:25–34.

Shannon, James A. Introduction. In *Science and the evolution of public policy*, ed. James A. Shannon, p. vii. New York: Rockefeller Univ. Press, 1973.

Silverberg, Edwin. Cancer statistics, 1977. *CA: Cancer J. for Clinicians* (1977), 27:26–41.

Sudhoff, Karl. Address delivered at the inauguration of the Department of the History of Medicine at the Johns Hopkins University, Baltimore, October 18, 1929. Trans. Fielding H. Garrison. *Bull. Johns Hopkins Hosp.* (1930), 46:101–16.

INDEXES

Name Index

A **boldface** page number refers to an illustration; an *italic* number refers to a note.

Subject Index

A **boldface** page number refers to an illustration; an *italic* number refers to a note.